LESLIE BECK'S
NUTRITION
ENCYCLOPEDIA

MANAGING OVER 75 HEALTH CONCERNS WITH DIET, VITAMINS, MINERALS AND HERBS

LESLIE BECK RD

ASSOCIATE RESEARCHER
ANNE VON ROSENBACH, B.A., M.L.S.

PENGUIN
CANADA

PENGUIN CANADA

Published by the Penguin Group

Penguin Group (Canada), 90 Eglinton Avenue East, Suite 700, Toronto, Ontario, Canada M4P 2Y3
    (a division of Pearson Penguin Canada Inc.)

Penguin Group (USA) Inc., 375 Hudson Street, New York, New York 10014, U.S.A.
Penguin Books Ltd, 80 Strand, London WC2R 0RL, England
Penguin Ireland, 25 St Stephen's Green, Dublin 2, Ireland (a division of Penguin Books Ltd)
Penguin Group (Australia), 250 Camberwell Road, Camberwell, Victoria 3124, Australia
    (a division of Pearson Australia Group Pty Ltd)
Penguin Books India Pvt Ltd, 11 Community Centre, Panchsheel Park, New Delhi – 110 017, India
Penguin Group (NZ), cnr Airborne and Rosedale Roads, Albany, Auckland 1310, New Zealand
    (a division of Pearson New Zealand Ltd)
Penguin Books (South Africa) (Pty) Ltd, 24 Sturdee Avenue, Rosebank, Johannesburg 2196, South Africa

Penguin Books Ltd, Registered Offices: 80 Strand, London WC2R 0RL, England

First published by Prentice Hall Canada, a division of Pearson Canada, 2001
Published in Penguin Canada paperback by Penguin Group (Canada), a division of Pearson Penguin Inc., 2003

(WEB) 10 9 8 7 6 5 4 3

Copyright © Leslie Beck, 2001

This publication contains the opinions and ideas of its author and is designed to provide useful information in regard to the
subject matter covered. The author and publisher are not engaged in health or other professional services in this publication.
This publication is not intended to provide a basis for action in particular circumstances without consideration by a competent
professional. The author and publisher expressly disclaim any responsibility for any liability, loss, or risk, personal or otherwise,
which is incurred as a consequence, directly or indirectly, of the use and application of any of the contents of this book.

Manufactured in Canada.

LIBRARY AND ARCHIVES CANADA CATALOGUING IN PUBLICATION

Beck, Leslie (Leslie C.)
    Leslie Beck's nutrition encyclopedia : managing over 75 health concerns with diet, vitamins, minerals
and herbs / Leslie Beck ; associate researcher, Anne Von Rosenbach.

Includes bibliographical references and index.

ISBN 0-14-301611-3

1. Nutrition—Encyclopedias. 2. Vitamin therapy. 3. Minerals in nutrition. 4. Herbs—Therapeutic use.
I. Von Rosenbach, Anne II. Title. III. Title: Nutrition encyclopedia.

RA778.B428 2003   613.2'03   C2003-902478-4

Visit the Penguin Group (Canada) website at **www.penguin.ca**
Special and corporate bulk purchase rates available; please see **www.penguin.ca/corporatesales**
or call 1-800-399-6858, ext. 477 or 474.

This book is dedicated to my personal fan club—my family…

Janet, Eoin, Kevin, Alex and Julien

———∞∞∞———

To your health, happiness and vitality.

Contents

Copyright Acknowledgments

Acknowledgments

I would like to express a sincere and heartfelt thank-you to the people whose contributions helped make this book possible.

To my researcher, Anne von Rosenbach, B.A., M.L.S., who literally spent hundreds of hours researching the 78 health conditions you will read about in this book. Without Anne's dedication, thoroughness and efficiency, writing this book would not have been possible. It was a pleasure working with her as she made my job so much easier.

To Dr. Michael Smith, M.R.Pharm.S., N.D., Associate Dean of Research at the Canadian College of Naturopathic Medicine, who reviewed my chapters on herbal medicine. His expertise as both a pharmacist and a naturopathic physician ensured that the information presented was scientifically accurate.

To Sandi Williams, M.Ed., a registered dietitian and certified diabetes educator, for reviewing my section on diabetes. Her years of clinical experience counselling clients with diabetes helped make the section accurate and relevant for Canadians.

To Sherry Torkos, B.Sc.Phm., a pharmacist whom I have had the pleasure of working with on a number of occasions, and whose willingness to answer my many questions about various prescription medications is very much appreciated.

And finally, I am forever grateful to my clients, who over the past 14 years have inspired me to search for answers and, in the process, continue my learning.

Introduction

Today we are witnessing a growing movement toward self-care. We are taking increased responsibility for managing our health. More and more people are incorporating complementary therapies into their health care regime. According to a national IPSOS-Reid poll conducted in 2000, 35 percent of us were using herbal supplements to treat a health condition, up from 23 percent in 1997.[1] And our interest in nutrition remains high. The National Institute of Nutrition's most recent survey determined that 85 percent of us rank nutrition important when choosing foods, a statistic that has remained fairly constant since 1989.[2] As media reports and new studies about nutrition and health continue to bombard us, an increasing number of us are expected to continue on this path.

We are faced with the task of trying to make sense of an overwhelming amount of health information. Conflicting news stories, new "cure-all" pills and potions and a growing number of supercharged foods can leave the head of even the savviest consumer spinning. There definitely is a need for sound, credible and up-to-date information about the role nutrition plays in our health.

This encyclopedia is the culmination of hundreds and hundreds of hours spent researching, reading and writing. It is a comprehensive guide that translates the latest scientific information from the worlds of nutrition, herbal medicine and complementary therapies into easy-to-implement strategies. The information contained within the chapters of this encyclopedia is for people of all ages. It can benefit you even if you are completely healthy. You'll find a wealth of information that can help you prevent disease, increase your energy level, boost your immune system and achieve optimal nutritional health.

And there are plenty of suggestions to help you manage or treat a health condition. If you are suffering from a certain medical condition, *the information in this book is not intended to replace conventional medicine.* It is intended for educational purposes only. Under no circumstances should you discontinue a medication or put off a surgical procedure without consulting your doctor. For that matter, any recommended treatment described in this book, whether it be a vitamin supplement, a herbal remedy or another natural health product, should be discussed with your doctor. Some of the therapies outlined in this book can be used effectively in place of drug treatment, while others can be used to complement conventional treatment. While there may be exceptions, most of the food and vitamin and mineral recommendations are safe and healthy.

How to Use this Book

Part 1: Diet and Nutrition gives you a crash course on nutrition. In Chapters 1 through 3, you'll learn about carbohydrates, protein and fat. You'll learn why they are important for health, how much you need of each and what types you should be eating more often. Chapter 4 is a comprehensive reference to vitamins and minerals. Not only will you find information about daily dietary requirements and the best food sources, but you'll also find information that will help you take vitamin and mineral supplements safely.

Chapter 5, Elements of a Healthy Diet, helps you put all your newfound knowledge into practice. Based on the latest scientific evidence for disease prevention, I tell you what foods you should be eating more often and how to incorporate them into your diet. You'll even find a healthy eating guide that outlines daily recommended servings from each food group. And of course, I wouldn't be doing my job if I didn't mention what foods you should be cutting back on.

Part 2: Herbs and Natural Health Products provides in-depth information about popular supplements. Chapter 6 gives an overview of the field of herbal medicine—herbal traditions around the world, ways to take herbal remedies, and guidelines to choosing a high-quality product. Chapter 7 discusses 17 popular herbs for which there is scientific evidence to support health claims. You'll learn what these herbs are used for and how they work in the body. Potential side effects and safety issues are mentioned for each. In Chapter 8, you'll read about supplements that are not considered vitamins or minerals, nor are they considered herbs. The natural health products discussed are supplements that are being actively studied for their ability to keep us healthy. I tell you what they are used for, how they work, how to take them, side effects and safety issues.

Part 3: The Health Conditions is where you'll find in-depth information on 78 health conditions, from A to Z. For each health condition, you'll find a description of the disorder, causes, symptoms, risk factors, conventional treatments, and of course, nutritional recommendations. The nutrition recommendations are categorized under the headings of dietary strategies, vitamins and minerals, herbal remedies and other natural health products. Once again, I provide you with information on how to safely take the supplements suggested, as well as details about who should not take certain supplements. Unless otherwise specified, the RDAs cited and dosages for supplements suggested in Part 3 are the amounts for adults; you'll find the RDAs and appropriate suggested dosages for children in Chapter 4. I also include a list of recommended resources, including Web sites to visit for more information. As you read through the nutrition strategies for managing your health, you'll sometimes be directed back to Parts 1 and 2 for a more detailed description of a certain food, vitamin, mineral or supplement.

The nutrition recommendations presented in this book are based on scientific evidence. Some recommendations are backed by stronger evidence than others, and I have tried to convey this to you in the text. If there is very little or no evidence to support using a food, nutrient or supplement, I have not included it in this book.

Choosing Between Supplements

If you have a certain health condition that's described in this book, it is not my intention for you to implement every nutrition recommendation I discuss. While the dietary strategies and vitamin and mineral supplements can all be put into practice (unless a contraindication is specified), this is not the case for the herbal remedies and natural health products. Very often, many of these supplements work in the same way, so you'll want to choose the one that 1) is not contraindicated for you and 2) has the strongest scientific evidence to support its use. To help you choose which supplement to take, I give you a brief Nutrition Strategy Checklist at the end of each health condition. This checklist tells you which strategies to implement first. If the evidence is equally good for a few supplements, you'll have to make a choice. For instance, if you have osteoarthritis, I recommend glucosamine *or* chondroitin supplements.

Once you have decided on a herb and/or natural health product (and be sure to discuss with your doctor first), take the supplement for at least three months to see if your symptoms improve. If you find no change after three to six months, try the next supplement on the list. It may sound like a lot of work, but it's the only way to determine if a product is working for you. Unlike conventional drugs, herbs and supplements are gentler and take longer to take effect. Be patient. At this point you're already halfway there—you've chosen a high-quality product and you've taken the correct dose. Now it's time to let healthy food and good nutrition do the rest.

I hope you find my encyclopedia a valuable reference for you and your family. Enjoy your journey to good health.

Leslie Beck, RD
Toronto, 2001

Part One

Nutrition and Diet

1

Carbohydrates: Sugar, Starch and Dietary Fiber

Carbohydrates often get a bad rap…they make you fat, they cause diabetes, they trigger hyperactivity in children. However, contrary to the claims of many fad diets, carbohydrate-containing foods are an important component of a healthy diet and do not cause health problems if eaten according to proper guidelines. Carbohydrates provide about half of all the energy used by your muscles, nerves and other body tissues. And carbohydrate is your brain's preferred fuel source—the brain relies on a steady supply of carbohydrate to function properly. In fact, carbohydrate-rich foods should be the major source of energy in your daily diet. And if you choose your carbohydrates wisely, these foods also supply a fair share of fiber, vitamins, minerals and protective plant chemicals.

What Is Carbohydrate?

Carbohydrate is composed of carbon, hydrogen and oxygen and is found almost exclusively in plant foods. Plants make the carbohydrate we eat from carbon dioxide, water and the sun's energy. Fruit, vegetables, whole grains, legumes and nuts are all sources of carbohydrate. The only animal foods with carbohydrate are dairy products, which contain a naturally occurring sugar called lactose. The carbohydrate family includes simple sugars, starches and dietary fiber.

Simple sugars are classified as either monosaccharides ("mono" meaning one and "saccharide" meaning sugar) or disaccharides (two sugars). Monosaccharides are the simplest form of carbohydrate because they consist of a single sugar molecule. The three monosaccharides important to nutrition are glucose (also called dextrose and blood sugar), fructose (found in fruit, honey and corn syrup) and galactose. Galactose rarely occurs by itself in foods; instead, it attaches to another sugar unit to form the disaccharide lactose. Disaccharides are pairs of monosaccharides linked together. Maltose (malt sugar), sucrose (table sugar) and lactose (milk sugar) are disaccharides we consume every day.

Starches are more complex arrangements of carbohydrate. Starches in foods are long chains of hundreds or thousands of glucose units linked together. These giant molecules are stacked side by side in a grain of rice, a slice of bread or a flake of breakfast cereal. Other starchy foods are potatoes, wheat, rye, oats, corn and legumes (including chickpeas, kidney beans and lentils).

Dietary fibers are the structural parts of vegetables, fruit, grains and legumes. Pectins, lignans, cellulose, gums and mucilages are all different forms of fiber found in these foods. Although our digestive enzymes are not able to break down the chemical bonds that link the building blocks of fiber, bacteria in our colon can digest some of these fibers.

Dietary fiber is made up of two types of fiber: *soluble* and *insoluble.* Both are present in varying proportions in the different plant foods; some foods may be rich in one or the other. Soluble fibers dissolve in water. Once consumed, they form a gel in the stomach and slow the rate of digestion and absorption. Dried peas, beans and lentils, oats, barley, psyllium husks, apples and citrus fruits are good sources of soluble fiber. Diets high in soluble fiber have been shown to stabilize blood sugar and reduce the need for insulin in some people with diabetes. And plenty of evidence supports the cholesterol-lowering effect of oat bran and psyllium.

Foods like wheat bran, whole grains and certain vegetables contain mainly insoluble fibers. These fibers have a significant capacity for retaining water and act to increase stool bulk and promote regularity. By reducing constipation, a diet high in fiber may prevent a condition called diverticulosis (see page 275). Since high-fiber diets are usually low in fat and calories, they also may help you achieve and maintain a healthy weight. To reap its health benefits, Canadians should be getting 25 to 35 grams of fiber in their diets each day. Here's a list of fiber-rich foods:

Food	Fiber (grams)
Legumes and Nuts	
Beans and tomato sauce, canned, 1 cup (250 ml)	20.7 g
Black beans, 1 cup (250 ml), cooked	13.0 g

Food	Fiber (grams)
Chickpeas, 1 cup (250 ml), cooked	6.1 g
Kidney beans, 1 cup (250 ml), cooked	6.7 g
Lentils, 1 cup (250 ml), cooked	9.0 g
Almonds, 1/2 cup (125 ml)	8.2 g
Peanuts, dry roasted, 1/2 cup (125 ml)	6.9 g
Cereals	
100% bran cereal, 1/2 cup (125 ml)	10.0 g
Bran Flakes, 3/4 cup (175 ml)	6.3 g
Grape Nuts, 1/2 cup (125 ml)	6.0 g
Kellogg's All Bran Buds, 1/3 cup (75 ml)	13.0 g
Quaker Corn Bran, 1 cup (250 ml)	6.3 g
Oat Bran, 1 cup (250 ml), cooked	4.5 g
Oatmeal, 1 cup (250 ml), cooked	3.6 g
Red River Cereal, 1 cup (250 ml), cooked	4.8 g
Shreddies, 3/4 cup (175 ml)	4.4 g
Bread and Other Grain Foods	
Pita pocket, whole wheat, 1	4.8 g
Whole wheat bread, 100%, 2 slices	4.0 g
Spaghetti, whole wheat, 1 cup (250 ml), cooked	4.8 g
Rice, brown, 1 cup (250 ml), cooked	3.1 g
Flaxseed, ground, 2 tbsp (30 ml)	4.5 g
Wheat bran, 2 tbsp (30 ml)	2.4 g
Fruits	
Apple, 1 medium with skin	2.6 g
Apricots, dried, 1/4 cup (60 ml)	2.6 g
Banana, 1 medium	1.9 g
Blueberries, 1/2 cup (125 ml)	2.0 g
Figs, 5 dried	8.5 g
Orange, 1 medium	2.4 g
Pear, 1 medium with skin	5.1 g
Prunes, 3 dried	3.0 g
Raisins, seedless, 1/2 cup (125 ml)	2.8 g
Strawberries, 1 cup (250 ml)	3.8 g
Vegetables	
Broccoli, 1/2 cup (125 ml)	2.0 g
Brussels sprouts, 1/2 cup (125 ml)	2.6 g
Carrots, 1/2 cup (125 ml)	2.2 g

Food	Fiber (grams)
Corn niblets, 1/2 cup (125 ml)	2.3 g
Green peas, 1/2 cup (125 ml)	3.7 g
Lima beans, 1/2 cup (125 ml)	3.8 g
Potato, 1 medium baked with skin	5.0 g
Sweet potato, 1/2 cup (125 ml), mashed	3.9 g

Nutrient Values of Some Common Foods, Health Canada, Ottawa, 1999.

Carbohydrate and Digestion

The process of carbohydrate digestion begins in your mouth, where an enzyme in saliva starts to break down starch once you have eaten a carbohydrate meal or snack. The food then makes its way into your small intestine, where digestive enzymes are released to break down starches into smaller units. Finally, vital enzymes on the surface of your intestinal cells dismantle disaccharides into their monosaccharide building blocks. (Inflammatory diseases, certain medications, hereditary factors and age can predispose us to deficiencies in some of these enzymes, most commonly, lactase deficiency. People who don't produce enough lactase cannot break down the milk-sugar lactose into its two components, glucose and galactose. The result is cramping, bloating, gas and diarrhea. See page 407 for more on lactose intolerance.)

Once digested, the three monosaccharides—glucose, fructose and galactose—enter the bloodstream and make their way to the liver. Here, fructose and galactose are converted to glucose. Some glucose is used immediately for energy, while some is stored as glycogen, the body's storage form of carbohydrate (glucose), which the liver breaks down and releases as glucose according to your body's need for energy. When your blood-sugar level falls because you haven't eaten for a while, glucose is released so body cells can use it to fuel metabolic reactions. But your liver is able to store only about one-third of your body's glucose. The rest is housed in your muscles as glycogen. During exercise, your body burns glycogen in order to keep muscles contracting. This is why low-carbohydrate diets can make exercise difficult: your muscles feel tired and you fatigue much sooner.

Carbohydrate and the Glycemic Index

By now it's apparent how important carbohydrate is for energy. All carbohydrate-rich foods ultimately end up as glucose in your bloodstream, where it's used to fuel your body's metabolic machinery. But the speed at which that glucose enters your bloodstream may affect your hunger, your weight, even your long-term health.

Carbohydrates do not raise your blood sugar all in the same way. Some carbohydrate-rich foods are digested and absorbed into your bloodstream quickly, while others are broken down and converted to blood glucose more slowly. What effect does this have on your feeling of energy? Let's say you eat two slices of toast for breakfast. Bread (both white and whole-wheat) is digested relatively quickly, causing your blood glucose to rise quickly. This rapid rise in blood glucose triggers your pancreas to release an excessive amount of insulin, the hormone that regulates blood sugar, causing your blood-glucose level to drop to a very low level. The result is that you'll feel sluggish and tired, not to mention hungry, not long after eating the toast. Moreover, studies suggest that regularly eating foods that cause high blood insulin levels may increase the risk of heart disease and cancer.

On the other hand, a bowl of high-fiber breakfast cereal with low-fat milk is digested and absorbed more slowly, causing a gradual rise in blood glucose. Because this meal does not result in a fast blood-sugar response, you don't get a surge of insulin. As a result, your blood-sugar level won't plummet. Instead you will experience a smooth, steady blood-sugar level, leading to more consistent energy levels.

The rate at which a food causes your blood sugar to rise can be measured and assigned a value. This measure is referred to as the food's glycemic index value. The glycemic index (GI) is a ranking from 0 to 100. The number indicates whether a food raises your blood glucose rapidly, moderately or slowly. Foods that are digested quickly and cause your blood sugar to rise rapidly have high glycemic index values. Foods that are digested slowly leading to a gradual rise in blood sugar are assigned low glycemic index values. All foods are compared to pure glucose, which is given a value of 100 (fast acting).

The glycemic index is used, and being studied, in athletics. After heavy exercise that depletes muscle carbohydrate stores (what muscles use for fuel during exercise), consuming a high glycemic index food such as a bagel or sugary drink is best since it will be more rapidly digested and converted to blood glucose. That means muscles will recover and rebuild their energy stores faster. A low glycemic index food such as yogurt is best for a preworkout snack since it will take longer to be converted to blood sugar. That means that when you start to exercise, your blood-glucose levels are starting to increase, giving your muscles energy for the workout.

To help prevent large increases in blood sugar, practice the following:

- Choose low GI foods for your meals.

- Avoid eating high GI foods as snacks as they can trigger low blood sugar; choose low GI foods instead.

- Combine a high GI food with a low GI food to result in a meal with a medium GI value.

Here's a list of foods ranked by their GI value; < 55 = low GI; 55–70 = medium GI; > 70 = high GI. Use this table to plan your meals.

Food	GI Value
Bread and Crackers	
Baguette, French	95
Kaiser roll	73
Melba toast	70
Pita bread, whole-wheat	57
Pumpernickel, whole-grain	51
Rice cakes	82
Rye bread	65
Soda crackers	74
Sourdough bread	52
Stoned Wheat Thins	67
White bread	70
Whole-wheat bread	69
Breakfast Cereals	
All Bran, Kellogg's	51
All Bran Buds with Psyllium, Kellogg's	45
Bran Flakes	74
Corn Bran, Quaker	75
Corn Flakes	84
Oat Bran	50
Oatmeal	49
Raisin Bran	73
Shredded Wheat, spoon size	58
Special K	54
Cookies, Cakes and Muffins	
Angelfood cake	67
Arrowroot	69
Banana bread	47
Blueberry muffin	59
Graham crackers	74
Oat bran muffin	60
Oatmeal cookies	55
Social Tea biscuits	55
Sponge cake	46

Food	GI Value
Pasta, Grains and Potato	
Barley	25
Bulgur	48
Corn, sweet	55
Couscous	65
Fettuccine, egg	32
Potato, french fries	75
Potato, new, unpeeled, boiled	62
Potato, instant, mashed	86
Potato, red-skinned, mashed	91
Potato, red-skinned, boiled	88
Potato, white-skinned, baked	85
Rice, basmati	58
Rice, brown	55
Rice, converted, Uncle Ben's	44
Rice, instant	87
Rice, long-grain, white	56
Rice, short-grain	72
Spaghetti, whole-wheat	37
Spaghetti, white	41
Sweet potato, mashed	54
Legumes	
Baked beans	48
Black beans	31
Black bean soup	64
Chickpeas, canned	42
Kidney beans	27
Lentils	30
Lentil soup, canned	34
Soy beans	18
Split pea soup	66
Fruit	
Apple	38
Apricot, dried	31
Banana	55
Cantaloupe	65
Cherries	22
Dates, dried	103

Food	GI Value
Grapefruit	25
Grapes	46
Mango	55
Orange	44
Peach, canned	30
Pear	38
Raisins	64
Watermelon	72
Dairy Products and Alternatives	
Milk, skim	32
Milk, whole	27
Milk, chocolate	34
Ice cream, low-fat	50
Soy beverage	31
Yogurt, flavored, low-fat	33
Snack Foods	
Corn chips	72
Peanuts	14
Popcorn	55
Potato chips	54
Pretzels	83
Sports Bar, PowerBar™, chocolate	58
Sugars	
Fructose (fruit sugar)	23
Glucose	100
Honey	58
Lactose (milk sugar)	46
Sucrose (table sugar)	65

Foster-Powell, K. and J. Brand Miller. "International tables of glycemic index," *American Journal of Clinical Nutrition* 1995; 62:871S-893S.

Carbohydrate and Weight Control

After reading about the importance of carbohydrate, you might be wondering why some diet books shun them. Books like *Dr. Atkins Protein Revolution, Sugar Busters* and *Protein Power Plan* recommend eliminating or drastically reducing carbohydrates from your diet for a period in order to help you lose weight. Many of these diets claim that carbohydrates make you fat. However, carbohydrate-rich foods will make you gain weight *only* if you're eating a lot of them, or if you're slathering them with high-fat spreads or sauces.

It is true, however, that many people today overeat carbohydrates—high-carbohydrate foods are often fast, portable and fat free. Yet, although they contain very little fat, dense bagels, fat-free muffins, baked pretzels and bowls of pasta all add calories to your diet. Often, fat-reduced foods are not much lower in calories than the original version. Did you know that a large bagel is the equivalent of five slices of bread? Or that 20 pretzel sticks are equivalent to two slices? Even that restaurant portion of pasta with tomato sauce is probably worth at least four slices of bread (not to mention the bread you might eat with it!). And here's a shocker: one slice of pizza from the street-corner shop can have as much carbohydrate as seven slices of bread. When it comes to weight control, portion size is what counts.

Carbohydrate and Diabetes

It is a common misconception that consuming too much sugar will cause diabetes. As you'll read on page 263, diabetes is a disease caused by genetic and lifestyle factors. It occurs when the body does not produce enough insulin, or does not use it properly. As a result, rather than entering blood cells, glucose builds up in the bloodstream and is excreted in the urine, thus not providing body cells with their main source of fuel.

People with diabetes must carefully manage their carbohydrate intake. Meals need to be regularly scheduled and contain measured portions of carbohydrate foods. However, people with diabetes are allowed to eat a little bit of sugar.

Carbohydrate and Dental Caries

Here's where sugar *is* a culprit. In the mouth, the enzyme amylase begins breaking down starch into smaller units of starch and the disaccharide maltose. Bacteria in the mouth then ferment these carbohydrates and, in the process, produce an acid that erodes tooth enamel. The longer carbohydrate foods stay in the mouth, the greater the chance that cavities will form. Sticky foods like candy adhere to the teeth and will keep acid-yielding bacteria in action longer. Snacking on carbohydrate-rich foods regularly throughout the day will keep the bacteria working, too.

Eating nonsugary foods can help remove carbohydrate from the surface of your teeth. This is why, as you may have heard, eating cheese can help prevent cavities. Rinsing your mouth and brushing your teeth after eating are important strategies to help prevent dental caries.

How Much Carbohydrate Should You Eat?

Here's what you should be striving for each day:

1. At least 55 percent of your daily calories should come from carbohydrate-containing foods. This means that foods like legumes, grains, vegetables and fruit should take up from two-thirds to three-quarters of your plate.

2. As often as possible, choose whole grains: starchy foods that have not been refined and retain important minerals, vitamins, antioxidants and fiber. (You'll read more about whole grains in Chapter 5.) Choose 100 percent whole-wheat bread, whole rye or pumpernickel bread, brown rice, whole-wheat pasta and breakfast cereals made from whole grains.

3. Limit your intake of sugary foods like candy, chocolate, soda pop, fruit drinks, desserts and other sweets. I advise my clients to "treat" themselves once a week.

4. Strive to include 25 to 35 grams of dietary fiber in your daily diet. If you, like the average Canadian, are getting only about half this amount, gradually work more fiber into your diet. The list of fiber-containing foods on page 3 will give you some ideas.

5. Remember that fiber needs fluid to work. Be sure to consume at least eight glasses of water each day. And always have a glass of water with a high-fiber meal or snack.

2

Protein and Amino Acids

It may be hard to believe that our ancient ancestors got most of their protein from vegetables. Animal foods entered our diet only 1.5 million years ago—a short time ago in our evolutionary history. Today, foods like steak, burgers, chicken breast, eggs and dairy products occupy a central part of our dinner plates. These foods are rich in protein and supply a fair share of our daily protein intake.

Protein is essential for life. It is used to make many critical body compounds. Proteins form structural components in the body—muscle tissue, connective tissue and the support tissue inside bones—are all derived from the protein we eat. Many of these body proteins are in a continual state of breakdown, repair and maintenance. If your diet is chronically low in protein, protein rebuilding slows down.

Body Proteins

Proteins are used by our bodies to produce hormones and enzymes. For example, thyroid hormones, which control metabolic rate, and insulin, which controls blood sugar, are made from proteins. Enzymes, functioning as catalysts, control virtually all chemical reactions in your cells.

Meeting your daily protein requirements also keeps your immune system in shape. Protein is used to make antibodies, white blood cells and other immune compounds that attack foreign invaders and prevent infection. Other proteins in your blood help maintain your body's fluid balance.

Your body uses protein for energy, too. In Chapter 1 I told you about the important role carbohydrate plays in providing glucose (energy) to all body tissues. If your diet doesn't supply enough carbohydrate, your liver is forced to use protein to make glucose. Metabolizing protein into glucose for energy is a normal process—it occurs when you skip a meal or don't eat for a long period. But if your usual diet is low in carbohydrate and calories, your body will break down muscle and other important proteins to make glucose. The result can be muscle wasting, a slower metabolism and a weakened immune system.

Dietary Protein

Proteins are made up of building blocks called amino acids. There are 20 amino acids, all of which are necessary for good health. Eleven of these can be synthesized by your body and are therefore called nonessential amino acids. The remaining 9, however, must be supplied by food as your body either cannot synthesize them on its own or cannot synthesize them in sufficient quantities. They are called essential amino acids.

Essential Amino Acids	Nonessential Amino Acids
Histidine	Alanine
Isoleucine	Arginine
Leucine	Asparagine
Lysine	Aspartic acid
Methionine	Cysteine
Phenylalanine	Glutamic acid
Threonine	Glutamine
Tryptophan	Glycine
Valine	Proline
	Serine
	Tyrosine

If your diet does not supply enough essential amino acids, your body's rate of protein building will slow down. Eventually your body will break down its own protein to get these amino acids.

Animal and plant proteins have very different amino-acid profiles. Animal protein foods contain all the essential amino acids in sufficient quantities to support growth, repair and maintenance of body tissues. For this reason, animal proteins are considered complete proteins, or high-quality proteins. Plant proteins, on the other hand, are always low, or limited, in one or more of the nine essential amino acids. In some cases, a plant food may even be lacking an essential amino acid completely. The proteins from plant foods are considered incomplete proteins, or low-quality proteins.

Complementary Proteins

Many of us eat enough protein to get ample amounts of essential amino acids. But what about those who follow a strict vegetarian (vegan) diet? Vegetarians must take care to combine their vegetarian protein foods so that the essential amino acid missing from one is supplied by the other. When two or more vegetarian protein foods are combined in this way, they are called complementary proteins. The following table lists limited amino acids, the amino acid that occurs in the shortest supply relative to the amount needed by the body, and offers some suggestions for complete protein meals. For instance, you'll see below that tofu (made from soybeans) does not provide enough methionine to cover the body's requirements. By eating tofu with brown rice (or nuts and seeds), which provide plenty of methionine, you'll end up with a complete protein meal.

Complementary Vegetarian Proteins

Food	Limiting Amino Acids	Food to Combine	Complete Protein Meal Ideas
Legumes, Soybeans	Methionine	Grains, nuts, seeds	Tofu and brown rice stir-fry
Grains	Lysine, threonine	Legumes	Pasta with white kidney beans
Nuts and seeds	Lysine	Legumes	Hummus with tahini (sesame seed paste)
Vegetables	Methionine	Grains, nuts, seeds	Bok choy with cashews
Corn	Lysine, tryptophan	Legumes	Black bean and corn salad

Nutritionists once thought it was important to combine protein foods in the same meal. We now know that as long as vegetarians eat a variety of vegetarian proteins over the course of the day, they'll meet their requirements for essential amino acids. A protein deficiency will develop, however, when fruits and vegetables make up the core of the diet, severely shortchanging the quantity and quality of protein.

However, it is important for children to have combined proteins in the same meal. To support growth and development, infants and preschoolers need 35 percent of their daily protein from essential amino acids. The meals of young vegetarians must be carefully planned to ensure they get all the essential amino acids they need.

How Much Protein Do You Need?

As adults, we need to consume enough protein each day to make up for the amount our bodies lose through urine, skin, hair and nails. However, eating more than your daily requirements will result in excess protein being stored as body fat (not muscle!). Here's a look at your daily protein requirements:

Daily Protein Requirements for Healthy Adults

No regular exercise	0.86 grams per kilogram body weight
Regular exercise	1.2–1.7 grams per kilogram body weight
Elderly adults	0.8–1.0 grams per kilogram body weight

To calculate your actual daily protein requirements, multiply your weight (in kilograms) by your RDA of protein. If you exercise regularly, you will need to eat more protein to compensate for that used up as energy. For example, a 135-pound (61 kg) woman who does not exercise needs 52 grams of protein each day (61 kg × 0.86). If that same woman jogged three or four times a week, she would need to eat 73 grams of protein (61 kg × 1.2). If you're a 180 pound (82 kg) male who works out with weights regularly, you need to consume 139 grams of protein each day (82 kg × 1.7).

Protein Content of Foods

Food	Protein (grams)
Meat, 3 oz (90 g)	21–25 g
Poultry, 3 oz (90 g)	21 g
Salmon, 3 oz (90 g)	25 g
Sole, 3 oz (90 g)	17 g
Tuna, canned and drained, 1/2 cup (125 ml)	30 g
Egg, 1 whole	6 g
Legumes, cooked, 1/2 cup (125 ml)	8 g
Milk, 1 cup (250 ml)	8 g
Yogurt, 3/4 cup (175 ml)	8 g
Cheese, cheddar, 1 oz (30 g)	10 g
Vegetables, 1/2 cup (125 ml)	2 g
Bread, 1 slice	2 g
Rice, pasta, cooked, 1/2 cup (125 ml)	2 g

Nutrient Values of Some Common Foods, Health Canada, Ottawa, 1999.

For most of us, getting too little protein is likely not a problem. It's estimated that the average North American male consumes 105 grams of protein each day while the average female consumes about 65 grams. Individuals at risk for protein deficiency include:

- those who live alone and don't often cook meat, chicken or fish
- those who frequently grab a quick meal during the day—bagels, pasta, low-fat frozen dinners
- vegetarians who don't eat animal foods and don't incorporate high-quality vegetable protein sources into their daily diet
- those who engage in heavy exercise and fall into any of the above categories

At certain stages in the life cycle, the body's protein needs will increase. During pregnancy, women must eat an additional 5 grams per day of protein during the first trimester, an extra 20 grams per day during the second trimester, and an extra 24 grams per day during the third trimester. Women who are breastfeeding need to consume 65 grams of protein each day during the first six months and more if they exercise regularly. In Chapter 5, you'll find a food guide that will help you choose the right amount of protein-rich foods each day.

3

─────※─────

Dietary Fats and Oils

You might be surprised to learn that, when it comes to health, dietary fat actually has some virtues. In fact, some types of fat may ward off heart disease and cancer while others may ease the symptoms of arthritis and depression. It's when our diet contains too little or too much fat that ill health occurs. Today, Canadians continue to consume too many unhealthy and too few healthy fats. However, we are doing better than we were 20 years ago. Over the years, as we are bombarded by news reports of cholesterol and heart disease, fat and obesity, our intake of unhealthy fats has decreased.

Triglycerides, made up of building blocks called *fatty acids,* are the major form of fats in our food and bodies. Fat, once consumed, is broken down into its fatty acid building blocks by digestive enzymes in the intestine. These fatty acids are then absorbed into the bloodstream, making their way to the liver, where they are repackaged into triglyceride molecules and transported to body tissues. Enzymes in cells break down these circulating triglycerides so that their fatty acids can enter the cells. Some fatty acids are used immediately for energy, while the remaining fatty acids are reformed into triglycerides and stored as body fat (adipose tissue).

Fat has many important roles. Body fat acts as a layer of insulation protecting our major organs. Stores of body fat provide a vital source of energy for the body. In fact, about half of our daily energy requirements are supplied by stored fat. Fatty acids released from muscle cells provide most of the fuel for light activity. The body's ability to store fat is almost unlimited. Fat cells can increase in size if we consume more fat than we need, and our bodies can also form new fat cells if our existing ones can't expand any further. Although stored body fat gives cells the energy they need, storing too much fat is not healthy.

Dietary fat supplies us with the fat-soluble vitamins—A, D, E and K. It also adds flavor to foods and helps us feel satisfied after eating a meal. Because dietary fat empties from the stomach slowly, it imparts satiety, or a feeling of fullness.

Fatty acids in food consist of long chains of carbon molecules linked together, which in turn are bonded to hydrogen atoms. Each type of fatty acid has a particular chemical structure that determines how it will behave in the body. For instance, when a fatty acid is completely full of hydrogen atoms, it is considered a saturated fatty acid. Animal fat contains mostly saturated fatty acids. Fatty acids not saturated with hydrogen atoms, found primarily in vegetable oils, are either *monounsaturated* or *polyunsaturated*. Food fats almost always contain both saturated and unsaturated fatty acids and are classified as saturated, monounsaturated or polyunsaturated depending on which fatty acids are present in the greatest concentration.

Saturated Fats

Animal foods—meat, poultry, eggs and dairy products—all contain saturated fat. Eating a diet high in saturated fat increases your risk for heart disease. Many studies have shown that high intakes of saturated fat are linked with high levels of blood cholesterol. Saturated fat inhibits the ability of your cells to clear cholesterol from the bloodstream.

There are many types of saturated fats, and researchers are learning that they don't all influence blood cholesterol to the same degree. For instance, the saturated fat in dairy products raises cholesterol higher than does that in meat. And the type of saturated fat found in chocolate (stearic acid) does not raise blood-cholesterol levels at all. It's not important that you know the different types of saturated fats. What *is* important is that you eat only a small amount of saturated fat. It should account for less than 10 percent of your daily calories. Choosing lower-fat foods will help you achieve that goal. But you also need to pay attention to portion sizes. A portion size of lean meat shouldn't exceed 3 ounces (90 grams).

Food	Lower-Fat Choices or Substitutes
Milk	Skim, 1% milk fat (MF)
Yogurt	Products with less than 1.5% MF
Cheese	Products with less than 20% MF
Cottage cheese	Products with 1% or less MF
Sour cream	Products with 7% or less MF
Cream	Evaporated 2% or evaporated skim milk
Red meat	Flank steak, inside round, sirloin, eye of round, extra-lean ground beef, venison

Food	Lower-Fat Choices or Substitutes
Pork	Center-cut pork chops, pork tenderloin, pork leg (inside round, roast), baked ham, deli ham, back bacon
Poultry	Skinless chicken breast, turkey breast, lean ground turkey
Eggs	Egg whites (two whites replaces one whole egg)

Polyunsaturated Fats

Vegetable oils supply us with most of our polyunsaturated fats. There are two types of polyunsaturated fats in foods. Omega-6 polyunsaturated fats are found in all vegetable oils, including soybean, sunflower, safflower, corn and sesame. Omega-3 polyunsaturated fats are found in certain oils (flaxseed, walnut and canola) as well as in fish and shellfish. Replacing foods high in saturated fats with those rich in polyunsaturated fats will have a blood cholesterol lowering effect—primarily because you are eating less saturated fat.

Essential Fatty Acids

The omega-3 and omega-6 oils in our diet provide our bodies with two very important fatty acids they cannot produce on their own. Omega-3 oils provide *alpha-linolenic acid,* while omega-6 oils give us *linoleic acid.* These two essential fatty acids help form vital body structures and cell membranes, aid in immune function and vision, and produce powerful hormone-like compounds called eicosanoids. Without them, we would not be able to maintain good health.

The ability of alpha-linolenic acid and linoleic acid to produce eicosanoids has researchers excited. Eicosanoids regulate our blood, immune system and hormones. Prostaglandins (you'll read about their role in health throughout the book), prostacyclins, thromboxanes and leukotrienes all belong to the eicosanoid family. The type of fat you eat determines which kind of eicosanoids your body produces. For instance, linoleic acid from omega-6 oils is used to synthesize so-called "unfriendly" eicosanoids that cause inflammation and pain. Alpha-linolenic acid in omega-3 oils, on the other hand, produces "friendly" eicosanoids that tend to decrease inflammation and blood clotting and are thought to help prevent heart disease, ease symptoms of rheumatoid arthritis and influence brain function. These two essential fatty acids compete with each other for the same metabolic pathways. So if you eat a diet that contains primarily omega-6 oils, the unfriendly eicosanoids will win. If your diet is rich in omega-3 oils, more health-enhancing eicosanoids will form. We should be consuming a ratio of 4:1 omega-6 to omega-3 fats. It's estimated that the average Canadian currently consumes 10 to 20 times more omega-6s than omega-3s.

Omega-3 Fats in Fish

Fish oils contain two omega-3 fatty acids: docosahexanaenoic acid (DHA) and eicos-apentaenoic acid (EPA). These can lower high levels of blood triglycerides and cholesterol and reduce the stickiness of platelets, the cells that form blood clots in arteries. They may also increase the flexibility of red blood cells, allowing them to pass more readily through tiny blood vessels. Many studies have found that populations that consume fish a few times a week have lower rates of heart disease.

The best sources of DHA and EPA are oily fish such as salmon, trout, sardines, mackerel and herring. The body also produces DHA and EPA from foods rich in alpha-linolenic acid such as flaxseed oil, canola oil, walnuts, soybeans, whole grains and leafy greens. But researchers believe that the body converts alpha-linolenic acid to DHA and EPA inefficiently, especially when the diet is rich in omega-6 fats, since these slow down the conversion process.

The health benefits of omega-3s and fish oil supplements are discussed in more detail in Chapter 8.

Monounsaturated Fats

Monounsaturated fats found in olive, canola and peanut oils are considered healthy fats. Substituting them for saturated fats can lower high levels of blood cholesterol, since your intake of saturated fat will decrease. Some studies suggest that extra-virgin olive oil helps prevent blood clots from forming and acts as an antioxidant to help protect against heart disease. Extra-virgin olive oil has been processed the least (hence the dark green color) and contains more protective compounds than regular or light olive oil.

Trans Fats

Trans fat is formed by hydrogenation, a chemical process in which hydrogen atoms are added to liquid vegetable oils. The oils become more solid and therefore more useful to food manufacturers. Packaged foods like cookies, crackers, pastries and muffins made with hydrogenated vegetable oils are more palatable and have a longer shelf life. Margarine made by hydrogenating a vegetable oil is firm like butter.

Not only does hydrogenation make vegetable oil saturated and destroy the oil's essential fatty acids, the process forms a new type of fat called trans fat. Consuming too much trans fat heightens the risk of heart disease by increasing low-density lipoproteins (LDL) cholesterol levels and decreasing high-density lipoproteins (HDL) cholesterol levels. Many researchers believe that trans fat is worse for our cholesterol levels than saturated fat.

The easiest way to reduce your intake of trans fat is to pay attention to food labels and ingredients lists:

- Look for the phrase "hydrogenated vegetable oils" and eat foods that contain these kinds of oils less often. As much as 40 percent of the fat in foods like french fries, fast food, doughnuts, pastries, snack foods and commercial cookies is trans fat.

- If you eat margarine, choose one made with nonhydrogenated fat. This is often stated right on the label. If it's not, add the values for polyunsaturates and monounsaturates listed on the nutrition information panel: they should add up to at least 6 grams. Anything less means there is more trans fat present.

In the fall of 2000, Health Canada announced new recommendations designed to improve nutrition labels on foods. Not only will all prepackaged foods be required to disclose nutrition facts on the label, but this information must also be presented for a greater number of nutrients, including trans fat. Once these recommendations become law, food manufacturers will have two years to fully conform to the new nutrition labeling laws. In the meantime, check ingredients lists for the terms hydrogenated or partially hydrogenated.

Dietary Cholesterol

This wax-like fatty substance is found in meat, poultry, eggs, dairy products and seafood. It's particularly plentiful in shrimp, liver and egg yolks. While high-cholesterol diets cause high blood cholesterol in animals, this is not the case in humans. Dietary cholesterol has little or no effect on most people's blood cholesterol. One reason for this is that our intestines absorb only half the cholesterol we eat. The rest is excreted in the stool. Our bodies are also very efficient at secreting cholesterol into bile stored in the gallbladder. This means there's less cholesterol available for transport in your blood.

Nevertheless, too much dietary cholesterol can raise levels of LDL cholesterol in some people, especially those with hereditary forms of high blood cholesterol. Health Canada recommends that we consume no more than 300 milligrams of cholesterol each day. Choosing animal foods that are lower in saturated fat will also help cut down on dietary cholesterol. Here's how various foods stack up in terms of cholesterol:

Food	Cholesterol (milligrams)
1 egg, whole	190 mg
1 egg, white only	0 mg
Beef sirloin, lean only, 3 oz (90 g)	64 mg
Calf's liver, fried, 3 oz (90 g)	416 mg
Pork loin, lean only, 3 oz (90 g)	71 mg
Chicken breast, no skin, 3 oz (90 g)	73 mg
Salmon, 3 oz (90 g)	54 mg
Shrimp, 3 oz (90 g)	135 mg
Milk, 2% MF, 1 cup (250 ml)	19 mg
Milk, skim, 1 cup (250 ml)	5 mg
Cheese, cheddar, 31% MF, 1 oz (30 g)	31 mg
Cheese, mozzarella, part skim, 1 oz (30 g)	18 mg
Cream, half and half, 12% MF, 2 tbsp (30 ml)	12 mg
Yogurt, 1.5% MF, 3/4 cup (175 ml)	11 mg
Butter, 2 tsp (10 ml)	10 mg

How Much and What Kind of Fat Should You Eat?

Nutrition guidelines emphasize the importance of cutting back on total fat and saturated fat. But you also need to ensure you are getting essential fatty acids and omega-3 oils found in fish. To meet these recommendations, practice the following:

- Consume no more than 30 percent of your daily calories from fat, or, no more than 3 grams of fat for every 100 calories. This doesn't mean that each food you eat must be low in fat. You can make up for eating one high-fat food by including plenty of low-fat foods in other meals.

- Reduce your intake of saturated fat—it should contribute no more than 10 percent of your daily calories. But don't worry too much about numbers and percents. Rather, when choosing animal foods, simply make a habit of opting for those that are lower in fat. Vegetarian protein foods such as legumes and soy foods have very little saturated fat; try to make more of your meals vegetarian.

- Keep your daily cholesterol intake at no more than 300 milligrams.

- Reduce your intake of foods containing trans fat. As often as possible, avoid products made with hydrogenated fat.

- Eat fish three times a week for its heart-protective omega-3 fats. The oilier the fish, the better.

- Meet your daily requirements for essential fatty acids. Including one or two tablespoons of an oil rich in alpha-linolenic acid in your diet each day will ensure this. Omega-6 oils are widespread in processed foods, so most people don't have a problem meeting daily requirements for linoleic acid.

4

—————◇◇◇—————

Understanding Vitamins and Minerals

Eat right, live well—so the saying goes. Your body needs more than 45 nutrients to stay healthy. A diet that's low in fat and rich in vegetables, fruit and whole grains will give you all the vitamins and minerals you need, while offering many other natural compounds, like fiber and phytochemicals, that help your body fight disease. Yet, despite the wealth of information available on the benefits of eating healthily, many Canadians aren't getting enough vitamins and minerals in their diets. The following guide will help you choose the foods and supplements that are brimming with protective vitamins and minerals. In Chapter 5, you'll read more about the benefits of supplementing your diet with a daily vitamin and mineral pill.

Because of the lack of data needed to calculate a *recommended dietary allowance (RDA)* of some vitamins, scientists have instead established a daily *adequate intake (AI)*. Some nutrients also have been assigned a *daily upper limit*, which is the highest level of intake likely to pose no risk of adverse health effects for almost all people (adults and children).

The Vitamins

Vitamins are essential substances needed by the body in small amounts for normal growth, function and maintenance of healthy tissues. Without vitamins, we would succumb to deficiency diseases such as scurvy, rickets, pellagra and beriberi. But as scientists are learning, vitamins may also ward off chronic diseases like heart disease, cancer and osteoporosis.

Since the body is not able to synthesize vitamins, they must be supplied from foods—plant or animal. Vitamins don't supply the body directly with energy. Instead, they participate in metabolic processes that generate energy for the body. Each of the 13 vitamins has its own special role to play in maintaining health. Some vitamins dissolve in fat, others dissolve in water. Fat-soluble vitamins like A, D and E are not readily excreted from the body. This means that large doses of fat-soluble vitamins have the potential to accumulate in the body and cause toxic reactions. The water-soluble vitamins, consisting of the family of Bs and vitamin C, on the other hand, are easily lost from the body. With the exception of vitamin B6, water-soluble vitamins have less potential to cause toxic reactions when taken in large doses because they are excreted from the body.

Cook and store your foods with care to preserve their vitamin content. Because vitamins are organic, they can break down and lose their effectiveness.

Vitamin A

Vitamin A has many important roles in the body. It supports cell growth and development; maintains healthy skin, hair, nails, bones and teeth; and supports the immune system. It is also needed for night and color vision.

Vitamin A is found preformed in certain animal foods and also is derived from plant foods that contain beta-carotene. Once consumed, beta-carotene is converted to vitamin A by the liver. Beta-carotene may prevent heart disease, cataracts, macular degeneration and possibly lung cancer. However, no official dietary requirement for beta-carotene has been established as it is not considered an essential nutrient.

Recommended Dietary Allowance (RDA) of Vitamin A

Age	RDA (micrograms)
1–3 years	300 mcg
4–8 years	400 mcg
9–13 years	600 mcg
Boys, 14–18 years	900 mcg
Girls, 14–18 years	700 mcg
Men, 19+ years	900 mcg
Women, 19+ years	700 mcg
Pregnancy	770 mcg
Breastfeeding	1300 mcg

Daily Upper Limits of Vitamin A

Age	Daily Upper Limit (micrograms)
1–3 years	600 mcg
4–8 years	900 mcg
9–13 years	1700 mcg
Boys, 14–18 years	2800 mcg
Girls, 14–18 years	2800 mcg
19+ years	3000 mcg

The best sources of vitamin A are calf's liver, oily fish, milk, cheese, butter and egg yolks. Beta-carotene is found in orange and dark produce such as carrots, sweet potato, winter squash, broccoli, collard greens, kale, spinach, apricots, cantaloupe, peaches, nectarines, mango and papaya.

Vitamin A Supplements

Except in special circumstances, taking vitamin A supplements is not recommended. In particular, people with liver disease should not take vitamin A supplements. High dose vitamin A supplements have also been linked with a greater risk of bone loss and hip fracture. Because vitamin A is fat-soluble, the body stores it, and taking too much vitamin A for a period of time can be toxic. Your diet and a multivitamin will provide all the vitamin A you need. Pregnant women should avoid taking too much vitamin A since high doses may increase the risk of birth defects. Prenatal multivitamin and mineral formulas are safe because they have less vitamin A than regular multis.

If you want to boost your intake of vitamin A, beta-carotene supplements are a safe alternative to vitamin A supplements. Many multivitamin and mineral supplements provide 1000 to 10,000 international units (0.5 to 5.5 milligrams) of beta-carotene. If you opt for a separate beta-carotene supplement, I recommend you choose a product that offers a mix of carotenoids including beta-carotene, lycopene and lutein. You'll read in other chapters how these carotenoid compounds may enhance each other's absorption in the digestive tract.

If you are a smoker, avoid beta-carotene supplements and get your daily fix from foods only. Use of beta-carotene supplements in doses of 20 milligrams per day for five to eight years has been associated with an increased risk of lung cancer in men who smoke. This potential health risk has not been found in smokers who eat a diet plentiful in beta-carotene-rich foods.

B Vitamins

Thiamin (Vitamin B1)

One of the eight vitamins in the B family, thiamin, also known as vitamin B1, is needed by our bodies for energy metabolism. Thiamin also maintains normal appetite and nerve function.

Recommended Dietary Allowance (RDA) of Thiamin

Age	RDA (milligrams)
1–3 years	0.5 mg
4–8 years	0.6 mg
9–13 years	0.9 mg
Boys, 14–18 years	1.2 mg
Girls, 14–18 years	1.0 mg
Men, 19+ years	1.2 mg
Women, 19+ years	1.1 mg
Pregnancy	1.4 mg
Breastfeeding	1.4 mg
Daily upper limit	*None established*

To add a boost of thiamin to your diet, reach for pork, calf's liver, whole grains, enriched breakfast cereals, legumes and nuts.

Thiamin Supplements

People taking strong diuretic drugs (such as Lasix®) for congestive heart failure may need extra thiamin, as such drugs deplete the body of this B vitamin. People with conditions that cause malabsorption of nutrients may also benefit from additional thiamin. Since the B vitamins work closely together in the body, I recommend taking a high-potency multivitamin and mineral formula or a B complex supplement. Both will offer between 25 and 100 milligrams of thiamin.

Riboflavin (Vitamin B2)

Like the other B vitamins, riboflavin, or vitamin B2, is needed for energy metabolism. This vitamin also supports normal vision and maintains healthy skin. There is evidence to suggest that riboflavin may prevent cataracts and migraine headaches.

Recommended Dietary Allowance (RDA) of Riboflavin

Age	RDA (milligrams)
1–3 years	0.5 mg
4–8 years	0.6 mg
9–13 years	0.9 mg
Boys, 14–18 years	1.3 mg
Girls, 14–18 years	1.0 mg
Men, 19+ years	1.3 mg
Women, 19+ years	1.1 mg
Pregnancy	1.4 mg
Breastfeeding	1.6 mg
Daily upper limit	*None established*

Riboflavin is found in milk, yogurt, cottage cheese, fortified soy and rice beverages, meat, whole grains and enriched breakfast cereals.

Riboflavin Supplements

Studies suggest that 400 milligrams of riboflavin taken once daily can reduce the frequency of migraine attacks. Riboflavin supplements are available in 25, 50, 100, 500 and 1200 milligram doses. These supplements are nontoxic and very well tolerated by the body. However, it may take up to three months to notice an improvement. Riboflavin supplements may be difficult to find at a drugstore; visit your local health food or supplement store.

For possible cataract prevention, take a high-potency multivitamin and mineral formula or a B complex supplement that supplies 25 to 100 milligrams of riboflavin.

Niacin (Vitamin B3)

Niacin, also known as vitamin B3, is needed for energy metabolism. As well, it maintains healthy skin and the digestive tract, while supporting nerve function. Studies suggest that niacin may lower high blood cholesterol and may also prevent type 1 diabetes in children.

Recommended Dietary Allowance (RDA) of Niacin

Age	RDA (milligrams)
1–3 years	6 mg
4–8 years	8 mg
9–13 years	12 mg

Age	RDA (milligrams)
Boys, 14–18 years	16 mg
Girls, 14–18 years	14 mg
Men, 19+ years	16 mg
Women, 19+ years	14 mg
Pregnancy	18 mg
Breastfeeding	17 mg

Daily Upper Limits of Niacin

Age	Daily Upper Limit (milligrams)
1–3 years	10 mg
4–8 years	15 mg
9–13 years	20 mg
14–18 years	30 mg
19+ years	35 mg

Meat, poultry, fish, calf's liver, eggs, dairy products, peanuts, almonds, seeds, wheat bran, whole grains and enriched breakfast cereals are all good sources of niacin.

Niacin Supplements

Taken in very high doses, niacin can cause liver damage. Therefore, *high-dose niacin supplements should be taken only under the supervision of a doctor.* If you want to boost your intake of niacin, take a high-potency multivitamin and mineral formula or a B complex supplement. Both offer anywhere between 25 and 100 milligrams of niacin.

When taken in doses greater than 35 milligrams per day, niacin could cause flushing of the face, neck and arms. This can be avoided by taking your supplement just after eating a meal. This symptom is harmless and goes away within 20 minutes, but some people find it uncomfortable. To avoid flushing, look for a formula that contains the non-flushing form of niacin called niacinamide.

Vitamin B6 (Pyridoxine)

The body uses vitamin B6, or pyridoxine, to form an important enzyme that's needed to create serotonin, a chemical in the brain that has a calming and relaxing effect. This vitamin is also necessary for protein and fat metabolism and the production of red blood cells.

Vitamin B6 is thought to help prevent heart disease. Studies also suggest that it may reduce PMS-related depression and may be useful in treating morning sickness during pregnancy.

Recommended Dietary Allowance (RDA) of Vitamin B6

Age	RDA (milligrams)
1–3 years	0.5 mg
4–8 years	0.6 mg
9–13 years	1.0 mg
Boys, 14–18 years	1.3 mg
Girls, 14–18 years	1.2 mg
Men and women, adults, 19–50 years	1.3 mg
Men, 51+ years	1.7 mg
Women, 51+ years	1.5 mg
Pregnancy	1.9 mg
Breastfeeding	2.0 mg

Daily Upper Limits of Vitamin B6

Age	Daily Upper Limit (milligrams)
1–3 years	30 mg
4–8 years	40 mg
9–13 years	60 mg
14–18 years	80 mg
19+ years	100 mg

Vitamin B6 in Foods

Food	Vitamin B6 (milligrams)
Beef, flank, cooked, 3 oz (90 g)	0.3 mg
Pork center loin, cooked, 3 oz (90 g)	0.3 mg
Chicken breast, cooked, 1/2 (140 g)	0.3 mg
Chicken leg, cooked, 1 (187 g)	0.2 mg
Salmon, sockeye, cooked, 3 oz (90 g)	0.2 mg
Tuna, canned and drained, 3 oz (90 g)	0.4 mg
100% bran cereal, 1/2 cup (125 ml)	0.5 mg

Food	Vitamin B6 (milligrams)
Cereal, whole grain flakes, 2/3 cup (160 ml)	0.5 mg
Avocado, California, 1/2 medium	0.2 mg
Avocado, Florida, 1/2 medium	0.4 mg
Banana, medium	0.7 mg
Potato, baked, medium with skin	0.7 mg

Nutrient Values of Some Common Foods, Health Canada, Ottawa, 1999.

Vitamin B6 Supplements

If you want to boost your intake of vitamin B6 beyond what you can get from food, take a high-potency multivitamin and mineral pill or a B complex supplement. Both formulas will supply between 25 and 100 milligrams of vitamin B6. Do not exceed 100 milligrams per day: too much B6 over an extended period can be toxic and may cause irreversible nerve damage.

People with Parkinson's disease who take the medication levodopa are advised to not take more than 5 milligrams of B6 a day as the vitamin can interfere with the action of the drug.

Folate (Folic Acid)

This B vitamin is called folate when it occurs naturally in foods. When it is an addition to foods or present in a supplement, it's referred to as folic acid. Folate supports cell division and growth. The body uses it to make DNA and red blood cells. It is extremely important that women have sufficient amounts of folate before and during pregnancy in order to prevent neural tube birth defects in the newborn. Folate may reduce the risk of heart disease and breast cancer.

Recommended Dietary Allowance (RDA) of Folate

Age	RDA (micrograms)
1–3 years	150 mcg
4–8 years	200 mcg
9–13 years	300 mcg
14–18 years	400 mcg
19–50 years	400 mcg
51+ years	400 mcg
Pregnancy	600 mcg
Breastfeeding	500 mcg

Daily Upper Limits of Folate

Age	Daily Upper Limit (micrograms)
1–3 years	300 mcg
4–8 years	400 mcg
9–13 years	600 mcg
14–18 years	800 mcg
19+ years	1000 mcg

Folate in Foods

Food	Folate (micrograms)
Chicken liver, 3.5 oz (100 g)	770 mcg
Black beans, cooked, 1/2 cup (125 ml)	135 mcg
Chickpeas, cooked, 1/2 cup (125 ml)	85 mcg
Kidney beans, cooked, 1/2 cup (125 ml)	120 mcg
Lentils, cooked, 1/2 cup (125 ml)	189 mcg
Peanuts, 1/2 cup (125 ml)	96 mcg
Sunflower seeds, 1/3 cup (75 ml)	96 mcg
Artichoke, 1 medium	64 mcg
Asparagus, 5 spears	110 mcg
Avocado, California, 1/2	113 mcg
Avocado, Florida, 1/2	81 mcg
Bean sprouts, 1 cup (250 ml)	91 mcg
Beets, 1/2 cup (125 ml)	72 mcg
Brussels sprouts, 1/2 cup (125 ml)	83 mcg
Romaine lettuce, 1 cup (250 ml)	80 mcg
Spinach, raw, 1 cup (250 ml)	115 mcg
Spinach, cooked, 1/2 cup (125 ml)	139 mcg
Orange, 1 medium	40 mcg
Orange juice, frozen, diluted, 1 cup (250 ml)	115 mcg
Orange juice, freshly squeezed, 1 cup (250 ml)	79 mcg

Nutrient Values of Some Common Foods, Health Canada, Ottawa, 1999.

Folic Acid Supplements

Many people find it a challenge to consume 400 micrograms of this B vitamin on a daily basis. If you want to ensure you are meeting your daily folate requirements, take a high-potency multivitamin and mineral pill or a B complex supplement. Both formulas will offer between 400 and 1000 micrograms of folic acid. Most regular-strength formulas provide 400 micrograms.

If you decide to take a folic acid supplement, be sure to choose one with vitamin B12 added. Supplementing with folic acid alone can mask a vitamin B12 deficiency, which could lead to irreversible nerve damage. Do not exceed 1000 micrograms of folic acid per day.

Vitamin B12

Vitamin B12 maintains healthy nerve function and is necessary in the body to make DNA and red blood cells. Scientists have learned that vitamin B12 may reduce the risk of heart disease and may also be beneficial in the treatment of male infertility.

Recommended Dietary Allowance (RDA) of Vitamin B12

Age	RDA (micrograms)
1–3 years	0.9 mcg
4–8 years	1.2 mcg
9–13 years	1.8 mcg
14–18 years	2.4 mcg
19–50 years	2.4 mcg
51+ years	2.4 mcg
Pregnancy	2.6 mcg
Breastfeeding	2.8 mcg
Daily upper limit	*None established*

Vitamin B12 is found in all animal foods, including shellfish and dairy. Some soy and rice beverages are fortified with B12. Here's a look at amounts of B12 in selected foods:

Vitamin B12 in Foods

Food	Vitamin B12 (micrograms)
Beef, lean, 3 oz (90 g)	2.8 mcg
Mussels, shelled, 3 oz (90 g)	20 mcg
Salmon, sockeye, cooked, 3 oz (90 g)	4.9 mcg

Food	Vitamin B12 (micrograms)
Milk, 1 cup (250 ml)	1.0 mcg
Yogurt, 3/4 cup (175 ml)	1.0 mcg
Cottage cheese, 1%, 1 cup (250 ml)	0.7 mcg
Cheddar cheese, 1.5 oz (45 g)	0.4 mcg
1 egg, whole	0.6 mcg
Fortified soy beverage, 1 cup (250 ml)	1.0 mcg

Nutrient Values of Some Common Foods, Health Canada, Ottawa, 1999.

Vitamin B12 Supplements

Anyone over the age of 50 should be supplementing his or her diet with vitamin B12. Up to one-third of older adults produce inadequate amounts of stomach acid and so can no longer properly absorb B12 from food (stomach acid is needed to release the vitamin from food proteins). For that matter, anyone taking medication to reduce stomach acid secretion should take a B12 supplement.

To boost your intake of this vitamin, take a high-potency multivitamin and mineral pill or a B complex supplement. Both will offer between 25 and 100 micrograms of B12. No adverse effects have been reported in healthy individuals taking B12 supplements.

Biotin

This B vitamin, like the others in the B family, is necessary for energy metabolism. Biotin is also used to synthesize fat, amino acids and glycogen (the form in which your body stores carbohydrate).

Adequate Intakes (AI) of Biotin

Age	AI (micrograms)
1–3 years	8 mcg
4–8 years	12 mcg
9–13 years	20 mcg
14–18 years	25 mcg
19+ years	30 mcg
Pregnancy	30 mcg
Breastfeeding	35 mcg
Daily upper limit	*None established*

The best sources of biotin are kidney, calf's liver, clams, oatmeal, whole grains, egg yolk, soybeans, nuts, brewer's yeast, cauliflower, mushrooms and bananas. It is also produced from bacteria in our intestinal tract. In fact, most of us likely get all the biotin we need from this source.

Biotin Supplements

There is little evidence to support taking supplemental biotin. Most regular multi-vitamin and mineral supplements provide close to 50 micrograms of the nutrient. High-potency or super-strength multivitamin formulas offer up to 100 micrograms.

Pantothenic Acid

The body uses pantothenic acid to metabolize fat and carbohydrate for energy. The nutrient is also used to make bile, a digestive aid, as well as hormones, neurotrans-mitters, red blood cells and vitamin D. Pantothenic acid is involved in more than 100 steps in the body's production of fats, brain chemicals (neurotransmitters), hormones, vitamin D and the iron-carrying compound called hemoglobin. It is also an important part of coenzyme A, an essential compound used by the cells to gener-ate energy.

Adequate Intakes (AI) of Pantothenic Acid

Age	AI (milligrams)
1–3 years	2 mg
4–8 years	3 mg
9–13 years	4 mg
14–18 years	5 mg
19+ years	5 mg
Pregnancy	6 mg
Breastfeeding	7 mg
Daily upper limit	*None established*

Pantothenic acid is found in many foods. The best sources are brewer's yeast, calf's liver, meat, fish, poultry, peanuts, soybeans, split peas, nuts, seeds, lentils, whole grains, oatmeal, buckwheat and mushrooms.

Pantothenic Acid Supplements

There is little evidence to support taking supplemental pantothenic acid, since a deficiency of this B vitamin is rare. Most regular multivitamin and mineral supple-ments provide 10 milligrams of the nutrient. High-potency or super-strength multi-vitamin formulas offer up to 100 milligrams.

Choline

Although not considered a true vitamin, choline is needed in the body for fat metabolism and to maintain healthy nerve function. It is also used to make cell membranes and acetylcholine, a brain neurotransmitter that is involved in memory.

Adequate Intakes (AI) of Choline

Age	AI (milligrams)
1–3 years	200 mg
4–8 years	250 mg
9–13 years	375 mg
Boys, 14–18 years	550 mg
Girls, 14–18 years	400 mg
Men, 19+ years	550 mg
Women, 19+ years	425 mg
Pregnancy	450 mg
Breastfeeding	550 mg

Daily Upper Limits of Choline

Age	Daily Upper Limit (milligrams)
1–8 years	1000 mg
9–13 years	2000 mg
14–18 years	3000 mg
19+ years	3500 mg

Egg yolks, calf's liver, kidney, meat, brewer's yeast, wheat germ, soybeans, peanuts and green peas are foods to include in your diet to ensure you're meeting your daily requirement of choline.

Choline Supplements

There is little evidence to support taking supplemental choline. However, if you are concerned that your daily diet does not contain choline-rich foods, consider taking a supplement of choline, lecithin or phosphatidylserine (see Chapter 8 for more information on lecithin and phosphatidylcholine). Not all multivitamin supplements contain choline; check the contents list on the label.

High doses of choline from supplements may cause a fishy body odor and sweating. People with liver or kidney disease or Parkinson's disease, as well as those who suffer from depression, are at greater risk for adverse effects associated with high intakes of choline from supplements.

Vitamin C (Ascorbic Acid)

This water-soluble vitamin supports collagen synthesis and wound healing, strengthens blood vessels, and helps the body absorb iron. Its antioxidant powers may prevent heart disease, cataracts and macular degeneration. It may also help prevent osteoporosis. By supporting the body's immune system, vitamin C may lessen the severity and duration of the common cold.

Recommended Dietary Allowance (RDA) of Vitamin C

Age	RDA (milligrams)
1–3 years	15 mg
4–8 years	25 mg
9–13 years	45 mg
Boys, 14–18 years	75 mg
Girls, 14–18 years	65 mg
Men, 19+ years	90 mg
Women, 19+ years	75 mg
Pregnancy	85 mg
Breastfeeding	120 mg

Note: smokers need an additional 35 mg

Daily Upper Limits of Vitamin C

Age	Daily Upper Limit (milligrams)
1–3 years	400 mg
4–8 years	650 mg
9–13 years	1200 mg
14–18 years	1800 mg
19+ years	2000 mg

Vitamin C in Foods

Food	Vitamin C (milligrams)
Cantaloupe, 1/4 medium	56 mg
Orange, 1 medium	70 mg
Orange juice, fresh, 1 cup (250 ml)	131 mg
Grapefruit, red or pink, 1/2	47 mg
Kiwi, 1 large	68 mg
Mango, 1	49 mg
Strawberries, raw, 1 cup (250 ml)	89 mg
Broccoli, raw, 1 spear	141 mg
Brussels sprouts, cooked, 1/2 cup (125 ml)	50 mg
Cauliflower, raw, 1/2 cup (125 ml)	38 mg
Potato, baked with skin, 1	27 mg
Red pepper, raw, 1/2 cup (125 ml)	95 mg
Tomato juice, 1 cup (250 ml)	47 mg

Nutrient Values of Some Common Foods, Health Canada, Ottawa, 1999.

Vitamin C Supplements

If you don't eat at least two vitamin-C-rich foods each day, taking a supplement is a good idea. Choose one labeled "Ester C." Studies in the laboratory have found that this form of vitamin C is more available to the body.

Timed-release, sustained-release or continuous-release vitamin C supplements are thought by some experts to be the best choice. In contrast to a regular vitamin C tablet, which releases all the nutrient within a short time, these supplements are purported to release small quantities over a prolonged period. This keeps cells and tissues saturated with the vitamin longer. As the water-soluble vitamin is used up in metabolic processes, vitamin C newly released from the timed-release tablet replenishes the supply.

If you choose a chewable supplement, make sure it contains calcium ascorbate or sodium ascorbate. These forms of vitamin C are less acidic to the enamel of your teeth.

Take a 500 milligram supplement once or twice a day. Research has determined that your body can use only about 200 milligrams at one time. I've recommended 500 milligrams because this is the most common dose you'll find on the market. If you prefer to take 1000 milligrams once daily, choose a timed-release formula.

People with a history of kidney stones or kidney failure should restrict their intake to 100 milligrams per day.

Vitamin D

This vitamin regulates body calcium and phosphorus levels and helps the intestine absorb these two minerals. By maintaining bones and teeth, it helps to prevent osteoporosis. Most of our vitamin D comes from sunlight. When ultraviolet light hits the skin, it forms a pre-vitamin D. This compound then makes its way to the kidneys, where it's transformed into active vitamin D.

The long winter months in Canada result in very little vitamin D being synthesized in your skin. Even in the summer, you might be low in this vitamin, since sun protection factor (SPF) in sunscreen blocks its production. To help meet your vitamin D needs, expose your hands, face and arms to the sun for 10 to 15 minutes, two or three times a week (don't wear sunscreen), but avoid the hottest times of day to prevent sunburn.

Adequate Intakes (AI) of Vitamin D

Age	AI (International Units)
1–3 years	200 IU (5 mcg)
4–8 years	200 IU (5 mcg)
9–30 years	200 IU (5 mcg) / 400 IU*
31–50 years	200 IU (5 mcg) / 400 IU*
51–70 years	400 IU (10 mcg) / 800 IU*
71+ years	600 IU (15 mcg) / 800 IU*
Pregnancy	200 IU (5 mcg)
Breastfeeding	200 IU (5 mcg)
Daily upper limit	*2000 IU (50 mcg)*

*Note: Canadians at risk for osteoporosis are advised to consume 400 or 800 IU of vitamin D, depending on their age.

Vitamin D in Foods

Food	Vitamin D (International Units)
Liver, chicken, 3.5 oz (100 g)	50–65 IU
Liver, pork, 3.5 oz (100 g)	84 IU
Liver, beef, 3.5 oz (100 g)	8–40 IU
Cod, 3.5 oz (100 g)	85 IU
Herring, 3.5 oz (100 g)	330 IU
Mackerel, 3.5 oz (100 g)	120 IU
Salmon, canned, 3.5 oz (100 g)	220–440 IU
Sardines, 3.5 oz (100 g)	1500 IU

Food	Vitamin D (International Units)
Shrimp, 3.5 oz (100 g)	150 IU
Milk, fluid, 1 cup (250 ml)	100 IU
Soy beverage, fortified, 1 cup (250 ml)	100 IU
Rice beverage, fortified, 1 cup (250 ml)	100 IU
Egg, 1 whole	24 IU
Butter, 1 tbsp (15 ml)	3 IU
Margarine, 1 tsp (5 ml)	15 IU

The Vitamins: Fundamental Aspects in Nutritional Health, 2nd ed., San Diego: Academic Press, 1992.

Vitamin D Supplements

Vitamin D supplements should be taken only under the advice of a doctor. Most multivitamin and mineral supplements supply between 200 and 400 IU of the vitamin. If you take calcium supplements, choose a product with vitamin D added.

Vitamin E (Alpha Tocopherol)

This antioxidant protects cell membranes and enhances the body's immune system. Vitamin E is also necessary for iron metabolism and to protect polyunsaturated fats in the body and vitamin A from oxidation (free radical damage). Research suggests that vitamin E may help prevent heart disease and prostate cancer and slow the progression of Alzheimer's disease.

Recommended Dietary Allowance (RDA) of Vitamin E

Age	RDA (International Units)
1–3 years	9 IU (6 mg)
4–8 years	10 IU (7 mg)
9–13 years	16 IU (11 mg)
14–18 years	22 IU (15 mg)
19–30 years	22 IU (15 mg)
31–50 years	22 IU (15 mg)
51–70 years	22 IU (15 mg)
71+ years	22 IU (15 mg)
Pregnancy	22 IU (15 mg)
Breastfeeding	28 IU (19 mg)
Daily upper limit	*1500 IU (1000 mg)*

Vegetable oils, almonds, peanuts, soybeans, whole grains, wheat germ, wheat germ oil, avocado and green leafy vegetables, especially kale, are all good sources of vitamin E.

Vitamin E Supplements

Take 200 to 800 IU per day. There's no evidence to warrant taking more if you're healthy. Buy a natural source vitamin E supplement (or look for "d-alpha-tocopherol" on the label; synthetic forms are labeled "dl-alpha-tocopherol"). Although the body absorbs both synthetic and natural forms equally well, your liver prefers the natural form, incorporating more natural vitamin E into carrier molecules. You might also consider choosing a natural vitamin E supplement labeled "mixed tocopherols." In addition to alpha-tocopherol, these supplements contain a form of vitamin E known as gamma-tocopherol, which has been shown in preliminary research to have potent anti-inflammatory effects in addition to its antioxidant properties. This may play a role in cancer prevention.

If you're taking a blood-thinning medication like warfarin (Coumadin®), don't take vitamin E without your doctor's approval, as it has slight anticlotting properties.

Vitamin K

Vitamin K is essential for blood clotting. It also plays an important role in the formation of new bone and may help prevent osteoporosis. Studies show that high dietary intakes of vitamin K are associated with lower risk of hip fractures.

Adequate Intakes (AI) of Vitamin K

Age	AI (micrograms)
1–3 years	30 mcg
4–8 years	55 mcg
9–13 years	60 mcg
14–18 years	75 mcg
Men, 19+ years	120 mcg
Women, 19+ years	90 mcg
Pregnancy	90 mcg
Breastfeeding	90 mcg
Daily upper limit	*None established*

The best sources of vitamin K are green peas, broccoli, spinach, leafy green vegetables, Brussels sprouts, romaine lettuce, cabbage and calf's liver. Bacteria in the intestinal tract also produce Vitamin K.

Vitamin K Supplements

Whether vitamin K supplements help prevent osteoporosis remains to be seen. One study did show that supplements of the nutrient reduced the amount of calcium lost through urine. Although the amounts that appear to protect the bones can easily be obtained from food, no adverse effects have been reported in healthy people taking vitamin K supplements.

Vitamin K supplements counteract the effects of blood-thinning medication such as heparin and warfarin (Coumadin®). Do not take vitamin K supplements if you take these drugs.

The Minerals

Minerals, like vitamins, are vital to health. Minerals are important players in many different metabolic reactions in the body. Many minerals enable enzymes (protein compounds that catalyze chemical reactions) to function. Other minerals are key components of body compounds such as hormones and hemoglobin found in red blood cells. Electrolyte minerals like sodium, potassium and chloride help maintain fluid balance throughout the body. Finally, some minerals have a critical role in the body's growth and development.

Minerals are categorized according to our daily dietary requirements. In general, if we need 100 milligrams or more (about 1/50 of a teaspoon), it is considered a major mineral. If we require less, it's referred to as a trace mineral.

The body is unable to make minerals on its own and so must get them from foods. Our diet provides a wide range of minerals, but they can vary in their availability to the body. Some foods contain naturally occurring binders that prevent much of a mineral from being released from the food. For example, phytic acid in spinach reduces the amount of calcium, iron and zinc that's available to the body. Nevertheless, a key factor in determining how much a mineral we absorb is our body's need for that mineral at the time.

Some minerals are roughly the same size and share the same electric charge. For instance, calcium, magnesium, iron and zinc have the same charge and so compete with each other for absorption. That's why calcium supplements can interfere with iron absorption. Mineral absorption will be discussed in more detail below.

Toxicity reactions are much more likely to occur with mineral supplements than they are with vitamin pills. Take great care when supplementing with minerals. As you will read below, single high-dose supplements of many minerals are potentially dangerous and should be avoided.

The minerals are presented below in roughly alphabetical order—first the three major minerals (calcium, magnesium and phosphorus), followed by the trace minerals and finally, the electrolyte minerals.

Calcium

Calcium is critical for building strong bones and teeth. It also helps muscles contract and relax, and it supports nerve function. Calcium plays an important role in blood clotting and maintaining blood pressure. Scientists have learned that it may help prevent osteoporosis, colon cancer and high blood pressure. It may also help ease symptoms of premenstrual syndrome.

Recommended Dietary Allowance (RDA) of Calcium

Age	RDA (milligrams)
1–3 years	500 mg
4–8 years	800 mg
9–13 years	1300 mg
14–18 years	1300 mg
19–50 years	1000 mg
51+ years	1200 mg / 1500 mg*
Pregnancy	1000 mg
Breastfeeding	1000 mg
Daily upper limit	*2500 mg*

*Note: Canadian adults over the age of 50 who are at risk for osteoporosis are advised to consume 1500 mg of calcium per day.

Calcium in Foods

Foods	Calcium (milligrams)
Dairy Foods	
Milk, Lactaid, 1 cup (250 ml)	300 mg
Milk (Neilson TruTaste), 1 cup (250 ml)	360 mg
Milk (Neilson TruCalcium), 1 cup (250 ml)	420 mg
Carnation Instant Breakfast, with 1 cup (250 ml) milk	540 mg
Chocolate milk, 1 cup (250 ml)	285 mg
Cheese, cheddar, 1.5 oz (45 g)	300 mg
Cheese, Swiss or Gruyere, 1.5 oz (45 g)	480 mg
Cheese, mozzarella, 1.5 oz (45 g)	228 mg
Cheese, cottage, 1/2 cup (125 ml)	75 mg

Foods	Calcium (milligrams)
Cheese, ricotta, 1/2 cup (125 ml)	255mg
Evaporated milk, 1/2 cup (125 ml)	350 mg
Light sour cream, 1/4 cup (60 ml)	120 mg
Pudding, low-fat Healthy Choice, 1/2 cup (125 ml)	110 mg
Skim milk powder, dry, 3 tbsp (45 ml)	155 mg
Yogurt, plain, 3/4 cup (175 ml)	300 mg
Yogurt, fruit, 3/4 cup (175 ml)	250 mg
Nondairy Foods	
Soybeans, cooked, 1 cup (250 ml)	175 mg
Soybeans, roasted, 1/4 cup (60 ml)	60 mg
Soy beverage, 1 cup (250 ml)	100 mg
Soy beverage, fortified (So Good), 1 cup (250 ml)	330 mg
Baked beans, 1 cup (250 ml)	150 mg
Black beans, 1 cup (250 ml)	102 mg
Kidney beans, 1 cup, cooked (250 ml)	69 mg
Lentils, cooked, 1 cup (250 ml)	37 mg
Tempeh, cooked, 1 cup (250 ml)	154 mg
Tofu, raw, firm, with calcium sulfate, 4 oz (120 g)	260 mg
Tofu, raw, regular, with calcium sulfate, 4 oz (120 g)	130 mg
Sardines, 8 small (with bones)	165 mg
Salmon, 1/2 can drained (with bones)	225 mg
Broccoli, raw, 1 cup (250 ml)	42 mg
Broccoli, cooked, 1 cup (250 ml)	94 mg
Bok choy, cooked, 1 cup (250 ml)	158 mg
Collard greens, cooked, 1 cup (250 ml)	357 mg
Kale, cooked, 1 cup (250 ml)	179 mg
Rutabaga, cooked, 1/2 cup (125 ml)	57 mg
Swiss chard, raw, 1 cup (250 ml)	21 mg
Swiss chard, cooked, 1 cup (250 ml)	102 mg
Okra, cooked, 1 cup (250 ml)	176 mg
Currants, 1/2 cup (125 ml)	60 mg
Figs, 5 medium	135 mg
Orange, 1 medium	50 mg

Foods	Calcium (milligrams)
Almonds, 1/4 cup (60 ml)	100 mg
Brazil nuts, 1/4 cup (60 ml)	65 mg
Hazelnuts, 1/4 cup (60 ml)	65 mg
Blackstrap molasses, 2 tbsp (30 ml)	288 mg
Fancy molasses, 2 tbsp (30 ml)	70 mg
Oasis Florida Premium orange juice, 1 cup (250 ml)	300 mg
Oasis Health Break (juice & milk cocktail), 1 cup (250 ml)	300 mg
Calcium-fortified orange juice, 1 cup (250 ml), Tropicana™	360 mg

Nutrient Values of Some Common Foods, Health Canada, Ottawa, 1999.

Our body does not absorb calcium from all foods equally well. While many plant foods contribute calcium to the diet, certain natural compounds in vegetables prevent some of this calcium from being absorbed. Studies show that dairy products contain the most absorbable form of calcium. The following strategies will help you enhance your body's absorption of calcium:

- Cook green vegetables in order to boost their calcium content by releasing calcium that's bound to oxalic acid.

- Don't take iron supplements with calcium-rich foods as iron competes with calcium for absorption.

- Drink tea between rather than during meals. Tannins, natural compounds in tea, inhibit calcium absorption.

- Make sure you're meeting dietary requirements for vitamin D each day (as you read earlier in this chapter, vitamin D stimulates the intestine to absorb dietary calcium).

Calcium Supplements

Recent surveys show that most Canadians get only 1.6 servings of milk products each day. (The recommended number of servings is 2 to 3.) That translates to 480 milligrams of calcium. Many people find it difficult to meet their calcium goals if they are lactose intolerant, if they follow a vegetarian diet or if they have poor eating habits. Supplements are often the only way they can ensure they meet their calcium needs.

To help you decide if you need a calcium supplement, use my 300 Milligram Rule. One milk serving supplies 300 milligrams of calcium. For each serving you miss without replacing with other calcium-rich foods, you need to get 300 milligrams of elemental calcium through a supplement. Here's how to choose a high-quality supplement, along with tips on taking it:

1. Look at the source of calcium. Many types of calcium supplements are available, including:

    - *Calcium carbonate* is about 10 to 30 percent absorbed by the body. The amount you absorb depends on how much stomach acid is present. As people age, their stomach produces less hydrochloric acid. Because of this, calcium carbonate is not the best choice for older adults or people on medications that block acid production. If you do take calcium carbonate pills, take it with meals to increase absorption. Do not take calcium carbonate at bedtime, unless you take it with a snack. Calcium carbonate can cause bloating and constipation. On the plus side, this is the most inexpensive type of calcium supplement.

    - *Calcium citrate* is about 30 percent absorbed by the body, making it a better choice for anyone over the age of 50. Studies suggest that this form of calcium is more effective than other forms for osteoporosis treatment. Calcium citrate malate is one of the most highly absorbable (and expensive) forms of calcium. Calcium citrate supplements are well absorbed either with meals or on an empty stomach.

    - *Calcium chelates (HVP chelate)* are supplements that contain calcium that's bound to an amino acid. In the case of HVP chelate, the amino acid is from vegetable protein. Some manufacturers claim that up to 75 percent of calcium in the chelate form is absorbed by the body, although this has not been proven.

    - *Effervescent calcium supplements* contain calcium carbonate and often other forms of more absorbable calcium. Because they get a head start on disintegrating, they may be absorbed in the intestinal tract more quickly. Dissolve these in water or orange juice.

    - *Bone meal* or *dolomite* or *oyster shell* is not recommended because some products have been found to contain trace amounts of contaminants such as lead and mercury.

2. Know how much elemental calcium each pill gives you. Look on the list of ingredients for this information. The amount of elemental calcium is what you use to calculate your daily intake. Some calcium supplements may not be 100 percent elemental calcium. The label may state 500 milligrams, but when you look carefully at the ingredients list you may find the product contains only 350 milligrams of elemental calcium. This will determine how many tablets you need to take to get your recommended dose.

3. Choose a formula with vitamin D and magnesium. These nutrients work in tandem with calcium to promote optimal bone health. For instance, vitamin D increases calcium absorption in your intestine by 30 to 80 percent.

4. Spread larger doses throughout the day. Since all calcium sources (including food sources) are not 100 percent absorbed, it makes sense to split a higher dose over two or three meals. If you've been advised to take 600 milligrams of calcium a day, take a 300 milligram tablet with breakfast and another one at dinner.

5. Take your calcium supplements with a large glass of water.

Do not exceed the daily upper limit of 2500 milligrams of calcium from food and supplements. The major risks from getting too much calcium include kidney stones in people with a history of stones, constipation and gas. Extremely high doses of calcium can cause calcium deposits in the body.

Magnesium

Important for bone growth, protein building, muscle contraction and the transmission of nerve impulses, magnesium is found in abundance in the body. This mineral may prevent migraine headaches, reduce high blood pressure, and ease symptoms of premenstrual syndrome.

Recommended Dietary Allowance (RDA) of Magnesium

Age	RDA (milligrams)
1–3 years	80 mg
4–8 years	130 mg
9–13 years	240 mg
Boys, 14–18 years	410 mg
Girls, 14–18 years	360 mg
Men, 19–30 years	400 mg
Women, 19–30 years	310 mg
Men, 31+ years	420 mg
Women, 31+ years	320 mg
Pregnancy	350–360 mg
Breastfeeding	310–320 mg

Daily Upper Limits of Magnesium*

Age	Daily Upper Limit (milligrams)
1–3 years	65 mg
4–8 years	110 mg
9+ years	350 mg

*from a supplement source

Magnesium in Foods

Food	Magnesium (milligrams)
Wheat bran, 2 tbsp (30 ml)	46 mg
Wheat germ, 1/4 cup (60 ml)	91 mg
Almonds, 1 oz (24 nuts)	84 mg
Brazil nuts, 1 oz (8 nuts)	64 mg
Peanuts, 1 oz (35 nuts)	51 mg
Sunflower seeds, 1 oz	100 mg
Black beans, cooked, 1 cup (250 ml)	121 mg
Chickpeas, cooked, 1 cup (250 ml)	78 mg
Lentils, cooked, 1 cup (250 ml)	71 mg
Kidney beans, cooked, 1 cup (250 ml)	80 mg
Navy beans, cooked, 1 cup (250 ml)	107 mg
Soybeans, cooked, 1/2 cup (125 ml)	131 mg
Tofu, raw, firm, 1/2 cup (125 ml)	118 mg
Dates, 10	29 mg
Figs, 10 dried	111 mg
Green peas, 1/2 cup (125 ml)	31 mg
Spinach, cooked, 1/2 cup (125 ml)	81 mg
Swiss chard, cooked, 1/2 cup (125 ml)	76 mg

Nutrient Values of Some Common Foods, Health Canada, Ottawa, 1999.

Magnesium Supplements

You may find it challenging to eat a magnesium-rich diet. In addition to including magnesium-rich foods in your daily diet, consider taking a magnesium supplement. If you take calcium supplements, buy one with magnesium added. Choose a 2:1 ratio supplement. (A 2:1 calcium citrate supplement will generally give you 300 milligrams of calcium and 150 milligrams of magnesium.) Calcium and magnesium pills with equal parts of each (a 1:1 ratio) are more likely to cause gastrointestinal upset. If you don't need supplemental calcium but need to boost your magnesium, buy a supplement made from magnesium gluconate, citrate, aspartate, succinate or fumarte. The body absorbs these forms of the mineral more efficiently. But be sure to meet your daily requirements for calcium, since magnesium supplements may reduce calcium absorption.

Taking more than the daily upper limit of supplemental magnesium can cause diarrhea, nausea and stomach cramps. Magnesium gluconate is the least likely form to cause diarrhea.

Phosphorus

The body uses this mineral in metabolic reactions. It is also part of a cell's genetic material (DNA). Phosphorus is necessary to maintain strong bones and teeth.

Recommended Dietary Allowance (RDA) of Phosphorus

Age	RDA (milligrams)
1–3 years	460 mg
4–8 years	500 mg
9–18 years	1250 mg
19+ years	700 mg
Pregnancy	700 mg
Breastfeeding	700 mg
Daily upper limit, 1–8 years	*3000 mg*
Daily upper limit, 9+ years	*4000 mg*

The best food sources of phosphorus are dairy products, meat, poultry, fish, egg yolks, legumes and wheat bran. Phosphorus is used as an additive in many processed foods, including bakery products, deli meats and soft drinks. Most people don't have a problem getting enough phosphorus in their daily diet.

Phosphorus Supplements

It is not necessary to take phosphorus supplements since the mineral is so common in foods. Too much phosphorus can interfere with calcium absorption and calcium balance in the body, especially if daily calcium requirements are not being met.

Boron

Research on this trace mineral shows that it may have several important roles in the body, including helping bones develop properly and assisting with calcium, magnesium and phosphorus absorption. It also may be necessary for cell membrane formation. Because of its possible role in bone health, boron may help prevent osteoporosis, as well as help in the treatment of osteoarthritis. It might also improve cognitive function in older adults.

Because of lack of evidence that boron is essential to humans, no recommended dietary intakes have been established. Boron intakes above the daily upper limit can cause nausea, vomiting, diarrhea and stomach pain. However, boron intake from a healthy diet does not pose a health risk. It's estimated that North Americans consume from 0.75 to 1.4 milligrams of this mineral each day from foods. Because of the part it might play in bone health, I encourage you to eat more boron-rich foods.

Daily Upper Limits of Boron

Age	Daily Upper Limit (milligrams)
1–3 years	3 mg
4–8 years	6 mg
9–13 years	11 mg
14–18 years	17 mg
19+ years	20 mg

Milk, legumes, peanuts, peanut butter, pecans, prunes, raisins, grapes, apples, avocado, potatoes, chocolate, wine and coffee all contain significant amounts of boron.

Boron Supplements

There is no evidence that boron supplements are necessary or beneficial for healthy people who eat a balanced diet. In Canada, the addition of boron to vitamin and mineral supplements is not permitted. This is not the case in the United States, where you can find boron-containing nutritional supplements.

Chromium

Chromium helps the hormone insulin regulate blood sugar. It may help people with type 2 diabetes (see page 263) manage their blood-sugar levels, as well as possibly reduce elevated blood cholesterol and triglycerides in people with type 2 diabetes.

Adequate Intakes (AI) of Chromium

Age	AI (micrograms)
1–3 years	11 mcg
4–8 years	15 mcg
Boys, 9–13 years	25 mcg
Girls, 9–13 years	21 mcg

Age	AI (micrograms)
Boys, 14–18 years	35 mcg
Girls, 14–18 years	24 mcg
Men, 19+ years	35 mcg
Women, 19+ years	25 mcg
Pregnancy	30 mcg
Breastfeeding	45 mcg
Daily upper limit	*None established*

To get a boost of this mineral, eat calf's liver, chicken breast, oysters, refried beans, brewer's yeast, wheat germ, wheat bran, whole grains, blackstrap molasses, mushrooms, green peas and apples (with skin). Processed foods and refined starchy foods like white bread, white rice and pasta, sugar and sweets all contain very little chromium.

Chromium Supplements

If you're concerned you're not getting enough chromium in your diet, check your multivitamin and mineral formula to see how much it contains. Most brands supply 25 to 50 micrograms. If you choose to take a separate chromium supplement, *do not exceed 200 micrograms* per day, the amount generally recognized as the safe upper limit. Higher doses (e.g., doses above 400 micrograms) of chromium can cause cognitive impairment, anemia and kidney damage.

Supplements made from chromium picinolate are thought to be absorbed more efficiently than those made from chromium chloride or chromium nicotinate.

Copper

Copper helps our bodies absorb iron. Copper also maintains nerve function and is used by the body to make connective tissue, red blood cells and enzymes.

Recommended Dietary Allowance (RDA) of Copper

Age	RDA (micrograms)
1–3 years	340 mcg
4–8 years	440 mcg
9–13 years	700 mcg
14–18 years	890 mcg
19+ years	900 mcg
Pregnancy	1000 mcg (1.0 mg)
Breastfeeding	1300 mcg (1.3 mg)

Daily Upper Limits of Copper

Age	Daily Upper Limit (micrograms)
1–3 years	1000 mcg (1 mg)
4–8 years	3000 mcg (3 mg)
9–13 years	5000 mcg (5 mg)
14–18 years	8000 mcg (8 mg)
19+ years	10,000 mcg (10 mg)

The best food sources of copper are calf's liver, meat, shellfish, legumes, nuts, prunes, whole grains, dark green vegetables and sweet potatoes.

Copper Supplements

There is no evidence that single copper supplements are necessary or beneficial for healthy people who eat a balanced diet. Copper deficiency is seldom seen in humans. Large amounts of iron or zinc can interfere with copper absorption, so if you take supplemental doses of either, you may want to increase your copper intake by taking a multivitamin and mineral supplement. Most brands supply 2000 micrograms (2 milligrams) of copper. Also pay attention to your copper intake if you take vitamin C supplements—those in the range of 1500 milligrams per day may decrease the activity of copper-dependent enzymes.

More than 10 milligrams of copper per day can cause nausea, vomiting, bloody diarrhea and anemia.

Fluoride

Fluoride plays a key role in the formation of healthy bones and teeth, and makes teeth resistant to decay.

Adequate Intakes (AI) of Fluoride

Age	AI (milligrams)
1–3 years	0.7 mg
4–8 years	1.0 mg
9–13 years	2.0 mg
14–18 years	3.0 mg
Men, 19+ years	4.0 mg
Women, 19+ years	3.0 mg
Pregnancy	3.0 mg
Breastfeeding	3.0 mg

Daily Upper Limits of Fluoride

Age	Daily Upper Limit (milligrams)
1–3 years	1.3 mg
4–8 years	2.2 mg
9+ years	10.0 mg

Fluoride is supplied to your diet through fluoridated water, beverages made with fluoridated water, black tea, green tea and fish. Many brands of toothpaste and mouthwash also contain fluoride.

Fluoride Supplements

Fluoride supplements are available by prescription for children who don't have access to fluoridated drinking water. The dosage is based on the concentration of fluoride present in the drinking water. (Call your local health department to find out if your water is fluoridated.) Fluoride supplements are rarely prescribed for adults.

Excessive consumption of fluoride causes fluorosis, a condition in which the teeth become yellow. Other symptoms of fluoride toxicity include nausea, vomiting, diarrhea, abdominal pain and numbness or tingling of the face and extremities.

Iodine

The body uses iodine to make thyroid hormones, which regulate growth, development, reproduction, body temperature and metabolism. Iodine may help treat fibrocystic breast conditions, especially mastaglia (cyclic breast pain).

Recommended Dietary Allowance (RDA) of Iodine

Age	RDA (micrograms)
1–8 years	90 mcg
9–13 years	120 mcg
14+ years	150 mcg
Pregnancy	220 mcg
Breastfeeding	290 mcg

Daily Upper Limits of Iodine

Age	Daily Upper Limit (micrograms)
1–3 years	200 mcg
4–8 years	300 mcg
9–13 years	600 mcg
14–18 years	900 mcg
19+ years	1100 mcg

Iodized table salt, seafood and plants grown in iodine-rich soil are good sources of iodine. Most foods provide from 3 to 75 micrograms of iodine per serving. Fish and shellfish tend to be better sources of the mineral since they concentrate iodine from the ocean. Processed foods also have higher iodine contents because of the added iodized salt.

Iodine Supplements

Most multivitamin and mineral supplements provide from 100 to 150 micrograms of iodine. If you use table salt and eat processed foods, you're getting more than enough iodine, perhaps even too much.

Kelp (kombu), a type of seaweed, contains very large amounts of iodine; in one study, 17 different types of kelp supplements were reported to contain anywhere from 45 to 57,000 micrograms of iodine. Taking kelp can increase your risk of iodine toxicity.

Excess intakes of iodine can interfere with the activity of your thyroid gland and cause hypo- or hyperthyroidism (see pages 367 and 356 for more information about these conditions). Chronic use of large amounts of iodine supplements can cause a metallic taste, sore teeth and gums, burning in the mouth and throat, increased salivation, eye irritation and headache.

Iron

Iron is used in the body to transport oxygen to all cells and tissues. It supports metabolism and is used to synthesize brain chemicals (neurotransmitters). Most of the body's iron is found in two proteins: hemoglobin in red blood cells and myoglobin in muscles. In both, iron helps accept, carry and then release oxygen to cells and tissues.

Iron is also needed by enzymes that make amino acids, hormones and brain chemicals (neurotransmitters) that regulate our attention span.

Recommended Dietary Allowance (RDA) of Iron

Age	RDA (milligrams)
1–3 years	7 mg
4–8 years	10 mg
9–13 years	8 mg
Boys, 14–18 years	11 mg
Girls, 14–18 years	15 mg
Men, 19+ years	8 mg
Women, 19–50 years	18 mg
Women, 51+ years	8 mg
Pregnancy	27 mg
Breastfeeding	9 mg
Daily upper limit, 1–13 years	*40 mg*
Daily upper limit, 14+ years	*45 mg*

Iron in Foods

Food	Iron (milligrams)
Lean beef, cooked, 3 oz (90 g)	3.0 mg
Beans in tomato sauce, 1 cup (250 ml)	5.0 mg
Kidney beans, 1/2 cup (125 ml)	2.5 mg
Apricots, dried, 6	2.8 mg
Prune juice, 1/2 cup (125 ml)	5.0 mg
Spinach, cooked, 1 cup (250 ml)	4.0 mg
All Bran, Kellogg's, 1/2 cup (125 ml)	4.7 mg
All Bran Buds, Kellogg's, 1/2 cup (125 ml)	5.9 mg
Bran Flakes, 3/4 cup (175 ml)	4.9 mg
Just Right, Kellogg's, 1 cup (250 ml)	6.0 mg
Raisin Bran, 3/4 cup (175 ml)	5.5 mg
Shreddies, 3/4 cup (175 ml)	5.9 mg
Cream of Wheat, 1/2 cup (125 ml)	8.0 mg
Oatmeal, instant, 1 pouch	3.8 mg
Wheat germ, 1 tbsp (15 ml)	2.5 mg
Blackstrap molasses, 1 tbsp (15ml)	3.2 mg

Nutrient Values of Some Common Foods, Health Canada, Ottawa, 1999.

The richest sources of iron are beef, pork, lamb, poultry and fish. These foods provide *heme* iron, the type that can be absorbed and utilized the most efficiently by your body. Sources of heme iron supply about 10 percent of the iron we consume each day. Even though heme iron accounts for such a small proportion of our intake, it is so well absorbed that it actually contributes a significant amount of iron.

The rest of our iron comes from plant foods such as dried fruits, whole grains, leafy green vegetables, nuts, seeds and legumes. These are sources of *nonheme* iron. The body is much less efficient in absorbing and using this type of iron. Vegetarians may have difficulty maintaining healthy iron stores because their diet relies exclusively on nonheme sources. The rate at which your body is able to absorb nonheme iron is strongly influenced by other factors in your diet. Practice the following to enhance your body's absorption of nonheme iron:

1. Add a little animal food to your meal if you're not vegetarian. Meat, poultry and fish contain MFP factor, a special component that promotes the absorption of nonheme iron from plant foods.

2. Add a source of vitamin C. Including a little vitamin C in your plant-based meal can enhance the body's absorption of nonheme iron fourfold. The acidity of the vitamin converts iron to the ferrous form that's ready for absorption (your stomach acid enhances iron absorption in the same way). Here are some winning combinations:

   • Whole-wheat pasta with tomato sauce

   • Brown rice stir-fry with broccoli and red pepper

   • Whole-grain breakfast cereal topped with strawberries

   • Whole-grain toast with a small glass of orange juice

   • Spinach salad tossed with orange or grapefruit segments

3. Don't take your calcium supplements with an iron-rich meal, since these two minerals compete with each other for absorption.

4. Drink tea between rather than during meals—tea contains tannins, compounds that inhibit iron absorption. Or add a little milk or lemon to your cup of tea, since both inactivate its iron-binding properties.

5. Cook your vegetables. Phytic acid (phytate), found in plant foods, can attach to iron and hamper its absorption. Cooking vegetables like spinach releases some of the iron that's bound to phytates.

Iron Supplements

To help you meet your daily iron requirements, a multivitamin and mineral supplement is a wise idea. Most regular formulas provide 10 milligrams, but you can find multivitamins that provide up to 18 milligrams of the mineral.

If you are diagnosed with iron-deficiency anemia, your doctor will prescribe single iron pills. Depending on the extent of your iron deficiency, you will take one to three iron tablets (each containing 50 to 100 milligrams of elemental iron) per day. If you are advised to take an iron pill, take it on an empty stomach to enhance absorption. Many people find that taking their iron supplement before bed rather than during the day reduces stomach upset.

A supplementation period of 6 to 12 weeks is usually sufficient to treat anemia. However, you may need to take the supplements for up to six months to completely restore your body's iron reserves. Your doctor will perform occasional blood tests to ensure that your iron supply has increased to a healthy level. Once your iron levels improve, discontinue the iron pills but continue taking a multivitamin and mineral supplement.

Too much iron may cause indigestion and constipation. Excessive doses of iron can be toxic, causing damage to your liver and intestines. An iron overload can even result in death. To avoid these problems, do not take single iron supplements without having a blood test to confirm that you have an iron deficiency.

Manganese

Used in the body to make many enzymes, manganese facilitates thyroid function and blood-sugar control. It also supports healthy bone growth.

Your body contains a tiny amount of manganese, most of it found in your bones, liver, kidneys and pancreas. Here, this trace mineral is used by enzymes to facilitate many different chemical reactions. It also helps protect fats in the body from free radical damage.

Adequate Intakes (AI) of Manganese

Age	AI (milligrams)
1–3 years	1.2 mg
4–8 years	1.5 mg
Boys, 9–13 years	1.9 mg
Girls, 9–13 years	1.6 mg
Boys, 14–18 years	2.2 mg
Girls, 14–18 years	1.6 mg

Age	AI (milligrams)
Men, 19+ years	2.3 mg
Women, 19+ years	1.8 mg
Pregnancy	2.0 mg
Breastfeeding	2.6 mg

Daily Upper Limits of Manganese

Age	Daily Upper Limit (milligrams)
1–3 years	2 mg
4–8 years	3 mg
9–13 years	6 mg
14–18 years	9 mg
19+ years	11 mg

Legumes, nuts, seeds, tea (but not herbal tea), green peas, leafy green vegetables, berries, pineapple, avocados, grape juice, whole grains, egg yolks and chocolate are good food sources of manganese.

Manganese Supplements

There is no evidence that single manganese supplements are necessary or beneficial for healthy people who eat a balanced diet. Deficiencies of manganese have not been seen in humans. Most multivitamin and mineral formulas provide 5 milligrams, more than twice the RDA.

Molybdenum

Molybdenum is used by the body to make many enzymes. It also helps the body mobilize iron stores. Deficiencies of this trace mineral are unknown, and as you'll see below, the amounts needed for good health are minuscule.

Adequate Intakes (AI) of Molybdenum

Age	AI (micrograms)
1–3 years	17 mcg
4–8 years	22 mcg
9–13 years	34 mcg
14–18 years	43 mcg
19+ years	45 mcg
Pregnancy	50 mcg
Breastfeeding	50 mcg

Daily Upper Limits of Molybdenum

Age	Daily Upper Limit (micrograms)
1–3 years	300 mcg (0.3 mg)
4–8 years	600 mcg (0.6 mg)
9–13 years	1100 mcg (1.1 mg)
14–18 years	1700 mcg (1.7 mg)
19+ years	2000 mcg (2.0 mg)

The best food sources are legumes, nuts, whole grains, liver and hard drinking water. The molybdenum content of plant foods depends on the molybdenum content of the soil in which they were grown. Animal foods, fruits and many vegetables tend to be low in molybdenum.

Molybdenum Supplements

There is no evidence that molybdenum supplements are necessary or beneficial for healthy people who eat a balanced diet. Most multivitamin and mineral formulas provide between 25 and 50 micrograms of the mineral.

Selenium

This trace mineral, with its antioxidant properties, works with vitamin E to protect cells from free radicals. (See Chapter 5 for more on antioxidants and their effects on free radicals.) Selenium also works closely with the enzyme that converts thyroid hormone to its active form. Research suggests that selenium may prevent prostate, colon and lung cancer.

Recommended Dietary Allowance (RDA) of Selenium

Age	RDA (micrograms)
1–3 years	20 mcg
4–8 years	30 mcg
9–13 years	40 mcg
14–18 years	55 mcg
19+ years	55 mcg
Pregnancy	60 mcg
Breastfeeding	70 mcg

Daily Upper Limits of Selenium

Age	Daily Upper Limit (micrograms)
1–3 years	90 mcg
4–8 years	150 mcg
9–13 years	280 mcg
14–18 years	400 mcg
19+ years	400 mcg

Seafood, meat, organ meats, wheat bran, whole grains, nuts (especially Brazil nuts), onion, garlic, mushrooms, Swiss chard and orange juice are good sources of this mineral. The selenium content of plant foods depends on the soil content in which they were grown.

Selenium Supplements

Selenium supplements come in both inorganic and organic forms. Studies indicate that organic forms of selenium (selenomethionine and high-selenium yeast) are absorbed better than inorganic forms. If you take a medication that blocks the production of stomach acid, pay attention to your selenium intake. These drugs can impair selenium absorption.

The typical supplemental dose for cancer prevention is 200 micrograms per day. Before you buy a separate selenium supplement, check your multivitamin and mineral formula. High-potency or super-strength formulas can contain up to 100 micrograms of the mineral. Daily doses of selenium greater than 400 micrograms can cause loss of hair and fingernails, nausea, depression and anxiety.

Sulfur

Sulfur is necessary to help stabilize the shape and form of protein compounds in the body. It also maintains healthy bones and teeth, activates enzymes and regulates blood clotting. It is used to make insulin and the B vitamins biotin and thiamin (B1).

No recommended daily allowance has been established for sulfur as it is not considered an essential nutrient. All protein-containing foods, such as meat, organ meats, poultry, fish, eggs, dairy products, legumes and nuts, provide sulfur. A daily upper limit has not been established for this mineral.

There is no evidence that sulfur supplements are necessary or beneficial for healthy people who eat a balanced diet. Sulfur deficiencies have not been seen in humans.

Zinc

This trace mineral has many key functions in the body. It is necessary for growth and reproduction, it supports immunity and it is used to make genetic material (DNA) and enzymes. Zinc also helps the body transport vitamin A. Studies suggest that zinc lozenges may reduce the severity and duration of the common cold.

Recommended Dietary Allowance (RDA) of Zinc

Age	RDA (milligrams)
1–3 years	3 mg
4–8 years	5 mg
9–13 years	8 mg
Boys, 14–18 years	11 mg
Girls, 14–18 years	9 mg
Men, 19+ years	11 mg
Women, 19+ years	8 mg
Pregnancy	11 mg
Breastfeeding	12 mg

Daily Upper Limits of Zinc

Age	Daily Upper Limit (milligrams)
1–3 years	7 mg
4–8 years	12 mg
9–13 years	23 mg
14–18 years	34 mg
19+ years	40 mg

Seafood (especially oysters), red meat, poultry, yogurt, wheat bran, wheat germ, whole grains and enriched breakfast cereals are rich in zinc. Drinking coffee with zinc-rich foods can decrease absorption of the mineral by 50 percent.

Zinc in Foods

Food	Zinc (milligrams)
Beef, cooked, 3 oz (90 g)	4.5 mg
Chicken, cooked, 3 oz (90 g)	1.5 mg
Turkey, cooked, 3 oz (90 g)	1.0 mg
Lamb, cooked, 3 oz (90 g)	1.0 mg
Pork, cooked, 3 oz (90 g)	2.3 mg
Crab, king, cooked, 3 oz (90 g)	6.8 mg
Oysters, eastern, 3 oz (90 g)	150.0 mg
Milk, 1 cup (250 ml)	1.0 mg
Cheddar cheese, 1 oz (30 g)	0.9 mg
Yogurt, 3/4 cup (175 ml)	1.4 mg
Egg, 1 whole	0.5 mg
Bran Flakes, 3/4 cup (175 ml)	1.2–3.7 mg
Wheat germ, 2 tbsp (30 ml)	2.3 mg
Baked beans, 1 cup (250 ml)	4.0–7.2 mg
Black beans, cooked, 1 cup (250 ml)	3.6 mg
Garbanzo beans, cooked, 1 cup (250 ml)	5.0 mg
Lima beans, 1/2 cup (125 ml)	1.9 mg
Lentils, cooked, 1 cup (250 ml)	5.0 mg
Soybeans, cooked, 1 cup (250 ml)	2.0 mg
Soy/rice beverages, fortified, 1 cup (250 ml)	1.0 mg
Tofu, 1/2 cup (125 ml)	2.0 mg
Veggie burger, 1	1.1–5.5 mg
Green peas, 1/2 cup (125 ml)	1.0 mg
Cashews, 1/4 cup (60 ml)	1.9 mg
Pumpkin seeds, 1/4 cup (60 ml)	2.6 mg
Sunflower seeds, 1/4 cup (60 ml)	1.8 mg

Nutrient Values of Some Common Foods, Health Canada, Ottawa, 1999.

Zinc Supplements

Your diet plus a good multivitamin and mineral supplement will give you all the zinc you need to stay healthy. Most multivitamin and mineral formulas provide 10 to 20 milligrams. Single zinc supplements are rarely appropriate. Too much zinc has toxic effects and can cause copper deficiency, heart problems and anemia. Consuming amounts greater than 40 to 50 milligrams per day can depress your immune system, making you more susceptible to infection. If you take separate zinc supplements, do not exceed 40 milligrams per day. Since large amounts of zinc can deplete the body's copper stores, buy a zinc supplement with a zinc to copper ratio of 10:1 (for every 10 milligrams of zinc, 1 milligram of copper is present).

To treat a cold, take a zinc gluconate lozenge, containing 10 to 20 milligrams of zinc per lozenge, every two hours to a maximum of five per day (see page 234 for more on treating colds).

Nickel, Silicon, Tin, Vanadium, Colbalt and Arsenic

These six trace minerals play important roles in maintaining our health, but they are not considered essential nutrients. Research to determine if such trace minerals are required from the diet is difficult because the quantities in the body are so small and human deficiencies are unknown.

Sodium

The electrolyte mineral sodium maintains normal fluid balance in the body and assists nerve impulse transmission. It also helps muscles to contract. No recommended dietary allowance has been established for sodium, although it is generally recognized that a daily intake of 1 to 3 grams is adequate to maintain health.

Table salt, soy sauce, processed foods, snack foods, dairy products and seafood all provide significant amounts of sodium. Sodium tablets are not recommended nor are they warranted. Excess sodium can exacerbate high blood pressure, heart failure and kidney disease. Sodium's role in a healthy diet is discussed in more detail in Chapter 5.

Potassium

This electrolyte mineral maintains normal fluid balance and nerve function, promotes normal muscle function and supports cell structure and integrity. It also may help prevent and treat high blood pressure.

No recommended dietary allowance has been established. A daily intake of 2 to 6 grams is adequate to maintain health. Meat, chicken, salmon, cod, lima beans, potatoes, bananas, oranges, orange juice, avocado, cantaloupe, peaches, tomatoes and tomato juice are good sources of potassium.

Healthy people who eat a balanced diet do not need potassium supplements. Potassium is widespread in foods and deficiency is rare. However, people with high blood pressure or a potassium deficiency (often caused by a disease or medication) may benefit from potassium supplements. In this case, your doctor will determine your dose of potassium based on your blood level of the nutrient.

Excessive intakes of potassium can cause stomach upset, nausea, diarrhea, vomiting, flatulence and potentially life-threatening levels of potassium in the bloodstream.

Chloride

Chloride maintains normal fluid balance. This electrolyte mineral is also used to make hydrochloric acid in your stomach, thereby aiding in digestion. No recommended dietary allowance has been established, but a daily intake of 2 to 5 grams is adequate to maintain health. Table salt, soy sauce, processed foods, salty snack foods, meat, milk, eggs and seafood will supply your diet with chloride. Healthy individuals who eat a balanced diet do not need chloride supplements. Chloride, like sodium, is widespread in foods, especially processed foods, and deficiency is rare in humans.

5

———— ❧ ————

Elements of a Healthy Diet

These days, we're bombarded with nutrition information. Often it can be confusing, even for a nutritionist. One day oat bran is in, the next day it's out (I'm pleased to say that it now seems to be back to stay). After reading the morning paper, you're left wondering if margarine really is better than butter. If you're feeling frustrated, you're not alone. A whopping 56 percent of Canadians say they are tired of the conflicting messages about how they should eat to be healthy.

The key is to not react to every single study. The media often pick up on sensational or controversial studies in order to make headlines. It's important to realize that nutrition science is evolving. As it advances, it seldom follows a straight path. For every positive study, there is usually a negative study. In spite of this, we are making progress. We know far more today about how diet affects health than we did 20 years ago.

In the first few chapters of this book, I discussed the important role nutrients—both macro (big) nutrients like carbohydrate, protein and fat, and micro (tiny) nutrients like vitamins and minerals—play in our health. But we don't eat nutrients in isolation. Rather, we consume them in whole foods that provide many other protective compounds. Fruits, vegetables, whole grains, legumes and other plant foods offer fiber and many types of naturally occurring compounds, known as phytochemicals. Some phytochemicals act as antioxidants, others trigger enzymes that inactivate cancer-causing substances and yet others boost the body's immune system. Some phytochemicals even mimic the beneficial effects of estrogen in our body.

Scientists are continually discovering that healthy eating means eating a variety of foods that contain these protective compounds, since phytochemicals likely work in concert with the vitamins and minerals in foods to exert their health benefits. We're also learning that certain foods, or components of them, may not be so good for our health. Sodium, alcohol and caffeine fall into this category.

So what does a healthy diet look like? I don't believe in a "one size fits all" approach. Each person has a unique metabolism, unique nutrient needs and unique food preferences. But given the scientific evidence to date, I do believe that a plant-based diet is the healthiest way to eat. Repeatedly, nutrition researchers are finding that an increased intake of vegetables, fruits, whole grains and other plant foods is associated with a lower risk for heart disease, stroke and many types of cancer.

Eating a plant-based diet does not mean following a strict vegetarian diet. Rather, it means that your meals focus on grains, vegetables, fruit and legumes, with less emphasis placed on animal foods like meat and poultry. For some people, making the transition to a plant-based diet means eating a 4-ounce portion of steak instead of their usual 10-ounce cut. For others it means adding lentils instead of ground meat to pasta sauce, or pouring a soy beverage over breakfast cereal instead of milk.

Here's a closer look at what foods make up a healthy diet.

Fruits and Vegetables

An overwhelming amount of research has found that a diet high in fruits and vegetables lowers the risk of many types of cancer. Despite our knowledge that these foods are good for us, many of us still fall short of the recommended daily five to ten servings. We tell ourselves we don't have time and grab a bagel instead of an apple. Or we throw together pasta with tomato sauce instead of preparing a salad and baked potato. Perhaps we think a strawberry cereal bar counts as a fruit serving. And when it comes right down to it, some people just don't like vegetables. Well, it's time to learn to love them!

Antioxidants

Fruit and vegetables provide us with plenty of antioxidants, compounds that protect our cells from damage caused by free radical molecules. Every day, as a consequence of normal metabolism, our bodies form free radicals from oxygen. Pollution and cigarette smoke increase the number of free radicals our bodies are exposed to. Free radicals roam the body and damage the genetic material of cells, which may lead to cancer development. They can also damage protein and fat molecules.

Each cell in our body has a defense mechanism against free radicals, consisting, in part, of a system of enzymes and antioxidants. Antioxidants act as scavengers, mopping up free radicals before they cause harm. Without continuous antioxidant protection, our cells would not survive. Dietary antioxidants like beta-carotene and vitamins C and E, as well as many phytochemicals, provide the body with extra ammunition against free radicals.

Choosing Fruits and Vegetables

When choosing your fruits and vegetables, consider their color. Many of the natural chemicals in a plant that offer health benefits are the same ones responsible for the plant's vibrant color. For instance, beta-carotene is found in orange-colored fruits and orange and dark green vegetables. Lycopene is plentiful in red-colored fruits, whereas lutein is found in dark green and orange vegetables. Other protective plant components include anthocyanins (abundant in deep red and purple fruits; see Chapter 8), cruciferous compounds (cancer prevention) and sulfur compounds (cancer and heart disease prevention). The following lists the fruits and vegetables you'll find them in:

Beta-Carotene	Lycopene	Lutein
Broccoli	Grapefruit, pink and red	Beet greens
Brussels sprouts	Guava	Collard greens
Carrots	Tomatoes	Kale
Rapini	Canned tomatoes	Okra
Spinach	Tomato sauce	Red pepper
Sweet potato	Tomato juice	Romaine lettuce
Winter squash	Watermelon	Spinach
Apricots		Zucchini
Cantaloupe		Grapes
Mango		Kiwi
Nectarines		Orange juice
Papaya		
Peaches		

Anthocyanins	Cruciferous Compounds	Sulfur Compounds
Blackberries	Bok choy	Garlic
Black currants	Broccoli	Green onions
Blueberries	Cabbage	Leeks
Boysenberries	Cauliflower	Onions
Cherries	Collard greens	Shallots
Cranberries	Kale	
Plums	Radish	

Anthocyanins	Cruciferous Compounds
Raisins	Rutabaga
Raspberries	Turnip
Red grapes	
Strawberries	

Beta-carotene, lutein and lycopene belong to the carotenoid family, a group of natural chemicals that act as antioxidants in many parts of our body. Dietary carotenoids aren't that well absorbed—our small intestine takes in roughly 10 to 30 percent of them from food. Because they are fat-soluble molecules, you'll absorb more if you eat these foods with a small amount of fat. Try a yogurt dip with carrot sticks, a splash of salad dressing on your roasted red pepper, or a little olive oil in lycopene-rich pasta sauce. Heat-processed tomato products (juice, sauce, ketchup) offer a much more accessible form of lycopene than do fresh tomatoes. You'll learn more about lycopene and lutein in Chapter 8.

Here are a few tips to help you add more fresh produce to your daily diet:

- Buy prechopped vegetables like baby carrots, broccoli and cauliflower florets. They're ready to throw in the microwave, steamer or salad bowl.

- Pick up fresh fruit or raw veggies from the salad bar at the local supermarket.

- Drink vegetable juice instead of soda pop at lunch.

- Eat salad for lunch (if ordering in a restaurant, ask for the dressing on the side).

- For a nutrient boost, use romaine and other dark green lettuces in salad.

- Ask for tomatoes, cucumbers and lettuce in your sandwich. When making a sandwich yourself, reach for spinach leaves as a change from lettuce.

- Add quick-cooking greens like spinach, kale, rapini or Swiss chard to soups and pasta sauces.

- Fortify soups, pasta sauces and casseroles with grated zucchini and grated carrot.

- Bake (or microwave) a sweet potato for a change from rice or pasta.

- Add slices of lemon, lime or orange to water for flavor and a little vitamin C.

- Top desserts (like chocolate cake) with a few spoonfuls of strawberries.

- Replace a cereal bar with a piece of fruit for a snack.

Whole Grains

Grains provide the fuel that our brain, nervous system and muscles rely on. They're naturally low in fat and an important source of dietary fiber, iron, folate, vitamin E and other protective compounds. Whole grain provides nutrition from *all* parts of the grain—the outer bran layer where nearly all the fiber is, the germ layer, rich in nutrients like vitamin E, and the endosperm, which contains the starch. When whole grains are milled, scraped, refined and heat-processed into flakes, puffs or white flour, all that's left is the starchy endosperm. Processed grains contain significantly less vitamins E and B6, magnesium, potassium, zinc and fiber than whole grains.

Many studies have found that whole grains offer protection from heart disease, stroke, diabetes and cancer. The Iowa's Women Health Study, which observed almost 35,000 women between the ages of 55 and 69, found that the more whole grains eaten, the lower the rate of heart disease.[1] The Nurses' Health Study followed almost 90,000 women and revealed a 33 percent lower risk of heart disease among women who ate the most whole grains compared to those who ate the least.[2] Until recently, the health benefits of whole grains were attributed mostly to their fiber content. While fiber may play an important role in protecting the heart, scientists have now identified other protective ingredients in whole grains. Antioxidant compounds like vitamin E, tocotrienols and flavonoids may reduce heart disease by preventing blood cells from clumping together. They may also prevent bad LDL cholesterol from sticking to artery walls. As well, whole grains are important sources of minerals like zinc, selenium, copper and iron, which may protect the heart.

Many studies have found a link between fiber from whole grains and a reduced rate of colon cancer. By absorbing water and adding bulk, fiber helps move food through the digestive tract fast. This may reduce the exposure of colon walls to cancer-causing substances, or, fiber may inactivate these harmful compounds in some way. The anticancer properties of whole grains might also come from the natural antioxidants found in these foods. Vitamin E, selenium and phytochemicals may protect the genetic material inside intestinal cells from damage.

Whole grains are digested and absorbed into the bloodstream more slowly than refined grains. A gradual rise in blood glucose means less insulin is secreted, putting less wear and tear on the body's pancreas. For this reason, whole grains are an important part of a diabetic diet. A large US study found that the women who consumed the most sugar and refined starches had a higher risk for type 2 (noninsulin dependent) diabetes than those who ate more whole grains.[3]

At least half of your daily grain servings should be whole grain. But knowing what's whole grain and what's not can be a challenge since this information isn't always printed clearly on packaging. When buying bread, look for the words "whole wheat flour" on the list of ingredients; wheat flour and unbleached wheat flour have been refined.

Whole Grain	Refined Grain
Barley	Cornmeal
Brown rice	Pasta
Bulgur	Pearled barley
Flaxseed	Unbleached flour
Kamut	White rice
Oat bran	
Oatmeal	
Quinoa	
Spelt	
Whole-rye bread	
Whole-wheat bread (100%)	

Flaxseed

These tiny whole-grain brown and golden seeds contain natural compounds called lignans. When we eat flaxseed, bacteria in our gut convert these plant lignans to human lignans, which, in the body, look very much like estrogen. Once in the body, lignans have a weak estrogen action and are able to bind to estrogen receptors on breast cells. This means that they are able to block the action of the body's own, more potent, estrogen by reducing the contact breast cell receptors have with the hormone.

Animal studies conducted at the University of Toronto found that flaxseed has anti-cancer properties.[4,5] Another Canadian study has shown that flaxseed may slow breast cancer growth in women.[6] Researchers at the Princess Margaret Hospital in Toronto and the Toronto General Hospital studied 50 women who had been recently diagnosed with breast cancer. While waiting for their surgery, the women were divided into two groups. One group received daily a muffin containing 50 grams of ground flaxseed (about two tablespoons); the remaining women were given an ordinary muffin. When the tumors were removed, the researchers found that the women who ate the flaxseed muffins had slower-growing tumors than the other women. This exciting finding suggests that a daily intake of flaxseed might offer protection against breast cancer.

Besides lignans, flaxseed is a source of soluble fiber and alpha linolenic acid, an essential fatty acid (Chapter 3 discusses essential fats in more detail). Aim to get one to two tablespoons of ground flaxseed in your diet each day. Grind your flaxseed in a clean coffee grinder or use a mortar and pestle. Flaxseed is also available preground at most health food stores. The natural fats in flaxseed go rancid quickly if exposed to air and heat, so store ground flaxseed in an airtight container in the fridge or freezer. Here are a few ways to add crunch and a great nutty flavor to your meals:

- Add ground flaxseed to hot cereals, muffin batters, and cookie mixes.
- Mix ground flaxseed into a single serving of yogurt.
- Sprinkle flaxseed on salads and soups.
- Add flaxseed to casseroles.
- Buy a loaf of flaxseed bread. Check your local bakery or supermarket.
- Try Red River cereal, a good source of flaxseed.

Soy Foods

You've probably heard plenty about the health benefits of soy. According to many of its proponents, this is one bean we should all be eating more of. A regular intake of soy foods may protect both our heart and bones and may even lower the odds of prostate and breast cancer. Soy foods may also be beneficial for women experiencing perimenopausal symptoms.

It's clear that a regular intake of soy foods can lower both total and LDL blood cholesterol levels. In fact, the US Food and Drug Administration has recently allowed manufacturers of soy foods to print a health claim on the label. Labels on tofu, soy beverages and veggie burgers can now tell American shoppers that eating a low-fat diet containing 25 grams of soy protein a day lowers the risk for heart disease. Studies also show that soy raises good HDL cholesterol, lowers blood pressure and keeps blood vessels healthy. In addition, soy can prevent free radical damage to LDL cholesterol. (Damaged LDL cholesterol sticks much more readily to artery walls.)

Research suggests that soy can delay bone loss and may even build bone density in both women and men. The interest in soybeans and osteoporosis began when researchers observed that populations that consume soy foods on a regular basis report much lower rates of hip fracture. Since then, soy foods and their naturally occurring phytoestrogens have been the focus of many studies. While some find no effect of soy on bone loss, others show a significant bone-sparing effect. Japanese researchers recently learned that soy protein was associated with high bone-density scores in postmenopausal women.[7,8] And a three-month study conducted at Iowa State University found that 40 grams of phytoestrogen-rich soy protein powder daily prevented bone loss in postmenopausal women.[9] Women in this study who were instead given whey protein powder (a protein made from milk) showed significant bone loss in the lower spine.

Diets rich in soy have been shown to reduce menopausal hot flashes, although the amount of improvement may not be helpful for all women. What does have researchers excited, though, is the ability of soy to lower blood estrogen levels in premenopausal women. In this way, a high-soy diet consumed for a long period might lower the risk for breast cancer. Scientists are also learning how a daily intake of soy might prevent and possibly even treat prostate cancer. A recent study conducted among 12,395 California Seventh-Day Adventist men found that drinking soy milk at least once daily was associated with a 70 percent lower risk of prostate cancer.[10]

Isoflavones

Soybeans contain naturally occurring compounds called isoflavones, a type of phyto-estrogen. Isoflavones have a structure similar to the hormone estrogen and, as a result, have a weak estrogen-like effect in the body. Even though isoflavones in soy are about 50 times less potent than estrogen, they are able to offer some of estrogen's protective effects on blood cholesterol and bones. This is an especially important finding for women, whose estrogen levels decline with menopause. Genistein and daidzein are the most active soy isoflavones and have been the focus of much research.

Some studies suggest that isoflavones protect from certain types of cancer. Since soy isoflavones are able to attach to estrogen receptors in the body, they are able to prevent the body's own estrogen from taking that spot. It's believed that long-term exposure to the body's own estrogen can lead to the development of breast and prostate cancer.

How Much Soy Should You Eat?

To ease menopausal complaints or lower blood cholesterol, aim for two or three servings of soy food each day. (Both soy isoflavones and soy protein play a role in cholesterol lowering, which explains why supplements containing only isoflavones have been found ineffective for this purpose.) The benefits of soy seem to be greatest if it is consumed at two or three meals over the day, rather than all at once. But if you're a healthy person who's simply looking for an overall benefit, aim for one serving of soy food each day. For most people, even that's a big leap. I recommend replacing three meat-based meals with soy each week in order to introduce soy into your diet. There are many ways to incorporate soy into your meals:

Soy beverages Last year Canadians consumed 24 million liters of soy beverage, and sales have grown by 116 percent over the past two years. Buy soy beverages fresh or in tetra packs and use them just as you'd use milk: on cereal or in smoothies, coffee and soups, and in cooking and baking. For a boost of calcium and vitamin D at the same time, choose a fortified product.

Soybeans Canned soybeans are convenient to use. Just open the can and rinse the beans before adding them to soups, casseroles, chili and curries. Or mash them and add them to burger mix. If you have the time, buy dried soybeans, soak overnight, then simmer for one hour until they're cooked.

Soy flour Available in health food stores and some supermarkets, soy flour can be substituted for up to half of the all-purpose flour in recipes for breads, muffins, loaves, cookies, cakes or scones.

Soy meats These ready-to-eat or frozen soy foods resemble meat and can be used to replace burgers, hot dogs, deli cold cuts and ground meat. You'll find them in the freezer, delicatessen or produce section of grocery stores.

Soy nuts This roasted snack food comes in flavored varieties and has less fat and more fiber than other nuts. Sprinkle on salads, stir into yogurt or enjoy them on their own.

Tempeh A cake of fermented soybeans mixed with grain, tempeh is good sliced and added to casseroles and stir-fries or grilled in kebabs and burgers. You'll find this soy food in health food stores, either refrigerated or frozen.

Texturized vegetable protein (TVP) Made from soy flour that's been defatted and dehydrated, TVP is sold in packages as granules. Rehydrate it with an equal amount of water or broth and then use it to replace ground meat in pasta sauces, lasagna, chili and tacos.

Tofu Use soft tofu in smoothies, dips, lasagna and cheesecakes. Firm tofu is best for grilling and stir-frying. Or add cubes of firm tofu to soup for a vegetarian protein boost.

Soy protein powders Make a morning "power shake" with 1 tablespoon (15 ml) of soy protein powder made from isolated soy protein. Buy a product that's made with Supro® brand soy protein. This extract of soy protein is manufactured by Protein Technologies International using a process that prevents isoflavone loss. It's also the soy protein isolate that's used in most of the scientific studies. Products that use Supro® include Genisoy, Twin Lab's Vege Fuel, SoyOne, JustSoy, GNC's Challenge 95% ISP, GNC's Challenge Soy Solution, Nutrel's Soy Serenity and Soy Strategy, and Naturade's Total Soy.

For recipes, information and free brochures on soy foods, visit **www.soybean.ca** or write to The Ontario Soybean Growers' Marketing Board, P.O. Box 1199, Chatham, Ontario, N7M 5L8.

Nuts

There's good reason to think that adding a handful of nuts to your daily diet will help keep you healthy. Populations that include nuts as a regular part of their diet, such as vegetarians and Mediterranean and Asian cultures, have lower rates of heart disease. So far, five large prospective scientific studies have examined the relationship between nut consumption and the risk for heart disease and all have found a protective effect. Harvard researchers discovered from the Nurses' Health Study that women who ate more than five ounces of nuts each week had a 35 percent lower risk for heart attack and death from heart disease compared with women who never ate nuts or ate them less than once a month.[11] Walnuts, pecans and pistachios have all been found to lower LDL cholesterol levels. Some findings even suggest that nuts might protect against certain cancers.

The protective effect of nuts may be due to ingredients that are similar to those in whole grains. Nuts and seeds are rich sources of potent antioxidants like vitamin E and many important minerals. Nuts are good sources of essential fatty acids (alpha linolenic acid and linoleic acid) as well as dietary fiber. Finally, nuts contain plant sterols, special fat compounds that have cholesterol-lowering properties.

Aim to get at least five servings of nuts a week, but keep your serving size to 1 ounce (30 grams), or about 1/4 cup (60 ml). Try the following:

- Toss in a handful of peanuts to an Asian-style stir-fry.
- Stir-fry collard greens with cashews and a teaspoon of sesame oil.
- Add walnuts to a green or spinach salad.
- Try walnut oil in your next salad dressing (use half olive oil and half walnut oil).
- Mix sunflower or pumpkin seeds into a bowl of hot cereal or yogurt.
- Snack on a small handful of almonds and dried apricots.
- Sprinkle your casserole with mixed nuts.

Fish

Fish contains a special type of fat called omega-3. You learned about the health benefits of these fatty acids in Chapter 3 and the protective role they play in our health.

They can lower blood cholesterol and triglyceride levels and can offer protection against heart disease. As well, omega-3 oils in fish may ease the symptoms of rheumatoid arthritis. Most experts agree that we should eat fish three times each week to reap its health benefits. Choose oilier fish for a boost of omega-3s—salmon, trout, sardines, herring, mackerel, sea bass and fresh tuna are good choices (canned tuna has very little omega-3 fat). In Chapter 8, I discuss fish oil supplements and the health benefits of omega-3s in further detail.

Green and Black Tea

You probably never thought that your afternoon cup of orange pekoe was a source of healthy antioxidants. Tea, as a plant food, contains natural chemicals that act as antioxidants. The antioxidants in tea leaves belong to a special class of compounds called catechins. By mopping up harmful free radical molecules in the body, catechins in tea may protect your blood cholesterol and your cell's genetic material from damage. A study at Tufts University in Boston compared tea's antioxidant ability to that of 22 vegetables (including broccoli, onions, garlic, corn and carrots). It found that 7 ounces (230 ml) of green or black tea brewed for five minutes had the antioxidant activity equivalent to the same amount of fruit or vegetable juice.

Researchers are now finding that green and black tea may lower our risk for heart attack and certain cancers. One study investigated the effect of tea, coffee and decaffeinated coffee in 340 people who had had a heart attack. Compared to non-tea drinkers, those who enjoyed at least one cup per day had a 44 percent lower risk of heart attack.[12]

There is also a growing body of evidence to suggest that tea protects from certain cancers, including breast cancer. The famous Nurse's Health Study from Harvard found that drinking 4 or more cups of tea per day (versus one or fewer) was associated with 30 percent lower risk of breast cancer.[13] Animal studies have also shown that clear tea, tea with milk and extracts of tea can suppress the growth of cancer cells.

There are three main types of tea: green tea, black tea and oolong. All three come from the same tea plant *(Camellia sinensis)* but they are processed differently.

Green tea leaves are steamed and dried immediately after picking.

Black tea leaves (there are many varieties, including the ever popular orange pekoe) are those that have been allowed to ferment or oxidize before steaming and drying.

Oolong teas have been partially fermented and have a flavor between that of green and black tea.

Herbal teas are not made from tea leaves and therefore don't have the antioxidant properties of green and black tea. The following suggestions will help you incorporate tea into your daily diet:

- If you drink coffee in the afternoon, replace it with tea.

- The next time you're at the grocery store, pick up a box of green tea bags.

- If you're preparing an Asian meal at home, serve it with a pot of green tea. Use tea bags or loose tea.

- Replace all regular and diet soft drinks with tea.

- Enjoy a cup of tea with your midday snack. Try different flavors like Earl Grey, orange spice, apricot or black current.

- The next time you're at your local coffee bar, try chai tea (tea brewed with Indian spices).

Water

It's easy to forget that water is an essential nutrient. While a deficiency of other nutrients can take weeks, months or even years to develop, you can survive only a few days without water. In the body, water becomes the fluid in which all body functions occur. The fluid in your bloodstream transports nutrients and oxygen to your cells. The fluid in your urine removes waste products from your body. And the fluid in your sweat allows your muscles to release heat during exercise.

If you drink too little fluid or lose too much through sweat, your body can't perform these tasks properly and you won't feel your best.

Symptoms of dehydration include early fatigue during exercise, cramping, headaches, dizziness, nausea and loss of appetite. The simplest way to tell if you're replacing the fluid you lose is to check the color and quantity of your urine. It should be clear and plentiful. If it's dark and scanty, you need to drink more fluids. However, if you're taking a multivitamin supplement containing the B vitamin riboflavin, your urine may be bright yellow, so in this case, quantity is a better indicator.

Don't rely on thirst to tell you when you need to drink. Feeling thirsty is an indication that you're already dehydrated—the sensation is triggered by a high concentration of salt in your blood. But the thirst mechanism does not work as well for infants and children, people who are sick and the elderly. Nor is thirst a good indicator during exercise in warm weather.

Water needs vary, depending on diet, exercise and the weather. A general guideline is to drink 1 liter of fluid (1.5 liters for children) for every 1000 calories consumed. This means about 2 to 3 liters of fluid each day for adults and 2 liters for kids. If you exercise or if you are outside in hot, humid weather, you need to drink even more (it's possible to lose as much as 6 liters of fluid through sweat during a long workout in warm weather). To meet your daily fluid needs, practice the following:

- Drink fluids with each meal and snack and throughout the day.

- Keep a bottle of water on your desk at the office; the water cooler may be close at hand but how many times do you get up to fill your glass?

- Fluid needs are best met by water, but other beverages and foods—milk, unsweetened fruit and vegetable juice, herbal tea, soup and fruits and vegetables with a high water content—can contribute to your daily intake. Caffeine and alcohol have a dehydrating effect.

- Bring a water bottle with you when you exercise; drink 1/4 to 1/2 cup (60 to 125 ml) of fluid every 10 to 15 minutes.

- For workouts longer than one hour, use a sports drink like Gatorade, All Sport or PowerAde. These beverages have sodium, which speeds their absorption, and carbohydrate, which your muscles use for fuel.

Do You Need a Multivitamin and Mineral Supplement?

Nutritionists have long argued that if you eat a well-balanced diet, there's no need for vitamin pills. It's true that a healthy diet is better for you than a handful of supplements, but there are a few reasons why taking a daily multivitamin is wise.

Many Canadians don't get enough vitamins and minerals in their diets, despite a constant barrage of information on the benefits of eating right. If you're on the go, under stress, or eat haphazardly, chances are you're not always eating right. Sometimes that fat-laden muffin is more convenient than a bowl of high-fiber cereal. Or pouring a jar of tomato sauce over pasta takes a lot less effort than preparing a vegetable stir-fry. Or perhaps you'd just rather eat french fries than broccoli. In our fast-paced life, we tend to reach for refined, processed foods that offer fewer nutrients than their whole-grain counterparts.

A recent national survey shows that many women's diets are falling short on folate, calcium, iron and zinc. And it seems that Canadian children, too, need a boost of good nutrition. A study by the Canadian Heart and Stroke Foundation found that only 20 percent of Canadian children eat the recommended daily minimum of five servings of fruits and vegetables. What's more, two out of every three kids eat refined grain products rather than nutritious whole-grain bread and cereals.

Even if you are getting Health Canada's recommended dietary allowance (RDA) of nutrients, you might want to consider taking a multivitamin. That's because some vitamins, in amounts greater than the RDAs, may reduce your risk for cancer, heart disease and certain age-related illness. For example, studies have linked use of daily vitamin C supplements to a lower risk of cataracts in women. And although the daily RDA for vitamin E, a powerful antioxidant, is 22 international units (IU), scientific evidence suggests that taking supplemental doses of 200 to 800 IU each day may help prevent heart disease. But it can be a challenge to consume the daily recommended intakes of some heart-protective vitamins, such as vitamin E and folate, from foods. And as we age, we absorb certain nutrients, such as vitamin B12, less efficiently. In fact, adults over the age of 50 are recommended to get their B12 from a supplement.

But make no mistake—supplements cannot make up for a high-fat diet lacking fruits, vegetables and whole grains. These foods provide nutrients, fiber and natural chemicals that most likely work together to keep you healthy. Nutritional supplements are meant to support and reinforce a healthy diet. So eat right first, then consider taking a multivitamin and mineral supplement. Consult your registered dietitian, doctor or pharmacist for more advice about supplementing safely.

What to Look For

Choose a broad-spectrum multivitamin and mineral supplement that provides 100 to 300 percent of the RDA for most vitamins and minerals (with the exception of calcium, magnesium and iron). Mega-, super- and high-potency formulas usually provide larger amounts of B vitamins and antioxidants (vitamins C and E, beta-carotene, selenium). Women's formulas offer extra folate, calcium and iron but do not always include all 13 essential minerals (those that have RDAs or AIs). Older adult formulas provide less iron and more B vitamins. Be sure to check the ingredients list on the label.

People who eat haphazardly, dieters, adults over 50, and seniors with a poor food intake could all benefit from a one-a-day formula. Buy a product that contains beta-carotene, vitamins A, D, B1, B2, niacin, B6, B12 and folic acid. It's not important to supplement biotin and pantothenic acid since they're both easily found in food. The supplement should also contain iron, copper, zinc, magnesium, selenium and chromium. Phosphorus and potassium are widely distributed in most diets and aren't necessary to supplement. I discuss vitamin and mineral supplements in detail in Chapter 4.

When the recommended dosage of a supplement you are taking is high (grams rather than milligrams), be sure to buy a product made by a reputable manufacturer. There is a greater risk for ill effects from contaminants when taking products in large doses, even if the contaminant is present in small amounts.

What You Need to Limit

Alcohol

Most nutrition and cancer experts recommend that we do not drink alcohol. Alcohol may make cells in the body more vulnerable to the effects of carcinogens or may enhance the liver's processing of these substances. It may also inhibit the ability of cells to repair faulty genes and increase hormone levels in the body that influence the development of cancer.

On the plus side, alcohol, whether it's wine, beer or liquor, raises the level of good HDL cholesterol and it may reduce blood clotting. There's also evidence that antioxidants in wine, especially red wine, may keep LDL cholesterol healthy. But the heart-healthy effects of alcohol are most apparent in people over the age of 50 and in those with more than one risk factor for heart disease.

Women who do enjoy the occasional alcoholic drink should limit their intake to one per day or seven per week. Men should limit their alcoholic drinks to two per day and no more than nine per week. A drink is considered 12 ounces (340 ml) of regular beer, 5 ounces (145 ml) of wine or 1 1/2 ounces (45 ml) of 80-proof (40 percent) distilled spirits.

If you need to lower your intake of alcohol, replace alcoholic beverages with sparkling mineral water, Clamato or tomato juice or soda with a splash of cranberry juice. Eliminate alcoholic beverages on evenings that you are not entertaining. Instead, save your glass of wine or cocktail for social occasions.

Sodium

Sodium is an essential nutrient that our body needs to maintain its fluid balance, but we need only a very tiny amount. For sedentary Canadians, all it takes is a mere 500 milligrams (1/5 of a teaspoon) of sodium to cover the body's requirement. If you sweat during exercise, you need a little more salt, but not much. You might have already guessed that we're getting much more sodium than we need—40 times more, to be precise. Each day the average Canadian consumes about 1 3/4 teaspoons of salt.

To help cut back on sodium, avoid the saltshaker at the table, minimize the use of salt in cooking and buy commercial food products that are low in added salt. Eating fewer processed foods is one of the key strategies to de-salt your diet. Most of the salt we consume each day comes from processed and prepared foods. Only one-fourth comes from the saltshaker!

The list below will help you cut down on foods high in sodium. Aim for no more than 2400 milligrams of sodium each day (1 teaspoon of salt). To season your foods without adding salt, use herbs, spices, flavored vinegars and fruit juices.

Sodium Content of Foods

Food	Sodium (milligrams)
Meat and Alternatives	
Fresh meat, poultry, fish, cooked, 3 oz (90 g)	Less than 90 mg
Shellfish, 3 oz (90 g)	100–325 mg
Tuna, canned, 3 oz (90 g)	300 mg
Sausage, 2 oz (60 g)	515 mg
Bologna, 2 oz (60 g)	535 mg
Frankfurter, 1.5 oz (45 g)	560 mg
Lean ham, 3 oz (90 g)	1025 mg
Egg white, 1	155 mg
Whole egg, 1	165 mg
Egg substitute, 1/4 cup (60 ml)	80–120 mg
Dairy Products	
Skim or 1% milk, 1 cup (250 ml)	125 mg
Swiss cheese, 1 oz (30 g)	75 mg
Cheddar cheese, 1 oz (30 g)	175 mg
Blue cheese, 1 oz (30 g)	395 mg
Low-fat cheese, 1 oz (30 g)	150 mg
Processed cheese and cheese spreads, 1 oz (30 g)	75 mg
Cottage cheese, low-fat, 1/2 cup (125 ml)	460 mg
Yogurt, flavored, 1 cup (250 ml)	120–150 mg
Yogurt, nonfat or low-fat, plain, 1 cup (250 ml)	160–175 mg
Vegetables	
Fresh or frozen, 1/2 cup (125 ml)	Less than 70 mg
Canned, no salt, 1/2 cup (125 ml)	Less than 70 mg
Canned, no sauce, 1/2 cup (125 ml)	55–470 mg
Canned, 1/2 cup (125 ml)	215–800 mg
Tomato juice, canned, 3/4 cup (175 ml)	660 mg
Tomato sauce, 1/4 cup (60 ml)	150–370 mg
Grain Foods	
Breads, 1 slice	110–175 mg
English muffin, 1/2	130 mg
Bagel, 1/2	190 mg
Baking powder biscuit, 1	305 mg
Cereal: shredded wheat, 3/4 cup (175 ml)	Less than 5 mg
Cereal: puffed wheat and rice, about 1 1/2 cups (375 ml)	Less than 5 mg
Cereal: granola-type, 1/2 cup (125 ml)	5–25 mg

Food	Sodium (milligrams)
Cereal: flaked, 2/3 to 1 cup (160–250 ml)	170–360 mg
Cereal, cooked, unsalted, 1/2 cup (125 ml)	Less than 5 mg
Cereal, cooked, instant, 1 packet	180 mg
Crackers, saltine type, 5	195 mg
Cooked rice and pasta, unsalted, 1/2 cup (125 ml)	Less than 10 mg
Rice and sauce mix, cooked, 1/2 cup (125 ml)	250–390 mg
Peanut butter, 2 tbsp (30 ml)	150 mg
Peanut butter, unsalted, 2 tbsp (30 ml)	Less than 5 mg
Dry beans, plain, canned, 1/2 cup (125 ml)	350–590 mg
Fats and Oils	
Butter, salted, 1 tsp (5 ml)	25 mg
Margarine, unsalted, 1 tsp (5 ml)	Less than 5 mg
Margarine, salted, 1 tsp (5 ml)	50 mg
Mayonnaise, 1 tsp (5 ml)	80 mg
Prepared salad dressing, low-calorie, 2 tbsp (30 ml)	50–310 mg
Prepared salad dressing, 2 tbsp (30 ml)	210–440 mg
Snack Foods	
Unsalted nuts, 1/4 cup (60 ml)	Less than 10 mg
Salted nuts, 1/4 cup (60 ml)	120–350 mg
Popcorn, microwave, 3 cups (750 ml)	135–500 mg
Popcorn, air popped, unsalted, 3 cups (750 ml)	1 mg
Unsalted potato chips and corn chips, 1 cup (250 ml)	Less than 5 mg
Salted potato chips and corn chips, 1 cup (250 ml)	170–285 mg
Pretzels, 1 oz (30 g)	500–700 mg
Tortilla chips, 1 oz (30 g)	150–300 mg
Frozen Desserts	
Ice cream, 1/2 cup (125 ml)	35–50 mg
Frozen yogurt, nonfat or low-fat, 1/2 cup (125 ml)	40–55 mg
Ice milk, 1/2 cup (125 ml)	55–60 mg
Condiments and Miscellaneous	
Baking powder, 1 tsp (5 ml)	400–550 mg
Bouillon, 1 cube	1200 mg
Garlic salt, 1 tsp (5 ml)	1480 mg
Mustard, chili sauce, hot sauce, 1 tsp (5 ml)	36–65 mg
Ketchup, steak sauce, 1 tbsp (15 ml)	100–230 mg
Salsa, tartar sauce, 1 tbsp (15 ml)	85–205 mg
Salt, 1/2 tsp (2 ml)	1370 mg

Food	Sodium (milligrams)
Pickles, sweet or dill, 1 large	330–830 mg
Soy sauce, low-sodium, 1 tbsp (15 ml)	600 mg
Soy sauce, 1 tbsp (15 ml)	1030 mg
Convenience Foods	
Canned and dehydrated soups, 1 cup (250 ml)	600–1300 mg
Regular pasta sauce, 1/4 cup (60 ml)	125–275 mg
Lower sodium versions	Read the label*
Canned and frozen main dishes	500–1570 mg
Lower sodium versions	Read the label*

* The sodium content of convenience foods labeled "low sodium" or "reduced salt" can vary, so be sure to check the nutrition information panel. And don't forget to rinse canned vegetables to remove excess salt.

From The Nephrogenic Diabetes Insipidus Foundation, 2000, available at www.ndif.org/na9/html

Caffeine

Health Canada recommends a daily maximum of 450 milligrams of caffeine. Too much caffeine depletes your bones of calcium, interferes with sleep and may affect fertility in women. Use the list below to help you keep your caffeine intake to a minimum.

Food or Medication	Caffeine (milligrams)
Beverage or Food	
Coffee, filter drip, 8 fluid oz (235 ml)	110–180 mg
Coffee, filter, Starbuck's, 8 fluid oz (235 ml)	200 mg
Coffee, instant, 8 fluid oz (235 ml)	80–120 mg
Coffee, decaffeinated, 8 fluid oz (235 ml)	4 mg
Espresso, 2 fluid oz (60 ml)	90–100 mg
Tea, black, 8 fluid oz (235 ml)	46 mg
Tea, green, 8 fluid oz (235 ml)	33 mg
Cola, regular, 12 fluid oz (350 ml)	35 mg
Dark chocolate, 1 oz (30 g)	20 mg
Milk chocolate, 1 oz (30 g)	6 mg
Chocolate cake, 1 slice	20–30 mg
Medication (2 tablets)	
Anacin®	64 mg
Excedrin®	130 mg
Midol®	64 mg

Putting It All Together: A Healthy Eating Plan

To make sure you get your daily share of nutrients, antioxidants and the many other protective chemicals plant foods have to offer, follow the food plan below. Adjust your daily number of servings according to your exercise level. If you work out every day, the number of servings you'll need to eat are those at the upper end of the recommended range. If you engage in heavy exercise, you may find you need to eat even more than that outlined below. Add more whole grains, fruits, vegetables and vegetarian foods to provide extra calories. If you are trying to lose weight, stick to the lower end of the range.

Before you start down the road to healthy eating, there are a few pointers to keep in mind:

• *Make one change at a time.* There's no need to do everything at once. You'll be surprised to find that small changes make a big difference. Set one new goal each week.

• *Plan ahead whenever you can.* Most of my clients report that their biggest roadblock to eating well is a lack of time. Plan your weekly meals in advance. Grocery shop once a week so you have healthy foods in your fridge and cupboards. You'll find that taking the extra time to plan ahead actually saves you time during the busy week.

• Remember that *all foods can be part of a healthy diet.* The occasional splurge on ice cream or deep-fried chicken wings won't upset your healthy eating plan. It's the overall picture that counts.

• *Periodic overeating or eating of junk food does not mean you have failed.* We're all human. Just return to your usual healthy diet at the next meal.

Food Group	Food Choices	Recommended Daily Servings
Grain Food		**5 to 12**
(Carbohydrate, iron, fiber;	Whole-grain bread, 1 slice	
choose whole-grain as often	Bagel, large, 1/4	
as possible)	Roll, large, 1/2	
	Pita pocket, 1/2	
	Tortilla, 6", 1	
	Cereal, cold, 3/4 cup (175 ml)	
	Cereal, 100% bran, 1/2 cup (125 ml)	
	Cereal, hot, 1/2 cup (125 ml)	
	Crackers, soda, 6	
	Corn, 1/2 cup (125 ml)	
	Popcorn, plain, 3 cups (750 ml)	

Food Group	Food Choices	Recommended Daily Servings
Grain Food		**5 to 12**
	Grains, cooked 1/2 cup (125 ml)	
	Pasta, cooked, 1/2 cup (125 ml)	
	Rice, cooked, 1/3 cup (75 ml)	
Vegetables and Fruits		**5 to 10**
(Carbohydrate, fiber, vitamins, minerals)	Vegetables, cooked or raw, 1/2 cup (125 ml)	
	Vegetables, leafy green, 1 cup (250 ml)	
	Fruit, whole, 1 piece	
	Fruit, small (plums, apricots), 4	
	Fruit, cut up, 1 cup (250 ml)	
	Berries, 1 cup (250 ml)	
	Juice, unsweetened, 1/2 to 3/4 cup (125 to 175 ml)	
Milk and Milk Alternatives		**2 to 4**
(Protein, carbohydrate, calcium, vitamin D, vitamin A, zinc)	Milk, 1 cup (250 ml)	
	Yogurt, 3/4 cup (175 ml)	
	Cheese, 1.5 oz (45 g)	
	Rice beverage, fortified, 1 cup (250 ml)	
	Soy beverage, fortified, 1 cup (250 ml)	
Meat and Alternatives		**6 to 10**
(Protein, iron, zinc)	Fish, lean meat, poultry, 1 oz (30 g)	
	Egg, whole, 1	
	Egg whites, 2	
	Legumes (beans, chickpeas, lentils), 1/3 cup (75 ml)	
	Soy nuts, 2 tbsp (30 ml)	
	Tempeh, 1/4 cup (60 ml)	
	Tofu, firm, 1/3 cup (75 ml)	
	Texturized vegetable protein, 1/3 cup (75 ml)	
	Veggie dog, small, 1	

Food Group	Food Choices	Recommended Daily Servings
Fats and Oils*		**4 to 6**
(Essential fatty acids, vitamin E)	Butter, margarine, 1 tsp (5 ml)	
	Mayonnaise, 1 tsp (5 ml)	
	Nuts/seeds, 1 tbsp (15 ml)	
	Peanut and nut butters, 1.5 tsp (7 ml)	
	Salad dressing, 2 tsp (10 ml)	
	"Light" salad dressing, 4 tsp (20 ml)	
	Vegetable oil, 1 tsp (5 ml)	

* To include sources of essential fatty acids, choose canola oil, walnut oil, flaxseed oil and nuts and seeds more often as your fat servings. As you read through the chapters in this book, you'll find many mentions of these health-enhancing fats.

Fluids	Water, 1 cup (250 ml)	**8 to 12**

All serving sizes are based on measures after cooking.

Part Two

Herbs and Natural
Health Products

6

———— ❧❧❧ ————

Herbal Medicine

Simply put, the term "herb" refers to a plant that is used for medicinal purposes (it may also be used for flavoring food and for its scent). Herbal medicine may be new to North America, but it is certainly not new to the rest of the world. According to the World Health Organization, 80 percent of the world's population rely on herbs to stay healthy. In countries such as Germany, France, Italy, China, Japan and India, herbal remedies have been integrated into the national health care systems. And in Africa, Latin America and North America, herbs have been used for hundreds of years as folk medicines.

North Americans are now returning to this alternative form of therapy. But there is a lot we still need to learn. Although we may know that a certain plant has a beneficial effect on our health, we might not know what compounds are responsible for those effects. Nor do we know all the possible ways an herb may interact with prescription medications. Most studies on herbal medicines have lasted less than a year, so the effects of taking herbs for a longer period are largely unknown. And very little research has been done on herbs and pregnant women and children.

Despite the unknowns, the use of herbs has boomed in Canada over the past five years. According to a recent national survey, 35 percent of Canadians used herbal supplements to treat health conditions, up from 23 percent in 1997.[1,2] As media reports on new studies continue to bombard us, more and more Canadians are expected to go the herbal route.

News stories aren't the only reason Canadians are turning to herbs, nor is it simply because herbs cost less than many drugs. In this day and age, an increasing number of people are taking a more active role in their health care. Many clients I see in my private practice are leery about taking prescription drugs and would rather first try an herbal remedy. They feel it's safer or more natural. Scientists are discovering that some herbal extracts may be just as effective as drug treatment. You'll read in the next chapter how black cohosh, an herb used to ease menopausal hot flashes, has been shown to be comparable to estrogen therapy in its short-term effect on hot flashes, without the uncomfortable side effects.

It's true that, in general, herbs have far fewer side effects than prescription drugs. They are gentler in their action and, as a result, take longer to work. But it's important to realize that just because something is deemed "natural" does not mean it is necessarily safe. Herbal therapies, just like drugs, must be treated with respect and taken wisely. As you'll read in the next two chapters, herbal remedies and natural health products can have side effects, they can interfere with medication and they can be dangerous for people with certain health conditions. Since herbs are largely unregulated in Canada, you'll also learn the importance of choosing a high-quality product. Before I tell you what you might use herbs for, and how to take them safely, let's take a closer look at the world of plant medicine.

Herbal Traditions Around the World

Herbs play an important role in the medical systems of many cultures and have done so for thousands of years. In traditional Chinese medicine (TCM), herbs have been used for more than 2000 years. In North America, interest in Chinese medicine is relatively recent and has been growing over the past 20 years. Ayurveda medicine developed on the Indian subcontinent some 3000 to 5000 years ago.

Traditional Chinese Medicine

This comprises four main disciplines: acupuncture, herbology, massage and manipulation (called Tui Na) and diet therapy. Doctors of TCM are concerned with the person as a whole. Both physical and psychological characteristics are viewed as important determinants of health and disease. From a detailed examination and the history of signs and symptoms, practitioners of TCM piece together a pattern of disharmony, which is used to make a diagnosis and develop a personalized treatment plan. TCM aims to alleviate symptoms and treat the underlying causes of disease. The goal of TCM is to return the body, mind and spirit to a balanced state.

Concepts important to TCM include yin and yang (cold/passivity/interior and heat/vigor/exterior); substances such as qi (energy), blood, jing (a congenital essence inherited from one's parents and vitality obtained from food) and other body fluids; organs such as the heart and spleen; meridians or channels that connect the organs and circulate blood and qi throughout the body; and conditions that cause disharmony in the body (wind, heat, cold, dampness). Mastering the art and science of TCM takes years of practice. Traditional Chinese herbal remedies, which are combinations of herbs, are called patent medicines and are used to treat specific syndromes. The doses are quite high and typically taken in the form of strong-smelling soups.

Ayurveda

This complex traditional Hindu healing system focuses on healing from within, rather than on treating individual symptoms. Ayurveda recognizes that there are unique constitutional differences between individuals and therefore different treatments are needed for different types of people: although two people may share the same symptoms, their energetic constitutions may differ and call for very different remedies.

Three fundamental principles guide an Ayurvedic practitioner in the diagnosis and development of a treatment plan: Vata (movement, breathing, activity), Pitta (energy released from biochemical process, digestion, vision) and Kapha (stability, mental strength, resistance to disease). According to Ayurveda, these three principles control all human biological and psychological functions.

Treatments include the use of herbal medicines, minerals, animal products, strict dieting, yoga, meditation, exercise and surgery. Ayurvedic herbal remedies involve the use of more than 1000 medicinal plants. The system has over 8000 recipes for medicines, the majority of which are made from herbs and minerals. Ayurvedic medicines are given as pills, infusions, tinctures, powders and oils. Both the choice and dose of an herbal medicine are influenced by the disease, the patient's constitution and the environment.

There are Ayurvedic practitioners in North America, but they can be difficult to find. Your local health food retailer that sells Ayurvedic herbal formulas may be able to help you locate one.

Herbalism and Phytotherapy

As I mentioned earlier, it's only recently that herbal medicine has come to be appreciated by the Western world. Over the past 20 years, there has been an enormous amount of research on herbs and their role as medicines. Today in North America, you'll find two distinct philosophies among practitioners who recommend herbal therapies. Traditional herbalists practice what is often referred to as "herbalism." They believe that the sum of the plant parts is greater than the individual part. Herbalists believe that the constituents of the plant work in synergy with each other. They also believe that the plant has both a drug-like and an energy aspect. Herbalists rarely prescribe one herb; rather, they prescribe a combination of herbs to treat a disorder.

Modern practitioners who prescribe herbs believe that a plant's medicinal action is determined solely by its active components. This approach is commonly referred to as "phytotherapy," the science of using herbs to treat illness. Countries such as Germany, Italy and France have adopted this model of herbal medicine and have combined it with conventional medical practice. It is in the field of phytotherapy that we are seeing an explosion of scientific research. Throughout the rest of this book, I discuss the use of herbal remedies using this model—remedies made from plants with active ingredients that can be used to treat or prevent a health condition.

Forms of Herbal Remedies

Like vitamins and minerals, herbs can be taken in several forms. Here's a look at the various ways an herbal remedy might be prepared:

Teas (infusions and decoctions) Infusions are made by steeping the delicate part of an herb (leaves, flowers) in hot water. Boiling roots, barks and stems results in a decoction. Some herbs taste unpleasant in tea form. As well, many herbs have components that are not soluble in water (saw palmetto and valerian are two examples). You're better off buying a standardized extract of those herbs in pill form. A variety of herbs, such as chamomile and echinacea, are available in tea bags at health food stores. Some stores also sell bulk herbs that you can steep in boiling water for a specified time, then strain. Bulk herbs are also available from reputable herbalists.

Tinctures These are made by soaking the herb in a mixture of alcohol and water for as little as a few hours or as long as a few weeks, depending on the plant. The herbal material is then removed—the remaining liquid is the tincture. Usually packaged in small bottles with droppers, tinctures are readily available in health food stores. They're great for people who don't like to swallow pills, especially children. Alcohol-free tinctures are also available and are recommended for children or anyone with a health condition for which alcohol in contraindicated. To take a tincture, add the specified amount to a glass of water.

The strength of a tincture is determined by its concentration. This information may be on the label, though manufacturers are not required to state it. Tinctures usually range in concentration from 1:3 to 1:10. This means that, for instance, one part herb was soaked with three parts solvent (water and alcohol), or, in the case of the weaker concentration, there is ten times the amount of solvent in the tincture as there is herb. Your health care provider should advise you on the concentration of tincture to buy.

Fluid extracts These liquid herbal remedies are more concentrated than tinctures. They are usually a 1:1 or 1:2 concentration.

Solid extracts The strongest form of herb you can buy, solid extracts are made by removing all the solvent, leaving only the solid material (which looks like thick molasses). Solid extracts of herbs are sold as capsules, pills and tablets, and their strength is expressed in concentration. A concentration of 4:1 means that one part of the extract is equivalent in strength, or potency, to four parts of the dried herb. The label's statement of concentration, however, does not tell you the amount of active ingredients present, often an important factor if the herb is to be effective.

Standardized extracts These are solid extracts guaranteed to have a specific amount of a specific ingredient(s) in the final product. This amount is expressed as a percentage. For example, the label on my bottle of echinacea says it contains 4 percent echinacosides. All the components of the plant may be present in a standardized extract but often not in the proportions in which they occurred naturally in the plant. Some manufacturers standardize their products to contain a certain amount of a marker compound. This compound is not the active ingredient but a characteristic component of the plant. By standardizing to such a marker, manufacturers can assure quality of the product, guaranteeing the correct plant was used to make the herbal remedy.

Clearly, the biggest advantage of buying a standardized herbal product is assurance of quality. Many proponents of standardized extracts also believe that they enable health care professionals to recommend a more accurate dose, based on a measured amount of specific ingredients, and that, in turn, standardized products are more likely to be effective in treating a health condition. But there are a few caveats. First, we don't yet know all the active ingredients responsible for an herb's effect. A case in point is feverfew, an herb used to prevent migraine headaches. Scientists isolated what they thought was the active ingredient and made a standardized extract from it, but the standardized extract turned out to be ineffective in preventing migraines. It turns out that, in order to be effective, feverfew products need to be made from the whole leaf, rather than from a standardized extract. And while standardized extracts do offer an assurance of quality, it's important to keep in mind that some unstandardized products may also be of high quality and effective.

How to Choose a High-Quality Product

The herbal supplement industry in Canada is largely unregulated. Currently, natural health products (herbs, vitamins, minerals, homeopathic remedies and other supplements) are regulated either as a drug or a food. In general, if no therapeutic claim is made for a product, it is classified as a food and regulated as such. Essentially, this means that these products do not have to undergo the rigorous testing that drugs do. These products also can be used as desired because they lack drug-like properties. But many natural health products are not meant to be consumed ad lib, and therefore this type of regulation does not ensure consumer safety. Most herbs fall into the food category.

If a health claim is made for an herb, or the product has a drug-like action that makes it more like a remedy than a food, it is classified as a drug. These products must pass tests of safety and effectiveness, and they must meet specific labeling criteria imposed by Health Canada. Their packaging must carry a drug identification number (DIN).

This system of regulation is expected to change over the next few years. In 1999, Health Canada established the Natural Health Product Directorate (NHPD) to ensure that Canadians have access to safe, high-quality and properly labeled natural health products. At the time of writing this book, the NHPD was busily defining exactly what will be considered a natural health product. Once that task is complete, the NHPD will develop regulations for manufacturing and labeling so that you, as a consumer, can feel satisfied that you are buying a safe and efficacious product.

In the meantime, this list will help you shop for a high-quality herbal supplement:

- Choose a supplement manufactured by a company with a strong reputation for producing high-quality products. Ask your dietitian, naturopath, doctor, pharmacist or health food retailer for a list.

- Consider buying an herbal remedy manufactured by a company that also produces pharmaceuticals, since it should have very high quality-control standards.

- If possible, always buy a standardized extract that clearly states the percentage of active ingredient or marker on the label.

- Ask the retailer or manufacturer if the product was manufactured according to good manufacturing practices (GMP) if this is not indicated on the label.

- Look for a product that discloses all the ingredients, including binders and fillers.

- Check the expiry date; make sure the product will not expire during the period you intend to use it.

- Check to see if the product has a safety seal.

- Don't be afraid to ask the supplement manufacturer or health food retailer questions, including, How is one product different from another? What measures does the retailer take to make sure it stocks high-quality products? How does the manufacturer ensure that it uses high-quality raw ingredients?

Another approach to buying high-quality herbs is to look for an herbal extract that has been used in scientific research. Some manufacturers will produce their herbal remedy using the specific extract that researchers found to be effective. However, most consumers are not privy to such information. If your health care provider makes a point of keeping up to date with the scientific literature, he or she may know this information. The following is a list of some of the most frequently researched herbs and their North American brand names:

Herb	Brand Name	Used For
Black cohosh	Remifemin Menopause by GlaxoSmithKline	Menopausal symptoms
Chasteberry	Femaprin by Nature's Way	PMS
Echinacea	Echinguard by Nature's Way	Colds, flu
Garlic	Kyolic by Wakunaga Kwai by Lichtwer Pharma	High cholesterol, circulation, immune enhancement
Ginkgo biloba	Ginkoba by Pharmaton Ginkogold by Nature's Way	Cognitive function, circulation
Ginseng	Ginsana by Pharmaton	Immune enhancement, stress
Horse chestnut	Venastat by Pharmaton	Varicose veins
Milk thistle	Thisylin by Nature's Way	Liver
Saw palmetto	Elusan Prostate by Plantes & Medicines Ltd.	Prostate enlargement
St. John's wort	Movana by Pharmaton Perika by Nature's Way	Mild to moderate depression

Consulting with an Expert

As you can see, there's a lot to consider before buying an herbal remedy. I certainly do not recommend self-diagnosing your condition and rushing off to the health food store to buy an herb that seems to match. Take the time to consult with a professional who can properly assess your symptoms and guide you in the right direction. Herbalists are not officially recognized as health professionals in Canada and so are not regulated. When choosing an herbalist, it is important to ask about his or her credentials, training and clinical experience. Here's what you need to know to choose a competent practitioner (the following applies to practitioners in both Canada and the United States):

- Herbalists with a science degree in phytotherapy have completed a four-year university or college program.

- Herbalists with the MNIMH designation (Member of the National Institute of Medical Herbalism) have completed a four-year university program.

- North American–trained herbalists with the Clinical Herbalist (ClH) designation have completed a three- or four-year university program.

- Master herbalists (MH) have usually completed a 6- to 12-month program, or a self-directed course through correspondence. Courses can vary, so ask questions!

- Naturopathic doctors (ND) have completed a four-year program that includes many courses on herbal medicine. Some naturopaths choose to specialize in this area and may have more expertise than others.

- Doctors of traditional Chinese medicine (DTCM) have completed at least four years of training.

Recommended Resources

www.altmed.com
A consumer Web site that contains plenty of information on alternative or complementary medical treatments. The herbal guide gives information on more than 50 herbal remedies.

www.herbalgram.com
American Botanical Council
Incorporated in November 1988 as a nonprofit education organization, the American Botanical Council (ABC) aims to educate the public about beneficial herbs and plants and promote the safe and effective use of medicinal plants. ABC disseminates responsible, science-based information on herbs and phytomedicines on a subscription or one-time basis.

www.herbsociety.ca
Canadian Herb Society
The Canadian Herb Society (CHS) is a national nonprofit association providing accurate information, education, networking and representation for all those with an interest in herbs.

www.herbs.org

Herb Research Foundation

The Herb Research Foundation (HRF) is an excellent source of accurate, science-based information on the health benefits and safety of medicinal plants. Founded in 1983 with a mission of herb research and public education, HRF has a vast storehouse of information resources, including a specialty research library containing over 300,000 scientific articles on thousands of herbs. HRF is a nonprofit organization.

7

⟨⟨⟨⟩⟩⟩

Popular Herbal Remedies

Scientific research suggests that the 17 herbs which are discussed in this chapter may be effective in helping to treat or prevent certain health conditions. These remedies are widely available in health food stores and pharmacies. Lesser-known herbs are discussed in Part 3.

Herbal remedies are not a substitute for other medical treatments. If you have a health condition that persists or worsens, seek the advice of your doctor. Many serious medical conditions are not appropriate for self-diagnosis and require the supervision of a qualified health professional. Never substitute an herbal supplement for a prescription medication without first consulting your doctor.

It is important to note that the safety of most herbal remedies has not been evaluated in children, in pregnant and breastfeeding women and in people with liver or kidney disease. Seek the advice of a health professional if you fall into one of these categories.

Some herbal remedies, including ginkgo biloba, can conflict with surgery because of their blood-thinning effect. You should stop taking such supplements two weeks prior to scheduled surgery.

Bilberry (*Vaccinium myrtillus*)

Used for visual acuity (macular degeneration [see page 420], eye complications of diabetes, night vision), menstrual cramps

A relative of the American blueberry, the bilberry plant grows in Canada, the United States and northern Europe. Bilberry is an excellent source of naturally occurring compounds called flavonoids, or, more specifically, of anthocyanins. These compounds help the body form strong connective tissue and blood capillaries.

Traditionally, bilberry has been used for diabetes and gastrointestinal disorders. It was during World War II that British pilots noticed that their night vision improved after eating bilberry jam. Since then, a handful of well-controlled studies found that, compared to placebo treatment, bilberry significantly improved eye health in people with diabetic eye complications.[1,2] One study revealed that the herbal extract improved night vision in air traffic controllers and pilots.

The anthocyanins in bilberry are thought to improve blood flow in the tiny capillaries of the eye. Bilberry's effect on circulation may also be responsible for its ability to reduce symptoms of dysmenorrhea, including breast tenderness, painful periods, nausea and headache.[3]

Bilberry Supplements

Only the ripe fruit of bilberry plants is used in medicinal extracts. Do not confuse bilberry extract with bilberry leaf or bog bilberry. If you are taking bilberry supplements to improve vision, choose a product standardized to contain 25 to 36 percent anthocyanins. Take 160 milligrams twice daily. Use for one to six months is usually recommended for improvement in visual disorders.

For dysmenorrhea, take 50 to 160 milligrams twice daily three days before your period and during your period. Stop on day seven. It may take up to three menstrual cycles for bilberry to have an effect on dysmenorrhea.

No adverse effects have been reported on the use of bilberry supplements, and no drug interactions are known to occur.

Black Cohosh (*Cimicifuga racemosa*)

Used for perimenopause (see page 464): hot flashes, mood swings, vaginal dryness
Also known as black snakeroot, bugbane and baneberry, black cohosh has a long tradition of being used to treat gynecological conditions. This perennial shrub is native to North America, growing up to two feet high, with white flowers. The root of the plant is used for medicinal purposes. The herb was first used by Native Americans, who introduced it to European colonists. In Germany, physicians have been prescribing this herb for more than 40 years to more than 1.5 million women.

Exactly how the herb works is still under scientific debate. While some studies suggest it may bind to estrogen receptors, others do not.[1,2] Black cohosh may exert its effect by interacting with certain brain receptors. The herb contains triterpene glycosides, naturally occurring compounds thought to be responsible for its effect. It may take up to four weeks to notice improvement in symptoms.

Eight randomized controlled clinical trials have found a standardized extract of black cohosh to be as effective as estrogen therapy in reducing the severity and frequency of menopausal hot flashes.[3] A recent study also suggests that the herb may have positive effects on bone density.

Black Cohosh Supplements

Buy a product standardized to contain 2.5 percent triterpene glycosides. The typical dose is 40 milligrams taken twice daily. The type of black cohosh used in virtually all the scientific research is sold under the name Remifemin® Menopause. This product is sold in 20 milligram strength, since a recent study has shown that a lower dose of the herb is equally effective.

Today, many menopausal supplements combine a number of herbs known to ease menopausal symptoms. You might try one of these products rather than taking black cohosh alone. Products include Estro-Logic™ (Quest® Vitamins), Menopause Formula (Natural Factors®), Meno+ (ehn®) and Life® Menopause Formula (Shopper's Drug Mart). The herbal formula for Estro-LogicTM was developed by an American gynecologist, Dr. Kathleen Fry, and a medical herbalist, Claudia Wingo. The product is being studied in a trial of 100 menopausal women. Preliminary findings look promising—the combination appears to be effective in easing a number of common menopausal complaints, including hot flashes.

Mild stomach upset and headache have been reported in a small number of women who have taken doses of black cohosh greater than 40 milligrams. The herb may be taken over the long term with the recommended dosage. However, it should not be used by pregnant or breastfeeding women.

Chasteberry (*Vitex angus-castus*)

Used for premenstrual syndrome (see page 480), amenorrhea, infertility (see page 378)
The use of chasteberry as a medicinal plant was first mentioned some 2000 years ago by a Greek physician, who noted the ability of a drink made from the plants' seeds to reduce sexual desires. The herb has also been reported to help medieval monks keep their vow of chastity. Its Latin name, angus-castus, means chaste lamb. In modern times, European physicians have been prescribing chasteberry to women for more than 40 years to regulate the menstrual cycle and ease symptoms of premenstrual syndrome (PMS).

The active ingredients in chasteberry are believed to act on the pituitary gland in the brain to cause the release of a neurotransmitter called dopamine. Herbalists believe that chasteberry increases the production of progesterone, leading to a normal balance of estrogen and progesterone. Through its action on dopamine in the brain, studies show that chasteberry also suppresses the release of prolactin, thereby lowering excessive levels. Its action on prolactin is considered the main reason for its effectiveness.

One German study, which followed more than 1600 women with PMS for three months, found that 93 percent of women taking chasteberry reported improvement of symptoms (mood swings, anxiety, food cravings and fluid retention) or complete relief.[1] Although a limited number of well-controlled clinical studies have assessed the effectiveness of chasteberry, the experience of physicians has long established the practical use of the herb in women with PMS. Less vigorous research has been done in the area of amenorrhea and infertility, though a few studies do support the use of chasteberry for these conditions.

Chasteberry Supplements

Choose a product standardized to contain 0.5 percent agnuside and 0.6 percent aucubin. The recommended dose is 175 to 225 milligrams once daily. It takes at least four weeks for noticeable effects. Mild side effects occasionally reported include nausea, headache and skin rash.

Historically, chasteberry has been used to promote lactation; however, since the herb inhibits prolactin secretion (prolactin is necessary for milk production), you should *not* use it if you are breastfeeding unless you have been advised to do so by a health care practitioner. The herb has not been evaluated in pregnant women.

If you are on a medication that interacts with the neurotransmitter dopamine (e.g., the antidepressants Wellbutrin® and Effexor®), be sure to tell your doctor that you are taking chasteberry. He or she should monitor you closely to ensure the herb doesn't interact with your medication and make it less effective. If you are taking birth control pills or hormone replacement therapy, use caution. Although there have been no case reports, theoretically, chasteberry could interfere with the effectiveness of these medications because of its hormone-regulating activity.

Dong Quai (*Angelica sinensis*)

Used for premenstrual syndrome (see page 480), menstrual cramps, infertility (see page 378), menopause (dong quai appears to help menopausal women only when used according to a traditional Chinese medicine diagnosis)

This aromatic herb has probably been the herb longest used in traditional Chinese medicine (TCM), which considers it a "blood tonic" that enriches and nourishes the blood and regulates the menstrual cycle. As such, it has been traditionally used to treat women with deficiency disorders related to menstruation. Often referred to as the "female ginseng," this herb is a member of the celery family and grows in south-western China.

The root of the herb contains coumarins, essential oils and a compound called ligustilide, all of which are thought to exert beneficial effects. Dong quai has been shown to dilate blood vessels, thin the blood and act as an antispasmodic. The herb may have a weak estrogen-like action in the body, binding to estrogen receptors.

Studies have found dong quai to be effective in treating amenorrhea, menstrual irregularities, infertility and PMS.[1-3] A recent American study found that when dong quai was given alone, it was not effective in relieving menopausal symptoms.[4] However, when taken in a combination TCM herbal formula, dong quai does appear to be effective for treating menopausal symptoms.

Dong Quai Supplements

Buy a product standardized to contain 0.8 percent ligustilide. Take 150 milligrams two or three times daily. For a 1:1 fluid extract, take 0.5 to 2 milliliters three times daily. For menopausal symptoms, use a TCM formula with a TCM diagnosis of "blood deficiency." One such formula is Si Wu Tang, which combines dong quai with four other herbs.

Adverse effects are rare but may include diarrhea and sun sensitivity. Dong quai should not be used during pregnancy unless given by a qualified practitioner of TCM. Avoid using this herb during breastfeeding, as there is insufficient information to evaluate its safety. Dong quai is contraindicated in cases of heavy menstrual bleeding. According to TCM, dong quai should not be taken during illness as it may cause diarrhea. The herb may interact with the blood-thinning medication warfarin (Coumadin®). If you are taking this drug and dong quai at the same time, be sure to inform your doctor.

Echinacea (*Echinacea purpurea, Echinacea angustifolia, Echinacea pallida*)

Used for colds (see page 233) and flu, ear infections (see page 278), candidiasis (see page 195), sinusitis (see page 511), urinary tract infections (see page 525)

This plant, also known as purple coneflower, is native to North America. You may even have this tall daisy-like flower growing in your summer garden. Historically, the herb was used by North American Natives and early settlers as a topical treatment for burns, wounds and snake and insect bites. The root of the herb was chewed to cure toothache, and preparations were ingested to cure a host of ailments. Today, three species of echinacea are found in products; all have medicinal benefits.

Many studies in the laboratory have shown the ability of echinacea to enhance the body's production of white blood cells, which fight infection. The herb also appears to prevent the recurrence of Candida albicans, the organism responsible for vaginal yeast infections.[1] Studies in humans have not been consistent in their findings. Despite the positive results in the laboratory, clinical trials in adults taking echinacea to treat a cold or flu have not conclusively shown that the herb is effective, perhaps because so many different brands were used.[2-5] However, a review of studies conducted to date finds that most studies report a positive effect on infection.[6]

Echinacea contains many different compounds, and the amounts present differ depending on which part of the plant is being used (flower, leaf or root). At this point, scientists are uncertain as to which particular plant components are most responsible for the herb's immune-stimulation effect. It is thought that these ingredients work together to exert their effects in the body.

Echinacea Supplements

To ensure quality, buy a product standardized to contain 4 percent echinacosides (*Echinacea angustifolia*) and 0.7 percent flavonoids (*Echinacea purpurea*), two of the herb's active ingredients.

You can choose from several forms of the herb to treat active colds, flu and infection:

- *Products made from echinacea root* a total of 900 milligrams three to four times daily.

- *Fluid extracts (1:1)* 0.25 to 1.0 milliliters three times daily.

- *Tinctures (1:5)* 1 to 2 milliliters three times daily.

- *Teas* 125 to 250 milliliters three to four times daily.

Take until symptoms are relieved, then continue taking two to three times daily for one week. Some experts recommend taking the herb once every two hours (300 milligram standardized extract or 3 to 4 milliliter tincture) until symptoms have subsided, then up to three times daily for a week. To prevent infection, take two to three times daily for two weeks of every month.

Doses for children are based on their body weight. For children under the age of 12, a general guideline is as follows:

- Adult dose (milligrams) $\times$ (age of child $\div$ 12) = child's dose, or

- Adult dose (milligrams) $\times$ (body weight in pounds $\div$ 150) = child's dose

For older children who are at acceptable percentiles for height and weight, half the recommended adult dosage can be used. Studies have not yet determined appropriate doses for children.

Daily use should be limited to eight consecutive weeks because of concern that long-term use of echinacea might depress the immune system.

Adverse reactions are rare but can include allergic skin and respiratory reactions. High doses of the herb can cause nausea and dizziness. Don't use echinacea if you are allergic to plants in the Asteracease/Compositae family (ragweed, daisy, marigold and chrysanthemum). Although controversial among experts, the herb is generally not recommended for use by people with autoimmune diseases (HIV, lupus), multiple sclerosis, diabetes or asthma. People on immune-suppressing drugs (corticosteroids, cyclosporin) should not take the herb.

Evening Primrose (*Oenothera biennis*)

Used for cyclic breast pain (mastalgia), (see fibrocystic breast conditions, page 279), premenstrual syndrome (see page 480), eczema, rheumatoid arthritis (see page 502), schizophrenia, alcoholism (see page 148), cystic fibrosis (page 247)

Also known as King's cure-all, evening primrose is a wildflower native to North America. Once its bright yellow flowers die, pods are left that contain brown seeds rich in oil. It is this oil that is used medicinally.

Evening primrose oil is rich in a special type of fatty acid called gamma-linolenic acid (GLA). The body uses GLA to make prostaglandins (PGs), powerful hormone-like compounds that regulate our blood, immune system and hormones. PGs can either increase or decrease inflammation. In the case of GLA, it is used to make friendly, or less inflammatory, PGs.

There is very little GLA in food and so GLA must be made from other types of fat in the diet, such as vegetable oils (the body converts linoleic acid in these oils to GLA). Some researchers think that women with PMS may have difficulty converting linoleic acid in food into GLA and that this can cause symptoms such as breast pain and tenderness, irritability, depression and headache. By taking supplemental evening primrose oil, women with PMS may get adequate GLA to produce friendly PGs, and a result, experience fewer uncomfortable symptoms.

Studies in the 1980s did show that daily supplements of evening primrose oil outperformed the placebo pill in improving PMS symptoms of breast tenderness, irritability and depression. In a few studies, the difference between evening primrose oil and placebo was statistically significant. However, studies performed over the past ten years have not found any beneficial effects for evening primrose oil treating PMS as a whole. Lack of an effect may be because these studies were of short duration (evening primrose oil may take up to eight months to reach its peak effectiveness).

Evening primrose oil appears to offer most promise in treating breast pain and tenderness. Some studies have found the supplement to be as effective as certain drugs used to treat cyclic breast pain. Researchers from the University of Wales in Great Britain concluded that evening primrose oil was the best first-line therapy for cyclic breast pain.[1]

GLA is used to make other anti-inflammatory PGs, one of which appears to ease the itchiness of atopic eczema. When British researchers analyzed the results from a number of studies, they found that evening primrose oil does relieve eczema symptoms.[2] However, two other studies found that evening primrose oil was no better than the placebo treatment. It is possible, however, that the duration of these studies was not long enough to detect effects.

A handful of studies show that evening primrose oil combined with fish oil may be a promising treatment for easing symptoms of rheumatoid arthritis.[3] In arthritis, painful and inflamed joints are caused by an excess production of inflammatory, or unfriendly, PGs. Consuming more GLA (and fatty acids in fish oil) may help the body make more anti-inflammatory PGs, thereby relieving joint swelling and pain.

Although preliminary, there is some research to suggest that people suffering with alcoholism may be deficient in GLA, and that supplementing with evening primrose oil may help improve their tolerance to alcohol. Studies show that alcohol administration changes the fatty-acid profile of brain cells and that evening primrose oil can reverse these effects.[4,5]

Evening primrose oil has also been shown to reverse a deficiency of PGs in brain cells in people with schizophrenia.[6] Increasing the levels of GLA and anti-inflammatory PGs may help improve symptoms in these patients.

Evening Primrose Supplements

Buy a supplement standardized to contain 9 percent GLA. For cyclic breast pain and PMS, take 3 to 4 grams per day, split in two equal doses. Start by taking three 500 milligram capsules at breakfast, and repeat at dinner. For eczema, adults should take 6 to 8 grams per day, split in two equal doses; children should take 2 to 4 grams per day, split in two equal doses. For rheumatoid arthritis, take 6 grams per day, split in two equal doses. For other conditions, the effective dose has not been determined. Treatment for at least three months is usually required to notice an effect.

Evening primrose supplements may cause indigestion, headache and soft stools in some people. Large doses can lead to diarrhea. Evening primrose oil may increase the risk of pregnancy complications and so should be avoided by pregnant women. However, the herb is safe to take while breastfeeding. People with epilepsy and those taking the schizophrenia medication phenothiazine should use evening primrose oil with caution.

Feverfew (*Tanacetum parthenium*)

Used for migraine headache prevention (see page 425)

This plant, once native to Europe, can now be found throughout most of the world. Its use dates back to ancient Greek times, when it was often used to treat a fever, headache, gynecological problems and stomach upset. The use of feverfew for migraines became popular in England in the 1970s after a doctor's wife noticed that her migraines were much improved once she started chewing fresh feverfew leaves. As the story goes, after one year of faithfully taking the leaves, she almost forgot that she ever suffered from migraines.

Researchers believe that feverfew reduces the frequency and intensity of migraines by preventing the release of prostaglandins, which dilate blood vessels and cause inflammation. It was once thought that parthenolide, one of the herb's active ingredients, was responsible for feverfew's beneficial effect. But an alcohol extract containing only parthenolide was found to have no effect on migraine headaches. It seems that parthenolide is only one of the compounds in feverfew leaf responsible for preventing migraines.

Feverfew has been the focus of a number of studies on people with migraines. In one, a randomized controlled trial from England, 76 people who experienced migraines were given either whole feverfew leaf or placebo for four months.[1] The treatments were then reversed for another four-month period. Without knowing which treatment they received when, 59 percent of the people taking feverfew identified the feverfew period as more effective, compared with 24 percent who chose the placebo period. The herbal remedy reduced the number of classic migraines (with aura) by 32 percent and common migraines (without aura) by 21 percent.

Feverfew Supplements

Don't buy an alcohol extract containing parthenolide only. Instead, buy capsules of powdered feverfew leaf. Take 80 to 100 milligrams daily. You can also try taking the herb at the onset of a migraine to ease the symptoms.

Feverfew rarely causes side effects other than mild gastrointestinal upset. The herb may cause an allergic reaction in people sensitive to members of the Asteracease/Compositae plant family (ragweed, daisy, marigold and chrysanthemum). The safety of feverfew has not been studied in pregnant or nursing women or those with liver or kidney disease. Feverfew should not be used during pregnancy (historically, it was used to induce abortions).

Garlic (*Allium sativum*)

Used for lowering blood cholesterol (see page 327) and blood pressure (see page 328), colds (see page 233) and flu, ear infections (see page 278), Helicobacter pylori infection (see Ulcers, page 520), colon cancer prevention (see page 227)

This herb has a long tradition of healing powers. Ancient Egyptians ate garlic as part of their daily diet. In fact, well-preserved cloves of garlic were found in King Tutankhamen's tomb. In Biblical times, garlic was thought to preserve strength and was given to slaves to increase their fitness. In ancient Greece, athletes took garlic before competing in the Olympic games to enhance strength and vigor. Historically, garlic has been used worldwide to fight bacterial infections. The French chemist Louis Pasteur was the first to describe the antibacterial effect of garlic. Today, garlic is still taken to fight infection, but it is also being praised by scientists for its protective effects against heart disease and cancer.

Garlic contains many different sulfur compounds, and one in particular, S-allyl cysteine (SAC), has been shown to lower LDL cholesterol by up to 10 percent in humans.[1-4] SAC is present in small amounts in raw garlic, but it increases in concentration as the garlic ages. The scientific studies that have found a cholesterol-lowering effect have used an extract of aged garlic extract (Kyolic® brand from Wakunaga).

Garlic may protect from heart disease in other ways. Studies have shown the herb can lower blood triglyceride levels and thin the blood by reducing the stickiness of platelets.[5] The sulfur compounds in aged garlic extract also act as an antioxidant and prevent damage to LDL cholesterol.[6,7] Aged garlic has been shown to have a modest blood-pressure-lowering effect.[8]

Much of the research on cancer prevention has looked at stomach and colon cancer. Population-based studies have found that eating raw and cooked garlic may reduce the risk of stomach cancer by as much as 60 percent. The Iowa Women's Health Study, which followed 42,000 women for five years, found that those who consumed 0.7 grams of raw or cooked garlic each day (less than one clove) had a 32 percent lower risk of colon cancer than women who did not consume garlic.[9] A

Swiss study found that men who consumed raw or cooked garlic had a 23 percent lower risk of colon cancer.[10]

Some research suggests that eating garlic may also offer protection from prostate cancer. A study from the United Kingdom found that, compared to men who never consumed garlic, those that consumed garlic in foods and supplements at least twice a week had a 40 percent reduced risk of prostate cancer.[11] Men who consumed garlic one to four times per month had a 30 percent reduced risk. The more garlic the men consumed, the greater the protection.

There are three possible reasons for the potential anticancer effect of garlic's sulfur compounds. First, these compounds help the liver detoxify and get rid of cancer-causing substances. Second, some sulfur compounds may have a direct toxic effect on certain cancer cells. And third, studies have shown that sulfur compounds in aged garlic extract can stimulate the body's immune system.

Helicobacter pylori (H. pylori) is a bacterium that's implicated in the development of stomach cancer and ulcers. Laboratory studies show that garlic, especially aged garlic extract, inhibits the growth of the organisms.[12,13]

Garlic Supplements

As little as half a clove of raw or cooked garlic each day is thought to offer general health benefits. Raw garlic contains very little SAC, but researchers at Pennsylvania State University found that allowing crushed garlic to sit at room temperature for ten minutes before using it in cooking will increase the concentration of SAC.[14]

When buying garlic supplements, choose a product made with aged garlic extract (e.g., Kyolic® brand). Aged garlic extract has been aged for up to 20 months. Take two to six capsules a day in divided doses throughout the day. Studies have used up to 7.2 grams per day. Aged garlic extract is odorless and less irritating to the gastrointestinal tract than other forms of garlic supplements (such as garlic oil capsules and garlic powder tablets). Kwai® garlic powder has also been used in clinical research.

When taken in large amounts, garlic may cause stomach upset, heartburn, flatulence, nausea and diarrhea. Certain people are more sensitive to the sulfur compounds in garlic, and these effects are more pronounced when eating raw garlic. Garlic supplements in high doses may be unsafe during pregnancy. Garlic (both fresh and supplements) may enhance the effects of blood-thinning medications like warfarin (Coumadin®). If you are taking this type of drug and garlic at the same time, be sure to inform your doctor. Since garlic can prolong bleeding time, stop taking it one week prior to scheduled surgery.

Ginger (*Zingiber officinale*)

Used for motion sickness (see page 430), morning sickness (pregnancy), post-operative nausea and vomiting

This perennial plant has been cultivated for thousands of years in China and has been a part of traditional Chinese medicine for more than 2500 years. Historically, ginger was prescribed for abdominal distension, vomiting, diarrhea and coughing. Ginger has also played an important healing role in the medical systems of India, Nigeria and the West Indies. Ginger became popular as an herbal remedy in the Western world in the early 1980s when a scientist with the flu noticed that taking capsules of ginger cured his nausea. Since then, ginger has been widely accepted as a treatment for nausea. The gingerroot you can buy at the supermarket is the underground stem (rhizome) of the plant and is what is used for medicinal purposes.

The precise active ingredient in ginger remains unknown. Ginger contains many ingredients, all of which may play a role in the herb's beneficial effects. Ginger owes its pungent smell to the compounds gingerols and shogoals. Scientists believe that ginger acts on the stomach and improves the motility of the intestinal tract. Gingerol compounds may improve appetite and digestion because of their ability to reduce gastric secretions and increase the release of important digestive aids.

A number of studies have found ginger an effective agent in reducing motion sickness. In one Swedish study of 79 naval cadets, ginger reduced vomiting and cold sweats.[1] Another study conducted among almost 1500 people aboard a ship found ginger to be just as effective as various medications for seasickness.[2] Despite these positive findings, a few studies have reported no effect of ginger on nausea associated with travel.[3,4]

Fewer studies have assessed the effectiveness (and safety) of ginger supplements in pregnant women with morning sickness. A recent study from Thailand gave 70 pregnant women experiencing nausea and vomiting 1 gram of ginger for four days, or a placebo pill.[5] Among the women receiving ginger, 87 percent had less nausea. As well, episodes of vomiting decreased significantly in the group taking ginger. Another study from Denmark looked at 27 pregnant women suffering from severe morning sickness and revealed that ginger taken four times a day significantly reduced nausea and vomiting.[6] The effects of ginger became apparent after four days of treatment.

Studies support the use of ginger for reducing nausea and vomiting that occurs after surgery. Two out of three studies found ginger to be superior to placebo and equally effective as metoclopramide, the standard medication given to patients.[7]

Ginger Supplements

Buy powdered ginger pills. Dose ranges from 1 to 4 grams daily, taken in two to four divided doses. For nausea and vomiting associated with pregnancy, try 1 cup of ginger tea four times daily (make from boiled gingerroot and dilute to desired taste). If using ginger pills, stay at the lower dosage range—250 milligrams four times daily (as was used in the clinical study I mentioned earlier).

Mild intestinal upset is the only adverse effect that has been reported from taking ginger at the recommended doses. Ginger does have a slight blood-thinning effect and may possibly interact with blood-thinning medications like warfarin (Coumadin®), though no studies have reported this effect. The safety of taking ginger supplements during pregnancy has not been proven and therefore its use during pregnancy remains controversial. The effect of ginger on the developing fetus is unknown. Ginger may also increase bleeding time and should not be taken before scheduled surgery.

Ginkgo (*Ginkgo biloba*)

Used for dementia, Alzheimer's disease (see page 155), age-related memory loss, sexual dysfunction (caused by taking certain antidepressant medications), intermittent claudication (peripheral vascular disease)

Ginkgo biloba is the world's oldest living species of tree—its fossil records date back more than 200 million years. The ginkgo tree lives as long as 1000 years and grows over 100 feet high. Ginkgo extracts used in herbal medicine come from the tree's characteristic fan-shaped, bilobed leaves. The use of ginkgo as a medicinal plant dates back almost 5000 years, to the beginning of Chinese medicine. Scientific research into ginkgo's active ingredients started in the late 1950s. A standardized extract of ginkgo was produced some 20 years later. It is this special extract, EGb 761, that continues to be used in much of the scientific research today.

The active ingredients responsible for ginkgo's beneficial effects are terpene lactones and ginkgo flavone glycosides. A number of studies suggest that ginkgo increases circulation and oxygen delivery to the brain. The herb's active ingredients also make platelets less sticky. By doing this, circulation becomes more efficient. Ginkgo also has a strong antioxidant effect in the brain. (Free radical damage to brain cells may be a contributing factor in Alzheimer's disease.)

Many clinical trials have demonstrated a significant improvement or delay in the progression of Alzheimer's disease when standardized extracts of ginkgo leaf were given over several weeks to one year. A 52-week American clinical trial conducted with 309 patients with mild to moderate dementia as a result of Alzheimer's disease or stroke compared the effects of 40 milligrams of ginkgo (EGb 761) taken three times daily to a placebo pill.[1] After one year, the placebo group showed a decline in cognitive function, whereas the ginkgo group did not. When the researchers looked at Alzheimer's patients only, there were modest but statistically significant changes in memory and other brain functions.

Ginkgo has been shown to be an effective treatment for relief from intermittent claudication, a condition in which the arteries supplying the legs with blood may become blocked because of hardening of those arteries. Because the muscles in the legs can't get enough oxygen, walking more than a short distance causes cramps and pain. One study of 79 patients suffering from this condition found that leg pain was reduced and walking distance increased after taking a standardized extract of ginkgo.[2] A smaller study found that ginkgo (the EGb 761 extract) improved the health of the blood vessels in people with intermittent claudication.[3]

If you are taking Prozac®, Effexor®, Paxil®, Zoloft® or Serzone® for depression and are experiencing sexual dysfunction, research suggests that ginkgo may be an effective remedy. In a study from California 63 men and women who complained of sexual dysfunction as a result of antidepressant medication were given 60 to 120 milligrams of ginkgo each day.[4] The herb was found to be 84 percent effective in treating sexual dysfunction. Women were more responsive than men, with success rates of 91 percent versus 76 percent.

Ginkgo Supplements

Choose a product that is standardized to contain 24 percent ginkgo flavone glycosides and 6 percent terpene lactones. The EGb 761 extract used in scientific research is sold as Ginkoba® (Pharmaton® Natural Health Products) in Canada and the United States. For dementia syndromes, take 120 to 240 milligrams daily, in divided doses. The typical adult dose is 40 milligrams three times daily. For intermittent claudication, take 120 to 240 milligrams daily, in divided doses. For reversing sexual dysfunction due to antidepressant drugs, start by taking 60 milligrams twice daily. Increase the dose if needed, but do so slowly to avoid stomach upset.

On rare occasions, ginkgo may cause gastrointestinal upset, headache or an allergic skin reaction in susceptible individuals. The herb's safety during pregnancy and breastfeeding has not been established. Ginkgo has a slight blood-thinning effect, so it has the potential to enhance the effects of other blood-thinning medications (warfarin, aspirin). If you're on blood thinners, let your doctor know if you start taking ginkgo.

Ginseng (*Panax ginseng, Panax quinquefolius*)

Used for stress (see page 515) and fatigue, immune enhancement (see Common Cold, page 233), type 2 diabetes (see page 263) (American ginseng only)

Ginseng is a perennial herb with a taproot. Panax ginseng goes by many names, including Asian ginseng, Korean ginseng and Chinese ginseng. It grows in northern China, Korea and Russia. American ginseng (Panax quinquefolius) grows in the United States. The herb takes five years to grow and, as a result, high-quality ginseng root is extremely expensive. White ginseng is ginseng root that has been dried and unprocessed; red ginseng refers to the herb when it has been steamed and heat-dried. Both are thought to have unique characteristics.

A part of Chinese medicine for more than 2000 years, ginseng root is known as an adaptogenic herb. That is, it increases the body's resistance to stress and balances functions of the immune, nervous and cardiovascular systems.

Evidence suggests that Panax ginseng has strong immune-enhancing properties. Studies done in test tubes, in animals and in humans found that ginseng increases the body's production of a number of different immune cells. Ginseng also seems to be able to help certain cells engulf foreign compounds that invade the bloodstream.

A well-designed Italian study tested the theory that regular use of Panax ginseng helps prevent colds and flus.[1] The researchers enrolled 227 people, giving half the participants 100 milligrams of a standardized ginseng extract (G115). The remaining volunteers were given a placebo pill. Four weeks later, all participants received a flu vaccine. Those individuals taking ginseng had significantly higher levels of antibodies in response to the flu shot compared with those who did not take the herb. Killer white blood cells (an important part of the body's defense against viruses and foreign molecules) were nearly twice as high in the ginseng group after eight weeks of supplementation. As well, the ginseng users had significantly fewer episodes of cold or flu compared with the placebo group.

Although more research needs to be conducted, American ginseng may help control blood-sugar levels in people with type 2 diabetes (adult onset, not requiring insulin injections). Researchers from the University of Toronto found that American ginseng effectively lowered the blood-sugar rise that resulted from drinking a sugar solution in people.[2] This effect was seen in both people with type 2 diabetes and healthy volunteers.

The active ingredients in Panax ginseng are thought to reduce stress by stimulating the body's adrenal glands. These triangular-shaped glands sit above the kidneys and regulate the release of stress hormones. Chronic fatigue or stress can compromise adrenal function, affecting the body's release of hormones and immune compounds, as well as diminishing one's overall feeling of energy.

The health benefits of Panax ginseng can be attributed to ginsenosides, active compounds in the root. Many ginsenosides have been identified, but ginsenosides Rg1 and Rb1 have received the most attention. Scientific research has focused on ginseng extracts standardized to contain 4 to 7 percent ginsenosides.

Ginseng Supplements

To ease stress and enhance the immune system, choose *Panax ginseng*. Buy a product with a statement of standardization or "G115" printed on the label. The product Ginsana® (Pharmaton® Natural Health Products) contains the G115 extract that's been used in clinical studies. The typical dose is 100 or 200 milligrams once daily. Take ginseng for three weeks to three months and follow with a one- to two-week rest period before you resume taking the herb.

Ginseng is relatively safe at the recommended dosage. In some people, it may cause mild stomach upset, irritability and insomnia. To avoid overstimulation, start with 100 milligrams a day and avoid taking the herb with caffeine. Ginseng should not be used during pregnancy or breastfeeding or by individuals with poorly controlled high blood pressure.

Siberian Ginseng (*Eleutherococcus senticosus*)

Unlike Panax ginseng, this herb has a much milder effect and fewer reported side effects. Pregnant and nursing women can safely take Siberian ginseng, and it is much less likely to cause overstimulation in sensitive individuals. To ensure quality, choose a product standardized for eleutherosides B and E. The usual dosage is 300 to 400 milligrams once daily for six to eight weeks, followed by a one- to two-week break.

Horse Chestnut (*Aesculus hippocastanum*)

Used for varicose veins (see page 529) and chronic venous insufficiency
This herb comes from trees that are native to Asia and northern Greece but are now grown in North America and other parts of Europe. The fruit of the tree consists of a capsule that contains up to three large seeds, known as horse chestnuts. It is these seeds that are used to make medicinal extracts of horse chestnut. Traditionally, the herb was used both internally and externally to treat a host of ills, from arthritis to varicose veins. Today, horse chestnut has received much attention from scientists as an effective remedy for discomfort caused by varicose veins.

The seed of the horse chestnut tree contains active compounds called saponins. One compound in particular, aescin, enhances circulation through the veins. Studies have demonstrated aescin's ability to constrict and promote normal tone in the veins so that blood returns to the heart. The compound also has anti-inflammatory properties and may reduce swelling in the legs.[1,2]

After a comprehensive review of all horse chestnut studies, researchers from the United Kingdom concluded that the use of the herb is associated with a "decrease of the lower-leg volume and a reduction in leg circumference at the calf and ankle."[3] The herbal remedy was found to ease symptoms such as leg pain, fatigue and tenseness. Five studies even found that horse chestnut was as effective as standard drug therapy for varicose veins.[4] Another study suggests that taking horse chestnut seed extract is as effective as wearing compression stockings.[5]

Horse Chestnut Supplements

Buy a product standardized to contain 16 to 21 percent aescin. Take one capsule up to three times per day. The extract used in the clinical studies is sold as Venastat® (Pharmaton® Natural Health Products) in Canada and the United States.

In rare instances, horse chestnut seed extract can cause stomach upset, nausea and itching. Use is not recommended during pregnancy and breastfeeding since there is insufficient information available about its safety at these times. Horse chestnut should not be taken by people with liver or kidney disease.

Kava Kava (*Piper methysticum*)

Used for anxiety disorders

The use of kava kava dates back to the 18th century, when Polynesians participated in kava-drinking ceremonies to produce a soothing, relaxing effect without altering consciousness. Captain Cook, encountering the plant in the South Pacific, called it "intoxicating pepper." Today, kava remains a popular social drink with Pacific Islanders and is still used for ceremonial purposes. In Western medicine, kava is slowly becoming accepted as an effective treatment for anxiety disorders.

Kava is extracted from the roots of this pepper plant.

The active ingredients, kavalactones or kavapyrones, have many effects on the central nervous system, but their exact mechanism of action remain unknown. Many scientists believe that kavalactones exert their effect by working on the limbic system of the brain, the center of emotion. People consuming kava report feeling more sociable, tranquil and happy.

A number of clinical studies have deemed kava effective in the treatment of anxiety disorders.[1] Anxiety is described as a feeling of apprehension, uncertainty and fear. It's also associated with physical changes—an increased heart rate, sweating and even tremors. Studies show that standardized extracts of the herb are superior to placebo, and possibly comparable to low-dose benzodiazepines, for the short-term relief of anxiety.[2-4] Two studies have found kava helpful in the management of menopause-related anxiety, without the negative side effects of traditional drugs like Valium®. In one study, significant improvement occurred after one week of treatment.[5]

Kava Kava Supplements

Most studies have been conducted using kava extracts standardized to contain 70 percent kavalactones. This is more than twice as concentrated as most products available in health food stores and pharmacies. Most products are standardized to 30 percent kavalactones (30 milligrams of kavalactones in each 100 milligram capsule). The recommended dose depends on the kavalactone content of the capsule.

Until recently kava was thought to have a wide margin of safety. The only side effects reported were mild stomach upset, headache, or dizziness. But that's all changed. If you are already taking kava, or have a bottle in your medicine cabinet, *read the following section very carefully*. There is growing concern over reports from Europe that describe liver damage in some people taking kava. Many of these reports note liver damage in those who have taken kava concurrently with alcohol or medication. Based on current information, individuals at particular risk for liver damage associated with use of kava include those who have compromised liver function due to liver disease, age factors, or prior or current drug/alcohol abuse.

So far in Canada, there have been four cases of liver toxicity associated with the use of kava-containing products. As a result of these reports and others, Health Canada issued a stop-sale for kava products in August 2002. Canadian manufacturers, distributors and importers were required to stop the sale of kava -containing products and all products were recalled from the market. If you have a bottle at home, I advise you to throw it out.

Milk Thistle *(Silybum marianum)*

Used for liver disorders: chronic hepatitis (page 339), acute hepatitis, alcoholic liver disease (see Alcoholism, page 148), liver cirrhosis (see page 222)

Often referred to as wild artichoke or holy thistle, this native European plant has characteristic spiny leaves and thistle-shaped flowers. It has a long history of use as both a food and a medicine. In the early 1900s, milk thistle leaves were tossed into salads and often substituted for spinach. The seeds and leaves were used to treat jaundice and promote the production of breast milk. It wasn't until 1960 that German researchers began the process of identifying the plant's active compounds. By 1986, milk thistle had become accepted by German physicians as a treatment for liver disease.

Milk thistle has three active ingredients, known collectively as silymarin. This active complex appears to protect the liver in a few ways. First, silymarin can prevent toxic substances from penetrating liver cells, possibly by preventing the binding of harmful compounds to the liver.[1,2] Second, silymarin has been shown to help liver cells regenerate more quickly. And finally, milk thistle may act as an antioxidant and, as such, protect liver cells from damage caused by unstable oxygen molecules (free radicals).[3]

Studies conducted in people with chronic viral hepatitis found that milk thistle can improve symptoms such as poor appetite, fatigue and stomach upset.[4-6] As well, liver-function blood-test results improve (liver enzyme levels are reduced) with milk thistle.[7] A handful of studies looking at the effects of milk thistle in alcoholic liver disease have found the herb able to improve both liver-function blood-test results and the health of the liver cells.[8,9]

Two studies suggest that milk thistle may improve survival in patients with cirrhosis of the liver.[10,11] One study looked at the effect of taking milk thistle for three to six years in 146 people with liver cirrhosis. At the end of four years, the survival rate was 58 percent in the herb-treated group compared with 38 percent in the placebo group. The herb might also inhibit liver damage caused by certain prescription drugs such as acetaminophen, Dilantin® (phenytoin) and phenothiazines.[12]

Milk Thistle Supplements

Buy a product standardized to contain 70 percent silymarin. The usual dose ranges from 70 to 210 milligrams, taken two or three times daily. If you buy a product that binds silymarin to phosphatidylcholine, take 100 to 200 milligrams twice daily (some research suggests that this form of milk thistle is better absorbed).

Milk thistle is very safe in the recommended doses. A mild laxative effect may occur in some individuals. Use milk thistle with caution if you are allergic to plants in the Astercease/Compositae family (ragweed, daisy, marigold and chrysanthemum). Safety during pregnancy and breastfeeding has not been established, although it is thought to have no harmful effects. However, pregnant and breastfeeding women should use milk thistle with caution. Milk thistle may reduce the effectiveness of oral contraceptives.

St. John's Wort (*Hypericum perforatum*)

Used for mild to moderate depression (see page 252); seasonal affective disorder
This plant is native to Europe but can be found growing in Canada and the United States along roadsides and in meadows and woods. It produces bright yellow flowers that are said to be the brightest in color on June 24, the birth date of St. John the Baptist. The medicinal use of St. John's wort dates back more than 2000 years, when it was used to ease pain and promote wound healing. Today, St. John's wort is regarded as an effective treatment for mild depression. As well, new research is emerging around its potential antiviral activity against HIV and herpes simplex virus. It is the above-ground parts of the plant that are used to make extracts of St. John's wort.

Many experts believe that St. John's wort works by keeping brain serotonin levels high for a longer period, just like the popular antidepressant drugs Paxil®, Zoloft® and Prozac®. Serotonin is a neurotransmitter, a natural brain chemical associated with feeling happy, relaxed and calm. St. John's wort also appears to alter levels of dopamine and norepinephrine in the brain, two other neurotransmitters involved in mood. Researchers believe the power of St. John's wort lies in a few active ingredients: hypericin, hyperforin, flavonoids and xanthones. Recently, scientists have attributed most of the herb's effect on serotonin to its hyperforin content.[1,2]

In 1997, British researchers analyzed 26 controlled studies conducted in over 2000 patients and concluded that the herb was superior to placebo and as effective as certain antidepressant drugs in the treatment of mild to moderate depression.[3] The herb was helpful in relieving fatigue, tiredness, anxiety and disturbed sleep, and it may improve cognitive functioning. Those taking St. John's wort experienced significantly fewer side effects compared with those taking prescription medications. The herb did not cause drowsiness or dampen libido.

St. John's Wort Supplements

Buy a product standardized to contain 0.3 percent hypericin and 3 to 5 percent hyperforin. Advanced St. John's wort formulas, such as Movana® (Pharmaton® Natural Health Products), contain hyperforin and are available in Canada. The effective dose is 300 milligrams, three times a day.

St. John's wort is generally well tolerated. When the herb is taken in high doses for a long period, it may cause sensitivity to sunlight in very light-skinned individuals. St. John's wort has the potential to interact with a number of medications. Do not take the herb if you are taking indinavir, cyclosporine, theophylline, warfarin, oral contraceptives or digoxin. St. John's wort is not recommended for use during pregnancy and breastfeeding. If you are taking a prescription antidepressant drug, do not take it concurrently with St. John's wort, and always consult your physician before stopping any medication.

Saw Palmetto
(*Serenoa repens, Sabal serrulata*)

Used for prostate enlargement (benign prostatic hyperplasia) (see page 494)
This plant, sometimes referred to as sabal in Europe, is native to North America and can be found growing in Atlantic Canada. Historically, the wrinkled dark-colored berries were used for food and to treat medical conditions affecting the bladder, urinary tract and prostate. It was once believed that saw palmetto increased sperm production and libido in men. Today, the berries of this plant are used to relieve symptoms associated with benign prostate enlargement.

Benign prostatic hyperplasia (BPH) affects roughly half of all men over 40 years of age. BPH is an enlargement of the prostate gland due to an overproduction of the hormone dihydrotestosterone (an active form of testosterone) in the prostate.

The active ingredients in saw palmetto berries are thought to be fatty acids (a group of fat-soluble compounds), sterols and esters. Saw palmetto berries have been shown to lower the level of dihydrotestosterone in the prostate. The active ingredients appear to block the conversion of testosterone to dihydrotestosterone and prevent the binding of dihydrotestosterone to prostate cells. As well, saw palmetto might have anti-inflammatory and antiestrogenic properties.

Extracts of saw palmetto berries have been found to be effective in 90 percent of patients within a four- to six-week period. In a recent review of 18 randomized controlled studies, American researchers concluded that compared with the standard drug treatment Proscar®, saw palmetto was equally effective at improving urinary tract symptoms and improving urinary flow.[1] And use of the herb was associated with fewer side effects.

Saw Palmetto Supplements

Buy a product standardized to contain between 85 and 95 percent fatty acids and sterols. Take 160 milligrams twice daily (320 milligrams per day). Continue for several months. Improvement may take up to two months of treatment. Teas made from saw palmetto berries are not likely to be effective, since adequate amounts of the fat-soluble active ingredients may not be released from the herb.

On rare occasions, saw palmetto may cause stomach upset and headache. No interactions with medications are known.

Valerian (*Valeriana officinalis*)

Used for insomnia (see page 390)

Over 200 species of valerian can be found growing around the world. The species used for medicinal purposes grows wild in Europe, but most of the plants used for making herbal extracts are cultivated. Ancient Greek physicians recommended valerian as a healing aid for stomach upset, liver problems and urinary tract disorders. The herb was not used to treat sleep problems until some time late in the 16th century. By 1940, mention of valerian could be found in American medical textbooks. Today, many European countries have approved its use as an over-the-counter medication for insomnia. It is starting to gain popularity in North America among consumers and the medical profession.

Valerian root acts like a mild sedative on the central nervous system. Scientists have learned that valerian promotes sleep by weakly binding to two brain receptors, GABA receptors and benzodiazepine receptors. Many active components, including volatile oils and valepotriates, are believed to be responsible for the herb's sedating effect. The herb also appears to have antianxiety and mood-enhancing properties.

Several small studies conducted among patients with sleep disorders have found valerian reduces the time to fall asleep and improves the quality of sleep. In one double-blind study conducted in Germany, 44 percent of patients taking valerian root reported perfect sleep and 89 percent reported improved sleep compared with those taking the placebo pill.[1] Another small study found that individuals with mild insomnia who took 450 milligrams of valerian before bedtime experienced a significant decrease in sleep problems.[2] The same researchers studied 128 individuals and found that compared with the placebo, 400 milligrams of valerian produced a significant improvement in sleep quality in people who considered themselves poor sleepers.[3]

Unlike commonly prescribed sleeping pills, valerian does not lead to dependency or addiction. Nor does it produce a morning drug hangover.

Valerian Supplements

Buy a product standardized to contain 0.5 percent essential oils or 0.8 percent valerenic acid. Take 400 to 900 milligrams in capsule or tablet form, 30 minutes to one hour before bedtime. For tinctures (1:5), take 1 to 3 milliliters (15 to 20 drops) in water several times per day, or try 5 milliliters before bedtime. The herb works best when used over a period of time.

Do not take valerian with alcohol or sedative medications. The herb is not recommended for use during pregnancy and breastfeeding.

8

———❦———

More Natural Health Products

Alpha-Lipoic Acid (Lipoic Acid)

Used for diabetes (see page 263)

Lipoic acid is a sulfur-containing fatty acid found in liver, yeast and, to a lesser extent, spinach, broccoli, potatoes and kidney. There is no dietary requirement for lipoic acid as the body is able to make its supply. However, supplements are necessary to achieve the amounts of lipoic acid used in clinical studies. Lipoic acid was first identified and isolated from food in 1950. Since then, it has been actively studied for its potential to help control blood-sugar levels and complications of diabetes.

Lipoic acid helps enzymes turn the carbohydrate we eat into a useable source of energy for the body. It is needed by cells to generate ATP (adenosine triphosphate), energy molecules used in all cellular reactions. Lipoic acid is also an antioxidant, able to neutralize free radicals, compounds naturally produced by the body that, if produced in excess, damage many types of body cells. Unlike other well-known antioxidants, such as vitamins C and E, lipoic acid works in both a water and fat environment, which allows it to have a broad effect. Because of antioxidant effects in fat tissue, lipoic acid is able to enter nerve cells, where it may offer protection. In addition, the body uses lipoic acid to regenerate vitamins C and E.

European studies have found intravenous injections of lipoic acid effective in improving symptoms of diabetes neuropathy (nerve damage caused by high blood-sugar levels), including pain, tingling and numbness of the arms and legs. Oral supplements of lipoic acid have been shown to help lessen the nerve damage caused by diabetes.[1-3] One study of people with diabetes suggests that lipoic acid supplements can also help reduce nerve damage caused to the body's internal organs. Two studies also found that when lipoic acid was combined with gamma-linoleic acid (GLA), it offered some relief for this conditiondiabetic nerve damage.[4,5] Lipoic acid also seems to help type 2 diabetics control their blood-sugar level. A few studies have found lipoic acid supplements improve insulin sensitivity and glucose clearance from the bloodstream after four weeks of treatment.[6]

Alpha-Lipoic Acid Supplements

For diabetes, take 600 milligrams three times daily on an empty stomach. For antioxidant protection, take 20 to 50 milligrams once daily on an empty stomach.

Lipoic acid supplements appear to have no significant side effects. On rare occasions, it may cause a skin rash. Some evidence suggests that high doses of lipoic acid may cause thiamine (vitamin B1) deficiency. Individuals at risk for thiamine deficiency (e.g., those with alcoholism) should consider supplementing with a B complex formula or a high-potency multivitamin and mineral pill.

If you have diabetes and you take lipoic acid, be sure to closely monitor your blood-sugar levels. Because of its potential to lower blood glucose, lipoic acid could have additive effects when taken together with diabetes medications, ginseng, garlic or psyllium.

Chondroitin Sulfate

Used for osteoarthritis (see page 447)
Chondroitin sulfate belongs to the glucosaminoglycan family of compounds. These compounds are a normal part of cartilage—a tough, elastic tissue in joints that covers the ends of bones, tendons and ligaments. Cartilage allows bones to glide smoothly over one another when they move. In osteoarthritis, the cartilage breaks down and disintegrates, the bones rub painfully against each other and movement is restricted.

Chondroitin sulfate supplements appear to have anti-inflammatory properties. Studies show that supplemental chondroitin sulfate can reduce the painful symptoms of hip and knee osteoarthritis.[1-6] When taken with pain relievers and compared with nonsteroidal anti-inflammatory drugs (NSAIDs), chondroitin sulfate is significantly better at reducing pain and improving walking ability than the medication alone. Some studies have found that people taking the supplement are able to reduce their dose of medication.

Scientists believe that chondroitin supplementation can slow the progression of this "wear and tear" disease. When researchers looked at the effects of chondroitin in people with osteoarthritis, they found that those using chondroitin experienced less joint damage over time compared with those not taking the supplement. Taking supplemental chondroitin may offer joints the building blocks they need to repair cartilage. Some experts believe that chondroitin increases the amount of hyaluronic acid in the joints. (Hyaluronic acid is the fluid that keeps the joints lubricated.) Chondroitin may also inhibit enzymes that break down cartilage.

Chondroitin Sulfate Supplements

Although some studies have seen favorable results with 1200 milligrams taken once daily, the normal typical dose for chondroitin sulfate supplements is 400 milligrams three times daily. Chondroitin sulfate and glucosamine sulfate are frequently sold together in combination products, but there is no evidence from studies on humans that this combination works better than either product alone. It may take two to four months of treatment to notice significant improvement in osteoarthritis symptoms.

Occasionally, chondroitin supplements may cause stomach upset and nausea. No serious side effects have been reported. There is a potential for allergic reaction in some individuals from chondroitin supplements made from animal sources.

Beware of chondroitin and glucosamine combination products that also contain manganese. When taken according to the manufacturer's directions, these products can sometimes supply greater than the tolerable upper limit for manganese of 11 milligrams per day. Consuming more than this amount of manganese might cause toxic effects to the central nervous system.

The potential risk of transmission of bovine spongiform encephalopathy (BSE, or mad cow disease) is raising people's concerns about products containing chondroitin, which is produced from bovine trachea. Although bovine trachea tissue does not seem to carry a high risk of BSE infection, in some cases, manufacturing methods might lead to contamination with diseased animal tissues. So far there are no reports of BSE or other disease transmission to humans from dietary supplements containing animal materials, and the risk of potential disease transmission is thought to be quite low. If you are concerned, call the manufacturer and ask what steps are being taken to ensure that its chondroitin is not contaminated.

Coenzyme Q10

Used for congestive heart failure (see page 238), angina (see page 165)

Coenzyme Q10 (CoQ10) is found in virtually all plant and animal cells. The human body manufactures CoQ10, so there is no official dietary requirement. CoQ10 works with many different enzymes in the body and, as such, is needed for many important metabolic reactions. One very important function of CoQ10 is the production of the body's energy compounds, ATP (adenosine triphosphate).

The compound was first identified in 1957 by researchers at the University of Wisconsin. In the 1960s, Japanese scientists began studying its health benefits. Today, CoQ10 is widely used in Japan, Europe and Russia. In fact, the Japanese government approved the use of CoQ10 for the treatment of congestive heart failure in 1974.

CoQ10 levels in the body decline with age and stress. Some medications can also interfere with the body's production of CoQ10 or may hamper its action. Studies have shown that CoQ10 levels are much lower in the heart cells of people with congestive heart failure than they are in healthy people. Many clinical trials have shown that CoQ10 supplements (along with medication) improve the quality of life of patients with congestive heart failure.[1-4] Supplementation with CoQ10 can decrease hospitalization and significantly decrease many of the symptoms associated with the condition.

CoQ10 also acts as an antioxidant, neutralizing free radicals before they cause harm. (See Chapter 5 for more on antioxidants and free radicals.) In the liver, CoQ10 is packaged into LDL cholesterol molecules and then transported on LDLs to other parts of the body. As part of the LDL molecule, CoQ10 is able to prevent damage to LDL cholesterol and may help reduce the risk of heart disease.[5,6] CoQ10 also prolongs the effects of vitamin E, another powerful antioxidant.

Cholesterol-lowering medications such as lovastatin (Mevacor®), simvastatin (Zocor®), pravastatin (Pravachol®) and cerivastatin (Baycol™) have been shown to reduce blood levels of CoQ10.[7-9] Whether this affects heart health is not yet known, but it may be wise to take CoQ10 supplements if you are on these drugs.

CoQ10 Supplements

CoQ10 supplements are made by fermenting beets and sugar cane with special strains of yeast. Buy a CoQ10 supplement in an oil base (instead of dry-powder tablets or capsules) as this is more available to the body.[10] For congestive heart failure, take 50 milligrams twice daily. For angina, take 50 milligrams three times a day.

CoQ10 supplements are very safe; no significant side effects have been reported. However, when taken in daily doses of 300 milligrams or more, CoQ10 can interfere with liver enzyme blood tests. Studies suggest that CoQ10 supplements might interfere with blood-sugar levels in people with diabetes.[11-13] The supplement may also interfere with the blood-thinning effects of warfarin (Coumadin®).[14,15] If you are taking this medication, don't take CoQ10 unless monitored by your doctor.

Conjugated Linoleic Acid (CLA)

Used for weight loss (see page 439)
Conjugated linoleic acid (CLA) is a naturally occurring fatty acid found in dairy products and red meat. It's also found in pork and chicken though in lesser amounts. It's estimated that nonvegetarians consume about 1 gram of CLA each day. Since the body does not manufacture CLA, the only way to get it is through foods or supplements. But because there is no evidence that CLA is essential to our body, no official daily recommended intake has been established.

The health benefits of CLA have been studied for some time. Research on animals and experiments using human breast cancer cells suggest that CLA may be protective from breast cancer.[1-4] CLA is also an antioxidant: it can protect cells from damage caused by free radicals and therefore may help ward off heart disease by keeping cholesterol levels in check. Recently, however, studies are indicating that CLA supplements may play a role in weight control.[5-8] CLA is thought to facilitate weight loss by inhibiting the action of lipoprotein lipase, an enzyme that breaks down dietary fat so it can be absorbed by the body. CLA is also believed to increase the activity of the enzyme responsible for breaking down body fat stores.

Two studies presented at the Research Conference of the American Chemical Society (August 2000) found that CLA supplements helped people lose weight and keep the extra pounds off. In one of the studies, Norwegian researchers studied 60 overweight people.[9] Half were given CLA and the others took a placebo pill. After three months, the CLA users lost more weight than those in the placebo group. A second study from the University of Wisconsin followed 80 overweight people for six months.[10] Subjects received either daily CLA supplements or a placebo pill. All subjects dieted and exercised, and most lost weight. After the study was finished, the people who were not taking the CLA regained weight in the typical pattern: 75 percent of their weight gain was fat. But the people in the CLA group put weight back on very differently: only half as fat, the other half as muscle. In both studies, participants were given 3 grams of CLA per day, an amount that is usually not accessible from your diet alone.

CLA Supplements

Because of its emerging role as a weight loss aid, CLA supplements are now easy to find in health food stores and pharmacies. Buy a high-quality supplement that's made with Tonalin® CLA or Clarinol®. These are manufactured under high-quality standards and have been used in clinical research. Take 1 gram (1000 milligrams) three times a day with meals.

CLA supplements may cause mild stomach upset in some people. Studies using CLA supplements have lasted no longer than six months, so effects of longer-term use are still unknown.

DHEA (Dehydroepiandrosterone)

Used for impotence (erectile dysfunction) (see page 373), adrenal insufficiency in women, lupus (see page 415)

DHEA (dehydroepiandrosterone) is a hormone produced by the adrenal glands, two small triangular-shaped glands that sit above the kidneys. DHEA levels are higher in men than they are in women, and they naturally decline with age: by the age of 60, we produce 5 to 15 percent of what we did when we were 20. Some experts attribute this decline in DHEA to the aging process, although this remains to be proven.

Once your adrenal glands secrete DHEA, it's used as a building block to make estrogen and testosterone. DHEA supplementation seems to change circulating levels of estrogen and progesterone. In men, DHEA supplements appear to increase estrogens, but not the male sex hormones. In women, the opposite is true: DHEA increases blood levels of androgens, but not estrogens. The effect of DHEA on circulating hormone levels may be responsible for its health benefits.

Researchers have found that compared to healthy volunteers, DHEA levels are lower in men with erectile dysfunction.[1] One study involving 40 men with erectile dysfunction revealed that a daily 50 milligram supplement of DHEA taken for six months was associated with improved sexual performance.[2]

Failure of the adrenal glands can occur because of an illness or surgical removal of the glands. People with adrenal failure are given medications that provide the body with the hormones the adrenal glands are no longer producing. Studies show that when DHEA supplements are taken along with standard medications, women with adrenal failure report increased energy, libido and feelings of well-being.[3,4] Keep in mind that adrenal failure is not the same as "tired adrenal glands," a condition often diagnosed by natural health practitioners. DHEA supplements are not warranted for so-called adrenal weakness.

A number of studies have shown DHEA supplements improve symptoms of lupus, an autoimmune disease that affects mostly women in their childbearing years.[5-11] DHEA may be helpful in easing symptoms of fatigue and sore joints. It may also reduce flare-ups of the disease.

DHEA Supplements

DHEA supplements consist of a hormone manufactured from compounds found in soybeans. It is sold as a dietary supplement in the United States but is not allowed for sale in Canada.

For impotence, take 50 milligrams per day. For adrenal failure, take 50 milligrams per day. For lupus, take 200 milligrams per day as an adjunct to conventional medication.

Short-term use of DHEA is considered safe. Long-term use in amounts that raise DHEA levels above normal might increase the risk of prostate cancer. Even at low doses, side effects can occur. DHEA has been shown to lower the level of good HDL cholesterol as well as cause acne and hair loss. DHEA may also increase or decrease your body's sensitivity to insulin, the hormone that regulates your blood sugar.[12] If you have diabetes, be sure to have your doctor closely monitor your blood-glucose levels.

Because DHEA is converted to estrogen and testosterone, women with an estrogen-sensitive disease (breast cancer, uterine cancer, endometriosis) should avoid using this supplement.

Fish Oils

Used for high blood cholesterol (see page 327) and high blood triglycerides, high blood pressure (see page 328), Crohn's disease and ulcerative colitis (see inflammatory bowel disease, page 385), attention deficit hyperactivity disorder (see page 173), clinical depression (see page 252), rheumatoid arthritis (see page 502), lupus (see page 415), psoriasis (see page 498)

Fish oils contain two omega-3 fatty acids: DHA (docosahexanaenoic acid) and EPA (eicosapentanoic acid). As you learned from reading Chapter 3, the body makes these two fatty acids from foods rich in alpha-linolenic acid, an essential fat found in flaxseed oil, canola oil, walnuts, soybeans, whole grains and leafy greens. You can also get DHA directly by eating oily fish.

The body needs fatty acids to make eicosanoids, a family of powerful compounds, including prostaglandins, prostacyclins, thromboxanes and leukotrienes, that regulate our blood, immune system and hormones. Omega-3 fatty acids like DHA and EPA are used to make friendly eicosanoids that reduce inflammation and blood clotting and are believed to offer a number of other health benefits. Animal fats and omega-6 fatty acids (found in corn, sunflower and safflower oils) are used to make inflammatory eicosanoids, compounds that have been linked to a number of ill-health effects.

Omega-3 and omega-6 fats compete with each other in the body. Many experts believe that it's important to eat several times more omega-3 fats than omega-6 fats so that healthy eicosanoids are formed. However, by some estimates, the typical North American diet provides 20 times more omega-6s than omega-3s. Although there is no official daily dietary requirement for omega-3 fats, many experts fear that, as we gobble up low-fat and fat-free foods, we are not getting enough of these important compounds. Fish oil supplements are one way to help balance your fat intake in favor of omega-3 fatty acids.

Fish oils may help lower the risk of heart disease in a number of ways. Studies find they can lower blood triglyceride levels by 20 to 50 percent.[1-4] They have also been found to decrease cholesterol absorption in the intestine and hamper the liver's ability to produce cholesterol.[5,6] In this way, fish oil supplements may help lower high blood cholesterol levels. Fish oils might even raise good HDL cholesterol levels. Fish oils also have a blood-thinning effect and may prevent blood clots that lead to heart attack and stroke. Studies conducted of people with mild hypertension have found that supplementation with fish oils provided a modest reduction in blood pressure.[7-9]

Omega-3 fats are important components of nerve and brain cell membranes, where they help cells communicate messages effectively. Omega-3 fats may also be crucial for the formation of brain hormones that help stabilize mood. Scientists have found that people with major depression have lower levels of omega-3 fats in their body.[10,11] Studies are beginning to suggest that fish oils might be useful in the treatment of manic-depressive illness.[12] As well, attention deficit hyperactivity disorder is thought to be linked with a deficiency of omega-3 fats.[13] Omega-3 fats are necessary for proper brain development and function in growing children.

By helping the body form friendly prostaglandins, DHA and EPA have anti-inflammatory effects. It is this effect that is thought to be responsible for their ability to help relieve joint pain, soreness and stiffness associated with rheumatoid arthritis and lupus. Studies have found that levels of these two fatty acids are lower in people with rheumatoid arthritis.[14] Studies show that when used in people with rheumatoid arthritis, fish oil supplements relieve morning stiffness and allow people to reduce their dose of nonsteroidal anti-inflammatory drugs (NSAIDs).[15-18]

The anti-inflammatory effects of fish oils are believed to help reduce symptoms and flare-ups of Crohn's disease and ulcerative colitis, conditions in which parts of the digestive tract are severely inflamed.[19-24] Studies have also found fish oils to reduce the severity of itching, redness and scaling in chronic psoriasis.[25,26]

Fish Oil Supplements

Buy a product with a combination of EPA and DHA (fish oil supplements vary considerably in the amount and ratio of DHA and EPA). Look for a supplement that has vitamin E added as it helps prevent the oils from going rancid. Avoid fish *liver* oil capsules. Fish liver oil is a concentrated source of vitamins A and D, which can be toxic when taken in large amounts for long periods.

The typical dosage is 2 to 9 grams of fish oil per day, often taken in divided doses. Check the product label to see how much each capsule provides (many products provide 500 milligrams of fish oil per capsule). In most clinical studies, participants took enough fish oil capsules to provide a minimum of 1800 milligrams of EPA and 900 milligrams of DHA.

Fish oil supplements can cause belching and a fishy taste. High doses can cause nausea and diarrhea. Because fish oil has a blood-thinning effect, use caution if you are taking blood-thinning medication such as aspirin, warfarin (Coumadin®) or heparin. If you take these drugs, consult your physician before taking fish oil supplements.

Glucosamine Sulfate

Used for osteoarthritis (see page 447)
The body uses glucosamine to make a family of compounds called mucopolysaccharides. These compounds are a normal part of cartilage—a tough, elastic tissue found in joints that covers the ends of bones, tendons and ligaments. Cartilage allows bones to glide smoothly over one another when they move. In osteoarthritis, the cartilage breaks down and disintegrates, the bones rub painfully against each other and movement is restricted.

Foods do not directly supply glucosamine. Instead, your body makes this compound from glucose found in foods. Studies show that glucosamine stimulates the production of glycosaminoglycons, important compounds of cartilage in your joints. Research suggests that glucosamine supplements stop and possibly even reverse this degenerative disease of the joints.

Findings from studies lasting from four weeks to three years have found that glucosamine significantly improved pain and mobility in people with osteoarthritis of the knee.[1-6] Some studies have found the supplement to be as effective as ibuprofen and piroxicam (Feldene®), two nonsteroidal anti-inflammatory drugs used to manage osteoarthritis.[7] Whereas conventional medications appear to take two weeks to improve symptoms, glucosamine takes four weeks to have an effect. In one study, glucosamine was superior to ibuprofen after eight weeks of use.

Glucosamine Supplements

Glucosamine supplements are made from chitin, a substance found in shrimp, lobsters and crab or produced synthetically. They are available in various forms, such as glucosamine sulfate, glucosamine hydrochloride and N-acetyl glucosamine. Glucosamine sulfate is the preferred form, since it has been used in most of the research. Some experts also believe it is the most stable form of glucosamine.

Take 500 milligrams three times daily. One three-year study found that 1500 milligrams taken once daily was effective.

No serious side effects have been reported. Glucosamine supplements may cause nausea, heartburn, diarrhea or constipation. It is possible that glucosamine might exacerbate diabetes by decreasing the body's sensitivity to insulin.[8-10] Until more research is done, people with diabetes should closely monitor their blood-sugar levels if taking glucosamine supplements.

There is concern that glucosamine supplements made from shellfish may cause allergic reactions in people with a shellfish allergy. If you have such an allergy, contact the manufacturer to determine the source of the glucosamine (this information is not always on the label).

Grapeseed Extract

Used for heart disease prevention (see page 327), chronic venous insufficiency (intermittent claudication), varicose veins (see page 529), hemorrhoids (see page 336)

Grapeseed extract is most often derived as a byproduct of wine manufacturing. Grapeseed is a rich source of anthocyanins, naturally occurring compounds also found in red wine, tea leaves, blueberries, cranberries, black currants and bilberry (see page 97, Chapter 7). In Europe, grapeseed extract is widely used to treat conditions related to fragile blood capillaries. It is also used to help reduce the risk of heart disease.

Anthocyanins are thought to keep blood vessels healthy by inhibiting the action of enzymes that break down connective tissue. A handful of studies have found that a daily supplement of grapeseed extract can significantly reduce symptoms of peripheral venous insufficiency, including leg pain and swelling.[1-6]

The heart-protective effects of grapeseed extract are inferred from the antioxidant powers of anthocyanins. While no study has looked at whether grapeseed extract can ward off heart attack, studies in the laboratory show that anthocyanins can prevent free radical damage to LDL cholesterol.[7,8] One study found grapeseed anthocyanins to be superior to vitamins C and E in their antioxidant capacity. Anthocyanins may also help reduce blood clots.[9,10]

Grapeseed Extract Supplements

For venous insufficiency, take 150 to 300 milligrams per day. Some experts recommend taking 150 to 300 milligrams for three weeks, followed by a maintenance dose of 40 to 80 milligrams daily. For a general antioxidant effect, take 50 milligrams once daily.

Grapeseed extract is considered extremely safe: no adverse effects are known.

A supplement with the same effects as grapeseed extract and which can be used to prevent or treat the same conditions is pycnogenol. Rich in anthocyanins, Pycnogenol™ is the US-registered trademark for an extract made from the bark of pine trees. However, it is more expensive than grapeseed extract. The usual dose is 50 milligrams once daily.

Inositol

Used for depression (see page 252), panic disorder, polycystic ovary syndrome (see page 475)
Although not recognized as a vitamin, inositol is closely related to the B vitamin family (see Chapter 4). It is found in foods mainly as phytic acid, a fibrous compound. Our diet provides approximately 1000 milligrams of inositol each day, mainly from citrus fruits, whole grains, legumes, nuts and seeds. When you eat these foods, bacteria in your intestine liberate inositol from phytic acid.

Once in the body, inositol is an essential component of cell membranes. It promotes the export of fat from cells in the liver and intestine. Inositol is also abundant in the central nervous system and contributes to the healthy functioning of nerves and muscles.

Researchers think that inositol might improve the sensitivity of serotonin receptors in the brain. Serotonin is a natural brain chemical that's associated with feelings of happiness, calmness and relaxation. Some evidence suggests that inositol may have benefits similar to serotonin-reuptake inhibitor drugs (Prozac®, Effexor®, Paxil®, Zoloft®, Serzone®) in conditions such as panic disorder and depression.[1]

One small study found that, compared to placebo treatment, daily inositol supplementation significantly improved depressive symptoms based on the Hamilton Depression Rating Score.[2] When the researchers followed up with these patients after the study, they found a rapid relapse in symptoms once inositol was discontinued.[3]

Inositol is thought to improve insulin sensitivity and has therefore been used to treat symptoms of polycystic ovary syndrome (PCOS). One study found that inositol taken once daily for six weeks decreased blood triglycerides and testosterone levels, reduced blood pressure and caused ovulation in obese women with PCOS.[4] Previous studies have suggested that people with insulin resistance and type 2 diabetes might be deficient in inositol.

Inositol Supplements

Inositol supplements may be difficult to find as few companies manufacture them. In Canada, the following products are available:

- Swiss Natural Sources® inositol, 250 milligrams per tablet
- NuLife® inositol powder, 550 milligrams per 1/4 teaspoon (mix into water)
- Seroyal® inositol (a Genestra® brand), 300 milligrams per capsule (each also contains 100 micrograms of chromium picinolate)

For depression and anxiety, take 12 grams per day. For polycystic ovary syndrome, buy D-chiro-inositol; take 12 milligrams per day.

No adverse effects have been reported from taking inositol supplements; however, no long-term studies have been conducted. Because the recommended dosage of inositol is high (grams), be sure to buy a product made by a reputable manufacturer. There is a greater risk for ill effects from contaminants when taking products in large doses, even if the contaminant is present in small amounts.

Lecithin (Phosphatidylcholine)

Used for liver disease (alcoholic fatty liver, alcoholic hepatitis, cirrhosis [see page 222], viral hepatitis), Alzheimer's disease (see page 155), manic depression (bipolar disorder illness) (see depression, page 252), Tourette syndrome, tardive dyskinesia

Lecithin is a natural substance consisting of phosphatidylcholine, fatty acids and carbohydrate. Phosphatidylcholine supplies the body with choline, an essential nutrient belonging to the B vitamin family (see Chapter 4). Choline is also found in foods; egg yolks, liver, soybeans, legumes, oatmeal and cabbage are good sources.

For years, lecithin supplements have been promoted to lower cholesterol levels. However, there are no well-controlled studies to support this claim. One small double-blind study found that lecithin had no effect on blood cholesterol levels.[1]

Lecithin and phosphatidylcholine supplements are thought to exert their health benefits by supplying the body with choline. Once ingested, choline becomes incorporated into the membranes of cells. In the body, choline donates a part of itself, a methyl group, to surrounding body tissues, especially the brain. Choline also acts as a building block for acetylcholine, a brain chemical involved in memory. Researchers believe that choline supplements will improve brain tasks only if you're deficient in the nutrient. (Stress and aging can deplete choline levels.) Although the evidence is preliminary at best (and conflicting), phosphatidylcholine supplements may be useful in treating Alzheimer's disease, manic depression, Tourette syndrome and tardive dyskinesia, a disorder of the nervous system.[2-8]

Phosphatidylcholine supplements are used by European physicians to treat a number of liver disorders. Some studies have shown benefit and others have not.[9-13]

Despite the popularity of lecithin, very few studies support its effectiveness in the treatment of any of the above conditions.

Lecithin Supplements

Most lecithin supplements are manufactured from soybeans and contain between 10 and 20 percent phosphatidylcholine. Others, however, are almost pure phosphatidylcholine and will be labeled as such. Most clinical studies have been done with phosphatidylcholine supplements, and I recommend that you choose a supplement labeled phosphatidylcholine. A typical dose is 1200 to 2220 milligrams per day, taken in divided doses.

Lecithin is considered to be very safe. Lecithin and phosphatidylcholine supplements may cause diarrhea, nausea, stomach upset and a feeling of fullness in some people. Unlike choline supplements, lecithin taken orally does not cause a fishy odor.

Lutein

Used for age-related macular degeneration (see page 420), cataracts (see page 203)
Lutein, Latin for "egg yolk" and "yellow," is a member of the carotenoid family, a group of chemicals found in dark green and orange vegetables. The best dietary sources of lutein include corn, egg yolks, spinach, kiwi, grapes, orange juice, zucchini, squash, broccoli, collard greens, kale and Swiss chard. Although lutein is not considered an essential nutrient, scientists are learning that this natural chemical may be very important to eye health.

High dietary intakes of lutein are associated with up to a 40 percent lower risk of age-related macular degeneration, the leading cause of blindness in adults over 65. Most cases of macular degeneration are dry macular degeneration, a condition that occurs when the tissues in the eye, called the macula, gradually thin out. Lutein is concentrated in the macula of the eye, the small part of the retina that's responsible for fine, detailed vision. In the macula, lutein acts as a filter, protecting structures of the eye from the damaging effects of the sun's ultraviolet (UV) light. Lutein contributes to the density, or thickness, of the macula. The denser the macula, the better they can absorb incoming light.

A handful of studies have shown that adding lutein-rich foods or a lutein supplement to your daily diet can increase the density of the macula.[1-7] In fact, researchers have noted significant increases in macular density within as little as three months.

In one study from the Veterans Administration Medical Center in Chicago, lutein in the form of 1/2 cup (125 ml) of sautéed spinach or a supplement, taken four to seven times per week, improved visual function in men with age-related macular degeneration.

Lutein also acts as an antioxidant, protecting the retina from oxidative damage caused by UV light. UV light can also lead to the development of cataracts, a disease in which the lens of the eye becomes yellow, making vision cloudy and blurry. Two large studies from Harvard University found that men and women with the highest intakes of lutein had a 20 percent lower risk of cataract compared with those who consumed the least.[8,9] Broccoli, spinach and kale were the foods most often associated with protection.

There's some evidence to suggest that lutein may also help protect from breast and colon cancer. Both low intakes and low blood levels of lutein are linked with a higher risk of these cancers. Studies have shown that a lutein extract from marigold flowers can halt the growth of cancer cells in animals.

Lutein Supplements

According to researchers, a daily lutein intake of 6 to 10 milligrams, the equivalent of five to seven servings of vegetables and fruit, can protect the eye. Choose a supplement made with FloraGlo™, a high-quality lutein extract made from marigold petals that's been used in clinical studies. Take 6 to 10 milligrams once daily with food. Lutein is best absorbed when consumed with fat in a meal. No adverse reactions or drug interactions have been reported.

Lycopene

Used for prostate cancer prevention (see page 488), cataracts (see page 203), age-related macular degeneration (see page 420), cervical dysplasia (see page 211)
Lycopene, belonging to the same family of carotenoid compounds as beta-carotene, is found in red-colored fruits and vegetables. It's the natural chemical that gives these foods their bright color. Tomatoes are the richest source of lycopene, but you'll also find some in pink grapefruit, watermelon, guava and apricots. There is no daily recommended intake for lycopene as it is not an essential nutrient.

Lycopene is an antioxidant, a compound that defends the body from free radical damage. Free radicals, toxic byproducts formed in the body from oxygen, can destroy the genetic material of cells, which in turn may lead to cancer development. Compared with its cousin beta-carotene, lycopene is twice as potent an antioxidant.[1,2]

A famous study from Harvard University followed 47,000 men for four years.[3] The investigators found that those men who consumed ten or more weekly servings of tomato-based foods had a 35 percent lower risk of prostate cancer compared with men who ate one or less weekly servings. Many studies have determined that low blood and tissue lycopene levels are linked with higher rates of prostate cancer.[4-6] Lycopene stores can be raised by eating foods rich in the antioxidant or by taking lycopene supplements.[7]

Researchers are also investigating lycopene's potential role as a treatment for prostate cancer. One study from the Karmanos Cancer Center Institute in Detroit found that 30 milligrams of supplemental lycopene given to men with prostate cancer was associated with smaller prostate tumors at the time of surgery.

Lycopene's ability to fight off free radicals may make it useful in the prevention of cataract and macular degeneration. Free radical damage from ultraviolet light, cigarette smoke and environmental pollution contribute to the development of these two eye diseases. To date there is some (although weak) evidence to suggest that lycopene might reduce the risk of both.[8]

A handful of studies have suggested that consuming foods rich in lycopene protects women from cervical dysplasia, a condition in which cells lining the surface of the cervix grow abnormally. One study from the University of Pennsylvania School of Medicine found that women with the highest intake of lycopene were one-third as likely to have dysplasia compared with those who consumed the least.[9]

Lycopene Supplements

Choose a supplement that's made with the Lyc-O-Mato™ or LycoRed™ extract. This source of lycopene comes from Israel and is derived from whole tomatoes. It's also the extract that has been used in clinical studies. Take 5 to 10 milligrams (usually this is one tablet or capsule) once daily with a meal.

Absorption of lycopene is enhanced by the presence of some dietary fat. Some experts recommend taking a supplement that combines lycopene with beta-carotene, since beta-carotene appears to increase lycopene absorption. Lycopene is considered very safe. No adverse reactions or serious side effects have been reported.

Lysine

Used for herpes simplex virus (cold sores, genital herpes) (see page 344)
Lysine is an essential amino acid, a building block of protein foods that the body must get from the diet. Lysine is found in animal protein foods, including meat,

poultry, dairy products and eggs. It's also found in dried peas, beans and lentils. It's estimated that the body needs about 1 gram (1000 milligrams) each day for good health. The body uses lysine to form collagen, a fibrous protein that holds together various structures in the body.

Studies in the lab show that lysine inhibits the growth of the herpes simplex virus.[1] Lysine seems to block the action of arginine, an amino acid the virus needs in order to replicate.

Herpes simplex remains dormant in nerve cells until periods of stress, when the virus can reappear, causing symptoms such as cold sores or genital sores. Studies lasting six months to one year found that supplemental lysine reduced the number of herpes flare-ups.[2-7] Lysine also lessened the severity of symptoms during a herpes attack and sped the rate of healing.

Lysine Supplements

Take 1000 milligrams three times daily. (Although one study found effects with 1000 milligrams taken only once daily.) Taking lysine with a calcium supplement may increase calcium absorption and prevent calcium loss in the urine.[8]

High daily doses (10 grams per day) of lysine may cause diarrhea, stomach pain, gallstones and elevated cholesterol levels. If you have gallbladder disease or high blood cholesterol, use caution when taking concentrated lysine supplements.

Melatonin

Used for insomnia (see page 390), jet lag

Melatonin is a hormone produced in the body's pineal gland, a tiny gland located in the brain. Melatonin regulates the body's wake-sleep cycles. Its release from the brain is stimulated by darkness: the darker the room, the more melatonin your body produces. The hormone induces sleep by interacting with melatonin receptors in the brain. Once into the bloodstream, melatonin lowers body temperature, alertness and performance. Contrary to popular belief, melatonin production does not appear to decline as we age.

However, studies have found decreased melatonin production in people suffering from insomnia.[1] Supplemental melatonin has been shown to produce rapid sleep-inducing effects without a hangover effect the next day.[2-9] Most of the research has found that melatonin supplements help elderly people with insomnia. The effect on younger people is unclear. Melatonin may also be helpful to people who are trying to discontinue prescription sleeping aids.

Research also suggests that melatonin is useful in preventing jet lag, especially when many time zones are crossed. A number of studies have determined that people who take melatonin before and during plane travel sleep better, take less time to fall asleep and wake up feeling more energetic afterward.[10-14] Whether melatonin supplements can help shift workers adjust to a new schedule is less clear.

Melatonin Supplements

These supplements are not natural health products; rather, they are hormones produced from the pineal gland of animals or synthetically in the lab. In Canada, melatonin supplements are not legally available. Melatonin is available by prescription from a doctor.

In the United States, melatonin supplements are available in quick-release and slow-release forms. Some experts believe that the quick-release form helps people fall asleep faster whereas slow-release helps people stay asleep.

For insomnia, take 0.3 to 0.5 milligrams 30 minutes before bed. For jet lag, take 5 milligrams before bed for one week, starting three days before travel.

Melatonin supplements can cause headache, depressed mood, daytime fatigue and drowsiness and stomach upset in some people. Do not drive or operate machinery for five hours after taking melatonin. People with depression should avoid this supplement as it can worsen symptoms.[15] Since melatonin is metabolized in the liver, people with liver disease should avoid using it.

The potential risk of transmission of bovine spongiform encephalopathy (BSE, or mad cow disease) is raising concerns about products containing melatonin, since melatonin is sometimes made from the pineal gland of animals. However, some melatonin products are made synthetically and are free of this potential risk. If the product label does not state the source of melatonin, ask the manufacturer. If animal products are used, ask what steps are being taken to ensure that the supplement is BSE-free.

Long-term use of melatonin supplements should be avoided. Studies have been brief in duration and long-term safety has not been evaluated. Because melatonin is a hormone, its effects, if any, may take years to develop.

Phosphatidlyserine

Used for Alzheimer's disease (see page 155), dementia, age-related memory impairment
Phosphatidylserine belongs to a family of chemical compounds known as phospholipids. Phospholipids are components of cell membranes and are essential to

their healthy functioning. Phospholipids derived from phosphatidylserine give cell membranes structural integrity. Phospholipids also regulate the nutrients and waste products that pass in and out of cells.

Phosphatidylserine is not an essential nutrient. A very tiny amount is found in foods. The body manufactures its own phosphatidylserine from other phospholipid building blocks. The only way to get the amounts of phosphatidylserine used in clinical studies is to take a supplement.

Phosphatidylserine is routinely used in European countries to help preserve mental function in patients with Alzheimer's disease and dementia. A number of studies that have lasted up to six months have shown that supplements of phosphatidylserine slow the progression of Alzheimer's disease.[1-4] Compared with patients taking placebo pills, phosphatidylserine users do significantly better on tests of cognitive function. These supplements also seem to help ease feelings of depression in people with Alzheimer's disease.

Memory loss is a normal part of the aging process. One study found that people with ordinary memory loss not caused by dementia benefited from phosphatidylserine.[5] Those with the greatest memory impairment had the most improvement.

Phosphatidylserine Supplements

Phosphatidylserine supplements are made from soybeans. Take 100 milligrams three times daily.

Phosphatidylserine is considered safe when used for up to six months (longer studies have not been conducted). The supplement may cause gastrointestinal upset in some individuals. Phosphatidylserine has a slight blood-thinning effect. If you are taking other supplements that have a similar effect (vitamin E, ginkgo biloba, garlic), be sure to inform your doctor so that he or she can monitor your blood. Phosphatidylserine is thought to enhance the effects of heparin, a prescription blood thinner.[6]

Probiotics (Lactic Acid Bacteria)

Used for diarrhea (see page 271), vaginal yeast infections and candidiasis (see page 195), irritable bowel syndrome (see page 399)
The term probiotic means "to promote life" and refers to living organisms that, upon ingestion in certain numbers, improve microbial balance in the intestine and exert health benefits. Such friendly bacteria are known collectively as lactic acid bacteria and

include L. acidophilus, L. bulgaricus, L. casei, S. thermophilus and bifidobacteria. These are often called "friendly" bacteria.

The human digestive tract contains hundreds of strains of bacteria, making up what is called the normal intestinal flora. Among the intestinal flora are the lactic acid bacteria, which inhibit the growth of unfriendly, or disease-causing, bacteria by preventing their attachment to the intestine. Lactic acid bacteria also produce lactic acid and hydrogen peroxide, substances that suppresses harmful bacteria and yeast.

Lactic acid bacteria are found in fermented milk products such as yogurt, kefir and acidophilus milk. But many natural health experts believe that taking a high-quality supplement is the only way to ensure that a sufficient number of friendly bacteria reaches the intestinal tract. Plenty of studies have shown that consuming probiotic foods or supplements increases the number of lactic acid bacteria in the intestinal tract and can exert a number of health benefits.

Several well-controlled clinical studies have shown that lactic acid bacteria, when taken as a supplement or as yogurt, speed recovery from diarrhea in children and adults. Bifidobacteria, L. acidophilus and L. casei have been shown to be particularly helpful in reducing diarrhea associated with antibiotic treatment.[1-4] (Antibiotics kill not only disease-causing organisms but also helpful lactic acid bacteria.) Probiotic supplements have also been found to help treat viral diarrhea and traveler's diarrhea (diarrhea caused by eating contaminated foods).[5-11]

Lactic acid bacteria can inhibit the growth of Candida albicans, a yeast organism responsible for vaginal yeast infections.[12] One American study found that women who consumed one cup (250 ml) of L. acidophilus yogurt each day for six months had a threefold decrease in Candida infections compared with women who did not eat yogurt.[13] Another study found that taking the probiotic supplement Kyo-Dophilus® once or twice daily resulted in 89 percent of women having lower Candida-symptom scores.

Irritable bowel syndrome may be partly caused by an imbalance of bacteria in the intestinal tract. Two studies found that individuals with irritable bowel syndrome experienced improvement and had less intestinal gas after taking a daily probiotic supplement.[14,15]

Probiotic Supplements

Buy a product that offers 1 to 10 billion live cells per dose. The strength of the product is determined by the number of living organisms in each capsule. For convenience, choose a product that is stable at room temperature and does not require refrigeration. This allows you to conveniently continue taking your supplement while traveling or at the office. Good manufacturers will test their products to ensure that they maintain their viability over a long period.

Many experts believe that supplements made from human strains of bacteria are better adapted for growth in the human intestinal tract. When choosing a product, you might ask the pharmacist or retailer if the formula contains human or nonhuman strains.

Take 1 to 10 billion viable cells, in three or four divided doses. If your product contains 1 billion cells per capsule, take one capsule three times daily. To reduce antibiotic-related diarrhea, take the supplement when you start your antibiotic therapy and continue taking it for five days after antibiotics are stopped.

Always take your probiotic supplement with food. After a meal, the stomach contents become less acidic because of the presence of food, allowing live bacteria to withstand stomach acids and reach their final destination in the intestinal tract.

Children's products are available. These usually contain one-quarter to one-half the adult dose, or 250 to 500 billion live cells.

Probiotic supplements may cause flatulence, which usually subsides as you continue treatment. There are no safety issues associated with taking these supplements.

SAMe (S-Adenosyl-Methionine)

Used for depression (see page 252), fibromyalgia (see page 301), osteoarthritis (see page 447), alcoholic liver disease (see alcoholism, page 148, and cirrhosis of the liver, page 222)
SAMe (S-Adenosyl-Methionine) is a compound our body makes naturally from certain amino acids in high-protein foods like fish and meat. It is found in virtually all body tissues and fluids. The production of SAMe is closely linked with folate and vitamin B12. Deficiencies in these two B vitamins can lead to depressed levels of SAMe in the brain and nervous system. In the body, SAMe is used to synthesize hormones, brain neurotransmitters, proteins and cell membranes. SAMe donates a part of itself, a methyl group, to surrounding body tissues, especially the brain.

SAMe is approved as a prescription drug in 14 countries, and is available as a dietary supplement in the United States. European physicians use SAMe to treat patients with depression. SAMe is associated with higher levels of brain neurotransmitters, natural chemicals that influence mood. It may also work by favorably changing the composition of cell membranes in the brain, enabling neurotransmitters and cell receptors to work more efficiently. The results of well-controlled studies show that SAMe is significantly better than a placebo in treating depression, with symptoms improving in as few as four to five days, and that it may even be more effective than tricyclic antidepressant medications.[1-7]

SAMe also has analgesic and anti-inflammatory properties, which are thought to be responsible for its beneficial effects in treatment of osteoarthritis and fibromyalgia. Some evidence even suggests that SAMe might stimulate the growth and repair of cartilage. Several studies lasting from two weeks to two years have found SAMe to be significantly better than a placebo and comparable to nonsteroidal anti-inflammatory drugs (NSAIDs) for decreasing symptoms of osteoarthritis.[8-16] Two studies also found that fibromyalgia patients who took SAMe had significant improvement in their symptoms.[17,18]

SAMe Supplements

Choose an enteric-coated supplement to help SAMe withstand the acidity of your stomach. There are several forms of SAMe available: sulfate, sulfate-p-toluenesulfonate (tosylate) and butanedisulfonate. Some experts believe butanedisulfonate is more stable than tosylate.

For depression, take 800 to 1600 milligrams per day in divided doses. Start with one 400 milligram tablet twice daily, working up to two tablets three times daily. It may take 30 days of treatment to notice significant improvements in mood. For osteoarthritis, take 200 milligrams three times daily. For fibromyalgia, take 400 milligrams twice daily. Be sure to take SAMe on an empty stomach.

The supplement is very well tolerated at the recommended doses, but daily doses greater than 1600 milligrams may cause nausea, gastrointestinal upset and headache. European studies have not found any long-term problems associated with taking SAMe.

If you are currently taking medication for depression and are thinking about trying SAMe, *do not discontinue your medication without first speaking to your doctor.* When taken with antidepressant drugs, SAMe may have an additive effect causing potentially dangerous side effects.

Part Three

---∞∞∞---

The Health Conditions

Acne

Acne is the most common skin disease to affect North Americans. Almost everyone experiences the annoying pimples and inflammation of acne to some degree during their lifetime. The condition flares up most often during the teenage years, but for some people, acne doesn't show up until adulthood. Women are particularly prone to developing adult acne because of hormonal changes associated with the menstrual cycle and pregnancy.

Common acne is not a serious threat to health and usually subsides after five or ten years. However, acne can cause vulnerable teenagers to suffer from embarrassment, social withdrawal and reduced self-esteem. With modern medical treatment, most symptoms can be alleviated.

What Causes Acne?

Acne is a disorder of the sebaceous glands of the skin. The sebaceous glands produce an oily substance called sebum. Normally, sebum empties onto the surface of the skin through microscopic canals called hair follicles. In acne, these canals become plugged with dead cells, trapping the sebum inside the follicle. This mixture of cells and oil provides just the right environment to encourage the growth of bacteria, resulting in an inflammation or irritation of the skin. This inflammation is called a pimple.

Acne is most often associated with puberty because it is stimulated by the production of androgens, male sex hormones. When children reach the ages of between 11 and 14 years, their bodies produce increased levels of androgens, which in turn causes the sebaceous glands to enlarge. Acne seems to develop when androgens overstimulate these glands, causing them to produce excess sebum. As sebum production increases, hair follicles become blocked more easily and pimples are the result.

Younger women often find that acne flare-ups coincide with their menstrual cycles. The hormonal changes of menstruation upset the normal relationship between sebaceous glands and androgen hormones. Acne tends to develop in the areas where sebaceous glands are most numerous—the face, neck, back, upper arms, shoulders and scalp.

For some people, women especially, acne does not start until age 30 or 40. If you develop acne at an older age, it will probably be a type known as *acne rosacea*. Rosacea does not cause the whiteheads and blackheads of common acne. Instead, you will experience redness, tiny pimples and broken blood vessels, usually on the central area of your face. Your nose may also become bumpy and your skin will flush much more easily.

The cause of rosacea is not known, but it is more common among women and in people with fair complexions. Acne rosacea becomes worse if you drink hot beverages or alcohol, eat spicy foods, smoke or are exposed to excessive sunlight or extreme temperatures. Symptoms tend to go in cycles, with periods of remission and flare-up. Rosacea is a chronic disorder that will become more severe without treatment.

Symptoms

There are several types of acne pimples. A plugged hair follicle is called a comedo or comedone. If the comedo stays beneath the skin, it appears as a small white or yellowish bump—a whitehead. If the comedo opens up onto the surface of the skin, it looks like a small speck of dirt and is called a blackhead. Other types of pimples include papules, small pink bumps on the skin; pustules, inflamed, pus-filled sores; and nodules, large pus-filled cysts or abscesses that extend deep into the skin.

In most cases, acne doesn't leave any scars. In more serious cases of acne, deep cysts or abscesses develop, which are much more likely to rupture and cause scarring. Squeezing, picking or opening pimples in some way can make the acne worse by promoting infection and inflammation. This will increase the risk of scarring.

Who's at Risk?

Acne affects people of all races and ethnic groups, but it seems to be more common among Caucasians. It's safe to say that nearly 100 percent of youths between the ages of 12 and 17 have an occasional pimple or acne breakout. If you are this age and have acne, you can expect it to last for five to ten years and to disappear sometime during your early 20s. Unfortunately, acne can sometimes persist well into adulthood.

Women are very likely to develop acne during their adolescent years as a response to the hormonal changes of menstruation. As well, the elevated hormone levels caused by pregnancy and birth control pills can stimulate acne symptoms. In general, adolescent boys are more likely to develop severe, long-lasting forms of acne than girls.

Some people are born with a predisposition to certain types of acne. If your parents or older siblings had severe acne, the chances are greater that you will get it too. Other factors that may influence the development of acne include:

- *Stress* Severe or prolonged emotional tension may aggravate acne, especially if medications are prescribed to alleviate your stress symptoms.

- *Diet* Chocolate, pizza or french fries do not cause acne. As a matter of fact, diet has little or no effect on acne symptoms. But, if you think you are sensitive to certain foods, try eliminating them from your diet for several weeks. Then add them back to see if they do have an effect on your acne. Eating a balanced diet always has a good effect on your general health.

- *Cosmetics* Certain cosmetics and toiletries may contain ingredients that can clog pores. To prevent this problem, look for products labeled "noncomedogenic."

- *Sunlight* The drying and scaling effect of sunlight can help lessen acne. Many people find that their acne symptoms improve during summer and worsen during winter.

- *Medications* Certain drugs, including lithium, barbiturates and androgens, can cause acne.

- *Friction* Rubbing the skin or pressure from bike helmets, backpacks or tight collars can irritate your skin and trigger acne breakouts.

- *Environmental irritants* Pollution, high humidity or scrubbing with harsh soaps may provoke acne symptoms.

Conventional Treatment

Your doctor will prescribe the appropriate treatment. If your acne is more severe or does not respond to basic treatment, you may be referred to a dermatologist, a doctor who specializes in skin disorders. However, acne usually responds well to treatment and almost every case can be improved or cleared completely with the right medication.

- Wash your skin gently with a good soap twice daily. Avoid overwashing or using antibacterial soaps that may cause irritation and aggravate the acne.

- Comedos can be carefully removed from the skin using a sterile needle or a specialized tool, but this should be done only with the approval of your doctor.

- For mild or moderate acne, there are many over-the-counter medications that will limit the formation of whiteheads and blackheads and reduce inflammation. The most common topical medications contain benzoyl peroxide, resorcinol, salicylic acid or sulfur. These products are applied either directly on the pimples or over the entire affected area. It can take four to eight weeks before you see improvement in your skin, so be patient.

- Women may benefit from prescription oral contraceptives as these medications contain female hormones that suppress the production of androgens.

For more severe cases, prescription antibiotics are usually the treatment of choice. These products can be applied directly onto the skin in a topical gel or lotion or may be taken orally, in pill form. Oral antibiotics are more effective in treating severe acne because they circulate through the body and penetrate the sebaceous glands.

Prescription medications usually contain antibiotics such as clindamycin, erythromycin or tetracycline and may also include retinoids, which are vitamin A derivatives. Using products with retinoids may increase your sensitivity to sunlight, making you prone to sunburn. Tetracycline is not usually given to pregnant women or children under 12, because it can cause discoloration in developing teeth. Since some antibiotics may reduce the effectiveness of oral contraceptives, it is wise to use a back-up form of birth control when you are taking these medications.

In the case of severe acne that doesn't respond to standard treatment, your doctor may prescribe an oral retinoid called isotretinoin (Accutane®). This drug is very effective in treating deep cysts and abscesses and will prevent extensive scarring. However, it has numerous side effects, including birth defects in the developing fetus of pregnant women. It is crucial that you do not become pregnant while taking this drug. You must use appropriate birth control one month before starting the treatment, during the entire course of your prescription and for at least one month after the treatment stops. Consult your doctor for further information on this medication.

Managing Acne
Dietary Strategies
A Healthy Diet

It has long been thought that certain foods cause acne, yet there's little scientific evidence to support this notion. It is true that oily foods and sugary foods may exacerbate acne symptoms. As well, foods high in iodine, such as shellfish, table salt and milk, can worsen some cases of acne. Alcohol and cigarette smoking can also worsen acne. A diet low in fat and refined sugars and high in nutrients can boost the body's immune system, reduce inflammation and improve symptoms. (Chapter 5 discusses overall dietary guidelines.) In some cases, food allergies may trigger acne. If you suspect this is the case, it may be worthwhile to speak to your doctor about allergy testing.

Essential Fatty Acids

It has been suggested that abnormalities in the body's metabolism of essential fatty acids may play a role in acne. Studies have shown that people with acne have lower levels of an essential fatty acid called linoleic acid in acne sebum.[1] Linoleic acid is needed to suppress the inflammatory effects of white blood cells involved in acne. One Japanese study found that linoleic acid significantly decreased inflammation and the production of free radical molecules by white blood cells (free radicals may worsen acne symptoms).[2]

Linoleic acid is an omega-6 fatty acid found in all vegetable oils. Some linoleic acid is also found in meat. The body cannot produce linoleic on its own so it must be supplied by the diet. With our high intake of processed foods, most Canadians are not at risk for getting too little linoleic acid. But you should pay attention to your intake of these fats if you suffer from acne or you eat a very low-fat diet. Aim to include 1 tablespoon (15 ml) of an oil rich in linoleic acid in your daily diet.

Alpha-linolenic acid is also very important for health. This omega-3 essential fatty acid is found in flaxseed, walnut and canola oils. Alpha-linolenic acid is used by the body to produce anti-inflammatory immune compounds that may help prevent or reduce acne symptoms. Aim to get 1 to 2 tablespoons (15 to 30 ml) of these oils per day. Other sources of alpha-linolenic acid include Omega-3 eggs, soybeans and leafy greens.

To get both essential fatty acids in one oil, consider adding Udo's Choice Ultimate Oil Blend to your daily diet. Udo's oil contains oils from organic flaxseed, sesame and sunflower seeds, wheat germ, rice germ and oat germ. It contains a balance of both alpha-linolenic and linoleic acid fatty acids. The oils are sensitive to light, air and heat, so it should not be used for frying, deep-frying or sautéing, but can otherwise replace most oils in food preparation. Use it for making salad dressings, serve it on steamed vegetables or baked potatoes, add it to soups after cooking or add it to fresh vegetable juices or homemade smoothies. You'll find this product in health food stores.

Vitamins and Minerals

Vitamin A

This vitamin may influence the activity of sebaceous glands in such a way as to reduce sebum production. To get plenty of vitamin A in your diet, reach for liver, oily fish, milk, cheese, and whole eggs. Beta-carotene, a compound found in orange and dark green produce, is converted to vitamin A in the body and helps you meet your daily requirements. Foods rich in beta-carotene include carrots, sweet potato, winter squash, broccoli, collard greens, kale, spinach, apricots, cantaloupe, peaches, nectarines, mango and papaya.

Keep in mind that most studies have investigated the effects of very high doses of vitamin A on acne. Because vitamin A is fat soluble, the body stores it, and too much vitamin A taken for a period can be toxic. If you take a supplement, do not exceed 10,000 international units (3.3 milligrams) per day unless supervised by your physician. Vitamin A supplements should not be taken with vitamin A derivative acne drugs as this will increase the likelihood of a toxic reaction. Pregnant women must avoid vitamin A supplements since high doses can cause birth defects.

Vitamins C and E

Because white blood cells involved in the inflammation of acne can produce free radical molecules, getting plenty of dietary antioxidants may help reduce inflammation. Vitamins C and E may also boost the body's immune system, which can help reduce the chances of infection. Vitamin C rich foods include citrus fruit, strawberries, kiwi, cantaloupe, broccoli, bell peppers, Brussels sprouts, cabbage, tomatoes and potatoes. Vitamin E is found in vegetable oils, almonds, peanuts, soybeans, whole grains, wheat germ, avocado and green leafy vegetables, especially kale.

It can be difficult to obtain large amounts of these nutrients from a normal diet, so supplements may be useful. Take 500 milligrams of vitamin C once or twice daily. Take 200 to 800 international units (IU) of a natural source vitamin E once daily. To learn more about vitamin C and E supplements, refer to Chapter 4.

B Vitamins

This family of vitamins helps to maintain healthy skin. Vitamin B6, found in animal foods, whole grains, avocado and potatoes, may help reduce acne associated with the menstrual cycle. Studies in women have used supplemental doses of 50 milligrams once daily.[3] Niacin (vitamin B3) can help improve blood flow to the skin and may be useful in acne management. Food sources of niacin include meat, poultry, dairy products, peanuts, almonds, seeds, whole grains, enriched breakfast cereals and wheat bran.

To ensure that you are meeting your daily requirements for the B vitamins, take a multivitamin and mineral supplement or a B complex formula. High-potency multivitamins provide the B vitamin in amounts similar to those found in a B complex supplement. One word of caution: high doses of vitamins B6 and B12 may aggravate symptoms of acne rosacea and should be used with caution in women with this form of acne.

Chromium

Some experts suggest that the mineral chromium may be effective in treating acne, although little research on this has been done. Since many dermatologists have reported that the diabetes medications insulin and tolbutamide have been effective in acne, it's been hypothesized that chromium might be beneficial, since chromium works with insulin to regulate the blood sugar. One study did find that a chromium supplement derived from yeast was effective.[4]

The best food sources of chromium include Brewer's yeast, calf's liver, blackstrap molasses, wheat germ, wheat bran, whole grains, mushrooms, apples with skin, green peas, chicken breast, refried beans and oysters. If you're concerned you're not getting enough chromium in your diet, check your multivitamin and mineral supplement to see how much it contains. Most brands supply 25 to 50 micrograms. If you choose to take a separate chromium supplement, do not exceed 200 micrograms per day. High doses of chromium can cause cognitive impairment, anemia and kidney damage.

Selenium

This trace mineral is an essential component of an antioxidant enzyme called glutathione peroxidase. As such, selenium helps the body fight free radicals that are formed during normal metabolism. Selenium works very closely with vitamin E in the body. Researchers have noted depressed levels of glutathione peroxidase in people with acne.[5] One study found that a daily supplement of selenium (200 micrograms) and vitamin E (10 milligrams) taken for 6 to 12 weeks increased glutathione peroxidase levels and improved pustular acne symptoms.[6]

To boost the selenium content of your diet, reach for seafood, meat, organ meats, wheat bran, whole grains, nuts, Brazil nuts, onion, garlic, mushrooms, Swiss chard and orange juice. If you decide to supplement, take 200 micrograms per day. Supplements made from organic forms of selenium (selenomethionine and high-selenium yeast) are absorbed more efficiently than inorganic forms. Since vitamin E and selenium work in tandem, consider buying a supplement that combines the two nutrients. Look for a broad-based antioxidant supplement that contains selenium, vitamin E and vitamin C.

Do not exceed 400 micrograms of selenium per day. Higher doses can cause loss of hair and fingernails, nausea, depression and anxiety.

Zinc

This nutrient may be useful in treating acne, especially in boys. Studies have shown that zinc levels in the skin cells and blood are often low in adolescent males who are more prone to acne.[7] Zinc has many roles in the body that may affect the symptoms of acne. This mineral helps transport vitamin A, assists in wound healing, supports immune function and regulates the activity of oil glands. High concentrations of zinc may reduce oil gland secretion by preventing the conversion of testosterone to its active form. Two studies found that 30 milligrams of supplemental zinc significantly reduced inflammation in patients with acne.[8,9]

The best food sources of zinc include oysters, seafood, red meat, poultry, yogurt, milk, wheat bran, wheat germ, whole grains and enriched breakfast cereals. A healthy diet and a good multivitamin and mineral supplement will give you all the zinc you need to stay healthy. Taking too much zinc from supplements has toxic effects including copper deficiency, heart problems and anemia. Excess zinc can also depress your immune system, making you more susceptible to infection. If you take a separate zinc supplement, do not exceed 40 milligrams per day.

Herbal Remedies

In addition to ensuring your diet contains adequate amounts of the vitamins and minerals listed above, you may want to use one of the following topical herbal creams to help improve acne symptoms. These creams may be sold over-the-counter in certain supplement stores or they may be made by compounding pharmacists. Contact your provincial pharmacist's association to locate a compounding pharmacist in your community.

Echinacea
Many studies in the laboratory have shown the ability of echinacea to enhance the body's production of white blood cells that fight infection. The herb has also been found to have weak antibacterial and antiviral activity. Three species of echinacea have been shown to have medicinal benefits: Echinacea purpurea, Echinacea angustifolia and Echinacea pallida. Echinacea purpurea may be effective in promoting healing of acne. Apply a cream or liquid preparation that contains 15 percent Echinacea purpurea juice to affected areas.

Goldenseal (Hydrastis canadensis)
Historically, this herb was used by Native Americans to treat a variety of skin disorders and wounds. The plant name is derived from the golden-yellow scars on the base of its stem. When the stem is broken, the scar resembles a gold letter seal. One of the active ingredients in goldenseal, berberine, possesses strong antibacterial

activity. The herb is most effective when used topically because the intestinal tract poorly absorbs the plant's active ingredients. Apply a sufficient amount of a goldenseal cream to affected areas.

Tea Tree Oil (Melaleuca alternifolia)
Many studies have demonstrated the antiseptic and antibiotic properties of tea tree oil.[10] It appears to kill many types of bacteria and fungi, including some that are resistant to antibiotic therapy. Tea tree oil comes from the aromatic leaves of a plant native to Australia, where the oil had been used for hundreds of years to prevent and treat wounds. A recent review of four well-controlled trials found the topical use of tea tree oil to be an effective treatment for acne.[11]

Buy a preparation that contains 5 to 15 percent tea tree oil. Tea tree oil can irritate the skin, so you may want to start with a lower concentration. High-quality products are made from the oil of the alternifolia species of the plant. They should be standardized to contain not more than 10 percent cineole and at least 30 percent terpinen-4-ol. Apply the oil two or three times per day to affected areas until the acne symptoms resolve. Avoid contact with the eyes. Do not ingest tea tree oil. Topical use of tea tree oil may cause allergic skin reactions in some individuals.

Nutrition Strategy Checklist for Acne

☐ Low-fat, low-sugar diet
☐ Limit alcohol and salty foods
☐ Healthy oils
☐ Vitamin A
☐ Vitamin B6, niacin
☐ Vitamin C

☐ Vitamin E
☐ Chromium
☐ Zinc
☐ Herbal creams/oils: Tea tree oil* OR Echinacea OR Goldenseal

*Strongest evidence—start here.

Recommended Resources

www.crha-health.ab.ca
Calgary Regional Health Authority
Communications
1035-7th Avenue SW
Calgary, AB, Canada T2P 3E9
Tel: 403-265-INFO (403-265-4636) or
1-800-860-2742 (Alberta only)
E-mail: publicweb@crha-health.ab.ca

www.nih.gov/niams/healthinfo/acne/acne.htm
National Institute of Arthritis and
Musculoskeletal and Skin Diseases
Information Clearinghouse
National Institutes of Health
1 AMS Circle
Bethesda, MD, USA 20892-3675
Tel: 301-495-4484 or 1-877-22-NIAMS
(1-877-226-4267)
Fax: 301-718-6366

www.skincarephysicians.com/acnenet
An online information resource on acne, this
Web site is a collaborative effort by Roche
Laboratories Inc. and the American Academy of
Dermatology.

Alcoholism

Drinking alcohol has become an integral part of
North American culture. Recent statistical surveys indicate that nearly 75 percent of Canadians
reported consuming alcohol over a 12-month
period.[1] Used in moderation, alcohol is not
harmful for most adults. Moderate alcohol use is
defined as no more than two drinks a day for
men and no more than one drink a day for
women and older adults. A standard drink is 12
ounces (340 ml) of regular beer, 5 ounces (145
ml) of wine or 1 1/2 ounces (45 ml) of 80-proof
(40 percent) distilled spirits.

However, because social drinking is such a
popular activity, it's easy to overlook the fact that
alcohol is a depressant drug with powerfully
addictive properties. If used excessively, it can
have harmful effects on almost every system in
the body. Despite its general acceptance, alcohol
is one of the most abused drugs in our society.
Sadly, it is estimated that more than 14 million
people in North America abuse alcohol or are
alcoholics.

Effects of Alcohol

Physical Effects

Alcohol is quickly absorbed into the bloodstream
through the stomach and the small intestine.
While even small amounts of alcohol will produce physical changes, the overall effects of alcohol on the body are dependent on several factors,
including the drinker's size, gender and metabolism. For example, after drinking the same
amount of alcohol, women will usually have
higher blood alcohol concentrations (BAC) than
men. Women may have lower levels of alcohol
dehydrogenase, a stomach enzyme that helps the
body metabolize alcohol. Female hormones may
also influence a woman's ability to metabolize
alcohol.

Alcohol slows down the nervous system and
alters the functions of almost every organ in the
body. It depresses centers in the brain that are
responsible for inhibiting or restraining behavior. After only one drink, people will report feeling more relaxed, friendly and self-confident.
Higher levels of alcohol consumption will impair
thinking, judgment and physical reaction time.
Even a small amount of alcohol in the bloodstream is enough to impair performance skills,
greatly increasing the risk of accident when driving a car or operating machinery.

Other short-term effects of alcohol use
include

- dilation of blood vessels in the skin, causing loss of body heat

- increased urine production

- increased stomach secretions

- accumulations of fat in the liver cells

Although moderate alcohol use has been reported to have a protective effect against heart disease, eating sensibly, exercising regularly and quitting smoking provide better alternatives to good heart health.

Excessive use of alcohol over an extended period can result in serious, long-term health problems, such as

- brain injury, resulting in severe dysfunction

- sleep disruptions

- movement disorders

- serious diseases of the liver (alcoholic hepatitis and cirrhosis)

- serious disease of the pancreas (pancreatitis)

- damage to the stomach and intestines

- nutritional deficiencies

- anemia

- deterioration of the heart muscle, leading to sudden death

- impotence, sterility and breast enlargement in men

- early menopause and menstrual irregularities in women

- osteoporosis

- increased risk of having babies with birth defects for women who drink during pregnancy, the most serious defect being fetal alcohol syndrome

- depression of the immune system, leading to pneumonia, tuberculosis and cancer

Alcohol has been proven to react negatively with over 150 medications. Death may occur when even moderate amounts of alcohol are combined with other depressant drugs, such as tranquilizers and sleeping pills. Excessive consumption of alcohol can also lead to death by overdose.

Social Effects

Drinking alcohol has the potential to interfere with interpersonal relationships. Problems that may develop include

- arguments with spouse or family members, eventually leading to violence

- difficult relationships with coworkers

- lateness or absence from work

- loss of employment because of decreased productivity

- becoming the victim of violence

- suicide

Symptoms of Alcoholism

Alcoholism, also known as alcohol dependence syndrome, is characterized by

- *craving*—the strong need or compulsion to drink

- *loss of control*—the inability to stop drinking once a person has begun

- *physical dependence*—the development of withdrawal symptoms, such as nausea, sweating, shakiness and anxiety, when heavy drinking is stopped

- *tolerance*—a need for increasing amounts of alcohol to obtain the desired effect or to get "high"

Alcohol abuse differs from alcoholism in that there is not a strong craving to drink, nor is there loss of control or physical dependence. Alcohol abuse is a pattern of drinking that is accompanied by one of the following for a 12-month period:

- failure to meet professional or family obligations

- drinking while driving or operating machinery

- recurring alcohol-related legal problems

- continued drinking despite ongoing relationship problems that are worsened by alcohol use

Who's at Risk?

Men are more likely than women to be heavy drinkers, and heavier drinking is more prevalent at lower education and income levels. Children of alcoholics are more likely to develop alcoholism than are children of nonalcoholic parents. Studies have found that women who suffer from bulimia nervosa are more susceptible to alcohol abuse, and that people who are single, separated or divorced drink more than do people with partners. Environmental influences, such as peer pressure and availability of alcohol, may increase risk.

Conventional Treatment

Alcoholism is a treatable disease, but at this time there is no cure. Treatment depends on the degree of alcohol abuse or alcoholism and the availability of community resources. Treatment may include

- sociobehavioral counseling on an in- or outpatient basis; psychotherapy

- family therapy and marital counseling

- detoxification in a hospital or residential treatment center or on an outpatient basis

- medications to ease withdrawal symptoms or to help prevent a return to drinking

- involvement in support groups, such as Alcoholics Anonymous

Nutritional Care for Alcoholism

Nutrient deficiencies are common in alcoholism and are caused by many different factors. Many people with the disease have nutritionally poor diets, which contributes to malnutrition. But alcohol-induced damage to the gastrointestinal tract and the liver affects the body's ability to absorb, process and store a wide range of nutrients. Heavy drinking also causes certain minerals to be lost from the urine. Alcohol inactivates some vitamins needed to metabolize energy. And finally, people who suffer from alcoholism have an increased need for many nutrients to detoxify and metabolize alcohol, as well as to help heal damaged body tissues. The nutritional strategies listed below are intended to prevent or correct nutrient deficiencies and reduce the severity and length of withdrawal symptoms.

Dietary Strategies

A Healthy Diet

The importance of eating a nutrient-dense, well-balanced diet cannot be overemphasized. Research shows that nutritional therapy helps in the recovery from alcoholism.[2] Follow the healthy eating guide outlined on page 83, Chapter 5. Not only does a regular intake of food supply energy, vitamins, minerals and protective plant chemicals, but it can also minimize the symptoms of alcohol withdrawal. Both appetite loss and a ravenous appetite are rebound symptoms of quitting alcohol. Food cravings, especially for carbohydrates, and insomnia can also occur during the alcohol-withdrawal stage. Heavy drinking may result in damage to the liver or pancreas, making people with alcoholism susceptible to fluctuations in blood sugar. The following strategies can help manage these symptoms.[3]

To stimulate appetite:

- Eat small meals, every two to three hours.

- Drink plenty of fluids such as juice, milk, sports drinks, even ginger ale.

- Use commercial meal replacement beverages such as Ensure® or Boost®. These provide protein, carbohydrates, vitamins and minerals in a relatively small volume.

- Limit your intake of fatty foods as these foods can depress appetite.

- Limit caffeine intake, which further depresses appetite; aim for less than 450 milligrams per day (see page 82, Chapter 5).

To control ravenous hunger and food cravings:

- Eat meals and snacks at regular intervals throughout the day.

- Consume protein-rich foods at each meal and snack as these foods are digested slowly and promote a feeling of fullness.

- Limit intake of sweets and caffeine.

To prevent blood-sugar fluctuations:

- Eat once every three to four hours.

- Include a source of protein with each meal and snack.

- Choose carbohydrates that are more slowly digested and converted to blood glucose. (For a list of these foods, refer to page 7, Chapter 1.)

- Consume plenty of chromium-rich foods, which can help regulate blood-sugar levels (see page 50, Chapter 4).

To combat insomnia:

- Eat a carbohydrate-rich snack (milk, toast) one hour before bed.

- Eliminate or limit caffeine intake five to eight hours before bed.

Alcohol in Foods

If you are taking a protective drug such as Antabuse or Temposil, you must avoid consuming foods made with alcohol. Studies have shown that very little alcohol is lost in the cooking process: as much as two-thirds may still be present after 20 minutes of cooking. If alcohol is added after cooking, all of the alcohol will be present. The following foods, food ingredients and supplements may contain alcohol and should be avoided:

- Flavor extracts
- Miran (used in mock crab)
- Cooking wines
- Cakes and pastries made with liqueur
- Angostura aromatic bitter
- Bernaise and bordelaise sauces
- Herbal tinctures
- Hollandaise, Madeira and marsala sauces
- Liqueur-filled chocolates and candies
- Some soups (black bean, onion)
- Nonalcoholic beer and wine
- Aspic
- Apple cider
- Fondues
- Malt vinegar, cider vinegar, red-wine vinegar
- Chocolate mousse
- Wine-flavored cheese and pâté
- Liquid vitamin supplements
- Some brands of Dijon mustard
- Flambé desserts
- Commercial eggnog
- Teriyaki sauce
- Wine sauerkraut
- Lobster bisque

Essential Fatty Acids

Chronic alcohol ingestion causes alterations in fat metabolism, and this is worsened if liver damage is present. Studies consistently find that individuals with alcoholism have depressed levels of important fatty acids in their blood cells, where these acids play a vital role in maintaining healthy cell membranes.[4-6] Some experts hypothesize that fatty acid deficiency, especially a deficiency of the omega-3 fatty acid DHA, may contribute to depression that occurs in alcoholism.

The omega-3 and omega-6 oils in our diet provide two essential fatty acids that our body cannot make on its own. Omega-3 oils (flaxseed, canola, walnut) provide alpha-linolenic acid, and omega-6 oils (corn, sunflower, safflower, soybean) give us linoleic acid. These two essential fatty acids are used to form vital body structures and cell membranes, aid in immune function and vision and produce powerful compounds called eicosanoids that help regulate inflammation, hormones and nerve and brain function.

Aim to include 2 tablespoons (30 ml) of some combination of the following oils in your daily diet: flaxseed, walnut, canola and Udo's Choice Ultimate Oil Blend (available in health food stores). With the exception of canola oil, these oils should not be used for high-heat cooking. Use them for salad dressings or add them to hot foods after cooking.

To increase your intake of DHA, eat fish three times a week. Salmon, trout, sardines, herring, pickerel and fresh tuna are the best choices.

Vitamins and Minerals

B Vitamins

Deficiencies of many B vitamins are common with chronic heavy drinking. Body levels of thiamin (B1), niacin (B3), folate, B6 and pantothenic acid have all been found to be lower in people with alcoholism.[7-12] B vitamin deficiencies are due to an inadequate dietary intake; the toxic effects of alcohol that reduce absorption, metabolism and storage of nutrients; and the increased amounts of these vitamins needed to metabolize large quantities of alcohol.

One of the most serious consequences of alcoholism is Wernicke-Korsakoff syndrome, a disease caused by thiamin deficiency. This disease is often seen in people who have consumed alcohol heavily for several weeks and eaten very little.[13,14] Symptoms of Wernicke-Korsakoff syndrome include confusion, stupor, memory impairment and vision abnormalities. If left untreated, it can lead to permanent brain damage and death. Because alcohol requires thiamin for its metabolism, this serves to only further deplete body stores.

The following is recommended to replenish body stores of the B vitamins during alcohol withdrawal:

- Take a 50 to 100 milligram thiamin supplement once daily.

- Take a multivitamin and mineral supplement once daily.

- Emphasize foods rich in B vitamins: whole-grain breads and cereals, lentils and lean protein foods. You'll find a list of each B vitamin and food sources in Chapter 4.

If a thiamin deficiency has caused nerve damage, B vitamin treatment may be necessary for months or years. If you have alcoholic liver damage, do not take doses of vitamins (except thiamin) or minerals beyond what is provided in a regular multivitamin and mineral supplement. Excessive consumption of certain nutrients (vitamin A, niacin, iron) can lead to toxicity in the presence of impaired liver function. Higher doses should be taken under the direction and supervision of your doctor.

Antioxidants

Chronic alcohol drinking increases free radical production in the body. Free radicals are unstable oxygen molecules that can harm virtually every cell in the body and promote the development of heart disease and cancer. Furthermore, alcoholism is associated with depressed blood levels of many important antioxidants—the very compounds that seek and destroy free radicals. Studies show that compared to healthy adults, levels of vitamins C and E, beta-carotene and selenium are lower in people with alcoholism.[15-19] To get more dietary antioxidants, focus on the following foods.

Vitamin C
The recommended dietary allowance (RDA) of this vitamin is 75 and 90 milligrams for women and men respectively (smokers need an additional 35 milligrams). Best food sources include citrus fruit, citrus juices, cantaloupe, kiwi, mango, strawberries, broccoli, Brussels sprouts, cauliflower, red pepper and tomato juice. To supplement, buy a 500 or 600 milligram supplement of Ester C; take once daily. The daily upper limit for adults is 2000 milligrams.

Vitamin E
The RDA for vitamin E is 22 international units (IU) from foods and/or natural source supplements. Best food sources include wheat germ, nuts, seeds, vegetable oils, whole grains and kale. To supplement, take 200 to 800 IU of natural source vitamin E. Buy a "mixed" vitamin E supplement if possible. The daily upper limit is 1500 IU.

Selenium
The RDA for this trace mineral is 55 micrograms. Best food sources are seafood, chicken, organ meats, whole grains, nuts, onions, garlic and mushrooms. To supplement, take 200 micrograms of selenium-rich yeast per day. Check how much your multivitamin and mineral formula gives you before you buy a separate selenium pill. The daily upper limit is 400 micrograms.

Beta-Carotene
There is no established RDA for beta-carotene. Best food sources are orange and dark green produce, including carrots, sweet potato, winter squash, broccoli, collard greens, kale, spinach, apricots, cantaloupe, peaches, nectarines, mango and papaya. Choose a multivitamin and mineral supplement with beta-carotene added.

Calcium and Vitamin D

Chronic alcohol consumption can induce bone loss, a risk factor for osteoporosis. Alcohol hampers the activity of vitamin D in the body, making it less effective at maintaining bone health. Heavy drinking also increases urinary excretion of magnesium, calcium and zinc, all important minerals in preserving bone mass.[20] It is especially important to be meeting your daily requirements for calcium and vitamin D to slow down bone loss.

The RDA for calcium is 1000 to 1200 milligrams; best food sources are milk, yogurt, cheese, fortified soy and rice beverages, fortified orange juice, tofu, salmon (with bones), kale, bok choy, broccoli and Swiss chard. If you take calcium supplements, buy calcium citrate with vitamin D and magnesium added.

The adequate daily intake for vitamin D is 200 to 600 IU; best food sources are fluid milk, fortified soy and rice beverages, oily fish, egg yolks, butter and margarine. Your multivitamin and mineral formula should provide 400 IU of vitamin D.

Magnesium

Alcohol causes a rapid loss of magnesium in the urine; alcoholism is associated with depleted body stores of this mineral. It is believed that magnesium deficiency induced by heavy drinking may increase the risk of high blood pressure, stroke, sudden death and osteoporosis.[21] Studies have shown that short-term magnesium supplementation can improve liver cell function, muscle strength and body fluid balance in chronic alcoholics.[22]

The RDA for magnesium is between 320 and 420 milligrams per day (refer to the RDA chart on page 47, Chapter 4). Best sources of magnesium include nuts, seeds, legumes, prunes, whole grains, leafy green vegetables, Brewer's yeast, cheddar cheese and shrimp. If you decide to supplement your diet and you don't take supplemental calcium with magnesium, buy a separate magnesium supplement made from magnesium citrate, aspartate, succinate, fumarte or gluconate. The body absorbs these forms of the mineral more efficiently. Taking more than 350 milligrams of magnesium in a supplement can cause diarrhea, nausea and stomach cramps.

Zinc

Chronic alcoholism is associated with low blood zinc levels. Some researchers hypothesize that low levels of zinc in the brain enhance susceptibility to alcohol withdrawal seizures.[23] Zinc deficiency can also promote nerve damage by increasing the formation of harmful free radicals.

To prevent a zinc deficiency, focus on choosing zinc-rich foods every day: oysters, seafood, red meat, poultry, yogurt, wheat bran, wheat germ, whole grains and enriched breakfast cereals. A multivitamin and mineral supplement will provide 10 to 20 milligrams of the mineral. If you choose to take a separate zinc supplement, buy one with added copper and do not exceed 40 milligrams of zinc per day. Too much zinc can cause a copper deficiency, heart problems and anemia.

Herbal Remedies

Milk Thistle (*Silybum marianum*)

The active ingredients of this herb, known collectively as silymarin, can support and enhance liver function. Silymarin can prevent toxic substances from penetrating liver cells, and it may even help liver cells regenerate more quickly.[24] Milk thistle also seems to act as an antioxidant, protecting liver cells from damage caused by free radicals.[25]

Buy a product that's standardized to contain 70 percent silymarin. The usual dose ranges from 70 to 210 milligrams, two or three times daily. Use milk thistle with caution if you are allergic to plants in the Asteracease/Compositae family (ragweed, daisy, marigold and chrysanthemum).

Other Natural Health Products

Lecithin (Phosphatidylcholine)

Lecithin and phosphatidylcholine supplements are thought to exert their health benefits by supplying the body with choline, a B vitamin. Once ingested, choline becomes incorporated into the membranes of cells. Phosphatidylcholine supplements are used in Europe to treat alcoholic liver disorders. Studies suggest that phosphatidylcholine supplements can oppose alcohol-induced liver damage.[26-28]

Most lecithin supplements contain 10 to 20 percent phosphatidylcholine. Others, however, are almost pure phosphatidylcholine and are labeled as such. Most clinical studies have been done with phosphatidylcholine supplements. Buy a supplement labeled phosphatidylcholine. Take 1200 to 2220 milligrams per day, in divided doses.

SAMe (S-Adenosyl-Methionine)

SAMe is a compound that our body makes naturally from certain amino acids in high-protein foods like fish and meat. It is found in virtually all body tissues and fluids. The production of SAMe is closely linked with folate and vitamin B12, so deficiencies of these B vitamins can lead to depressed levels of SAMe. In the body, SAMe is used to synthesize hormones, brain neurotransmitters, proteins and cell membranes.

It's thought that SAMe acts as an essential nutrient by restoring biochemical compounds that are depleted in people with alcoholic liver disease.[29,30] People with liver disease lose the ability to form SAMe, and this leads to deficiencies in choline, a B vitamin, and glutathione, an enzyme that plays a critical role in liver detoxification and antioxidant reactions.

To supplement, take 300 to 400 milligrams three times daily. Buy an enteric-coated supplement product and take SAMe on an empty stomach.

Nutrition Strategy Checklist for Alcoholism

- ☐ Low-fat, high-fiber diet
- ☐ Avoid alcohol in foods
- ☐ Healthy oils
- ☐ Fish
- ☐ Multivitamin/mineral
- ☐ B complex supplement
- ☐ Thiamin
- ☐ Antioxidants: C, E, selenium, beta-
- carotene
- ☐ Calcium
- ☐ Vitamin D
- ☐ Magnesium
- ☐ Zinc-rich foods
- ☐ Milk thistle
- ☐ (Lecithin) Phosphatidylcholine

Recommended Resources

www.aadac.com
Alberta Alcohol and Drug Abuse Commission
200-10909 Jasper Avenue
Edmonton, AB, Canada T5J 3M9
Tel: 780-422-7319
Fax: 780-422-5237

www.alcoholics-anonymous.org
Alcoholics Anonymous World Services
475 Riverside Drive, 11th Floor
New York, NY, USA 10115
Tel: 212-870-3400

www.camh.net
Centre for Addiction and Mental Health
33 Russell Street
Toronto, ON, Canada M5S 2S1
Tel: 416-535-8501 or 1-800-463-6273

www.nacoa.net
National Association for Children of Alcoholics
Tel: 1-888-554-2627

www.health.org
National Clearinghouse for Alcohol and Drug Information
P.O. Box 2345
Rockville, MD, USA 20847-2345
Tel: 1-800-729-6686

www.niaaa.nih.gov
National Institutes of Health
The National Institute on Alcohol Abuse and Alcoholism
Scientific Communications Branch
6000 Executive Boulevard, Suite 409
Bethesda, MD, USA 20892-7003

Alzheimer's Disease

Alzheimer's disease is the leading cause of dementia in older people. In Canada, 364,000 people over the age of 65 are suffering from the condition. It's projected that by 2031, more than three-quarters of a million Canadians will be victims of Alzheimer's disease.[1] Unfortunately, as our population ages, the situation is expected to only become worse. Alzheimer's disease is likely to become one of the greatest public health problems in the coming decades.

What Causes Alzheimer's Disease?

Although Alzheimer's disease is often associated with getting older, it is not a normal part of the aging process. Rather, it's a medical condition that disrupts brain function by destroying vital nerve cells. Alzheimer's disease develops slowly, resulting in a gradual loss of motor skills and a general decline in intellectual ability. The disease targets the centers in the brain that control memory, thought and language. It causes changes in mood and behavior, as well as loss of memory, judgment and reasoning. The massive brain-cell death associated with Alzheimer's disease is permanent, and at this time there is no known cure.

Alzheimer's disease causes abnormal clumps or plaques and tangled bundles of fibers to develop in the brain. A build-up in the brain of a protein called beta amyloid has been associated with the disease. While the exact cause of Alzheimer's disease is still unknown, researchers are investigating a number of different possibilities, including genetic factors, viruses, vitamin and hormone deficiencies and head injuries. An accumulation of toxic substances in the brain (aluminum is a primary suspect) may also contribute to the degenerative brain changes associated with the disease.

Scientists have identified two types of Alzheimer's disease. Sporadic Alzheimer's disease is the most common type and is responsible for over 90 percent of the cases diagnosed. The second type, Familial Autosomal Dominant (FAD) Alzheimer's disease, has a genetic basis and is clearly passed from generation to generation. If a parent has the mutated gene responsible for this type of the disease, each child has a 50 percent chance of inheriting it. People with the mutated gene will inevitably develop Alzheimer's disease at some point in their lives. FAD accounts for 5 to 10 percent of all cases of Alzheimer's disease.

Symptoms

Symptoms of Alzheimer's disease include changes in intellectual abilities. Those with the disease

- gradually become unable to learn new things and make decisions
- forget how to do simple, familiar tasks

- have trouble remembering names, appointments, daily routines
- have difficulty understanding what has been said
- have difficulty communicating, forget simple words, use words inappropriately
- lose track of time and place; become lost and disoriented easily
- may remember past events more clearly than current events
- are no longer interested in normal activities; demonstrate no initiative

The disease also affects mood. Those with Alzheimer's disease

- have less expression; may eventually have little or no reaction to people or surroundings
- are more withdrawn
- have difficulty controlling moods and emotions
- have rapidly changing moods and emotions
- may worry excessively over small things
- may become suspicious or easily angered

Changes in behavior and physical functioning may include

- pacing, agitation, wandering and restlessness
- repetitive actions
- physical outbursts
- swearing, arguing and aggressiveness
- hiding things; constantly searching
- difficulty feeding, dressing and bathing
- loss of bowel and bladder control
- loss of mobility

The symptoms of Alzheimer's disease vary from person to person. So too does the speed at which the condition progresses. Some people with the disease live relatively normal lives for many years, whereas others experience rapid progression of their symptoms. No matter what the speed of onset, Alzheimer's disease will eventually lead to complete dependence on caregivers and, inevitably, death.

Who's at Risk?

Twice as many women as men have Alzheimer's disease. The risk of Alzheimer's disease increases as you age. After the age of 65, risks double every five years; by the age of 80, 20 percent of men and women suffer from the disease. Those with a family history of Alzheimer's disease are also at higher risk.[2] As well, an individual with a family history of Alzheimer's disease may face an increased risk of developing the condition when exposed to suspected trigger factors, such as viruses or environmental toxins.

Conventional Treatment

The management of Alzheimer's disease may include

- medications (usually tacrine, donepezil or rivastigmine) that treat memory loss and cognitive symptoms by increasing the brain's supply of acetylcholine, a nerve-communication chemical

- modification of the home environment to eliminate factors that may trigger behavior problems (noise, colors, lighting)

- establishment of daily routines

- creative leisure activities to improve behavior and mood

- antipsychotic or antidepressant medications to treat behavior and mood changes

- family education and counseling to help both the patient and caregivers deal with the symptoms of the disease

Managing Alzheimer's Disease

Dietary Strategies

A Healthy Diet

Ensuring that a loved one with Alzheimer's disease eats a nutritious diet can be a challenge. People with Alzheimer's often have difficulty staying focused on the task of eating. As well, the ability to use utensils deteriorates because of the progressive loss of cognitive function and motor skills. To help patients maintain good nutrition, it is important to alter the eating environment and provide a variety of foods.

People with Alzheimer's disease are at risk for developing protein and calorie malnutrition because of poor food intake and increased energy needs. As the disease progresses, a loss of weight and muscle mass is common. One study found, however, that patients were able to maintain their weight if they were given a diet that provided 35 calories per kilogram of body weight.[3] Emphasis must be placed on providing meals and snacks that supply adequate calories throughout the day.

Fish and Fish Oils

The brain is especially rich in DHA (docosahexaenoic acid), a polyunsaturated fat. This fat is also plentiful in oily fish. DHA contributes to the fluidity of brain cell membranes, allowing nutrients to pass in and out. DHA is also used to produce eicosanoids, powerful compounds that regulate the blood, hormones and immune system. Free radical molecules can damage DHA in cell membranes, so it is important to constantly supply the body with these fatty acids.

Omega-3 fatty acids (alpha-linolenic acid) from vegetable oils can be converted to DHA in the body, but this conversion is thought to be inefficient and can be sluggish with high intakes of animal fat and processed, oily foods. In fact, one study found that a diet high in saturated animal fat increased the risk of Alzheimer's disease, whereas fish consumption reduced it.[4] Studies suggest that an optimal balance of omega-3 and omega-6 fats can help improve mood, cooperation, appetite, sleep and short-term memory in people with Alzheimer's disease.[5]

To increase your intake of the omega-3 fats, especially DHA, eat fish three times a week. Salmon, trout, mackerel, sardines, herring, pickerel and fresh tuna are the best choices. Aim to include 2 tablespoons (30 ml) of one or a combination of the following oils in your daily diet: flaxseed, walnut, canola and Udo's Choice Ultimate Oil Blend (available in health food stores). With the exception of canola oil, these oils should not be used for high-heat cooking. Use in salad dressings and smoothies or add them to hot foods after cooking.

Vitamins and Minerals
Vitamin B12 and Folate
Studies consistently find that low levels of these two B vitamins are associated with Alzheimer's disease.[6,7] Vitamin B12 is crucial for maintaining healthy nerves. Some of the signs of a B12 deficiency are similar to those of Alzheimer's disease. Without adequate B12, the body is unable to use folate (folic acid) and, eventually, a folate deficiency will occur.

All animal foods contain B12: meat, poultry, fish, clams, eggs and dairy products. Fortified soy and rice beverages are also a good source of the vitamin. Adults over the age of 50 are advised to get their vitamin B12 from a supplement or fortified foods, since these are well absorbed by the body. Folate-rich foods include spinach, lentils, orange juice, whole grains, fortified breakfast cereals, asparagus, artichoke, avocado and seeds. In addition to choosing foods rich in B vitamins, take a high-potency multivitamin and mineral pill or a B complex supplement. Both formulas will supply anywhere from 25 to 100 micrograms of B12 and from 400 to 1000 micrograms of folic acid.

Vitamin E
This potent antioxidant nutrient appears to prevent free radical damage to the brain caused by beta-amyloid, the protein structures found abundantly in the brains of patients with Alzheimer's disease. It is thought that this free radical damage contributes to the progressive decline in brain function seen in Alzheimer's patients and, therefore, antioxidants may be an important tool in the prevention and treatment of the disease. A number of studies, including one that lasted two years, have found that vitamin E supplements helped slow the progression of Alzheimer's disease.[8-10]

The daily dose of vitamin E used in studies with Alzheimer's patients is 2000 international units (IU) of synthetic vitamin E or 1340 IU of natural vitamin E. If you do not have Alzheimer's disease, 200 to 800 IU of natural source vitamin E per day is recommended for antioxidant protection. Although vegetable oils, almonds, peanuts, soybeans, whole grains, wheat germ, avocado and green leafy vegetables provide vitamin E, it is not possible to consume much more than 50 IU through a normal diet. High-dose vitamin E may increase the risk of bleeding when taken with blood-thinning medications. Be sure to inform your physician if you are taking high-dose vitamin E.

Vitamin D and Calcium
Patients with Alzheimer's disease have lower bone mass and are at increased risk for falls and hip fractures.[11] The fact that most patients are deprived of sunlight and do not get adequate vitamin D in their diet puts them at a high risk for vitamin D deficiency. Elderly patients require 1200 milligrams of calcium and 400 to 600 IU of vitamin D each day. For a detailed list of food sources of these two nutrients, see Chapter 4.

Supplements are recommended to help prevent bone loss caused by poor intakes of vitamin D and calcium. Most multivitamin and mineral supplements supply 400 IU of vitamin D. Choose a calcium supplement made from calcium citrate, and be sure to buy a product with vitamin D added. Take 300 milligrams of calcium one to three times per day, depending on your calcium intake from foods. To determine the need for separate vitamin D supplements, ask your doctor to measure your blood vitamin D levels.

Herbal Remedies

Ginkgo Biloba

This herb is said to improve memory loss and slow the progression of Alzheimer's disease. A 52-week study looked at the effects of ginkgo in 309 patients with mild to moderate dementia as a result of Alzheimer's disease or stroke.[12] Patients were given either 40 milligrams of ginkgo (a special extract called EGb 761) three times daily or a placebo pill. After one year, the placebo group showed a decline in cognitive function whereas the ginkgo group did not. When the researchers looked at Alzheimer's patients only, there were modest but significant changes in memory and other brain functions. Other studies lasting three to six months have also found ginkgo to be an effective treatment in mild to moderate Alzheimer's dementia.[13,14]

A number of studies suggest that ginkgo increases circulation and oxygen delivery to the brain.[15] The herb's active ingredients make blood cells called platelets less sticky. By doing so, circulation becomes more efficient. Ginkgo also has a strong antioxidant effect in the brain, which may also have a positive effect in Alzheimer's disease.

Choose a product that is standardized to contain 24 percent ginkgo flavone glycosides and 6 percent terpene lactones. The EGb 761 extract used in scientific research is sold as Ginkoba® (Pharmaton® Natural Health Products) in Canada and the United States. For dementia, the recommended dose is 120 to 240 milligrams daily, in three divided doses.

Ginkgo biloba has slight blood-thinning effects. When combined with medications (aspirin) and/or supplements with similar effects (vitamin E, garlic), there is a potential for bleeding problems. Be sure to inform your primary care giver about any supplement you are taking.

Gotu Kola (*Centella asiatica*)

This herb may help improve memory, although it has not been studied in Alzheimer's disease to the same extent as has ginkgo biloba. Some evidence suggests that the herb's active ingredients, asiaticosides, can protect nerve cells from the toxic effects of beta-amyloid structures and therefore may have a role in treating Alzheimer's dementia.[16]

Buy a product standardized to 40 percent asiaticoside and 30 percent asiatic acid. The usual dosage is 20 to 60 milligrams three times daily. To make the herbal tea, steep 600 grams of dried leaves in 150 milliliters of boiling water for five to ten minutes. Drink three times daily. High doses of gotu kola may cause sun sensitivity and high blood pressure in some individuals. Pregnant women should not use this herb.

Other Natural Health Products

Acetyl-L-Carnitine

Carnitine is an amino acid found in all body cells, where it is used to metabolize fatty acids into energy. Carnitine also clears toxic accumulations of fatty acids from cells and serves as a building block for acetylcholine, a memory neurotransmitter. A number of studies involving more than 1400 people have found that one form of carnitine, acetyl-L-carnitine, can slow the progression of Alzheimer's disease.[17-21] It seems to have a small beneficial effect on short-term memory, especially in patients under 65 years of age.

The typical dosage is 1000 milligrams (1 gram) taken two or three times daily. Be sure to buy acetyl-L-carnitine and not one of its other chemical forms (L-carnitine or propionyl-carnitine). Acetyl-L-carnitine is available in the United States but it is not legally available in Canada. However, some health food stores do stock it. Do not take D-carnitine or DL-carnitine, which can cause heart and muscle dysfunction.

Lecithin (Phosphatidylcholine)

Lecithin and phosphatidylcholine supplements supply the body with choline, a member of the B vitamin family. Once ingested, choline becomes incorporated into the membranes of cells. In the brain, choline also acts as a building block for acetylcholine, a brain chemical involved in memory. People with Alzheimer's disease have been found to have lower levels of the enzyme needed to convert choline into acetylcholine. Extra consumption of lecithin or phosphatidylcholine may assist in the production of memory neurotransmitters. Although studies suggest that such a supplement may provide only a small benefit, lecithin and phosphatidylcholine are very safe and pose no risk to health.[22,23]

To get the most choline, buy a supplement labeled phosphatidylcholine. A typical dose is 1200 to 2220 milligrams per day, taken in divided doses.

Phosphatidylserine

Phosphatidylserine belongs to a family of chemical compounds known as phospholipids, important structural components of all cell membranes. Phospholipids also regulate the passage of nutrients and waste products in and out of cells.

The evidence for using this supplement in Alzheimer's disease is quite good. A number of studies that have lasted up to six months have shown that supplements of phosphatidylserine slow the progression of Alzheimer's disease.[24-26] Compared with patients taking placebo pills,

phosphatidylserine users do significantly better on tests of cognitive function. These supplements also seem to help ease feelings of depression in people with Alzheimer's disease. The standard dosage is 100 milligrams taken two or three times daily.

Nutrition Strategy Checklist for Alzheimer's Disease

- ☐ Three meals plus two to three snacks to maintain weight
- ☐ Fish
- ☐ Healthy oils
- ☐ Multivitamin/mineral
- ☐ B complex supplement
- ☐ Vitamin E
- ☐ Vitamin D
- ☐ Calcium
- ☐ Ginkgo biloba* OR Gotu kola
- ☐ Lecithin (phosphatidylcholine)
- ☐ Phosphatidylserine

*Strongest evidence; start here

Recommended Resources

www.alz.org
Alzheimer's Association
919 N Michigan Avenue, Suite 1100
Chicago, IL, USA 60611-1676
Tel: 312-335-8700 or 1-800-272-3900
Fax: 312-335-1110

www.alzheimer.ca
Alzheimer Society of Canada
20 Eglinton Avenue W, Suite 1200
Toronto, ON, Canada M4R 1K8
Tel: 416-488-8772 or 1-800-616-8816 (Canada only)
Fax: 416-488-3778

www.alz.co.uk/
Alzheimer's Disease International
45/46 Lower Marsh
London, UK SE1 7RG
Tel: 44-20-7621-3011
Fax: 44-20-7401-7351

Anemia

Anemia, a Latin word, literally means "too little blood." It refers to any condition in which too few red blood cells are present, or the red blood cells are too small or contain too little hemoglobin, the pigment that transports oxygen throughout the body. Anemia lowers the oxygen-carrying capacity of the blood and starves tissues in your body of the energy they need to function properly. Anemia affects the whole body, causing fatigue, shortness of breath, lack of energy and many other complications.

What Causes Anemia?

There are several kinds of anemia, but the most common and severe type is iron-deficiency anemia. The mineral iron is essential for making hemoglobin, the main component of red blood cells. Your body uses its iron supply very efficiently. It recycles the mineral from dead red blood cells to produce new ones. If you eat a healthy, well-balanced diet, chances are you are getting enough iron to ensure healthy red blood cell production.

There are, however, circumstances when normal dietary intake is not sufficient to maintain your iron stores. In adults, the main cause of iron deficiency is blood loss. Conditions that result in chronic or repeated bleeding, such as nosebleeds, hemorrhoids, certain cancers, ulcers or other gastrointestinal problems, will deplete iron stores and may eventually lead to anemia. Anemia can also develop because of a sudden blood loss caused by an injury or surgery.

Anemia is often a side effect of chronic disease, especially in the elderly. Health conditions such as infection, inflammation and cancer will suppress red blood cell production and deprive the developing cells of much needed iron. Deficiencies of folate and vitamin B12 can also cause anemia. Shortchanging your body of these vitamins affects your red blood cells differently than does a lack of iron.

Symptoms

Iron-deficiency anemia is a progressive condition. It usually develops in stages, so it can be months or even years before symptoms appear. Anemia ranges from mild to severe, and the symptoms also vary accordingly. The main symptoms of anemia include fatigue, weakness, loss of appetite, loss of energy, shortness of breath and increased susceptibility to infection. It's important to keep in mind that you may feel these symptoms even if you are not classified as "anemic." A marginal iron deficiency can affect your energy levels too, although not as severely.

Tongue irritation, cracks at the side of the mouth and spoonlike deformities in the fingernails also may result from iron deficiency. Some people with anemia develop pica, a craving for nonfood substances such as ice, dirt or pure starch. In young children, iron deficiency may cause irreversible abnormalities in brain development, resulting in impaired attention span, cognitive function and learning ability.

Who's at Risk?

If you fall into any of the following categories, you're at risk for developing iron-deficiency anemia:

- You're a female
- You're pregnant
- You engage in regular endurance exercise (e.g., long-distance running, triathlons)
- You follow a low-calorie diet (less than 1300 calories daily)
- You're a vegetarian

All women of reproductive age are at risk of developing iron deficiency, even more so if their diet lacks iron-rich foods. Women who are pregnant or breastfeeding are also predisposed to anemia because of the additional demands of the growing baby and placenta. Female runners or triathletes lose iron through sweat and can become iron deficient, especially if their diet lacks iron. Any woman who reduces her calorie intake to lose weight or eats an unbalanced vegetarian diet is also at risk.

Infants are born with sufficient stores of iron, but this iron supply becomes depleted during the first few months of life. For this reason pediatricians recommend that infants receive additional iron from iron-fortified cereals or formulas from the time they are six months of age.

Conventional Treatment

Anemia is treated by stopping the source of blood loss and rebuilding the body's nutrient stores through the use of supplements and diet. In most cases, iron supplements are prescribed as a short-term therapy for iron deficiency (you'll read more about this below).

When anemia is severe or the blood loss is rapid, a blood transfusion may be required to immediately replenish iron supplies. If excessive menstrual bleeding or another uterine problem is causing your anemia, your doctor may prescribe oral contraceptives to reduce your monthly blood flow.

The other types of vitamin-deficiency anemia are treated with a daily regimen of vitamin supplements. People with vitamin B12 and folic acid deficiency must take supplements for their entire life. Anemia caused by medical disorders or chronic disease usually disappears once the underlying cause of the condition is addressed.

Preventing and Treating Iron-Deficiency Anemia

Vitamins and Minerals

Iron

You learned above how iron helps carry oxygen throughout the body and releases it to tissues, where it is used for energy. To help prevent the signs and symptoms of an iron deficiency, it is critical that everyone, especially women, consume adequate amounts of iron every day. To learn your daily requirements, refer to page 55, Chapter 4.

The richest sources of iron are beef, fish, poultry, pork and lamb. These are heme sources of iron, the type that can be absorbed and utilized the most efficiently by your body. Heme sources of iron contribute about 10 percent of the iron we consume each day. Even though heme iron accounts for such a small proportion of our intake, it is so well absorbed that it actually contributes a significant amount of iron.

The rest of our iron comes from plant foods such as dried fruits, whole grains, leafy green vegetables, nuts, seeds and legumes. These are nonheme sources of iron, and the body is much less efficient in absorbing and using this type of iron. Vegetarians may have difficulty maintaining healthy iron stores because their diet relies exclusively on nonheme sources.

Iron Supplements
To help you meet your daily iron requirements, a multivitamin and mineral supplement is a wise idea. Most formulas provide 10 milligrams, but you can find multivitamins that provide up to 18 milligrams of the mineral.

If you are diagnosed with iron-deficiency anemia, your doctor will prescribe single iron pills. Depending on the extent of your iron deficiency, you may take one to three iron tablets (each containing 50 to 100 milligrams of elemental iron) per day. If you are advised to take an iron pill, take it on an empty stomach to enhance absorption. A supplementation period of 6 to 12 weeks is usually sufficient to treat anemia. However, you may need to take the supplements for up to six months to completely restore your body's iron reserves.

When it comes to iron supplements, more is *not* better. Excessive doses of iron can be quite toxic, causing damage to the liver and intestines, even death. Do not take iron supplements without having a blood test to confirm that you are suffering from an iron deficiency.

Enhancing Absorption of Nonheme Iron

Animal Foods   Meat, poultry and fish contain not only the most bio-available heme iron but also a special component, called MFP factor, that promotes the absorption of nonheme iron from other foods eaten with them. So, to absorb more iron from your brown rice stir-fry, throw in a little lean beef.

Vitamin C   Adding a vitamin-C-rich food to a plant-based meal can enhance the body's absorption of nonheme iron fourfold. Vitamin C is the most potent promoter of nonheme iron absorption. The acidity of the vitamin converts iron to the ferrous form that's ready for absorption (your stomach acid enhances iron absorption in the same way).

Calcium   Calcium and iron are absorbed the same way in the gut, so they compete with one another for transport across the intestinal tract. However, research has shown that taking a calcium supplement with meals for up to six months does not affect iron levels in healthy adults. But if you are taking calcium supplements *and* iron pills to treat anemia, it is advisable to take them at separate times.

Tea   Natural compounds in teas called tannins can bind with iron and make it unavailable for absorption. If you are a tea drinker, enjoy your cup of tea between meals rather than during. Or add a little milk or lemon to your cup of tea, since both inactivate the iron-binding properties of tannins.

Phytate-Rich Foods   Phytates are found in dietary fiber, nuts, spinach and other leafy vegetables and can bind to iron, inhibiting its absorption. The recommended intake for dietary fiber (25 to 35 grams per day) is not associated with impaired iron absorption. You would have to be eating a diet that is extremely high in fiber (50 grams or more each day) before you would interfere with the body's absorption of minerals. Cooking vegetables like spinach releases some of the iron that's bound to phytates. For this reason, cooked vegetables are always a better source of minerals than their raw counterparts.

Preventing and Treating Other Types of Anemia

Vitamins and Minerals

Folate

An ongoing deficiency of this important B vitamin leads to what is known as macrocytic or megaloblastic anemia. When your body lacks folate as a result of poor diet, impaired absorption or an unusually high need for the vitamin, metabolism of rapidly dividing red blood cells is slowed down. The red blood cells that do form are immature and cannot efficiently carry oxygen and travel through the tiny blood vessels.

To help prevent anemia associated with a folate deficiency, aim to meet your recommended dietary allowance (RDA) for folate (see page 31 Chapter 4). The best food sources include spinach, lentils, orange juice, whole grains, fortified breakfast cereals, asparagus, artichoke, avocado and seeds.

Folic Acid Supplements

Folate refers to the B vitamin in its natural form in foods. Folic acid describes the synthetic vitamin found in supplements or fortified foods like breakfast cereal. It can be challenging to meet your daily folate requirements through diet alone. To make sure you are meeting your requirements, take a daily multivitamin and mineral pill. Select a product that has 0.4 to 1.0 milligram (400 to 1000 micrograms) of folic acid. Vitamin B complex supplements provide all eight B vitamins in one pill and will also give you this amount of folic acid.

If you decide to take a separate folic acid supplement, buy one with vitamin B12, since these two nutrients work closely together (that's why I prefer a high-potency multi or a B complex). The body uses folic acid to activate B12 and vice versa. So a deficiency of one vitamin will eventually lead to a deficiency of the other. If you supplement with folic acid and don't pay attention to meeting your B12 requirements, you can hide an underlying B12 deficiency.

Vitamin B12

A lack of B12 can lead to an anemia called pernicious anemia. It's caused by impaired B12 absorption, rather than a poor dietary intake. After you consume B12 from your diet, the acid in your stomach helps to release the vitamin from proteins in food. B12 then binds to an intrinsic factor that enables B12 to be absorbed into the bloodstream. Some people produce an insufficient amount of hydrochloric acid in their stomach. This condition is particularly common in older adults. Without enough stomach acid, B12 can't be released from food proteins, and it won't be absorbed into the blood.

Some people inherit a defective gene for intrinsic factor and don't produce this necessary factor that attaches to B12 and delivers it into the bloodstream. A B12 deficiency caused by a lack of intrinsic factor leads to pernicious anemia, which is characterized by a deficit of red blood cells, muscle weakness and nerve damage. Most doctors prefer to treat pernicious anemia with injections of vitamin B12, although oral supplements may also be effective. A recent study found that taking a B12 supplement that dissolved under the tongue, twice daily, was as effective as shots in restoring B12 levels.[1]

Vitamin B12 is found naturally exclusively in animal foods: meat, poultry, fish, clams, eggs and dairy products. Fortified soy and rice beverages also supply vitamin B12.

B12 Supplements

If you are a strict vegetarian who eats no animal products and you don't drink fortified soy or rice beverages, take a B12 supplement. Anyone over the age of 50 should be getting vitamin B12 from a supplement or fortified foods, since up to one-third of older adults are inefficient at absorbing B12 from food.

If you take certain medications, you should consider taking extra B12. If you suffer from reflux or ulcers and take acid blockers (e.g., Tagamet®, Zantac®, Pepcid®), your body may not absorb enough B12 (as well as iron). Metformin® used to manage type 2 diabetes and polycystic ovary syndrome can also deplete B12 levels. If you take these medications, your doctor should monitor your blood periodically for signs of anemia.

To get adequate B12, take a good multivitamin and mineral supplement or a B complex supplement that contains the whole family of B vitamins. If you take a single B12 supplement, take 500 to 1000 micrograms once daily. If you are taking a high-dose B12 supplement to correct a deficiency, don't take it with a vitamin C pill. Large amounts of vitamin C can destroy B12. Take your vitamin C supplement one hour after you take your B12.

Nutrition Strategy Checklist for Preventing Anemia

- ☐ Iron-rich foods
- ☐ Vitamin-C-rich foods with nonheme iron
- ☐ Animal foods with nonheme iron (nonvegetarians)
- ☐ Multivitamin/mineral
- ☐ Foods rich in folate
- ☐ Foods rich in vitamin B12
- ☐ B complex supplement

Recommended Resources

www.familydoctor.org
American Academy of Family Physicians
11400 Tomahawk Creek Parkway
Leawood, KS, USA 66211-2672

www.merckhomeedition.com
Merck & Co., Inc.
One Merck Drive
P.O. Box 100
Whitehouse Station, NJ, USA 08889-0100

Angina

As heart disease narrows the arteries that feed the heart, the flow of oxygen-rich blood is gradually reduced. One of the first indications that your heart is not receiving enough oxygen is often a recurring pain. This pain is known as angina. Angina feels like a squeezing, pressing or aching pressure that starts behind your breastbone. The pain may travel to your left shoulder, down your left arm or through your back. Some people feel the discomfort of angina in their jaw, throat or teeth. There are two types of angina: stable and unstable. These are discussed in more detail below. (See also Heart Disease and High Blood Cholesterol.)

What Causes Angina?

Angina is usually triggered by physical activity. The pain usually lasts less than five minutes and eases off when you rest or stop exerting yourself. Emotional stress, heavy meals, alcohol, cigarette smoking or rapid changes in temperature can also provoke angina.

Although angina pain may be worrisome, it does not mean that you are having a heart attack. Episodes of angina rarely cause permanent or irreversible damage to your heart muscle. However, angina does indicate that you are feeling the early effects of coronary heart disease and that fatty deposits may be building up on your coronary arteries.

When angina symptoms are mild to moderate and develop fairly predictably at a certain level of exertion, you have what is known as stable angina. If your angina symptoms change, becoming more frequent, lasting longer or affecting you even when you are at rest, your condition has become unstable. Unstable angina is a sign that your coronary heart disease has progressed rapidly and may indicate that an artery is blocked or ruptured. Under these circumstances, the risk of heart attack is quite high, and you should seek medical attention immediately.

Symptoms

Symptoms of angina include

- squeezing pressure in the chest, behind the breastbone
- discomfort in the left arm, left shoulder, back, throat, jaw or teeth
- pain during exercise or physical activity
- pain that becomes worse after heavy meals, changes of temperature, drinking alcohol, smoking cigarettes or during times of emotional stress

- pain lasting only a few minutes and easing off when you rest

There is some indication that men and women experience angina symptoms quite differently. Men tend to describe angina pain as crushing or squeezing, while women feel it more as a vague discomfort that doesn't go away, even with rest. Women may also experience fatigue or shortness of breath during exercise or exertion, rather than feeling actual pain or discomfort. As a result, heart disease in women is harder to detect and often is not diagnosed until the disease is advanced.

Who's at Risk?

People with elevated levels of blood cholesterol and triglycerides are at risk for angina, as are those who smoke cigarettes. People with a family history of heart disease are also at greater risk.

Conventional Treatment

Any lifestyle modification that helps lower the risk of heart disease can help treat angina—quitting smoking, reducing alcohol intake, eating a low-fat diet, controlling your weight and controlling diabetes. Following a moderate exercise program will improve heart function. Keep in mind that you should increase exercise gradually and avoid sudden bursts of effort. Medications may be prescribed to reduce blood pressure. Medications to reduce angina pain include

- nitroglycerin to relieve pain by widening blood vessels

- beta-blockers to slow the heart rate and reduce the force of the heart's pumping action

- calcium channel blockers to reduce the frequency and severity of angina attacks

Managing Angina
Dietary Strategies
Dietary Fat
Eating a diet that's low in animal fat can help prevent the build-up of fatty deposits on artery walls. Diets high in animal fat raise your risk for heart disease by increasing your level of blood cholesterol. Animal foods contain mostly saturated fat, a type of fat that inhibits the activity of receptors on cells so that cholesterol is not cleared efficiently from the bloodstream. To reduce your intake of saturated fat, choose lean cuts of meat, poultry breast, 1 percent or skim milk, yogurt with less than 2 percent milk fat and cheese with less than 20 percent milk fat.

The other type of fat to avoid is trans fat, found in foods made with hydrogenated vegetable oils. The chemical process of hydrogenation makes a fat more saturated and forms trans fats. Many researchers believe that trans fat is worse for our cholesterol levels than saturated fat. (See Chapter 3 for more on trans fat.) The easiest way to reduce your intake of trans fat is to pay attention to food labels and ingredients lists. Look for the words "hydrogenated vegetable oils." Eat foods that contain such oils less often. As much as 40 percent of the fat in foods like french fries, fast food, doughnuts, pastries, snack foods and commercial cookies is trans fat. If you eat margarine, choose one that's made with nonhydrogenated fat. You'll find more dietary strategies to keep your cholesterol levels in check on page 327, Heart Disease and High Blood Cholesterol.

Vitamins and Minerals
B Vitamins
These nutrients won't lower your cholesterol, but they will help keep your homocysteine level at a healthy level. (A high level of homocysteine is

associated with a higher risk of heart attack.) To prevent homocysteine from accumulating and damaging blood vessels, the body uses three B vitamins—folate, B6 and B12—to convert it into other harmless compounds. One simple strategy to lower elevated homocysteine levels is to boost your intake of these three B vitamins. You'll learn your daily requirements and good food sources of B6, B12 and folate in Chapter 4.

If you have difficulty eating a varied diet, I recommend taking a good-quality multivitamin and mineral supplement to ensure you're getting your daily B vitamins. If you're looking for more B vitamins than a regular multi will give, choose a high-potency or super formula that contains 25 to 100 milligrams of B vitamins (or micrograms in the case of folic acid and B12).

Vitamin C

Vitamin C may protect from heart disease by acting as an antioxidant. The vitamin is able to neutralize harmful free radical molecules before they can damage your bad LDL cholesterol. This means that LDL cholesterol is less likely to accumulate on artery walls. Studies also suggest that vitamin C may inhibit the formation of blood clots by reducing the stickiness of platelets.

The recommended dietary allowance (RDA) is 75 and 90 milligrams for women and men respectively (smokers need an extra 35 milligrams). The best food sources include citrus fruit, citrus juices, cantaloupe, kiwi, mango, strawberries, broccoli, Brussels sprouts, cauliflower, red pepper and tomato juice. To supplement, buy a 500 or 600 milligram supplement of Ester C. Take once or twice daily. The daily upper limit for vitamin C is 2000 milligrams.

Vitamin E

This vitamin is a potent antioxidant that protects LDL cholesterol particles from oxygen damage caused by free radicals. Vitamin E may also inhibit blood clot formation and preserve the health of blood vessels that feed the heart. Large studies have found that vitamin E supplements can lower the risk of heart attack in healthy men and women, but the evidence for its protective effect is less clear in individuals with heart disease.[1,2] One large study has found that vitamin E had no effect on future heart attacks in people with advanced heart disease.[3]

Despite the conflicting findings, adding vitamin E to your daily regime certainly can't hurt, and it may help. To get the amount of vitamin E deemed protective, you must take a supplement. Take 200 to 800 international units (IU) per day. Buy a natural source vitamin E supplement. Although the body absorbs both synthetic and natural source vitamin E equally well, the liver prefers the natural form and incorporates more of it into LDL particles.

If you're taking a blood-thinning medication like warfarin (Coumadin®), don't take vitamin E without your doctor's approval, since it has slight anticlotting properties.

Magnesium

Many studies have reported lower magnesium levels in people with angina. Some studies have even found that the greater the degree of deficiency, the more severe the angina attacks.[4] While most studies have given patients magnesium through intravenous administration, a few have used oral supplements and reported fewer angina attacks and improved exercise tolerance.[5-7] Magnesium is thought to act like a calcium channel drug (a prescription heart medication), although much less powerfully. Magnesium is able to block calcium from entering heart cells.

The best food sources of magnesium are nuts, seeds, legumes, prunes, whole grains, leafy green vegetables, Brewer's yeast, cheddar cheese and shrimp. To supplement, buy a product made from magnesium citrate, aspartate, succinate, fumarte or gluconate. The body absorbs these forms of the mineral more efficiently. Taking

more than 350 milligrams of magnesium in a supplement can cause diarrhea, nausea and stomach cramps. If you have severe heart disease, do not take magnesium without your doctor's approval.

Herbal Remedies

Hawthorn (species *Crataegus*)

The active components in this plant, flavonoids and procyanidins, act on the heart by increasing the force of contraction, lengthening the period between heartbeats, reducing oxygen use and increasing nerve transmission.[8] The herb may also improve blood flow by dilating blood vessels.

There is a substantial amount of evidence for hawthorn's beneficial effects in congestive heart failure, and some experts believe it is also useful in angina. To supplement, buy a product standardized to contain between 2 and 3 percent flavonoids or 18 to 20 percent procyanidins. Take 100 to 300 milligrams three times daily. It may take six to eight weeks for the herb to reach its full effect. Hawthorn can interact with certain heart medications; check with your pharmacist. If you are on certain heart drugs, take hawthorn only under your physician's supervision. *Do not* take hawthorn with digitalis.

Other Natural Health Products

Coenzyme Q10

This substance, manufactured by the body, is found inside virtually every cell. Coenzyme Q10 (CoQ10) helps cells produce important molecules of energy called ATP (adenosine triphosphate). Research has found that supplemental CoQ10 can improve exercise tolerance in people with stable angina.[9]

Buy a CoQ10 supplement in an oil base (rather than dry-powder tablets or capsules) as these are more available to the body. Take 50 milligrams, three times a day. Cholesterol-lowering medications such as lovastatin (Mevacor®), simvastatin (Zocor®), pravastatin (Pravachol®) and cerivastatin (Baycol™) have been shown to reduce blood levels of CoQ10. Whether this affects heart health is not yet known, but it may be wise to take CoQ10 supplements if you are on these drugs.

L-Propionyl-Carnitine

Carnitine is an amino acid found in all body cells, where it is used to metabolize fatty acids into energy. Carnitine appears to help the heart produce energy more efficiently and, as a result, use less oxygen. A number of studies have found that individuals with angina who took L-propionyl-carnitine supplements improved in several measures of heart function, including the ability to exercise without chest pain.[10-16] Some studies found that people were able to reduce the dose of their heart medications.

Most studies use the form of carnitine called L-propionyl-carnitine. Look for this one in a good health food or supplement store. If you can't find it, use L-carnitine. L-carnitine is available in the United States but is not legally available in Canada. However, some health food stores do stock it. Take 1000 milligrams, two or three times daily. The supplement is considered to be very safe. Do not take D-carnitine or DL-carnitine, which can cause heart and muscle dysfunction.

Nutrition Strategy Checklist for Angina

- ☐ Low saturated- and trans-fat diet
- ☐ High-potency multivitamin/mineral OR B complex
- ☐ Vitamin C
- ☐ Vitamin E
- ☐ Magnesium
- ☐ Coenzyme Q10
- ☐ L-propionyl-carnitine

Recommended Resources

www.americanheart.org
American Heart Association
7272 Greenville Avenue
Dallas, TX, USA 75231
Tel: 1-800-AHA-USA1 (1-800-242-8721)

www.heartandstroke.ca
Heart and Stroke Foundation of Canada
222 Queen Street, Suite 1402
Ottawa, ON, Canada K1P 5V9
Tel: 613-569-4361
Fax: 613-569-3278

www.nhlbi.nih.gov
National Institutes of Health
National Heart, Lung and Blood Institute
Information Center
P.O. Box 30105
Bethesda, MD, USA 20824-0105
Tel: 301-592-8573

Asthma

Asthma is one of the most commonly diagnosed illnesses in North America, affecting 13 percent of all Canadians aged 5 to 19.[1] It is a chronic lung condition that causes breathing difficulties, such as wheezing, coughing and shortness of breath. There is no cure for asthma, although it can be effectively controlled with medication and other management strategies.

What Causes Asthma?

People with asthma have very sensitive airways that become swollen and inflamed when exposed to irritants. During an asthmatic episode, the airways or bronchial tubes tighten, making it difficult for the lungs to force air in and out. This tightening and narrowing of the airways is known as bronchoconstriction and can be caused by contraction of the small muscles surrounding the bronchial tubes, swelling of airway linings or the production of excess mucus.

Asthma attacks are often provoked by triggers or stimuli that irritate the airways. These triggers usually vary from person to person and can include

- cold air or changes in weather or temperature
- exercising, crying, laughing
- food allergies
- stress or emotional upset
- cigarette smoke
- strong odors, strong fumes or other inhaled irritants

Although triggers may irritate the bronchial tubes, they usually don't cause the airways to become inflamed. Asthma symptoms that result from exposure to triggers tend to be immediate, short-lived and easy to reverse.

Asthmatic episodes may also be provoked by factors that cause both irritation *and* inflammation in the airways. Symptoms resulting from inflammation will usually last longer and are harder to reverse than those caused by triggers. The most common causes of airway inflammation are allergens: pollen, especially from grasses, weeds and trees; animal dander and secretions; molds and dust mites. Some allergens provoke an immediate asthmatic reaction by irritating the overly sensitive airways. However, in most cases, exposure to allergens is also accompanied by inflammation, which tends to develop over a longer period. This delay can make it very difficult to identify the factors causing the asthma. Asthmatic symptoms may not appear until four to eight hours after initial contact with the allergen or may reappear several hours after the initial asthma attack has been successfully treated. Respiratory infections such as colds and flu can also inflame the airways and cause an asthma attack.

Symptoms

Signs of an asthma attack include

- wheezing
- coughing
- shortness of breath or labored breathing
- chest tightness

Who's at Risk?

Asthma can develop at any age. The following people are more susceptible to developing the condition:

- individuals with a family history of asthma
- children—asthma affects up to 10 percent of children[2]
- young boys—during childhood, asthma affects twice as many boys as girls
- teenage girls—during adolescence, more girls than boys develop asthma
- babies born to women who smoke during pregnancy

Conventional Treatment

It is very important to minimize exposure to triggers of asthma. Washing sheets and blankets weekly in hot water, enclosing your mattress and box spring in plastic, not smoking in the house, not allowing pets in the house, reducing humidity in the house to keep dust mites and molds under control and avoiding the outside air during times of high pollen counts all help reduce the chance of an asthma attack.

A variety of medications are often used to relieve asthma symptoms. Bronchodilators (e.g., Ventolin®, Berotec®, Bricanyl®, Atrovent®, Theo-Dur®) relax the muscles around the airways and may be used just before exercising or before exposure to known triggers. These medications are not intended for long-term use, and they may cause asthma to worsen if they're used too often. Bronchodilators may produce side effects, such as trembling, nervousness and flushing.

Anti-inflammatory drugs are used to reduce and prevent airway inflammation, swelling and mucus production. These include both steroid (e.g., Beclovent®, Vanceril®, Becloforte®, Pulmicort®, Flovent®) and nonsteroidal (e.g., Intal®, Tilade®) drugs. They do not have an immediate effect and will not help in an asthma emergency. Steroid drugs may cause side effects, such as hoarseness and sore throat and yeast infections (thrush), which can be prevented by rinsing the mouth or gargling after use.

Leukotriene receptor antagonists (e.g., Accolate®, Singulair®) are the newest oral asthma medications on the market. These help prevent inflammation and protect against bronchoconstriction when taken before exercise or exposure to a trigger.

Managing Asthma

Dietary Strategies

Fruits and Vegetables

Be sure to eat at least five to ten servings of fruits and vegetables each day and include at least one citrus fruit in your daily diet. Evidence is mounting for the protective effects of fruits and vegetables on lung function.[3] One survey of over 46,000 people aged 15 and older determined that those with the highest intake of fruits and vegetables had a 30 percent lower risk of asthma compared with those who had the lowest intake of such foods.[4] It appears that fruits rich in vitamin C are especially helpful in reducing wheezing in children with asthma.[5] A study of 12-year-old asthma sufferers revealed that a vegetarian diet followed for one year provided a significant decrease in asthma symptoms and allowed medication to be drastically reduced or discontinued.[6]

Eating plenty of fruits and vegetables may prevent asthma in a few ways. These foods offer important vitamins, minerals and antioxidants that are needed for healthy lung function. But people who eat more produce also tend to eat more fiber and less fat, two habits that can help maintain a healthy body weight. Studies conducted among women found that weight gain in early adulthood significantly increases the risk of developing adult-onset asthma.[7,8] What's more, researchers have learned that when obese individuals with asthma lose weight, their asthma symptoms improve.[9] To learn what a healthy body weight is for adults, refer to page 439, Obesity and Weight Loss.

Fish Oils

Eating oily fish may also help prevent asthma and improve symptoms of asthma. Fish contains the omega-3 fatty acid DHA (docosahexaenoic acid), which is used by the body to produce anti-inflammatory compounds. Studies show that populations that consume fish as a regular part of their diet have improved lung function and lower rates of asthma.[10] Aim to eat fish three times a week. The best choices are salmon, trout, herring, mackerel, sardines and fresh tuna.

Sodium

A low-salt diet may also help provide symptom relief, since many asthmatics, especially males, appear to be salt-sensitive.[11] Evidence suggests that a high intake of salt may trigger spasm of bronchial smooth muscle and that a low-salt diet may even reduce the need for asthma medications.[12,13] But, be careful to consume no more than 2400 milligrams of sodium (1 teaspoon worth of salt) each day (see page 79, Chapter 5). As often as possible, avoid eating processed foods and adding salt to foods.

Food Allergies

Studies on food allergies reveal that reactions to certain foods can cause asthma symptoms, especially in children. To determine if food allergies trigger your or your child's asthma, try an elimination/challenge diet as outlined below. You may want to seek the help of a registered dietitian (**www.dietitians.ca**) to help determine food allergies.

1. *Elimination phase* For a period of two weeks, eliminate common food allergens—dairy products, soy foods, citrus fruits, nuts, wheat, shellfish, fish, eggs, corn and sulfite food additives.

2. *Challenge phase* After two weeks, start introducing one food every three days. Keep a food and symptom diary, in which you record everything you eat, amounts eaten and what time you ate the food or meal. Document any symptoms, the time of day you started to feel the symptom and the duration of time you felt the symptom. If symptoms recur when a particular food is added back, you or your child may be allergic. Consult your doctor for further food allergy testing.

Vitamins and Minerals

Vitamin B6

This vitamin may help lessen asthma symptoms in children. One study found that a B6 supplement provided significant improvement after the second month of treatment, and the children were able to reduce their dosage of asthma medication.[14,15] Studies in adults have not found such benefits. The best food sources of B6 include meat, poultry, fish, liver, legumes, nuts, seeds, whole grains, green leafy vegetables, bananas and avocados. A multivitamin and mineral supplement will provide extra B6. If you take a separate B6 pill, be sure to not exceed the daily upper limit (see page 30, Chapter 4). Taking high doses of vitamin B6 for an extended period has toxic effects and can cause irreversible nerve damage.

Vitamin B12

Since a deficiency of vitamin B12 may increase the body's reactivity to sulfite preservatives in food, this vitamin has been proposed as a possible treatment for asthma. To prevent a deficiency, ensure you are meeting your daily requirements by eating animal foods such as meat, poultry, fish, clams, eggs, dairy products and fortified soy and rice beverages and taking a multivitamin and mineral supplement. Separate B12 pills are very safe. The recommended dose for vegetarians who consume no animal products is 500 to 1000 micrograms per day.

Vitamin C

A number of studies point to the protective effects of vitamin C in asthma. This antioxidant vitamin is concentrated in the fluid that surrounds the lungs, where it acts to protect the lungs from free radical damage. Studies show that people with asthma tend to have lower levels of vitamin C in their lung fluid.[16,17] One study found that 2 grams of supplemental vitamin C reduced exercise-induced asthma in children and young adults.[18]

The best food sources of vitamin C include citrus fruit, strawberries, kiwi, cantaloupe, broccoli, bell peppers, Brussels sprouts, cabbage, tomatoes and potatoes. To supplement, take 500 milligrams of Ester C twice daily or a 1000 milligram time-released vitamin C pill once daily. For more information on vitamin C, see page 37, Chapter 4.

Magnesium

This mineral plays an important role in lung function by influencing the contraction-relaxation state of bronchial smooth muscle. Studies show that low dietary intakes of magnesium are linked with impaired lung function, spasms of the bronchial passageway and wheezing.[19] In one study, 40 percent of patients with asthma were deficient in magnesium.[20] Another study found that supplementing the diet with magnesium can help reduce asthma symptoms in people who are magnesium deficient.[21]

To prevent a magnesium deficiency, include the following foods in your diet: nuts, seeds, legumes, prunes, whole-grain cereals, leafy green vegetables, Brewer's yeast and dairy products. Keep in mind that much magnesium is lost in refining foods, so a diet high in refined or processed food will be lacking magnesium.

To supplement, take 150 to 200 milligrams of magnesium citrate, aspartate, succinate, fumarte or gluconate once or twice daily. Refer to page 47, Chapter 4, to learn the daily upper limits for children and adults. Taking more than your daily upper limit can cause diarrhea.

Herbal Remedies

Boswellia (*Boswellia serrata*)

This herbal product is derived from the resin of the Indian Boswellia tree. Although very few studies have been conducted using this herb, one double-blind trial did find that it reduced the frequency of asthma attacks and improved breathing capacity in adults with mild asthma when taken for six weeks.[22] Seventy percent of people taking the herb experienced improvement. Boswellia is thought to work by reducing inflammation.

The effective dosage was 300 milligrams three times daily. Buy a product standardized to contain 37.5 percent boswellic acids. It may take up to eight weeks to notice improvement in asthma symptoms once you start taking the herb. Boswellia has not been evaluated for safety in children or in pregnant or breastfeeding women.

Other Natural Health Products

Fish Oil Supplements

A handful of studies have found that fish-oil-enriched diets have a positive effect on asthma symptoms.[23-25] Fish oil capsules are a concentrated source of DHA and EPA, two omega-3 fatty acids that have anti-inflammatory functions in the body. Some research suggests that fish oil may help lessen asthmatic symptoms resulting from airborne triggers. Fish oil appears to benefit children with asthma more than it benefits adults with the condition.

The typical dosage is at least 3 grams of fish oil per day, taken in divided doses. Buy a product with a combination of DHA and EPA. Look for a supplement that has vitamin E added as it helps prevent the oils from going rancid. Avoid fish *liver* oil capsules. Fish liver oil is a concentrated source of vitamin A and D, which can be toxic when taken in large amounts for long periods.

Nutrition Strategy Checklist for Asthma

☐ Fruits and vegetables
☐ Fish
☐ Low-sodium/salt diet
☐ Identify food allergies
☐ Vitamin-B6-rich foods
☐ Vitamin C
☐ Magnesium
☐ Fish oil capsules

Recommended Resources
www.lungusa.org/asthma
American Lung Association
1740 Broadway
New York, NY, USA 10019
Tel: 212-315-8700

www.asthmasociety.com
www.asthma.ca
The Asthma Society of Canada
130 Bridgeland Avenue, Suite 425
Toronto, ON, Canada M6A 1Z4
Tel: 1-800-787-3880
Fax: 416-787-5807

www.lung.ca/asthma
The Canadian Lung Association
3 Raymond Street, Suite 300
Ottawa, ON, Canada K1R 1A3
Tel: 613-569-6411
Fax: 613-569-8860

www.nhlbi.nih.gov/health/public/lung/asthma
US Department of Health and Human Services
National Heart, Lung and Blood Institute
Information Center
P.O. Box 30105
Bethesda, MD, USA 20824-0105
Tel: 301-592-8573

Attention Deficit Hyperactivity Disorder (ADHD)

Attention deficit hyperactivity disorder (ADHD) is a neurobiological disability that can have a profound and disruptive effect on daily life. People with ADHD have difficulty sitting still, paying attention and controlling impulsive behavior. They tend to be hyperactive and easily distracted, and they often act before they think. These negative and persistent behavior patterns can create long-term problems at home, work and school, as well as in social settings.

The disorder affects up to 5 percent of school-age children and is one of the most commonly diagnosed childhood illnesses.[1] Children rarely outgrow ADHD. Statistics indicate that nearly 2 to 4 percent of the North American population exhibits ADHD symptoms throughout their adult years.[2] In adults, the disorder is referred to as attention deficit disorder residual type (ADD-RT).

What Causes ADHD?

While considerable research has been conducted into ADHD, the cause of the condition is still unknown and no cure has been found. ADHD frequently runs in families. Chemical changes that affect brain function, exposure to toxins before birth and brain injuries are other possible explanations that are currently under investigation.

Symptoms

ADHD can be difficult to pinpoint because nearly everyone experiences periods of restless behavior and a short attention span during his or her lifetime. The diagnosis is further complicated by the fact that ADHD symptoms are very similar to those of other disorders, such as anxiety, depression and certain learning disabilities. As a result, the guidelines for identifying ADHD are quite specific. Symptoms must be long lasting, occur with more-than-normal frequency, persist from childhood and affect the ability to function in at least two areas of life (home, school, work or social life).

There are three main types of ADHD, and the symptoms of each type may vary from person to person.

Primarily inattentive:

- makes careless mistakes
- does not seem to listen when spoken to
- does not maintain an attention span
- is disorganized
- is easily distracted
- has difficulty following instructions
- is forgetful

Primarily hyperactive/impulsive:

- fidgets or squirms constantly
- runs around excessively
- has difficulty sitting still for any length of time
- has difficulty behaving quietly
- talks excessively
- has difficulty waiting or taking turns
- interrupts others

Combined:

- exhibits characteristics of both inattentive and hyperactive/impulsive types of ADHD

Children with ADHD usually do not perform well at school, have trouble making friends and experience family conflicts. With adolescents, the problems become more severe, often causing low self-esteem, mood swings, higher injury rates, drug abuse, poor school performance and early pregnancy. Adults with ADHD often experience career difficulties, are disorganized, have difficulty planning ahead and struggle with interpersonal relationships.

Who's at Risk?

Research indicates that there is a genetic basis to ADHD; children are at increased risk for ADHD if the disorder has been diagnosed in other close relatives. ADHD may be more common in very low birth-weight infants (1500 grams or less). As well, boys are three times more likely than girls to develop ADHD.

On average, one child in every classroom in North America needs treatment for ADHD. While the number of children identified and treated for ADHD has risen in recent years, this is most likely the result of increased media attention and heightened awareness of the condition. There is no scientific evidence to prove that the prevalence of ADHD has actually increased.

Conventional Treatment

Conventional treatments for children with ADHD include

- behavior management
- educational assistance in the classroom
- educational program modification

- special placement outside regular classrooms
- parent education
- psychostimulant medications
- antidepressant and antihypertensive medications
- psychotherapy
- vocational counseling for adults

Although many children continue to demonstrate symptoms of ADHD into adulthood, studies indicate that those who receive adequate treatment at an early age will have fewer problems at school, will interact more appropriately with their peer group and will generally function better in their daily life.

Many parents have tried a number of nutritional interventions claimed to improve ADHD symptoms in their children. Unfortunately, at this time, there are no well-established nutritional treatments that have been consistently demonstrated to be effective in helping a large number of children with the condition. Below, I describe nutritional approaches that studies suggest may benefit some children.

Managing ADHD

Dietary Strategies

Amino Acids and Protein

Since many amino acids in protein foods provide the building blocks for neurotransmitters, it has been hypothesized that supplementing the diet with some of these could improve ADHD symptoms. Indeed, some research has found that compared with healthy children, those with ADHD have lower levels of tyrosine and tryptophan, two amino acids which help the brain synthesize neurotransmitters that regulate mood and cognitive function.[3] However, studies find no effect on symptoms when children and adults with ADHD were given large doses of these amino acids.[4,5]

Although supplement studies have not shown positive results, it is crucial that children and adults with ADHD meet their daily protein requirements. Tryptophan is considered an essential amino acid because it cannot be made by the body and so must be supplied by the diet. Once inside the brain, tryptophan is used to make serotonin, a brain chemical believed to have a calming, relaxing effect. Tyrosine serves as a building block for dopamine, a neurotransmitter associated with improved alertness and sharpened thinking. In Chapter 5, you'll find a food guide that will help you choose the right amount of protein-rich foods each day.

Breakfast

Many studies of both children and adults have shown that compared with breakfast eaters, individuals who skip the morning meal do not score as well on tests of mental performance that same morning.[6] What seems to be affected the most is the speed of information retrieval (a component of memory). Breakfast foods supply glucose in the bloodstream, which the brain cells use for energy. After a night of sleeping, we wake up in a fasting state. That means blood-glucose levels are low and need to be replenished.

Breakfast also supplies key nutrients in the diet, including important B vitamins, calcium and iron. Research has shown that when breakfast is skipped, these missing nutrients are usually not made up for later in the day. Below you'll read about the important role that iron plays in brain function.

The best breakfast includes carbohydrates for blood glucose and a little protein to help sustain energy levels longer. This is partly because protein takes longer to digest. That means the carbohydrate you eat with protein gets converted to glucose more slowly. Here are a few combinations to ensure your diet provides both nutrients:

- Whole-grain cereal with low-fat milk or calcium-fortified soy beverage. Top with fruit or have a small glass of citrus juice.

- Whole-grain toast with a poached or hard-boiled egg and a fruit salad.

- Homemade breakfast smoothie made with soy beverage or milk, orange juice and a banana. Add soy protein powder or egg whites for a protein boost.

- If breakfast is usually consumed while you're dashing out the door, grab a piece of fruit, a cereal bar and a low-fat yogurt for protein.

Essential Fatty Acids

It has been suggested that children with ADHD have altered fatty acid metabolism, since some of the symptoms of ADHD are similar to those observed in people with a fatty acid deficiency. The omega-3 and omega-6 oils in our diet provide two essential fatty acids that our body cannot make on its own. Omega-3 oils (flaxseed, canola, walnut) provide alpha-linolenic acid, and omega-6 oils (corn, sunflower, safflower, soybean) give us linoleic acid. These two essential fatty acids are used to form vital body structures and cell membranes, aid in both immune function and vision and produce powerful compounds called eicosanoids that help regulate inflammation, hormones and nerve and brain function.

Sixty percent of our brain's solid matter is composed of essential fatty acids, especially an omega-3 fatty acid called DHA that is derived from alpha-linolenic acid in the diet. These fats make up a large portion of the communicating membranes of the brain. Based on the knowledge that essential fatty acids are needed for proper brain development in growing children, a number of studies have investigated their relationship to ADHD.

Research has revealed that children with ADHD have lower concentrations of these important fats in their blood.[7-9] Studies have also shown that children with lower levels of essential fatty acids demonstrate significantly more behav-

ioral problems, temper tantrums and learning and sleep problems. It is unclear why some children with ADHD are lacking essential fatty acids. Factors such as poor dietary intake and faulty metabolism of these fats in the body have been proposed.

Children and adults should consume 2 tablespoons (30 ml) of oil rich in alpha-linolenic acid per day. Flaxseed, walnut and canola oil are the best sources. A commercial product called Udo's Choice Ultimate Oil Blend is available in health food stores. Udo's oil contains a balance of both alpha-linolenic and linoleic fatty acids from organic flaxseed, sesame and sunflower seeds, wheat germ, rice germ and oat germ. Flaxseed oil, walnut oil and Udo's oil should not be used for sautéing or frying as their essential fatty acids are easily destroyed by heat. Store the oil in the refrigerator and use in salad dressings, dips and smoothies or add to foods like pasta sauces and soups after cooking.

It is also important to minimize intake of saturated fats by choosing lean meat, poultry breast, lower-fat dairy products and processed foods made without hydrogenated vegetable oils, since the fatty acids in these foods can impede essential fatty acid metabolism.

The Feingold Diet and Food Additives

A food-additive-free diet has long been proposed for children with ADHD. The diet was initially developed by Dr. Benjamin Feingold for the treatment of aspirin sensitivity in adults, and it was later extended to manage hyperactivity and learning disability in children. Most studies have failed to find improvements in learning and attention problems in children on the Feingold Diet.[10-13] A few studies, however, suggest that eliminating food additives may be beneficial for some children, particularly with respect to irritability, restlessness and sleep disturbances.[14-17] Given that there is little harm in following such a diet, a trial period may serve to determine if food additives do, in fact, trigger or exacerbate symptoms of ADHD in your child.

The Feingold Diet promotes the elimination of most food additives and certain natural compounds in foods called salicylates. These substances resemble aspirin and are produced by plants as a natural pesticide. A few studies do suggest that salicylates influence the activity of phenolsulfotranserfase, an enzyme needed by the brain but also used in the gut to metabolize artificial colors and flavors.[18-20] Salicylates can be found in natural flavoring, natural coloring and aspirin. In addition, they occur naturally in a number of foods, including almonds, apples, apricots, berries, cherries, chili powder, cider, cloves, coffee, cucumbers, currants, grapes, nectarines, bell peppers, tea and tomatoes.

The Feingold Diet also recommends the elimination of synthetic food coloring and flavoring agents, as well as food preservatives. Foods, toiletries, cleaning supplies and art supplies that contain any such ingredients are to be avoided. As a first step, advocates of the diet recommend avoiding perfume, corn syrup, molasses, caramel color, MSG (monosodium glutamate), HVP (hydrolyzed vegetable protein), natural flavoring, processed foods containing oil, processed foods containing fruit concentrates, nitrites and sulfites.

For more information about the Feingold Diet, log on to **www.feingold.org**. This Web site defines the diet and food restrictions and lists a number of books that you may find useful.

Sugar and Sweeteners

Whether eliminating sugars and artificial sweeteners can help reduce ADHD symptoms remains controversial. In fact, the evidence does not support the notion that sugar causes hyperactivity.[21,22] In studies in which children were given high amounts of refined sugar and aspartame (NutraSweet®), behavior was not negatively affected.[23,24] Despite the fact that sugar does not seem to trigger or worsen symptoms, there

may be a small number of children who react to sugary foods. One study did find that sugar, but not aspartame, exacerbated inattention in children with ADHD but had no effect in children without the disorder.[25] In this study, sugar did not worsen aggressive behavior.

For overall good nutrition, it is wise to minimize the consumption of table sugar, soft drinks, fruit drinks, fruit leather, candy and other sweets. Parents should help children understand that these foods are considered treats and so should not be eaten on a regular basis.

Vitamins and Minerals

Iron

Iron is needed by the body to carry oxygen to the brain cells. It is also used to make brain neurotransmitters, especially the ones that regulate the ability to pay attention, which is crucial to memory and learning. A deficiency of iron can also directly affect mood, attention span and learning ability.

Existing data suggest that iron-deficiency anemia is a risk factor for poor educational performance in schoolchildren. Studies have shown that even when children have an iron deficiency that is not severe enough to be diagnosed as anemia, they score better on tests of verbal learning and memory when they're given extra iron.

Whether iron deficiency is involved in ADHD remains to be seen, but it is extremely important for children and adults to meet their daily requirements (see page 55, Chapter 4). Good food sources of iron include lean beef, whole-grain breakfast cereal, whole-grain breads, raisins, dried apricots, legumes, bean dips and bran muffins. Iron in plant foods (nonheme iron) is not absorbed as well as iron in animal foods (heme iron). To enhance the body's absorption of nonheme iron, include a vitamin-C-rich food with the meal. A children's multivitamin and mineral supplement taken once daily will also help ensure your child's iron needs are met. Avoid single iron pills unless your doctor has prescribed them to treat anemia.

Magnesium

Based on a number of studies that show depressed magnesium levels in the red blood cells and hair of children with ADHD, it's been suggested that magnesium supplements may be useful in treatment.[26] In one study, 50 children with ADHD and magnesium deficiency were given 200 milligrams of supplemental magnesium daily for six months.[27] At the end of the trial, the researchers noted an increase in magnesium levels in hair and a significant decrease in hyperactivity.

Good food sources of magnesium include nuts, seeds, legumes, prunes, whole grains, leafy green vegetables, Brewer's yeast, cheddar cheese and shrimp. For a detailed listing and daily requirements, refer to Chapter 4. If you opt for a supplement, buy one made from magnesium citrate, aspartate, succinate, fumarte or gluconate. The body absorbs these forms of magnesium more efficiently. Taking more than 350 milligrams of supplemental magnesium can cause diarrhea, nausea and stomach cramps.

Zinc

A zinc deficiency may play a role in the development of ADHD. Low levels of zinc may in some way contribute to essential fatty acid deficiency seen in some children with ADHD.[28] Some research also suggests that a zinc deficiency may cause children to be less responsive to certain medications used to treat ADHD.[29]

To prevent a zinc deficiency, reach for the following foods: oysters, seafood, red meat, poultry, yogurt, wheat bran, wheat germ, whole grains and enriched breakfast cereals. You'll find daily recommended intakes and a detailed food list in Chapter 4. Single zinc supplements are rarely appropriate for adults and should not be taken by

children. Too much zinc has toxic effects, including copper deficiency, heart problems, anemia and depressed immunity.

Herbal Remedies

Evening Primrose Oil
(*Oenothera biennis*)

The oil of evening primrose contains a fatty acid called gamma-linolenic acid (GLA) that might help children with ADHD. The essential fatty acid called linoleic acid is converted in the body to GLA with the help of an enzyme. GLA is then transformed into prostaglandins, compounds that regulate our blood, immune system and hormones. Some researchers believe that children with ADHD may have difficulty carrying out this conversion. Dietary components such as animal fat and hydrogenated vegetable oils can interfere with this conversion. The enzyme responsible for making GLA requires zinc, magnesium and vitamins B6 and C to function properly. A high-fat diet that's missing important vitamins and minerals can hamper GLA production and contribute to low levels of fatty acids in the body. It's also thought that the amount of GLA actually made may not be enough to cope with the requirement for prostaglandin formation.

Evening primrose oil is a concentrated source of GLA. Two studies found no effect on ADHD symptoms with a daily evening primrose oil supplement, possibly because the dosage used was too low and/or the duration of the study too short (only four weeks) to notice improvements.[30,31] However, findings from a recent double-blind study suggest that a supplement containing a mixture of fish oil and evening primrose oil might improve ADHD symptoms.[32] Evening primrose oil is very safe; very few side effects are reported in studies. Buy a product standardized to 9 percent GLA. The dosage for children is 1 to 2 grams taken twice daily.

Herbal Teas

The use of herbal teas may have a calming effect in children and adults with ADHD. Lemon balm, lavender and chamomile all have mild sedative and relaxing properties. Tea bags can be purchased at health food stores or you can obtain dried herbs from a licensed herbalist.

To make herbal tea, use 1 teaspoon (5 ml) of dried herb per 1 cup (250 ml) of hot water. Steep, covered, for 5 to 10 minutes for leaf or flowers, 10 to 20 minutes for roots. Drink one cup of tea two or three times a day. If the taste of the tea is a deterrent, speak to your natural health care provider about the availability of these herbs as alcohol-free tinctures. (See Chapter 6 for more on teas and tinctures.)

Nutrition Strategy Checklist for ADHD

- ☐ Eat breakfast daily
- ☐ Healthy oils
- ☐ Fish
- ☐ Avoid food additives
- ☐ Limit sugar and sweeteners
- ☐ Iron-rich foods
- ☐ Magnesium-rich foods
- ☐ Zinc-rich foods
- ☐ Evening primrose oil

Recommended Resources

www.add-toronto.org
ADD/ADHD Toronto
This site lists resources for adolescents, adults and the parents of children with ADHD. The resources include psychiatrists, pediatricians, psychologists, educators and ADD (attention deficit disorder) coaches. Listings are limited to Greater Toronto and southern Ontario.

www.chadd.org
Children and Adults with Attention Deficit/Hyperactivity Disorder (CHADD)

8181 Professional Place, Suite 201
Landover, MD, USA 20785
Tel: 301-306-7070
Fax: 301-306-7090

www.camh.net/CLARKEPages/index.html
Clarke Institute of Psychiatry
Communications Department
250 College Street
Toronto, ON, Canada M5T 1R8
Tel: 416-595-6878

www.nimh.nih.gov/publicat/adhd.cfm
National Institute of Mental Health
NIMH Public Inquiries
6001 Executive Boulevard, Room 8184, MSC 9663
Bethesda, MD, USA 20892-9663
Tel: 301-443-4513
Fax: 301-443-4279

www.ninds.nih.gov/health_and_medical/disorders/adhd.htm
National Institute of Neurological Disorders and Stroke

Breast Cancer

Breast cancer is the most common type of cancer among Canadian women. Over her lifetime, a woman has a 10.6 percent chance of getting breast cancer. This lifetime risk represents the average risk for the population of Canadian women. If you have certain risk factors for breast cancer, like a family history or a poor diet, this number underestimates your risk. If you have no risk factors at all for the disease, this lifetime risk overestimates your chances of getting breast cancer.

Sadly, 15 Canadian women die every day from breast cancer. But the good news is that the death rate from breast cancer has decreased by 10 percent over the past 15 years. This is largely because more and more women are having mammograms, allowing for earlier detection.

What Causes Breast Cancer?

Simply put, cancer is a disease in which abnormal cells grow out of control. When enough of these cells accumulate, a tumor forms. Finally, if the cancer cells are able to break away from the tumor, they can circulate through the body and take up residence in another organ, a process called metastasis.

Every cell has a genetic blueprint, called DNA (deoxyribonucleic acid). The DNA of cells contains genes that program cell reproduction, growth and repair of all body processes. Sometimes genes can become damaged by a mutation that occurs during normal cell division or by exposure to cancer-causing agents (carcinogens). Such damage can result in cancer. Flawed genes can be inherited from your parents. However, very few cancers are the result of inherited genes.

Cancer is not explained by genetics alone. Experts agree that cancer is the result of an interaction between genes and environmental factors. For instance, you might have a mutated gene that predisposes you to breast cancer, but, because you eat a low-fat diet with plenty of fruits and vegetables, the cancer may never express itself.

Who's at Risk?

The clearest risk factors for breast cancer are associated with hormonal and reproductive factors. It is thought that estrogen promotes the growth and development of mutated breast cells. It seems that the longer breast tissue is exposed to the body's circulating estrogen, the greater the risk for breast cancer.

- *Age* Breast cancer is more common in women over 50 years of age.

- *Previous breast cancer* A history of breast cancer increases the odds that a woman will get breast cancer again, in the same and in the opposite breast.

- *Family history of breast cancer* If you have a first-degree relative (a mother or a sister) with breast cancer, your risk is approximately doubled. There is an even greater risk if more than one close relative is affected or if the cancer has occurred in a family member at a young age.

- *Age of first pregnancy* Women who have children before 30 years of age have a lower risk of breast cancer. Women who have their first child after 30 have a higher risk, and women who never have children are at an even greater risk.

- *Age of first period (menarche)* Onset of your period before 12 years of age is associated with a slightly higher risk of breast cancer.

- *Late menopause* Women who menstruate for longer than 40 years have a slightly higher risk of breast cancer.

The list below describes factors that also may play a role in the development of breast cancer, but they are not as well understood:

- *Exposure to radiation* Ionizing radiation from X-rays taken at a young age may increase the risk for breast cancer later in life.

- *Use of hormones* Animal studies show the use of estrogen is associated with an increased occurrence of breast cancer. In women, however, this relationship is less clear. Studies have failed to show an increased risk of breast cancer in younger women who take birth control pills. Short-term use of hormone replacement therapy (HRT) for menopausal symptoms is considered safe. But if HRT is taken for more than ten years or taken by women with a family history of breast cancer, the risk of breast cancer has been found to increase by 30 to 60 percent. The pros and cons of HRT need to be discussed with your family doctor.

- *Diet* A growing body of research is finding a link between certain dietary factors and the risk of breast cancer. Diet may affect breast cancer development by either initiating cancer growth or promoting the growth of cancerous cells.

Preventing Breast Cancer

By the age of 40, all Canadian women should be performing monthly breast self-exams to detect physical changes in their breasts. Use the pads of your fingers to examine the tissue in your breasts and in your armpits. Be sure to also look carefully at your breast for any noticeable physical changes, such as a lump in the breast or underarm area, unusual breast swelling, change in color or texture of skin on the breast, blood leakage from the nipple or inversion of the nipple. Any of these changes should prompt a visit to your family doctor.

All Canadian women between the ages of 50 and 69 years are recommended to have a mammogram every two years in combination with a physical exam of the breasts by a trained health professional. A mammogram is a special X-ray of the breast that can catch breast cancer early and lead to a significant improvement in the chance of survival.

Dietary Strategies

Dietary factors such as fat, alcohol, fiber, fruits and vegetables have all been well studied. Below I list nutrition recommendations based on the current body of scientific evidence. Some of these strategies have strong research to support their adoption; others have evidence to suggest that they *may* be helpful.

Dietary Fat

It is believed that dietary fat may increase breast cancer risk by affecting estrogen metabolism. Studies have found that vegetarian women who follow a low-fat, high-fiber diet have lower levels of estrogen and less breast cancer.[1] A high-fat diet

may lead to breast cancer by promoting weight gain and body fat accumulation, which in turn increases the risk of breast cancer.

A large Canadian study is underway to determine if a very low-fat diet can prevent breast cancer. So far, one report from this trial found that women who ate a 21 percent fat diet for two years had significantly reduced dense breast areas seen by mammogram (dense breast areas are a risk factor for cancer), compared with women on a 30 percent fat diet.[2] Another report from this research group revealed that women who followed a 15 percent fat diet for two years had lower levels of circulating estrogen, which could offer protection over the long term.[3]

Saturated Fat

Some studies show that higher meat intakes are linked with a greater risk of breast cancer. The harmful effect of meat may be because of its saturated fat content, or it may be because of the way it's prepared. Cooking meat at high temperatures forms compounds called heterocyclic amines, which have been shown to cause breast tumors in animals. This may hold true for women, too. A University of Minnesota study found that women who ate hamburger, steak and bacon cooked well done were more than four times as likely to have breast cancer than women who enjoyed their meat cooked rare or medium done.[4] Until we know more about the effect of cooked meat, breast cancer experts advise that we consume no more than 3 ounces (90 grams) of meat each day.

Omega-3 Fats

Studies show that consuming plenty of fish for many years is associated with a lower risk of breast cancer. While no trials have been done in women, one animal study did find that omega-3 fats from fish oil actually suppressed human breast cancer cell growth and metastases in female mice (scientists inject human breast cancer cells into mice to study the effects of different carcinogens).[5] Despite the lack of strong evidence for the protective effect of fish, the existing studies do suggest that you get more omega-3 fats in your diet. Aim to eat fish three times a week.

Soy Foods

Populations that consume the largest amount of soy in their diet have the lowest rates of breast cancer. Researchers attribute soy's possible protective effect to naturally occurring compounds called isoflavones. Once in the body, isoflavones behave like weak estrogen compounds and are able to attach to estrogen receptors in the breast. In so doing, they can block the ability of a woman's own estrogen from taking that spot. This means that breast cells have less contact with estrogen.

So far, no study has been conducted to show what years of eating a high-soy diet does to breast cancer risk. A handful of studies have shown that a regular intake of soy isoflavones may lower circulating levels of estrogen, and this might reduce a woman's future risk of breast cancer. Other studies show that consuming a soy-rich diet can lengthen a woman's menstrual cycle, thereby influencing how much estrogen her breast cells are exposed to. Based on what we know today, most experts believe women must consume soy foods over their lifetime to realize the potential benefits of soy isoflavones on breast health.

However, the estrogen-like properties of isoflavones have led some experts to be concerned about the use of soy by women with breast cancer. Some preliminary studies show that soy has protective effects for breast cancer while others suggest soy might increase breast cell growth. Because we lack sufficient reliable information about the effect of soy foods in women with breast cancer, a history of breast cancer or a family history of breast cancer, soy should be used cautiously. Until more is known, avoid consuming large amounts of soy each day, and avoid using soy protein powders and isoflavone supplements. Consuming soy foods three times a week as part of a plant-based diet is considered safe. For ways to include soy in your diet, refer to page 72, Chapter 5.

Flaxseed

These tiny whole-grain brown and golden seeds contain natural plant estrogens called lignans. Once in the body, phytoestrogens from flaxseed have a weak estrogen action, and they are able to bind to estrogen receptors (just like soy isoflavones). In so doing, they appear to block the action of our body's own estrogen on breast cells. Animal studies conducted at the University of Toronto found that flaxseed has anticancer properties.[6,7] And a recent Canadian study suggests that 50 grams (about 2 tablespoons) of ground flaxseed can slow breast cancer growth in women.[8]

Aim to get 1 to 2 tablespoons (15 to 30 ml) of ground flaxseed each day. Grind your flaxseed in a clean coffee grinder or use a mortar and pestle. You can also buy flaxseed preground at health food stores. Once you grind flaxseed, store it in an airtight container in the fridge or freezer, since the natural fats in flaxseed go rancid quickly if exposed to air and heat. For tips on adding flaxseed to your foods, refer to page 71, Chapter 5.

Fruits and Vegetables

Over 200 studies from around the world have shown that a diet high in fruit and vegetables lowers the risk of many cancers, including breast cancer. Researchers from Harvard University studied more than 89,000 women and found that those who ate more than 2.2 servings of vegetables a day had a 20 percent lower risk of breast cancer compared with those who ate less than one serving a day.[9] Another study in premenopausal women found that high total vegetable intake lowered the risk of breast cancer by 54 percent.[10]

It appears that dark green vegetables are the most protective. Spinach, kale, rapini, collard greens, Swiss chard and romaine lettuce are good sources of beta-carotene, an antioxidant nutrient that might protect breast cells from damage caused by harmful free radical molecules.

Make sure you get at least five to ten servings of fruits and vegetables each day. Aim for a minimum of three fruits and three vegetables. That may seem like a lot, but it's actually not: one serving is only 1/2 cup (125 ml) of cooked vegetable, 1 cup (250 ml) of raw greens or one piece of whole fruit.

Dietary Fiber

Evidence suggests that a high-fiber diet may offer protection from breast cancer. Toronto researchers found that 20 grams of fiber per day was associated with lower risk.[11] Fiber may help lower the risk of breast cancer by binding to estrogen in the intestine and causing it to be excreted in the stool. Every day, your intestine reabsorbs estrogen from bile, the compound that's released into your intestine from your gallbladder to help digest fat. If dietary fiber can attach to this estrogen and facilitate its removal from the body, your body has to take estrogen out of your bloodstream to make more bile. The net result is a lower level of circulating estrogen. It's possible that following a high-fiber diet for many years could lower your risk for breast cancer.

High-fiber diets also tend to be higher in antioxidant vitamins and lower in fat, both of which might protect from breast cancer. People who eat plenty of fiber also tend to maintain a healthy weight. The studies suggest that dietary fiber works best if you follow a low-fat diet. So adding a little wheat bran to a diet that's high in fat and low in fruits and vegetables probably won't do you much good.

Foods like wheat bran, whole grains and some vegetables contain mainly insoluble fibers (see Chapter 1 for more on insoluble fiber). Wheat bran has been studied the most in relation to breast cancer risk. To boost your intake of insoluble fiber and wheat bran, try the following:

- Strive for at least five servings of fruits and vegetables every day.

- Leave the peel on fruits and vegetables whenever possible.

- Eat at least five servings of whole-grain foods each day.

- Buy a high-fiber breakfast cereal. Gradually add 1/2 to 1 cup of 100 percent bran cereal to your morning meal.

- Add 2 tablespoons (30 ml) of natural wheat bran or oat bran to cereals, yogurt, casseroles and soup.

- Add nuts and seeds to salads.

- Reach for high-fiber snacks like popcorn, nuts, dried apricots or dates.

To avoid intestinal distress, build up your fiber intake gradually. Be sure to drink 8 ounces of fluid with every high-fiber meal and snack.

Tea

There is a growing body of evidence to suggest that tea protects from certain cancers, including breast cancer. The famous Nurses' Health Study from Harvard University found that drinking four or more cups of tea per day (versus one cup or fewer) was associated with 30 percent lower risk of breast cancer.[12] Animal studies have also revealed that clear tea, tea with milk and extracts of tea can block breast cancer development.

Like fruits and vegetables, tea is a plant food, and as such it contains natural chemicals that act as antioxidants. The antioxidants in tea leaves belong to a special class of compounds called catechins. By mopping up harmful free radical molecules in the body, catechins in tea may prevent damage to the genetic material of breast cells. Aim to drink one to three cups of tea each day. To learn more about tea, see page 75, Chapter 5.

Alcoholic Beverages

In a review of 38 studies conducted up until 1992, researchers concluded that having one, two or three drinks a day all increased the risk of breast cancer.[13] The more alcohol a woman consumed, the higher her risk. Alcohol may make breast cells more vulnerable to the effects of carcinogens or it may enhance the liver's processing of these substances. Alcohol may inhibit the ability of cells to repair faulty genes and may also increase estrogen levels in the body.

Nutrition and cancer experts recommend that women do not drink alcohol. If consumed at all, alcoholic drinks should be limited to one a day or seven per week.

Weight Control

Gaining weight after menopause is linked with a higher risk of breast cancer.[14-17] Obesity may influence breast cancer risk by increasing circulating estrogen levels, since estrogen is produced in body fat cells. If you are overweight or you have gained some weight since menopause, I strongly advise that you take steps to lose weight. Start by determining your body mass index to get a sense of how your current weight is affecting your health (see page 439, Obesity and Weight Loss).

Vitamins and Minerals

Carotenoids

Toronto scientists have estimated that women who get the most beta-carotene in their diet reduce their risk of breast cancer by 15 percent.[18] Researchers have also learned that a diet rich in beta-carotene fruits and vegetables may improve breast cancer survival.

Beta-carotene has two roles in the body. It has an antioxidant effect, which can help protect our genes from oxidative damage caused by free radicals. But beta-carotene is also converted to vitamin A inside the body. This vitamin is essential for proper cell growth and development. It also enhances our body's immune system. Both roles may help keep breast cancer at bay.

More than 600 types of carotenoid compounds exist in plants, beta-carotene being the most plentiful. Other important carotenoids include lutein and lycopene. Researchers are investigating the link between these carotenoids and breast cancer risk. The Harvard Nurses' Health Study found that premenopausal women who ate five or more servings of high-carotenoid fruits and vegetables had a lower risk of breast cancer than women who ate less than two servings a day.[19]

To help boost your intake of carotenoid-rich fruits and vegetables, use the list on page 67, Chapter 5. Aim for at least three servings per day.

Vitamin C

Although the research findings on vitamin C are less consistent than they are for beta-carotene, there is evidence to suggest you should be getting more vitamin C in your diet. This vitamin may keep women healthy by acting as an antioxidant, or it may work by enhancing the body's immune system. Vitamin C also plays an important role in collagen synthesis, an important tissue in the breast.

The best food sources of vitamin C are citrus fruit, strawberries, kiwi, cantaloupe, broccoli, bell peppers, Brussels sprouts, cabbage, tomatoes and potatoes. To supplement, take 500 milligrams of Ester C once or twice daily. Vitamin C is discussed in more detail in Chapter 4.

Vitamin B12

Although preliminary, research suggests that a deficiency of vitamin B12 may increase the risk of breast cancer.[20] It's thought that depleted levels of vitamin B12 can cause damage to DNA molecules. In the body, vitamin B12 works very closely with folate, an important B vitamin that's needed to synthesize DNA in cells. Folate is needed to activate B12 and vice versa.

Most B12 deficiencies are caused by impaired absorption, not a poor diet. After we consume B12 from foods, the acid in our stomach releases B12 from proteins in the food. The vitamin then binds to intrinsic factor, a compound that enables B12 to be absorbed into the bloodstream. You can develop a B12 deficiency if your stomach produces an insufficient amount of hydrochloric acid. This is common in older adults. Some people may also inherit a defective gene for intrinsic factor. Because they are unable to produce intrinsic factor, they are unable to absorb B12 into their bloodstream and so become deficient in the vitamin.

To prevent a B12 deficiency, ensure you are meeting your daily requirements by eating animal foods such as meat, poultry, fish, clams, eggs, dairy products and fortified soy and rice beverages and by taking a multivitamin and mineral supplement. Separate B12 pills are very safe. The recommended dose for vegetarians who consume no animal products is 500 to 1000 micrograms per day.

Folate

If you drink alcohol, be sure to meet your daily requirements for the B vitamin folate. A Harvard study found that, among women who consumed 15 grams of alcohol per day (about a glass and a half of beer or wine), those with the highest daily intake of folate (600 micrograms a day) had a 45 percent lower risk for breast cancer compared with women with the lowest folate intake (150 to 299 micrograms a day).[21] It's thought that alcohol interferes with the transport and metabolism of folate and may deprive body tissues of this B vitamin, which is essential to DNA synthesis.

The best food sources of folate include spinach, lentils, orange juice, asparagus, artichokes and whole-grain breads and cereals. To supplement, take a multivitamin and mineral or a B complex supplement. If you take separate folic acid supplements (folic acid is the synthetic form of folate found in vitamin pills and fortified foods; folate

refers to the vitamin as it occurs naturally in foods), choose one that has vitamin B12 added.

Nutrition Strategy Checklist for Preventing Breast Cancer

☐ Eat a low-fat diet
☐ Limit meat intake; avoid well-cooked meat
☐ Fish
☐ Soy foods
☐ Flaxseed
☐ Fruits and vegetables
☐ Beta-carotene-rich foods
☐ Dietary fiber
☐ Tea
☐ Avoid alcohol
☐ Manage your weight
☐ Multivitamin/mineral once daily OR B complex

Recommended Resources

www.cbcf.org
(This Web site is primarily advocacy related; however, it does provide useful links and bulletin boards for women to access.)
Canadian Breast Cancer Foundation
790 Bay Street, Suite 1000
Toronto, ON, Canada M5G 1N8
Tel: 416-596-6773 or 1-800-387-9816
Fax: 416-596-7857

www.cbcn.ca
(This Web site is primarily advocacy related; however, it does provide useful links and bulletin boards for women to access.)
Canadian Breast Cancer Network
331 Cooper Street, Suite 602
Ottawa, ON, Canada K2P 0G5
Tel: 613-230-3044
Fax: 613-230-4424

www.cancer.ca
Canadian Cancer Society
10 Alcorn Avenue, Suite 200
Toronto, ON, Canada M4V 3B1
Tel: 416-961-7223 or 1-888-939-3333 (Cancer Information Service)
Fax: 416-961-4189

www.cancernet.nci.nih.gov
National Cancer Institute (www.nci.nih.gov)
31 Center Drive, MSC 2580 Building 31, Room
10A16
Bethesda, MD, USA 20892-2580
Tel: 1-800-332-8615 or 1-800-422-6237
Fax: 301-330-7968

www.womenshealthmatters.ca
Sunnybrook and Women's College Health
Sciences Centre and The Centre for Research
in Women's Health
E-mail: info@womenshealthmatters.ca

Bronchitis

Bronchitis is a common respiratory condition
that affects most people at least once in their
lives. It's caused by viruses or bacteria and often
develops after a bout of common cold (see page
233). Normally, bronchitis is a mild illness that
heals completely in a few weeks. However, it can
be a serious problem for the elderly or for people
with heart or lung disease.

What Causes Bronchitis?

Bronchitis results from an inflammation of the
tiny bronchial tubes that line the main air passages of the lungs. Infections produced by viruses
or bacteria will damage these tubes, causing
swelling and excess mucus production. The
inflammation narrows the airways, which rapidly
become clogged with mucus. These obstructions
reduce the movement of air in and out of the
lungs, limiting the amount of oxygen that can
enter the bloodstream to nourish vital organs.
The swollen bronchial tubes also are responsible
for the telltale wheezing and coughing that is so
characteristic of bronchitis.

Most cases of infectious, or acute bronchitis,
clear up within a few days, though the cough may
linger for three weeks or longer. The bronchial
tubes will take longer to heal if there is additional damage caused by cigarette smoking. Allergies,
inhaled irritants, air pollution and chronic conditions such as sinusitis may also cause recurring
bronchial infections.

For some people, bronchitis develops when
stomach acids back up into the esophagus and
enter the lungs, a condition known as gastroesophageal reflux disease (see page 348, Hiatal
Hernia). In children, bronchitis may be the result
of enlarged tonsils and adenoids.

Sometimes, inflammation of the bronchial
tubes becomes a permanent condition. This is
known as chronic bronchitis and is a serious
health problem that endangers the lungs and can
be potentially life threatening. Unlike acute bronchitis, chronic bronchitis does not clear up in a
matter of a few days or weeks. It is caused by
inflammation that scars the lungs, limiting the
exchange of old air for new. Chronic bronchitis is
characterized by an ongoing, irritating cough and
excessive mucus production that can last for
months at a time, sometimes requiring hospitalization. Cigarette smoking is the most common
cause of chronic bronchitis.

Symptoms

Symptoms of bronchitis include

- persistent cough that lasts for less than six
  weeks
- coughing up sputum (which may be clear,
  yellow or green, indicating a secondary bacterial infection, or blood-streaked)
- shortness of breath
- wheezing
- chest pain, soreness or rattling in the chest
- slight fever
- sore throat

- tiredness
- back and muscle aches

The symptoms of acute bronchitis can also be confused with those of asthma or pneumonia. If coughing and wheezing persist or are accompanied by a high fever and weakness, specific testing by your doctor may be necessary to determine which condition is responsible for your respiratory problems.

Who's at Risk?

People who smoke are more likely to get bronchitis and take longer to recover from it than nonsmokers. Children of cigarette smokers are also more prone to bronchitis. Others at risk include

- people who are exposed to others suffering from acute bronchitis
- people suffering from chronic conditions that compromise the immune system
- people suffering from gastroesophageal reflux disease
- people who are exposed to lung irritants at work, especially dust particles and chemical fumes

Conventional Treatment

There are several ways to treat bronchitis, including

- bed rest
- increased fluid intake
- over-the-counter cough medicine
- use of a humidifier to loosen mucus and relieve coughing
- antibiotics if a bacterial infection is present (evidenced by yellow or green sputum) or in cases of pre-existing lung disease

- acetaminophen or aspirin to reduce fever
- avoidance of exposure to cold, damp environments
- avoidance of exposure to air pollution and inhaled irritants
- reduction or cessation of cigarette smoking

Managing Bronchitis
Dietary Strategies
Fruits and Vegetables
Fruits and, particularly, vegetables contain many vitamins, minerals and antioxidants that may protect the lungs. One study conducted among 46,000 people over the age of 15 found that those who had the highest intake of vegetables had a 31 percent lower risk of bronchitis compared to those who ate the least.[1] Aim to consume at least three vegetable servings per day. Evidence suggests that vegetables rich in vitamin C may offer the most protection. Aim to include at least two 1/2 cup (125 ml) servings of broccoli, Brussels sprouts, cabbage, bell peppers, tomato juice or potatoes in your daily diet.

Food Allergies
Chronic bronchial infections may be caused by food allergies. In one study, patients with bronchitis who eliminated problematic foods identified by allergy testing experienced a 70 percent improvement in symptoms.[2] To determine if food allergies trigger ongoing bouts of bronchitis, try an elimination/challenge diet as outlined below. You may want to seek the help of a registered dietitian (**www.dietitians.ca**) to help determine food allergies.

1. *Elimination phase* For a period of two weeks, eliminate common food allergens: dairy products, soy foods, citrus fruits, nuts, wheat, shellfish, fish, eggs, corn and sulfite food additives.

2. *Challenge phase* After two weeks, start introducing one food every three days. Keep a food and symptom diary in which to record everything you eat, amounts eaten and time you ate the food or meal. Document any symptoms, the time of day you started to feel the symptom and the duration of time you felt the symptom. If symptoms recur when a particular food is added back, you or your child may be allergic. Consult your doctor for further food allergy testing.

Vitamins and Minerals

Vitamin A
This vitamin plays an important role in maintaining healthy lung tissue and immune function. Some research suggests that a diet poor in vitamin A increases the risk of airway obstruction.[3] To prevent this, ensure you are meeting your daily vitamin A requirements by including liver, oily fish, milk, cheese and egg yolks in your diet. Beta-carotene, a natural chemical found in dark green and orange produce, is converted to vitamin A in the body. Consuming foods rich in beta-carotene also contributes to your daily vitamin A. Reach for carrots, sweet potato, winter squash, broccoli, collard greens, kale, spinach, apricots, cantaloupe, peaches, nectarines, mango and papaya.

Your diet and a multivitamin and mineral will provide all the vitamin A you require each day. High-dose vitamin A supplements are not recommended, since too much vitamin A taken for a period can produce toxic effects. If you want to get more vitamin A, beta-carotene supplements are a safe alternative for nonsmokers. To boost your intake, buy a multivitamin and mineral with added beta-carotene or buy a separate supplement that provides a mix of carotenoids (e.g., beta-carotene, lycopene, lutein).

Vitamin C
Oxidative damage to the lungs caused by air pollution and cigarette smoke can contribute to bronchitis. Consuming adequate amounts of the antioxidant vitamin C can reduce such damage. Vitamin C is also needed for the production of infection-fighting compounds in the body. Studies have revealed that lower levels of vitamin C in the body were associated with bronchitis symptoms in adults.[4,5] Researchers have also found that supplementing with vitamin C can help treat symptoms of acute bronchitis, especially in the elderly, who may have low dietary intakes of the vitamin.[6]

The best food sources of vitamin C are citrus fruit, strawberries, kiwi, cantaloupe, broccoli, bell peppers, Brussels sprouts, cabbage, tomatoes and potatoes. To supplement, take 200 to 500 milligrams of Ester C once or twice daily (or a 1000 milligram time-released vitamin C pill once daily). For more information on vitamin C, see Chapter 4.

Magnesium
It is thought that a low intake of magnesium is somehow related to the development of chronic bronchitis. Magnesium appears to influence the contraction-relaxation state of bronchial smooth muscle. One study conducted in over 2600 adults found that individuals who consumed the most magnesium from foods reported less wheezing in the previous year.[7] Higher magnesium intakes were also associated with a reduction in hyperactivity of the bronchial passages.

To prevent a magnesium deficiency, include the following foods in your diet: nuts, seeds, legumes, prunes, whole-grain cereals, leafy green vegetables, Brewer's yeast and dairy products. Magnesium is lost when grains are refined, so a diet high in refined or processed foods will be lacking magnesium.

To supplement, take 150 to 200 milligrams of magnesium citrate, aspartate, succinate, fumarte or gluconate once or twice daily. If you take calcium supplements, buy one with added magnesium. See page 48, Chapter 4, to learn more about magnesium supplements.

Zinc

This mineral plays an important role in maintaining a healthy immune system, and a deficiency can increase the chances of respiratory infections. One large study found that a lower level of zinc in the bloodstream was associated with bronchitis in adults.[8]

The best food sources of zinc include oysters, seafood, red meat, poultry, yogurt, wheat bran, wheat germ, whole grains and enriched breakfast cereals. Your diet and a good multivitamin and mineral supplement will give you all the zinc you need to stay healthy. Single supplements of zinc in high doses can have toxic effects, including copper deficiency, heart problems and anemia. Consuming more than 40 milligrams of zinc per day can depress your immune system, making you more susceptible to infection. If you do take a separate zinc supplement, be sure it has copper added and do not exceed 40 milligrams of zinc per day.

Herbal Remedies

Echinacea

Many studies in the laboratory have shown the ability of echinacea to enhance the body's production of white blood cells, which fight infection. To treat acute bronchitis, buy a product made from echinacea root. To ensure you're buying a high-quality product, look for a statement of standardization.

Take a total of 900 milligrams three to four times daily. For tinctures (1:5), take 1 to 2 milliliters three times daily. Take echinacea until your symptoms are relieved, then continue taking two

to three times daily for one week. Some experts recommend taking the herb once every two hours (300 milligram standardized extract or 3 to 4 milliliters of a tincture) until symptoms have subsided, then up to three times daily for a week.

Garlic (*Allium sativum*)

Garlic contains many different sulfur compounds, and one in particular, S-allyl cysteine (SAC), has been shown to stimulate the body's immune system and help ward off infection. Use one-half to one clove of garlic per day in cooking. If raw garlic irritates your stomach, use aged garlic extract supplements. This type of garlic is concentrated in S-allyl cysteine and has lost the irritating sulfur compounds in the aging process. Take two to six capsules per day in divided doses.

Myrtol (Essential Oils)

This standardized combination of three essential oils has been studied for its effectiveness in acute and chronic bronchitis. The product contains cineole from eucalyptus, d-limonene from citrus fruit and alpha-pinene from pine. Short-term use of this essential oil supplement in acute bronchitis has been shown to result in a more rapid recovery compared with placebo pills and to be comparable to standard prescription medications.[9,10] In chronic bronchitis, four weeks of Myrtol use has been associated with a reduced frequency and severity of coughing and expectoration and a reduced need for antibiotics. The usual dose is 300 milligrams taken three or four times daily.

Other Natural Health Products

N-Acetyl Cysteine

This supplement is a modified form of cysteine, an amino acid found in protein-rich foods. Studies suggest that it may be very helpful for cigarette smokers with chronic bronchitis. A review of nine well-controlled studies on N-acetyl cysteine and bronchitis concluded that the supplement could indeed reduce flare-ups.[11] It was originally believed that N-acetyl cysteine may help break up mucus; however, scientists now feel that it may work in other ways to help treat bronchitis.[12]

The recommended dose is 400 to 1200 milligrams per day. The supplement is well tolerated but occasional side effects may include nausea and diarrhea. Safety of this supplement has not been evaluated in young children or pregnant and breastfeeding women.

Nutrition Strategy Checklist for Bronchitis

- [ ] Vegetables and fruits
- [ ] Identify food allergies
- [ ] Foods rich in vitamin A and beta-carotene
- [ ] Vitamin K
- [ ] Magnesium
- [ ] Zinc
- [ ] Echinacea
- [ ] Garlic
- [ ] N-acetyl cysteine

Recommended Resources

www.familydoctor.org
American Academy of Family Physicians
11400 Tomahawk Creek Parkway
Leawood, KS, USA 66211-2672
Tel: 913-906-6000

www.lung.ca
(This site provides information on chronic bronchitis.)
The Lung Association of Canada
3 Raymond Street, Suite 300
Ottawa, ON, Canada K1R 1A3
Tel: 613-569-6411
Fax: 613-569-8860

www.mayoclinic.com
Mayo Foundation for Medical Education and Research

Burns

The entire surface of your body is covered with a vital, sensitive tissue that we know as skin. Composed of three main layers—the epidermis, the dermis and the subcutis—skin acts as a protective barrier against toxins, bacteria and injury. Although skin is normally a strong defender of the body, skin cells and tissue can be easily burned and damaged when exposed to heat at temperatures higher than 50°C (120°F). The most common causes of burn are contact with fire, hot liquids and steam, but contact with sun exposure, electricity and chemicals can also result in burn.

When skin tissue is burned, the blood vessels in the tissue leak fluid, causing swelling. If burns are extensive, large amounts of fluid may be lost, triggering the body to go into shock. Shock can be a life-threatening condition because it causes a dangerous drop in blood pressure, which restricts blood flow to the brain and other vital organs.

In some cases, internal organs can be burned, even when the skin is not affected. For example, inhaling smoke or hot air during a fire can burn the lungs. Swallowing hot liquids or chemical substances can injure the esophagus and stomach. Electrical burns are particularly deceiving. While burning of the skin may be quite minimal, the damage to tissue and organs underneath the skin may be extensive. Electrical shocks can also injure the heart and may paralyze breathing or disturb the heart rhythm, leading to cardiac arrest.

The severity of a burn depends on the amount of tissue affected and the depth of the injury. Burns are classified as first, second or third degree, depending on the amount of damage to body tissues. Healing depends on the location and the depth of the burn. Approximately 85 percent of all burns are minor and can be treated at home or at a doctor's office.

Symptoms

First Degree Burns

This is the least serious type of burn. Only the outer layer of skin (epidermis) is affected. The skin may redden and there may be swelling and pain. First degree burns heal quickly; the dead layers of skin drop off in a few days and the epidermis regrows to cover the layers of tissue below the skin surface. Little or no scarring results from first degree burns.

Second Degree Burns

These burns cause deeper damage than first degree burns. They affect the epidermis and some of the underlying dermis layer of skin. The skin becomes intensely reddened and splotchy. Blisters, severe pain and swelling develop. A minor second degree burn covers an area no larger than 2 to 3 inches (5 to 7.5 cm) in diameter. It is not serious and will heal in a short time. A major second degree burn covers a larger area or is on the hands, feet, face, groin, buttocks or a major joint. It is serious and requires immediate medical attention.

Third Degree Burns

This type of burn is always serious as it involves all three layers of the skin. Nerves, fat tissue, muscle and bone may also be affected. The burned area may appear white and soft or black, charred and leathery. Generally these burns aren't painful because nerve endings in the skin have been destroyed. Deep burns injure the dermis and may be life threatening. Healing is very slow and scarring is considerable.

Burned areas are more susceptible to infection. Signs of infection include increased pain, fever, redness, swelling or oozing. If infection develops, medical attention is necessary.

Who's at Risk?

Children and the elderly are most likely to experience serious burns because their skin is thinner. In fact, children account for more than 35 percent of all fire and burn injuries and deaths. Fires and burns are the second-leading cause of accidental death for children under age four, and the third-leading cause of death for all children under age 19.

Conventional Treatment

First Degree Burns

- Cover the burned area with cold water or cold, wet cloths for 10 to 15 minutes or until the pain lessens.

- Apply a topical anesthetic cream if the skin is not broken; this will minimize discomfort.

- Do not apply pressure to the burned area. Cover it with a light, dry, sterile dressing.

- Nonprescription pain relievers, such as aspirin, ibuprofen or acetaminophen, may help relieve temporary discomfort.

Second Degree Burns

- Follow the same procedures as for first degree burns (above).

- Do not apply creams or lotions to the area as they may interfere with medical treatment.

- Do not attempt to remove burned clothing that has become stuck to the skin.

- Do not break blisters or peel off damaged skin. Exposing tissues underneath the burned area increases the risk of infection.

- If blisters break, wash the area with mild soap and water, then apply an antibiotic cream and cover with a dry, sterile dressing. Change the dressing daily.

- Seek medical attention.

Third Degree Burns

- Call 911 for emergency medical services.

- Before the tissues swell, remove tight clothing that is not stuck to the skin, plus all jewelry, belts and shoes.

- Cover the burned area with a clean, dry dressing.

- Do not apply ointments or antiseptic creams.

- Elevate injured areas higher than the heart to reduce swelling.

- If breathing has stopped, check for blocked airways and perform CPR.

- To prevent a life-threatening loss of body fluids, intravenous fluids are essential. If medical assistance is delayed, give the burn victim frequent, small cold drinks to replace fluid loss.

- Skin grafting, plastic surgery and physical therapy may be necessary to complete the healing process.

Prevention Strategies

Burns are frequently caused by preventable accidents in the home. Studies indicate that death from fires is less common in homes equipped with smoke detectors. Take the following safety precautions to protect yourself and your family from injury:

- Equip each floor in your home with a smoke detector.

- Check smoke detector batteries annually.

- Practice fire drills and escape routes regularly.

- Keep a fire extinguisher in the kitchen.

- Keep hot foods and drinks out of reach of young children.

- When cooking, turn pot handles toward the back of the stove.

- Avoid holding young children in your lap when drinking hot liquids or smoking cigarettes.

- Keep young children safe by covering electrical outlets and blocking access to electrical devices.

- Check appliances regularly for frayed electrical wiring.

- Store potentially dangerous chemicals in childproof cabinets.

Managing Burns

Dietary Strategies

Nutrition plays a very important role in burn treatment. A healthy diet is needed to provide an adequate amount of nutrients in order to replace losses, promote the healing of burns and reduce the chances of infection. Diet should also provide enough calories and protein to minimize the muscle wasting associated with serious burns.

A High-Calorie, High-Protein, Low-Fat Diet

Burns cause the body to go into a hypermetabolic state (in which the body burns calories at a much faster rate than normal). It has been reported that adults who are severely burned need to increase their daily calorie needs by twice the normal amount, and young children suffering from serious burns can need up to four times more calories.[1,2] The more serious the burn, the faster the body uses nutrients. In the case of major burns, muscle protein tissue is used by the body for energy, and this leads to a progressive loss of muscle mass.

Many studies show that low-fat diets (where fat makes up only 15 percent of daily calories) can help promote healing and shorten the length of hospital stays.[3-5] Too much fat can depress the body's immune system, increasing the likelihood of infection. It is also important that a large portion of daily fat comes from omega-3 fats found in oily fish.[6,7] Once consumed, these fats are used by the body to produce anti-inflammatory immune compounds that help speed healing.

Major burns require hospitalization. A registered dietitian working in the burn unit will ensure that burn patients receive the appropriate amount of protein, carbohydrate and fat from a special diet or, in cases when eating by mouth is not possible, by tube feeding or intravenous feeding. Often, liquid supplements such as Ensure or Boost and nutrient-dense snacks are necessary to maintain a high calorie intake during the day.

Vitamins and Minerals

Multivitamin and Mineral Supplement

Since wound healing increases the body's need for many nutrients, a multivitamin and mineral supplement is recommended for adults and children suffering from minor or major burns.

Vitamin A

This fat-soluble vitamin is important for wound healing as it helps the layers of the skin fight infection by preventing the invasion of bacteria and viruses. Vitamin A also promotes cell division in the skin. The best sources of vitamin A include liver, oily fish, milk, cheese, butter and egg yolks. Foods rich in beta-carotene, such as orange and dark green produce (carrots, sweet potato, winter squash, broccoli, collard greens, kale, spinach, apricots, cantaloupe, peaches, nectarines, mango, papaya), also provide the body with some vitamin A.

For major burns, a daily vitamin A supplement is advised: 10,000 international units (IU) for adults and 5,000 IU for children. High-potency multivitamin and mineral supplements often provide 5,000 IU per day.

Vitamins C and E

Vitamin C has three important roles in wound healing: it is needed for healthy scar formation, it protects the body from inflammatory damage caused by burn wounds and it enhances the immune system. Research in patients with major burns shows that vitamin C can decrease free radical damage caused by burns and reduce tissue swelling.[8]

Some of the best food sources of vitamin C are citrus fruit, strawberries, kiwi, cantaloupe, broccoli, bell peppers, Brussels sprouts, cabbage, tomatoes and potatoes. Include at least two of these foods in your daily diet to promote healing of minor and major burns. In the case of major burns, take a vitamin C supplement: adults, 500 milligrams twice daily and children, 250 milligrams twice daily.

Like vitamin C, vitamin E also acts as an antioxidant and can protect cell membranes from damage induced by burns.[9] Food sources include vegetable oils, almonds, peanuts, soybeans, whole grains, wheat germ, avocado and green leafy vegetables. To get higher amounts of vitamin E, a supplement is necessary. Take 200 to 800 IU natural source vitamin E per day.

Zinc, Selenium and Copper

These trace minerals are involved in scavenging harmful free radicals and are needed in increased amounts following a burn. They also play an important role in supporting the body's immune system. Studies suggest that treatment of major burns with these minerals can reduce infection and shorten hospital stays.[10-12] Good food sources are as follows:

Zinc Oysters, seafood, red meat, poultry, yogurt, wheat bran, wheat germ, whole grains, enriched breakfast cereals.

Selenium Seafood, meat, organ meats, wheat bran, whole grains, nuts, Brazil nuts, onion, garlic, mushrooms, Swiss chard, orange juice.

Copper Liver, meat, shellfish (especially oysters), legumes, nuts, prunes, whole grains, dark green vegetables, sweet potatoes.

For minor first degree burns, diet and a multivitamin and mineral pill will provide you with adequate amounts of these minerals. For major burns, research suggests that supplemental doses help speed healing: 40 milligrams of zinc with 4 milligrams of copper once daily; 200 micrograms of selenium once daily.

Herbal Remedies

Gotu Kola (*Centella asiatica*)

This herb has long been used in India and Indonesia to promote wound healing. It seems to promote the formation of healthy connective tissue. Although no randomized controlled studies have been conducted, a number of clinical reports and small studies suggest that the herb does help burns heal.[13]

Buy a product standardized for 40 percent asiaticoside, 30 percent Asiatic acid, 30 percent madecassic acid and 1 to 2 percent madecassoside. Take 20 to 60 milligrams three times daily. The herb is not associated with any side effects other than the occasional skin rash. Safety in pregnant and breastfeeding women and young children has not been established.

Aloe Vera

The gel made from this plant has a long history of use in wound and burn healing; however, current science suggests it should be used only for the treatment of minor burns.[14-16] One study suggests that aloe vera gel may actually worsen the healing of severe burns.

The active ingredients in the aloe vera inhibit the activity of bradykinin, a pain-producing substance. Aloe vera also seems to reduce inflammation and possess antibacterial and antifungal properties.

For minor burns, buy a gel or cream that contains 0.5 percent aloe. Apply liberally as needed three to five times per day.

Calendula (*Calendula officinalis L.*) and Chamomile (*Matricaria recutita L.*)

Both of these herbs have an anti-inflammatory action and creams made from them have been used to promote the healing of minor burns. Apply one of these creams to the affected area one to four times daily.

Other Natural Health Products

Ornithine Alpha-Ketoglutarate (OAK)

This compound is made in the body from two amino acids: ornithine and glutamine. These amino acids are found in high-protein foods such as meat, poultry, fish, eggs and dairy products. Studies in burn patients show that when taken as a supplement, OAK results in reduced muscle breakdown and better wound healing.[17-19] This supplement is not intended for the treatment of a major burn—an injury that causes the body to go into a catabolic, or tissue breakdown, state.

Based on the research, the recommended dose for adults is 10 grams taken twice daily. Be sure to buy a product from a reputable manufacturer.

Nutrition Strategy Checklist for Burns

- ☐ High-calorie, high-protein, low-fat diet (major burns)
- ☐ Multivitamin/mineral
- ☐ Foods rich in vitamin A and beta-carotene
- ☐ Vitamin C
- ☐ Vitamin E
- ☐ Zinc and copper
- ☐ Selenium
- ☐ Aloe vera gel (for minor burns only)
- ☐ Ornithine alpha-ketoglutarate (for minor burns only)

Recommended Resources

**www.cps.ca/english/carekids/safety&
prevention/Safety.htm**
(This site offers good general tips on safety in
the home.)
Canadian Paediatric Society
100-2204 Walkley Road
Ottawa, ON, Canada K1G 4G8
Tel: 613-526-9397
Fax: 613-526-3332

**www.shrinershq.org/Prevention/BurnTips/
index.html**
Cincinnati Shriners Hospital
3229 Burnet Avenue
Cincinnati, OH, USA 45229-3095
Tel: 513-872-6000
Fax: 513-872-6999

A free copy of the booklet *Burn Tips* is available
through:
International Shrine Headquarters
Public Relations Department
2900 Rocky Point Drive
Tampa, FL, USA 33607
Tel: 813-281-8162

www.mayoclinic.com
The Mayo Foundation for Medical Education
and Research provides one of the best patient-
education sites on the Internet. The information
is reliable, thorough and clearly written.

Candidiasis

Your body is home to a wide variety of micro-
organisms. Invisible to the naked eye, microscopic colonies of bacteria and fungi live on or in your
skin, intestines and genitals—actually, they can
be found almost anywhere in the body. Many of
these micro-organisms are essential to maintaining good health. An intricate system of checks
and balances keeps the size of the colonies under
control and ensures that all the normal flora in
your body live in harmony.

If something disturbs this natural harmony,
certain bacteria or fungi colonies can grow out of
control, overwhelming your immune system and
causing infections or other health problems. The
Candida group of fungi is a prime example of a
harmless micro-organism that can cause persistent health problems if its growth is not kept in
check.

Candida is a type of yeast that normally lives
in the mouth, vagina and gastrointestinal tract
and on the skin. Bacteria that live in the same
areas of the body as Candida control growth of
this yeast. If these bacteria are harmed or
destroyed in any way, Candida colonies can grow
to unusually high levels. The overgrowth of
Candida disrupts natural bodily functions, causing a fungal infection known as candidiasis.

Candida albicans, a common type of Candida,
is the usual culprit behind candidiasis, but the
infection can also be caused by several other
types of Candida. Candida albicans is considered
an opportunistic organism because it spreads
only when the conditions for growth are ideal.
The most common types of candidiasis are

1. *Oral,* affecting the mucous membranes of the
   mouth and tongue, commonly known as oral
   thrush

2. *Vaginal,* such a yeast infection often develops
   during pregnancy or when taking oral contraceptives with high estrogen content

3. *Cutaneous,* an infection of the skin; in infants, it
   is often the cause of diaper rash

But candidiasis can develop on the surface of
almost any mucous membrane. In most cases,
the infection does not penetrate very far into the
body. However, under certain conditions, the
Candida fungus can enter the bloodstream,
where it causes a condition known as invasive or
systemic candidiasis. Once in the bloodstream,
the fungus is carried to all parts of the body,

spreading deep into organs such as the liver, heart, muscles, kidneys, joints or eyes. If not properly treated, it can cause serious health problems, such as blindness, heart damage, eating problems and organ failure. In rare instances, it may even lead to death. People at risk of developing invasive candidiasis are surgical patients, low-birth-weight babies and people with malfunctioning immune systems, particularly those with HIV, AIDS or leukemia.

Scientists are beginning to explore the possibility that candidiasis may be linked to chronic fatigue syndrome (see page 216), a serious medical condition that has been associated with other systemic infections, such as Epstein-Barr syndrome. At this time, however, there is no evidence to prove that the two conditions are connected.

What Causes Candidiasis?

Factors that have been blamed for candidiasis include intestinal disorders such as "leaky gut syndrome," inadequate stomach acid and digestive enzymes, vitamin and mineral deficiencies and a weakened immune system. Until further research has been completed, it is difficult to say for certain that these factors result in Candidiasis.

What *is* becoming clear, however, is the strong association between yeast infections and antibiotic use. Antibiotics disrupt or destroy the healthy bacteria that naturally keep the Candida fungus under control. By changing the normal balance between these two organisms, antibiotics encourage the overgrowth of Candida.

There is also a strong connection between yeast infections and the hormone estrogen. Over 75 percent of all women experience a yeast infection at least once during their reproductive years. Vaginal infections are a common complaint among pregnant women and among women who take oral contraceptives with a high estrogen content. An increased level of estrogen produces changes in the internal environment of the vagina, creating conditions that encourage Candida to grow and flourish.

Like all types of fungi, Candida thrives in warm, moist environments. It flourishes under diapers, in the folds of skin (particularly the skin of obese people) and in the areas between fingers and toes. Candida is an infectious condition and can be passed from one person to another. A pregnant woman with a vaginal yeast infection may transfer the infection to her newborn baby, leaving the baby with oral thrush or a yeast diaper rash. A vaginal yeast infection may also be transferred to a male sexual partner, where the organisms can cause an itchy rash on the penis. Swimming pool surfaces, showers, clothing or combs all provide easy routes for transferring the infection. In some cases, invasive candidiasis may enter the bloodstream through medical instruments or other devices used in surgical or hospital treatment.

While most episodes of candidiasis can be cleared up fairly easily with medications or over-the-counter treatments, sometimes the infection can be very persistent and recur frequently. Candida organisms that have become resistant to antibiotic treatment may cause such infections.

Symptoms

Vaginal Candidiasis (Vaginal Yeast Infection):

- abnormal vaginal discharge, which may be white and watery or thick and chunky, like cottage cheese

- itching and burning sensations in the vaginal area

- red, inflamed skin around the vagina area

- pain during intercourse and urination

Oral Candidiasis (Thrush):

- cracks in the corner of the mouth

- white patches on the mouth and tongue and inside the cheeks

- small pinpoints of bleeding when patches are rubbed

- if in an infant, fussiness and irritability and possibly difficulty feeding

Cutaneous Candidiasis (Skin Infection/Diaper Rash):

- itching that may be quite intense

- red, tender rash

- spots or lesions may be scaly or blistered and pimple-like

- rash usually develops in skin folds or around the buttocks or genitals or under the breasts

Systemic Candidiasis:
Symptoms are not specific and will vary depending on which area of the body is affected. They may include

- fever and chills that don't improve after antibiotic treatment (these are the most common symptoms)

- fatigue and a general feeling of ill health

- memory loss, short attention span

- depression, mood swings

Who's at Risk?

- females, especially those who use high-estrogen oral contraceptives

- pregnant women

- people taking broad-spectrum antibiotics

- elderly individuals

- people in poor general health

- people with diabetes

- people with a medical condition that compromises the immune system, such as HIV, AIDS or leukemia

- patients undergoing chemotherapy

- infants born to mothers with vaginal yeast infections

- obese people (cutaneous candidiasis)

- people who have been hospitalized (systemic candidiasis is the fourth most common bloodstream infection among hospitalized patients in the United States)

Conventional Treatment

Topical antifungal treatments, used directly on the skin or inside the vagina or mouth, are the most common way to clear up a Candida infection. These include mouthwashes, lozenges, shampoos and creams or vaginal inserts. Topical treatments may be messy to use and may take slightly longer to produce results but they have almost no side effects. Oral antifungal medications or injections also may be prescribed to treat candidiasis. They are more convenient and act faster but may cause side effects. Invasive candidiasis is treated with intravenous or oral medications.

Improving the health of the immune system, particularly for people with diabetes, may help control the infection and prevent recurrences.

Preventing Candidiasis

Because the Candida fungus lives naturally in our bodies, it is impossible to avoid. However, the following suggestions may help keep the fungus under control and prevent future infections.

Vaginal Candidiasis:

- Wear underwear and pantyhose with a cotton crotch; synthetic fabrics don't breathe as well as cotton and keep moisture trapped in the genital area.

- Avoid wearing tight-fitting slacks, which block air circulation and keep the genital area excessively moist.

- Don't wear wet bathing suits or sweaty exercise clothes for long periods; wash them after every use.

- Keep the vaginal area clean by washing with unscented soap. Avoid using vaginal sprays or douches.

Cutaneous Candidiasis:

- Follow good hygiene practices to keep the skin clean, dry and clear of infection.

- Wear loose-fitting clothing made of natural fibers to allow air to circulate over the skin.

- Wash hands thoroughly after contact with any fungal infection.

- Obese people may find that exercise and weight loss reduce the number of skin infections.

To Prevent Diaper Rash:

- Always change wet or soiled diapers immediately.

- Rinse cloth diapers several times to remove traces of soap, and avoid using fabric softeners that can irritate the skin.

- If possible, let your baby go without diapers for a few hours every day to allow the skin to dry thoroughly.

- Protect your baby's skin with a diaper cream or ointment.

Dietary Strategies

Natural health practitioners recommend many of the nutritional strategies listed below. With the exception of fermented milk products, no published studies could be found to show that the following foods and supplements are effective in the treatment and/or prevention of Candida yeast infections. Most of the recommendations below are based on laboratory studies and clinical experience. The rational and appropriate use of nutritional supplements for managing candidiasis should be determined in consultation with your health care provider.

Dietary Sugar

Since the Candida organism thrives on sugar, the first step to recovering from a Candida infection is to eliminate all simple sugars and refined starchy foods from your diet.[1,2] Avoid table sugar, cookies, cakes, desserts, candy, chocolate, fruit drinks, soda pop, syrup, corn syrup, jam, fruit juice, dried fruit and large portions of sweet fruit such as bananas and grapes. Refined foods made with white flour should also be avoided, including white bread, crackers, low-fiber breakfast cereals, cereal bars, granola bars and white pasta.

Dietary Fiber

An anti-Candida diet should consist of whole grains (brown rice, whole-wheat pasta, whole-grain breads and cereals), legumes (lentils, kidney beans, chickpeas) and vegetables and whole fruits in small quantities. These foods provide dietary fiber, which will help ease bloating, constipation, diarrhea and gas. As you increase your fiber intake, be sure to drink at least eight to ten glasses of water per day.

Psyllium-seed-husk powder is a water-soluble fiber that helps keep the intestinal tract healthy. It is available in health food stores. Mix 1 to 2 tablespoons into 2 cups (500 ml) of water before consuming to prevent bloating and constipation.

Fermented Milk Products

Yogurt, kefir and acidophilus milk are referred to as probiotic foods because they all contain friendly lactic acid bacteria that are normally resident in the intestinal tract. There they prevent the attachment of disease-causing microbes by taking up space and producing substances that prevent their growth. A number of studies have shown that women who consume yogurt or fermented milk beverages each day have a significant reduction in vaginal yeast infections.[3-7] (Some studies have found a yogurt douche to help treat these yeast infections.)

Consume 1 cup of plain yogurt or kefir each day to restore the microbial balance of your intestinal tract. You can also take a daily supplement that contains lactic acid bacteria (see page 138 for information on probiotic supplements).

Eat foods that contain fructo-oligosaccharides (FOS), a type of carbohydrate that promotes the growth of lactic acid bacteria, especially bifidobacteria, in the gut. Jerusalem artichokes, asparagus and soybeans contain these compounds, which pass undigested through the small intestine to the colon, where they are fermented and exert their health effects. Supplements of FOS are available. A typical dose is 4 to 10 grams per day.

Food Allergies

Candida infections are often associated with food allergies, especially allergies to foods containing yeast or fermented foods that contain fungi, such as cheese, breads and beer. Alternative health practitioners frequently suggest avoiding these foods to help clear up symptoms of Candida infections. Despite a great deal of discussion and several books on the subject, there is still no scientific proof to support these claims or to establish a clear link between candidiasis and food allergies.

Despite this, many people do find that avoiding certain foods reduces symptoms, especially gastrointestinal discomfort from bloating, constipation, diarrhea and gas. Try avoiding yeast and mold-containing foods (e.g., leavened breads, Brewer's yeast, beer, cheese, tomato paste) to see if you feel better. Caffeine-containing foods and beverages and alcohol may also aggravate symptoms.

You might consider getting tested for food allergies. ELISA and RAST blood tests are used by many nutritional physicians to assess food sensitivities.

Vitamins and Minerals

The following nutrients are important for a healthy immune system and may help treat and prevent Candida infections:

- *Vitamin C* Food sources include citrus fruit, strawberries, kiwi, cantaloupe, broccoli, bell peppers, Brussels sprouts, cabbage, tomatoes and potatoes. To supplement, take 500 milligrams of vitamin C once or twice daily.

- *Vitamin E* Food sources include vegetable oils, almonds, peanuts, soybeans, whole grains, wheat germ, avocado and green leafy vegetables, especially kale. To supplement, take 400 international units (IU) of natural vitamin E per day. Buy a vitamin E supplement made with "mixed tocopherols."

- *Zinc* Food sources include oysters, seafood, red meat, poultry, milk, yogurt, wheat bran, wheat germ, whole grains and enriched breakfast cereals. To supplement, take a multivitamin and mineral once daily. Most brands supply 10 to 15 milligrams of zinc.

Herbal Remedies

Garlic (*Allium sativum*)

A daily intake of fresh garlic and its accompanying sulfur compounds has been used to enhance the body's immune system and kill many types of bacteria and fungi.[8-11] One-half to one clove per day is recommended. Crushed garlic can also be used in combination with yogurt to treat Candida infections.

Supplements made from aged garlic extract have been shown to have immune-stimulating activity. You can purchase liquid drops or capsules of aged garlic (Kyolic® brand) at health food stores and drug stores. Take 300 to 600 milligrams three times daily with meals. If you don't like to swallow pills, add drops of aged garlic to your foods.

Echinacea

Laboratory studies have shown that active compounds in echinacea called polysaccharides have anti-Candida activity. The herb may prevent the recurrence of Candida once it is treated with antifungal drugs. Echinacea also enhances the body's production of white blood cells that fight infection.

To treat a Candida infection, choose a standardized extract of echinacea to ensure quality. For products made from echinacea root, take a total of 900 milligrams three to four times daily. For tinctures (1:5), take 1 to 2 milliliters three times daily. For teas, take 125 to 250 milliliters three to four times daily. Take until symptoms are relieved, then continue taking two to three times daily for one week.

Don't use echinacea if you are allergic to plants in the Asteracease/Compositae family (ragweed, daisy, marigold and chrysanthemum). Although the issue is controversial among experts, the herb is not recommended for use by people with autoimmune diseases (HIV, lupus), multiple sclerosis, diabetes or asthma.

Other Natural Health Products

Acidifying Supplements

These products are thought to help treat Candida infections by enhancing the acidity of the stomach. Try *one* of the following supplements with each meal (do not take on an empty stomach):

- *grapefruit seed extract*

- *betaine hydrochloride,* 325 to 650 milligrams taken with each meal

- *apple cider vinegar,* 1 tablespoon (15 ml) mixed into water, sipped with each meal

- *glutamic acid*

- *vitamin C,* 500 milligrams three times per day with meals

Excess stomach acid can lead to heartburn and possibly ulcers. Try these supplements only after consultation with your natural health care provider.

Digestive Enzymes

Digestive enzymes help break down carbohydrate, protein and fat. They may help people who suffer from gastrointestinal distress after eating. But they may also help digest Candida in the intestinal tract, thereby controlling its growth. Take one capsule after each meal, for three days. If your symptoms don't improve, increase your dose to two capsules. Some people require three capsules per meal. I highly recommend Sisu® brand digestive enzymes. Sisu products are plant-based enzymes that are active in a wide pH range.

Do not take digestive enzymes if you have ulcers or an inflammatory bowel disease (Crohn's disease, ulcerative colitis).

Nutrition Strategy Checklist for Candidiasis

- ☐ Eliminate sugars and sweets
- ☐ Fiber-rich foods
- ☐ Psyllium seed husks
- ☐ Fermented milk products
- ☐ Probiotic supplement
- ☐ Vitamin C
- ☐ Vitamin E
- ☐ Zinc
- ☐ Multivitamin/mineral
- ☐ Garlic
- ☐ Echinacea
- ☐ Digestive enzymes

Recommended Resources

www.askdrkoop.com
An Internet-based consumer health care network founded by Dr. Everett Koop, former US Surgeon General.

www.candida-society.org.uk
National Candida Society (UK)
This site is not scientifically based and is member-run, but you may find it helpful.

Canker Sores

Canker sores are small, shallow infections or ulcers that appear on the inside of the mouth. Irritating and painful, they usually develop on the tongue, the inside of the cheeks or on the soft palate. Canker sores are not considered to be contagious. They are quite different from cold sores, which are highly contagious and caused by the herpes simplex virus (see page 344).

Simple canker sores are the most common type of mouth ulcer. They appear singly or in clusters and typically last four to seven days. You may develop simple canker sores as often as three or four times a year. Complex canker sores are less common but more problematic. People suffering from complex canker sores will have ulcers in their mouths almost constantly, with new sores developing as old ones heal.

What Causes Canker Sores?

In any given year, up to 50 percent of the population will experience at least one outbreak of canker sores. Yet, despite the fact that it afflicts so many people, the cause of this annoying ailment is still unknown. Current thinking indicates that the following factors may be responsible for depressing the body's immune system and triggering an outbreak:

- stress
- tissue injuries caused by biting the tongue or the inside of the mouth, dental appliances, sharp tooth surfaces, hot food, toothbrushes or eating utensils
- food allergies or reactions to specific types of food, such as citrus fruits, tomatoes and some types of nuts
- nutritional deficiencies
- disease of the gastrointestinal tract

Symptoms

A tingling or burning sensation will be felt at the affected spot before the actual sore develops. A sore then appears as a round, white spot with a red border. Canker sores can be very painful, and the discomfort can become worse if you rub the sore with your tongue or eat hot or spicy food. Complex canker sores may cause fever, fatigue and swollen lymph nodes.

The following symptoms may be signs of more serious conditions that require medical treatment. Contact your doctor if:

- Your sores last more than 14 days;
- You have persistent, multiple mouth sores;
- You have signs of spreading infection or spreading sores;
- You develop high fever with new canker sores.

Who's at Risk?

Females are twice as likely as males to develop canker sores. Teenagers suffer from canker sores more often than do adults, possibly because their immune systems are not fully developed. As well, those with a family history of canker sores are at higher risk—susceptibility to the ailment seems to run in families. People who are under stress and run down are also at higher risk.

Conventional Treatment

Canker sores will usually heal by themselves; there is no really effective treatment. But there are some things you can do to help ease the pain:

- Avoid spicy, acidic or abrasive foods.
- Brush teeth carefully to avoid irritating the sores.
- Apply ice to the affected area.
- Apply an ointment containing topical anesthetic.

- Apply an ointment that provides a protective coating, such as glycerin.

Severe outbreaks may be treated with a prescription mouthwash, corticosteroid ointment, prednisone tablets or a lidocaine anesthetic solution.

Managing Canker Sores

Dietary Strategies

Food Allergies

Since food sensitivities may trigger the development of canker sores, it may be helpful to be tested for allergies if you have recurring sores.[1] If you suspect certain foods may be causing your mouth sores, speak to your doctor about food allergy testing. If you have already determined likely culprits in your diet, follow the elimination/challenge diet below to confirm your suspicions. Keep in mind though that some foods may trigger a canker sore only in the presence of stress or some other factor that contributes to canker development.

1. *Elimination phase* For a period of two weeks, eliminate suspected food allergens, such as citrus fruits, nuts, wheat or corn.

2. *Challenge phase* After two weeks, start introducing one food every three days. Keep a food and symptom diary, in which you record everything you eat, amounts eaten and what time you ate the food or meal. Document any symptoms. If the food causes a canker to develop, omit it from your diet.

Some people with recurrent mouth ulcers may benefit from a gluten-free diet. In fact, mouth sores may be the only presenting symptom of celiac disease, a condition in which the gluten protein in wheat is toxic to the body.[2,3] For more information about the gluten-free diet, refer to page 207, Celiac Disease.

Vitamins and Minerals

B Vitamins

Several studies have shown that deficiencies of a number of B vitamins, including B1, B2, B6, B12 and folate, are associated with recurring canker sores.[4-7] To determine if such a deficiency is the cause of your canker sores, ask your doctor about testing your blood for these nutrients. In the meantime, ensure that your daily diet contains adequate amounts of these B vitamins:

B1 (thiamin): pork, liver, whole grains, enriched breakfast cereals, legumes and nuts

B2 (riboflavin): milk, yogurt, cottage cheese, fortified soy and rice beverages, meat, whole grains and enriched breakfast cereals

B6: meat, poultry, fish, liver, legumes, nuts, seeds, whole grains, green leafy vegetables, bananas and avocados

B12: animal foods such as meat, poultry, fish, eggs and dairy products; fortified soy and rice beverages

Folate: spinach, lentils, orange juice, whole grains, fortified breakfast cereals, asparagus, artichoke, avocado and seeds

To ensure you are meeting your daily requirements (see Chapter 4), take a multivitamin and mineral supplement. You may also take a B complex supplement that contains the whole family of B vitamins in higher amounts than a regular multivitamin pill.

Iron

Some research shows that an iron deficiency may trigger canker sores.[8] To prevent a deficiency of this mineral, make sure you are eating iron-rich foods such as lean red meat, seafood, poultry, eggs, legumes, whole grains, enriched breakfast cereals and blackstrap molasses.

A daily multivitamin and mineral will usually supply 10 milligrams of iron. If a blood test reveals that you are deficient in this mineral, your doctor will recommend single iron supplements for 6 to 12 weeks to replenish your body's stores. For more information on iron-deficiency anemia, see page 161.

Herbal Remedies

Licorice (*Glycyrrhiza glabra*)

This herb may be useful in treating canker sores as it has anti-inflammatory and antiallergic properties. Licorice contains many active ingredients, but one, called glycyrrhin, can cause fluid retention, high blood pressure and potassium loss when taken in high amounts. However, an altered form of licorice, deglycyrrhizinated licorice (DGL), does not appear to have these negative side effects and is believed to be safe. Studies have shown that DGL can reduce the pain and speed the healing rate of canker sores.[9]

To treat cankers, chew one to three 380 milligram DGL tablets before each meal and at bedtime. Be forewarned: the taste may be unpleasant to some people.

Other Natural Health Products

Probiotics

Supplements of friendly bacteria known collectively as lactic acid bacteria may help clear up and prevent canker sores. Lactic acid bacteria such as L. acidophilus and bifidobacteria normally reside in the intestinal tract, where they prevent the attachment of disease-causing microbes. Many studies have found that supplementing with these bacteria protects the gastrointestinal tract and boosts the body's immune system.

To supplement, take 1 to 10 billion viable cells, in three or four divided doses, with meals. For more information about probiotic supplements,

see Chapter 8. Lactic acid bacteria are found in fermented dairy products such as yogurt, kefir and acidophilus milk.

Nutrition Strategy Checklist for Canker Sores

- [ ] Identify food allergies
- [ ] Multivitamin/mineral
- [ ] B-vitamin-rich foods
- [ ] Iron-rich foods
- [ ] Deglycyrrhizinated licorice
- [ ] Probiotic supplement

Recommended Resources

www.mayoclinic.com

This site is produced by a team of writers, editors, health educators, nurses, doctors and scientists. The Web site is part of the Mayo Clinic's commitment to provide health education to its patients and the general public. MayoClinic.com provides access to the experience and knowledge of the over 2000 doctors and scientists of the Mayo Clinic.

Cataracts

Imagine processing over one and a half million messages, all at the same time. Your eyes—those complex, sensory organs hard-wired to your brain—are capable of accomplishing this difficult feat. Containing over 70 percent of the body's sensors, your eyes gather visual images and send them directly to the brain, providing you with much of the information you need to perceive and understand the world around you.

Your eyes are designed to be extremely light sensitive because they need light to create clear, sharp visual images. Light enters through the cornea, the transparent outer surface of the eye, and passes through the pupil to reach the lens. The lens then focuses the light on the retina at the back of the eye, creating a visual message that is transmitted to the brain. To keep the light properly focused on the retina, the lens changes shape, becoming flatter or rounder depending on the distance between the eye and the viewed object.

Normally, the lens of the eye is clear and transparent, allowing light to travel directly to the retina. When a cataract develops, the lens becomes cloudy and foggy. This obstructs the passage of light into the eye, distorting your eyesight and causing vision to become blurry. Cataracts can develop in one or both eyes and usually progress very slowly and painlessly. They are the leading cause of blindness throughout the world, especially among older people.

What Causes Cataracts?

Cataracts are a natural part of the aging process and are most common in people over 65 years of age. Most cataracts are caused by a change in the chemical composition of the lens. Proteins within the lens become damaged and clump together, producing the characteristic clouding of vision. Some of these chemical changes are caused by free radicals, unstable oxygen molecules that are created through normal bodily functions. Free radicals can damage proteins in the eye and are thought to play a major role in cataract development.

Other factors that can contribute to cataracts include

- diabetes, atopic dermatitis or prolonged eye inflammation
- injuries or blows to the eye
- prolonged use of corticosteroid medications
- a hereditary predisposition to cataracts
- prolonged exposure to sunlight, ultraviolet light or infrared rays
- a diet lacking in protective nutrients

The degree of vision loss that accompanies a cataract depends on where the cataract occurs and how mature or dense it is. If the cataract develops on the outer edge of the lens, it may not cause any vision problems for a long time. If it develops in the center of the lens, then your vision will become hazy, fuzzy and blurry. Eventually, a cataract will interfere with your ability to read, drive or work. Some people reach this stage faster than others, depending on their sensitivity to the changes in their vision.

With improvements in technology and surgical techniques, cataracts can usually be successfully removed and replaced with a clear, artificial lens. More than 90 percent of people who have cataract surgery end up with improved vision.

Symptoms

Symptoms of cataracts include

- blurry or hazy vision; double vision
- sensitivity to light and glare
- seeing halos around lights
- poor night vision
- need for brighter light when reading and working
- frequent changes in eyeglass prescriptions
- change in pupil color from the normal black to yellowish or white

Occasionally, swelling in the lens and increased pressure in the eye may develop.

Who's at Risk?

Adults 65 years of age or older are at greater risk of developing cataracts, as are those people with a family history of cataracts. Other factors that may increase risk are, as I mentioned above, eye injuries or blows to the eye; prolonged use of medications, such as corticosteroids; excessive exposure to sunlight, ultraviolet light or radiation; cigarette smoking and alcohol consumption.

Conventional Treatment

Surgery is the most effective treatment. Two types of cataract surgery are most common:

1. *Phacoemulsification* involves a special instrument that breaks up the cataract with ultrasound waves; the fragmented pieces are then vacuumed out of the eye.

2. *Extracapsular* through a small incision in the lens capsule, the central portion of the lens is removed and smaller portions are vacuumed out.

After the cataract is removed, an artificial lens implant (intraocular lens) is inserted into the eye to focus the light on the retina. Vision improves within one to two days and improvement continues for approximately four weeks. Most people still need eyeglasses after cataract surgery. In some cases, contact lenses or glasses are used to replace the natural lens, instead of an implanted intraocular lens. The procedure is usually very safe and quite successful.

Preventing Cataracts

Since cigarette smoking generates free radicals, one of the most important ways to prevent cataracts is to quit smoking. Research has shown that compared to nonsmokers, those who smoke at least 20 cigarettes per day have almost a threefold higher risk for cataracts.[1] Giving up the habit may reverse some of the damage to the lens of the eye. Researchers from Harvard University found that compared to male smokers, past male smokers had almost a 25 percent reduced risk for cataract.[2]

It is also important to protect your eyes from sunlight whenever possible by wearing a hat and sunglasses that offer UVA and UVB protection.

Dietary Strategies

Weight Control

Studies find that people who are overweight have a higher risk of cataract formation.[3-5] People with a body mass index (BMI) of 27.8 or greater have twice the risk for cataract compared with those whose BMI is 22 or less. Even being moderately overweight with a BMI of 25 to 27 appears to increase one's risk. And carrying extra weight around the middle seems to be more predictive of cataracts than lower body fat. To calculate your BMI, refer to page 439, Obesity and Weight Loss. Researchers believe that restricting your calorie intake may in some way slow the development of cataract.

Sodium

Research suggests that high-salt diets can increase the risk of cataracts by as much as twofold.[6] Aim to consume no more than 2400 milligrams of sodium (about 1 teaspoon of salt) per day by avoiding processed foods and salty snacks and by limiting your use of the saltshaker. Refer to page 80, Chapter 5, to learn the sodium content of selected foods.

Alcohol

For reasons that aren't clear, drinking alcohol is linked with a higher risk of cataracts, particularly in men. Studies show that compared with non-drinkers, daily drinking or consuming more than seven drinks a week is associated with a significantly higher likelihood of cataract.[7-9] A recent study conducted in almost 80,000 women did not find that drinking up to two drinks per day was associated with cataract.[10] Limit your intake of alcohol to no more than one drink per day.

Lutein-Rich Foods

Lutein is related to beta-carotene, the carotenoid found in carrots. Once consumed in the diet, lutein is concentrated in the eye, where it protects proteins from damage caused by ultraviolet light. Two large studies from Harvard University found that men and women with the highest intakes of lutein had a 20 percent lower risk of cataract compared with those who consumed the least.[11,12] Broccoli, spinach and kale were most often associated with protection.

Lutein is found in egg yolks and a variety of fruits and vegetables. The best sources include beet greens, broccoli, Brussels sprouts, collard greens, corn (yellow), grapes, endive, kale, kiwi, mustard greens, okra, orange juice, red peppers, spinach, Swiss chard, watercress and zucchini.

Vitamins and Minerals

Multivitamin and Mineral Supplements

A handful of studies have linked regular use of a multivitamin pill to a lower risk of cataracts.[13-15] These broad-based supplements help you meet your recommended daily intake for antioxidant nutrients, including vitamins C and E and selenium. Take one multivitamin and mineral pill each day with a meal.

Vitamin C

This antioxidant nutrient is concentrated in the eye, where it protects the lens from oxidative damage caused by free radicals. Studies show that low blood vitamin C levels are linked with cataract disease.[16,17] A Harvard study of 80,000 American women found that long-term use of vitamin C supplements offered substantial protection from cataracts.[18] Compared with non–vitamin C users, those who took vitamin C pills for at least ten years had a 77 percent lower prevalence of early cataract formation and an 83 percent lower prevalence of moderate cataract development.

Based on the evidence available, it appears that supplemental doses of vitamin C are required to help prevent cataracts. Take 500 milligrams of vitamin C once or twice daily, or a 1000 milligram time-released vitamin C pill once

daily. There is some concern that high-dose vitamin C supplements might induce kidney stones in people with a history of stones or in individuals with kidney disease. In these cases, it is prudent to limit your dose to 100 milligrams per day.

Vitamin E

Diets rich in vitamin E and vitamin E supplements may also help lower the odds of cataract development. Vitamin E works with vitamin C and other antioxidant compounds in the eye to ward off free radical damage. Research has shown that low blood levels of vitamin E are linked with almost a fourfold increase in the risk of early cataract formation.[19,20] One study determined that regular use of a vitamin E supplement reduced the risk of cataract by one-half.[21] Vitamin E may not help you, however, if you are a current smoker. A study from Finland found that extra vitamin E made no difference to cataract risk in older men who smoked at least 20 cigarettes per day.[22]

To supplement, take 400 international units (IU) of natural vitamin E per day. Buy a product with "mixed tocopherols," since research suggests this form of vitamin E may have additional health benefits.

Herbal Remedies

Bilberry (*Vaccinium myrtillus*)

This herbal remedy contains anthocyanins, antioxidant compounds that may help preserve eye health. The anthocyanins in bilberry are thought to improve blood flow in the tiny capillaries of the eye. A handful of well-controlled studies found that compared with the placebo treatment, bilberry significantly improved eye health in people with diabetic eye complications.[23,24]

Buy a product standardized to 25 to 36 percent anthocyanins. Take 160 milligrams twice daily. For more information on bilberry, see Chapter 7.

Other Natural Health Products

Grapeseed Extract and Pycnogenol™

Like bilberry, both grapeseed extract and Pycnogenol™ contain potent antioxidants called anthocyanins that may be helpful in protecting the eye. Grapeseed extract is more readily available than pycnogenol and it's less expensive. For general antioxidant protection, take 50 milligrams once daily.

Lutein

If you don't eat five to seven servings of fruits and vegetables each day, you may want to consider taking lutein supplements. Buy a high-quality product that's made with the FloraGlo® extract. Take 10 milligrams once daily with a meal that contains some fat (carotenoids are best absorbed in the presence of dietary fat). See Chapter 8 for more on this carotenoid.

Lycopene

This carotenoid compound is found in certain red fruits and vegetables, but it is especially abundant in heat-processed tomato products such as tomato juice and pasta sauce. There is some evidence to suggest that lycopene helps to prevent cataracts. If your daily diet does not include tomato-based foods, consider taking a lycopene supplement made from the Lyc-O-Mato™ extract. Take one 5 milligram tablet per day with a meal that contains some fat. I discuss lycopene in more detail in Chapter 8.

Nutrition Strategy Checklist for Cataracts

- ☐ Quit smoking
- ☐ Maintain a healthy weight
- ☐ Limit sodium
- ☐ Limit alcohol
- ☐ Multivitamin/mineral
- ☐ Vitamin C
- ☐ Vitamin E
- ☐ Lutein
- ☐ Lycopene
- ☐ Bilberry
- ☐ Grapeseed extract

Recommended Resources

www.eyenet.org
American Academy of Ophthalmology
655 Beach Street
San Francisco, CA, USA 94109-7424
Tel: 415-561-8500

www.eyesite.ca
Canadian Ophthalmological Society
610-1525 Carling Avenue
Ottawa, ON, Canada K1Z 8R9
Tel: 613-729-6779 or 1-800-267-5763
Fax: 613-729-7209
E-mail: cos@eyesite.ca

www.nei.nih.gov
National Eye Institute, NIH, HHS
Building 31, Room 6A32, 31 Center Drive, MSC 2510
Bethesda, MD, USA 20892-2510
Tel: 301-496-5248
Fax: 301-402-1065

Celiac Disease (Gluten Intolerance)

The simple pleasures that most of us take for granted, such as enjoying a slice of bread, a plate of pasta or the sweet temptation of cookies, can be the source of acute discomfort for people suffering from celiac disease. This autoimmune digestive disorder is caused by sensitivity to gluten, a protein found in wheat, barley, rye and oats. Even a small indulgence in forbidden foods can trigger cramps, diarrhea, abdominal pain and fatigue. A lifetime of vigilance is necessary to keep the debilitating effects of celiac disease under control.

Celiac disease, also known as celiac sprue or nontropical sprue, is considered a malabsorption syndrome because it deprives the nervous system and vital organs of essential nourishment. There is no cure for celiac disease, but it can be effectively treated and controlled by following a gluten-free diet.

What Causes Celiac Disease?

When people with celiac disease eat foods containing gluten, the protein triggers a malfunction in the immune system. Normally, the nutrients from digested food are absorbed into the bloodstream through thousands of tiny projections, called villi, which line the surface of the small intestine. In celiac disease, gluten in the diet can provoke the immune system to attack the intestinal lining. The resulting swelling and inflammation damages the small intestine by causing the hair-like villi to shrink and flatten. This reduces the surface area of the intestinal lining, interfering with digestion and limiting the absorption of vitamins, minerals and other vital nutrients.

There is clear evidence that celiac disease is an inherited condition. Five to 10 percent of the immediate relatives (parents, children, siblings) of people diagnosed with this condition also eventually develop the disease. For those with a genetic predisposition, the onset of the disease is often stimulated by specific triggers, such as pregnancy, severe stress, viral infections or a physical injury. Celiac disease is difficult to diagnose, which makes it hard to determine how widely it affects the general population. Estimates vary from one in 500 to one in 2500 people being affected throughout North America.

Symptoms

Symptoms of celiac disease include

- anemia
- gas, bloating, abdominal pain and cramping
- diarrhea
- weight loss
- fatigue
- irritability
- pale, foul-smelling, bulky stools
- loss of menstrual periods
- unexplained infertility
- dermatitis herpetiformis, which causes severe rashes on the arms, elbows, back, knees and buttocks

Children with the disease may stop growing normally and may have abnormally bowed long bones, wasted buttocks and potbellies.

There is no typical case of celiac disease. Symptoms and reactions vary considerably from person to person and may develop at any age. Gluten intolerance does not always cause severe symptoms. In fact, some people may have the disease for years without knowing it. They may experience mild indigestion that's not serious enough to prompt a visit to a doctor. Often it's only when gluten is eliminated from the diet that a person will feel better and make the connection between grains and their symptoms.

The only way to know for sure if you have an intolerance to gluten is to have a doctor who specializes in gastrointestinal disorders take a biopsy of your small intestine. The specialist will look for signs of damage to your intestinal lining. Blood tests can be done to screen for the disease, but they do not confirm that you actually have it. Even when there are no obvious symptoms of the condition, there may still be damage to the intestinal lining. It is essential to get a confirmatory diagnosis from a physician.

Who's at Risk?

Women are at greater risk of celiac disease than men. The condition is also more prevalent in children, though an increasing number of adults, especially between the ages of 30 and 60, are being diagnosed with it.

People of northwestern European descent or with a family history of celiac disease are at greater risk. Individuals with type 1 diabetes or thyroid disease are also at greater risk.

Conventional Treatment

Following a gluten-free diet for life is the only effective treatment. Once gluten is removed from the diet, healing of the intestinal lining begins fairly quickly, though full recovery of the villi can take several months to years in adults with celiac disease. Consultation with a registered dietitian (**www.dietitians.ca**) will help ensure the nutritional quality of a gluten-free diet.

Gluten is widely used in the production of processed and packaged foods. As well, many commercial foods contain hidden sources of gluten, such as hydrolyzed vegetable protein (HVP) or hydrolyzed plant protein (HPP), malt, spelt and kamut. Because it is such a pervasive ingredient in our food supply, eliminating gluten from the diet can be a challenging task. People with celiac disease must pay careful attention to the ingredients list on food labels in order to avoid inadvertently consuming gluten. And since ingredients of commercial foods change frequently, labels must be checked with each purchase. If an ingredients list is not present, contact the manufacturer for product information.

People with celiac disease who do not maintain a gluten-free diet have a greater chance of developing osteoporosis and certain types of cancer, especially intestinal lymphoma.

Managing Celiac Disease

Dietary Strategies

A Gluten-Free Diet
Lifelong adherence to a gluten-free diet is essential for managing celiac disease. Use the following list to avoid gluten-containing grains:

Not Allowed	Allowed
Barley	Amaranth
Bulgur	Arrowroot
Couscous	Buckwheat
Eikorn	Corn
Emmer	Corn bran
Faro	Flaxseed
Kamut	Legumes
Mir	Millet
Oat bran	Nuts
Oats	Plantain
Rye	Potato
Semolina	Psyllium
Spelt	Quinoa
Triticale	Rice, rice bran, rice polishings
Wheat, wheat flour, wheat starch	Sweet potato

Gluten can also be a hidden ingredient in many foods such as soups, sauces and salad dressings. In addition to the grains listed above, the following should be avoided: bran, cereal binding, durum, edible starch, filler, food starch, germ, graham flour, gum base, hydrolyzed plant protein (HPP), hydrolyzed vegetable protein (HVP), icing sugar, malt, malt extract, malt flavoring, malt syrup, wheat germ and wheat starch.

For more information about gluten-containing foods, obtain a copy of *Acceptability of Foods and Food Ingredients for the Gluten-Free Diet*, a pocket dictionary available from the Canadian Celiac Association (see contact information below).

Gluten-Free Commercial Foods
The following organizations specialize in producing or selling gluten-free foods. Their product lists are posted on their Web sites.

Glutino	1-800-363-3468	**www.glutino.com**
El Peto	1-800-387-4064	**www.elpeto.com**
Kingsmill Foods	416-755-1124	**www.kingsmillfoods.com**

Kinnikinnick	877-503-4466	**www.kinnikinnick.com**
Liv-N-Well	877-270-8479	**www.liv-n-well.com**
Specialty Food Shop	1-800-737-7976	**www.specialtyfoodshop.com**

Dietary Fiber

A gluten-free diet may be low in fiber, since wheat bran and oat bran must be avoided. Some people might experience constipation. However, many of the allowed grains are good sources of fiber and should be added to your daily diet to promote bowel regularity.

Psyllium seed husks, flaxseed, corn bran, rice bran and rice polishings are all gluten-free sources of fiber. Legumes such as kidney beans, black beans, navy beans, chickpeas and lentils are very good sources of fiber and should regularly be included in the gluten-free diet. Drinking 8 to 12 glasses (2 to 3 liters) of fluid per day and getting regular exercise will also help prevent constipation.

Lactose

In the initial stages of celiac disease, avoidance of lactose-containing foods can help minimize symptoms of abdominal pain, bloating, gas and diarrhea. Lactose is a natural sugar found in dairy products and some commercial foods. It is digested by an enzyme called lactase that is present on the intestinal villi. Damage to the intestinal tract caused by gluten can impair lactose digestion and absorption.

Lactose intolerance usually normalizes within a few months of starting the gluten-free diet, once the intestinal lining has healed. However, some people find that a lactose intolerance persists; they will benefit from a lactose-free diet (see page 408, Lactose Intolerance).

Vitamins and Minerals

Multivitamin and Mineral Supplements

Untreated celiac disease causes malabsorption of many nutrients, including calcium, magnesium, fat-soluble vitamins (A, D, E, K), folate, vitamin B12 and iron.[1] In cases of severe malabsorption, vitamin and mineral supplements may be required for several months until the intestinal cells regenerate. Taking a multivitamin and mineral supplement is a good way to get the recommended daily amounts for most nutrients. It is wise to continue taking a multivitamin and mineral supplement even after the intestine has healed, since many gluten-free grains tend to be lower in B vitamins.

Your registered dietitian will assess the need for additional vitamin or mineral supplements based on the degree of malabsorption and resulting nutrient deficiencies.

Calcium, Magnesium and Vitamin D

Osteoporosis is a common condition in adults with celiac disease.[2] Impaired absorption of calcium, magnesium and vitamin D may all play a role in developing low bone density. Studies do show, however, that following a gluten-free diet promotes recovery of bone loss.[3-6] Despite this, it is crucial to ensure you are meeting your daily requirements for these bone-building nutrients. Young children, teens and women should pay very close attention to the adequacy of their diets, especially if they are lactose intolerant. The following are good food sources of these nutrients.

Calcium: milk, yogurt, cheese, fortified soy and rice beverages, fortified orange juice, tofu, salmon (with bones), kale, bok choy, broccoli and Swiss chard

Magnesium: nuts, seeds, legumes, prunes, leafy green vegetables, Brewer's yeast, cheddar cheese and shrimp

Vitamin D: fluid milk, fortified soy and rice beverages, oily fish, egg yolks, butter and margarine

If you determine that you need to supplement to meet your daily calcium needs, buy a calcium citrate pill, since calcium in this form is absorbed more efficiently. Choose a product with added vitamin D and magnesium. Take 300 milligrams, one to three times daily, depending on the amount of calcium provided by your diet. For a detailed list of calcium, magnesium and vitamin D in foods, see Chapter 4.

Nutrition Strategy Checklist for Celiac Disease

- ☐ Gluten-free diet
- ☐ Dietary fiber
- ☐ Low lactose
- ☐ Multivitamin/mineral
- ☐ Calcium
- ☐ Vitamin D
- ☐ Magnesium

Recommended Resources

www.celiac.ca
Canadian Celiac Association
5170 Dixie Road, Suite 204
Mississauga, ON, Canada L4W 1E3
Tel: 905-507-6208 or 1-800-363-7296
Fax: 905-507-4673

www.celiac.org
Celiac Disease Foundation
13251 Ventura Boulevard, Suite #1
Studio City, CA, USA 91604-1838
Tel: 818-990-2354
Fax: 818-990-2379

www.csaceliacs.org
Celiac Sprue Association/USA Inc.
P.O. Box 31700
Omaha, NE, USA 68131-0700
Tel: 402-558-0600
Fax: 402-558-1347

Cervical Dysplasia

If you are diagnosed with cervical dysplasia, it means that abnormal changes are beginning to take place in the cells lining the surface of your cervix, the part of your reproductive system that forms the entrance to your uterus. If left untreated, cervical dysplasia could progress to become cervical cancer. The only reliable way to detect this precancerous condition is to have an annual Pap smear, a laboratory test of a small sample of your cervical tissue.

What Causes Cervical Dysplasia?

Scientists don't know what causes the cell changes of cervical dysplasia, but they suspect that it is something spread through sexual contact. Current research indicates that the human papillomavirus (HPV), a virus that causes sexually transmitted genital infections, may trigger abnormal cell growth.[1,2]

There are three stages of cervical dysplasia. If abnormal cells are found only on the surface of the cervix, the condition is considered mild. But unfortunately, these precancerous cells often spread deeper into the tissue of the cervix lining. When this happens, cervical dysplasia is labeled as moderate or severe, depending on the extent of the tissue penetration. Up to 60 percent of women with mild cervical dysplasia find that these cell changes are only temporary. Within 6 to 12 months, the cells of the cervix return to normal and health is no longer at risk. However, once cervical dysplasia reaches the moderate or severe stage, there is a much greater chance that the condition will progress to cervical cancer within the next ten years.

Symptoms

There are no warning signs of cervical dysplasia. Without the appropriate medical testing, you probably won't realize that anything is wrong until the disease is well advanced. If you have regular medical check-ups, your doctor may notice a growth, sore or suspicious area on your cervix during a routine pelvic examination.

In most cases, identifiable symptoms don't appear until the cervical dysplasia has progressed to cervical cancer. At that time, a woman may experience some pain or some intermittent bleeding or spotting between menstrual cycles. To prevent cervical cancer, it is critical that you get tested for cervical dysplasia by having a Pap smear on an annual basis. The Pap smear identifies precancerous changes of cervical cells and also indicates the presence of invasive cancer cells. But an abnormal result does not always mean your health is at risk. Sometimes a virus may cause temporary cell changes that will disappear in a short period of time.

Who's at Risk?

Women who begin having sexual intercourse at an early age (16 years or younger) and those who have multiple sexual partners are at higher risk for developing cervical dysplasia. So are women who have a history of sexually transmitted disease, especially HPV infection. Other conditions that may increase the risk for cervical dysplasia include

- smoking cigarettes or exposure to second-hand smoke

- using oral contraceptives for more than five years

- having a history of a gynecological cancer

- following a diet that's low in vitamin A, beta-carotene and folate

Women who are sexually active and do not have regular Pap smears to test for cervical dysplasia have a greater chance of developing cervical cancer.

Conventional Treatment

The treatment for cervical dysplasia varies, depending on the extent and severity of the dysplasia. If a woman is diagnosed with mild dysplasia and has no other risk factors for cervical cancer, her doctor will probably monitor the condition and wait to see if the affected cells return to normal. A second Pap smear will be performed in four to six months and, if cell growth is normal at that time, no treatment will be necessary. It is recommended that women with mild dysplasia return for a pelvic examination and Pap smear twice a year for at least two years.

A diagnosis of moderate or severe dysplasia is treated differently. The surface of the cervix is examined for abnormalities in a procedure called a *colposcopy*. Using a viewing tube with a magnifying lens, your doctor will inspect your cervix and take a biopsy of tissue from the abnormal area. The tissue samples are then sent to a laboratory to determine the extent of changes to cervical cells.

Once the severity of the cervical dysplasia is known, the treatment will involve removing all the abnormal growth that can turn into cervical cancer. Your doctor may perform a surgical procedure called *cervical conization*, which removes a cone-shaped area of tissue. Other ways of removing the abnormal area include cauterizing the tissue with heat, freezing it with cryosurgery, vaporizing it with lasers or removing it with an electrified wire loop procedure known as LEEP. Because cervical dysplasia can return, it is important for women to have Pap smears every three months for the first year after surgery and every six months after that.

In more severe cases, a hysterectomy to remove the uterus may be necessary.

The sooner cervical dysplasia is detected and treated, the lower a woman's risk for developing cervical cancer. The following dietary and nutritional strategies may help prevent cervical dysplasia from developing in the first place. Some of the strategies I discuss below might even reverse the dysplasia.

Preventing Cervical Dysplasia

Vitamins and Minerals

Antioxidants

Many studies have found a link between cervical dysplasia and low blood levels of antioxidant nutrients, especially beta-carotene and vitamin C. Women with cervical dysplasia are also more likely to have poor dietary intakes of these and other antioxidants. Antioxidants are vitamins, minerals or natural plant chemicals that protect cells in the body from damage caused by free radicals—highly reactive oxygen molecules produced by normal body processes. Excess free radicals can also be formed by pollution, cigarette smoke and heavy exercise. These compounds can damage the genetic material of cells, which in turn may lead to cancer development. Antioxidants neutralize free radicals, preventing them from causing damage to cells.

The body has built-in antioxidant enzymes for keeping free radical activity in check, but levels decline as we age. Scientists are learning every day that a daily supply of dietary antioxidants is important for reducing the risk of certain cancers. When it comes to cervical dysplasia (a precursor to cervical cancer), a handful of dietary antioxidants have been identified that may prevent free radical damage to cervical cells.

Beta-Carotene

This antioxidant is plentiful in dark green vegetables and orange fruits and vegetables. It's been hypothesized that beta-carotene may protect from cervical dysplasia and cervical cancer in a few ways. First of all, we know that beta-carotene is a potent antioxidant and may therefore protect cervical cells from free radical damage. Beta-carotene is also used to make vitamin A in the body. Vitamin A is essential for normal cellular growth and development. A number of laboratory studies have shown the ability of vitamin A to prevent abnormal cell growth. Researchers have found that compared with women free of cervical dysplasia, those with the condition have significantly lower blood levels and dietary intakes of beta-carotene.[3]

This does not necessarily mean that beta-carotene can reverse the course of dysplasia once you are diagnosed with the condition. To date, two randomized control trials have compared women taking a 30 milligram beta-carotene supplement with women taking a placebo.[4,5] The researchers found no difference in regression of dysplasia in either group of women. It is possible that these studies, which lasted nine months and two years, respectively, were too short to notice an effect.

At the time of writing this book, there is a two-year trial nearing completion in the United States. The study involves 120 women with moderate to severe dysplasia who were randomized to receive either 30 milligrams of beta-carotene each day or a placebo. It is hoped that this trial will be long enough to find a protective effect of beta-carotene supplements.

Currently there is no daily recommended intake for beta-carotene, but many experts believe that 5 to 15 milligrams (9000 to 27,000 international units [IU]) per day offers plenty of protection.

Orange and dark green produce, including carrots, sweet potato, winter squash, broccoli, collard greens, kale, spinach, apricots, cantaloupe, peaches, nectarines, mango and papaya, contain the most beta-carotene. However, the body does not absorb the beta-carotene in raw foods efficiently. To enhance absorption, cook the vegetables and eat them along with a little fat in your meal.

Beta-Carotene Supplements To boost your intake, buy a multivitamin and mineral with added beta-carotene. Most brands provide 1000 to 10,000 IU (0.5 to 5.5 milligrams). If you opt for a separate beta-carotene supplement, choose a product that offers a mix of carotenoids including beta-carotene and lycopene. But keep in mind that taking a supplement is likely ineffective in preventing cervical cancer when a diet high in beta-carotene is consumed.

The use of beta-carotene supplements in doses of 20 milligrams per day for five to eight years has been associated with an increased risk of lung cancer in men who smoke. While these findings may not apply to women, it makes sense to be cautious. If you are a smoker, avoid beta-carotene supplements and instead eat at least two foods rich in beta-carotene per day. This potential health risk has not been found in smokers who eat a diet plentiful in beta-carotene-rich foods.

Lycopene
This antioxidant belongs to the same family of carotenoid compounds as beta-carotene. But compared with beta-carotene, lycopene is twice as potent an antioxidant. A few studies have suggested that lycopene protects women from cervical dysplasia. A study from the University of Pennsylvania School of Medicine found that women with the highest intake of lycopene were one-third as likely to have dysplasia compared with those who consumed the least.[6]

Lycopene is found in red-colored fruits and vegetables. It's the natural chemical that gives these foods their bright color. Heat-processed tomato products such as tomato juice, pasta sauce and cooked tomatoes are the richest source of lycopene, but you'll also find some in fresh tomatoes, pink grapefruit, watermelon, guava

and apricots. Based on the research that has been conducted in the area of heart disease, it appears that an intake of 5 to 7 milligrams offers protection. Lycopene is a fat-soluble compound and is better absorbed in the presence of a little fat.

Lycopene Supplements These are available in health food stores and drug stores. Choose a brand that's made with the Lyc-O-Mato™ or LycoRed™ extract. This source of lycopene comes from Israel and is derived from whole tomatoes. It is also the extract that has been used in clinical studies. Most supplements offer 5 milligrams of lycopene per tablet. Take 5 to 10 milligrams once daily with a meal.

Vitamin C
Less research has been done on this antioxidant vitamin and its potential role in protection from cervical dysplasia. A few studies have determined that women with low blood levels of vitamin C have a greater risk of cervical dysplasia compared with women with higher levels. Furthermore, cigarette smoke decreases the level of vitamin C in the body. One American study found a strong association between a woman's history of smoking and her level of vitamin C, whether or not she had cervical dysplasia.[7]

Citrus fruit, strawberries, kiwi, cantaloupe, broccoli, bell peppers, Brussels sprouts, cabbage, tomatoes and potatoes are all good sources of vitamin C. Mango, cantaloupe, red grapefruit and tomato juice also contain beta-carotene and/or lycopene. Aim to eat at least two foods rich in vitamin C per day.

Vitamin C Supplements If you decide to supplement your diet, choose a brand labeled Ester C. Studies in the laboratory have found that this form of vitamin C is more available to the body. Take 500 milligrams once or twice a day. There's little point in swallowing much more than that at once, since your body can use only about 200 milligrams at one time.

Vitamin E

As with vitamin C, less research has been done in the area of vitamin E and cervical dysplasia. Nevertheless, observational studies have found a link between the risk of dysplasia and blood levels of this vitamin. For instance, one study from the Cancer Research Center of Hawaii revealed that women with the highest blood vitamin E levels had a 70 percent lower risk of cervical dysplasia compared with women with the lowest blood levels of the vitamin.[8] The researchers also noticed what's called a dose response effect. That means the higher the level of vitamin E, the lower the risk of dysplasia.

Wheat germ, nuts, seeds, soybeans, vegetable oils, corn oil, whole grains and kale are all good sources of vitamin E. To supplement, take 200 to 800 IU of a natural source vitamin E per day. Consider choosing a vitamin E supplement labeled mixed tocopherols. Preliminary research shows that one form of vitamin E called gamma-tocopherol has potent anti-inflammatory effects in addition to its antioxidant properties. This may play a role in cancer prevention.

Folate

This B vitamin, although not an antioxidant, appears to have a very important role in preventing the development of dysplasia. Research shows that as one's intake of folate-rich foods decreases, the risk of cervical dysplasia increases. An American study found that women consuming less than 400 micrograms of folate each day were 2.6 times more likely to develop dysplasia than women who consumed more than 400 micrograms.[9]

A lack of folate may promote the development of dysplasia in a number of ways. Folate may act in some way to protect cervical cells. Studies have found that many women with dysplasia have normal blood levels of folate but low levels of the vitamin in cervical tissue.[10] A deficiency of folate may also enhance the harmful effect of human papillomavirus (HPV) infection on cervical cells.

Folate is critical for the synthesis of DNA (deoxyribonucleic acid), the genetic material of cells. Low levels of folate in cervical tissue can make cellular DNA more susceptible to damage. Even a marginal folate deficiency can cause damage to DNA in cells, damage that resembles cervical dysplasia. It is possible that this alteration to DNA is an early step in the progression of cervical dysplasia and cervical cancer. Furthermore, this damage to a cell's genetic material may be stopped or reversed if given supplements of the B vitamin. Two trials have found that folic acid supplements improved dysplasia in women taking birth control pills.[11,12] However, trials conducted in women not taking oral contraceptives did not find folic acid supplements to alter the course of dysplasia. The researchers concluded that a deficiency of this B vitamin may be involved in the initiation of dysplasia, but once you have the disease, supplements do not appear to reverse it.

The best sources of folate are spinach, lentils, orange juice, whole grains, fortified breakfast cereals, asparagus, artichoke, avocado and seeds.

Folate Supplements

For many women, consuming the recommended daily intake of 400 micrograms can be challenging. To supplement your diet, take a multivitamin and mineral supplement or a B complex formula once daily. Look for a brand that gives between 0.4 and 1.0 milligrams of folic acid. (Folic acid is the synthetic form of folate, whether in a supplement or enriched foods.) If you take a separate folic acid supplement, buy one that has vitamin B12 added. High doses of folic acid taken over a period of time can hide a B12 deficiency and result in progressive nerve damage.

Nutrition Strategy Checklist for Cervical Dysplasia

☐ Beta-carotene   ☐ Vitamin E
☐ Lycopene   ☐ Folate
☐ Vitamin C

Recommended Resources

www.askdrkoop.com
This site was founded by former US Surgeon General Dr. Everett Koop.

www.cancernet.nci.nih.gov
The gateway to recent and accurate cancer information from the National Cancer Institute.

www.hopkinsmedicine.org
The Johns Hopkins University School of Medicine
Barbara A. Biedrzycki, Adult Nurse Practitioner
1650 Orleans Street
Baltimore, MD, USA 21231

www.mayoclinic.com
Mayo Foundation for Medical Education and Research

Chronic Fatigue Syndrome (CFS)

Chronic Fatigue Syndrome (CFS) is an enigma— a largely misunderstood illness that saps vitality and steals mental acuity. Very little is known about the causes of CFS and even less about the possible cures. CFS is a disease characterized by a profound fatigue that is not improved with bed rest. People with CFS are easily exhausted by the slightest physical or mental activities. Because there is no known cure, CFS can persist for years, dramatically altering the lives of those who suffer from it.

What Causes CFS?

There doesn't seem to be one single cause for CFS. Instead, research indicates that there could be a number of different factors, working alone or in combination, that might cause CFS. Initially, CFS was thought to be produced by a virus infection. Scientific attention was focused on the Epstein-Barr virus, herpes-type viruses and infections that cause polio. But extensive studies were unable to establish a direct connection between CFS and these or any other infectious agents. Despite this, scientists still speculate that a virus may help trigger the disease.

There is little argument among experts that a disturbed immune system plays an important role in CFS. Scientists believe that CFS is caused when an infection or virus attacks someone with a weakened immune system. Once the infection has passed, the immune system doesn't return to its normal state. Instead, it remains active, continuously producing excess immune-activating factors. As these factors circulate through the bloodstream, they may cause profound fatigue. Studies do find that many people with CFS have chronically over-active immune systems, with white blood cells that are less able to fight off viruses.

Often people with CFS have a history of allergies, which, for some unknown reason, seems to predispose them to the disease. There is also the possibility that a severe metabolic dysfunction may be the culprit behind CFS. Many CFS sufferers show evidence of extreme shifts in metabolism that limit heart and lung functions, making it difficult and even physically damaging to carry out normal activities. Research has also linked brain abnormalities with CFS, especially those associated with sleep-related disorders.

In the hunt for the cause of CFS, research is beginning to assign an important role to the central nervous system. Certain malfunctions of the nervous system can produce racing heartbeats or sudden drops in blood pressure. These conditions seem to be associated with the development of CFS in ways that are not yet fully understood. Periods of physical or emotional stress also have an impact on the nervous system. Stressful events stimulate the brain to produce cortisol and other stress hormones. These hormones affect the immune system by suppressing inflammation. Because stress may be a trigger for the development of CFS, it's possible that there is a connection between the disease and altered levels of stress hormones.

Most recently, developments in CFS research have led to the exciting discovery of a new human enzyme. This abnormal enzyme may affect the body's ability to control common viruses and maintain energy in body cells. Early studies indicate that the enzyme is present in most people with CFS and may be the cause of low energy levels.

Symptoms

The most obvious symptom of CFS is an extreme fatigue that interferes with your ability to carry out daily activities. This level of fatigue goes far beyond the exhausted, overtired feelings that we all get from time to time. The fatigue that characterizes CFS is relentless and does not go away for weeks, months or years at a time, despite your best efforts to get adequate rest and relaxation.

CFS sufferers may also have a variety of other symptoms. Muscle weakness, sleep disturbances, lightheadedness, fainting and dizziness are all common problems associated with the disease. CFS may cause impaired thinking, forgetfulness, confusion, difficulty concentrating, depression and anxiety. Because the disease involves a faulty immune system, it's common for people with CFS to experience food allergies, other fungal infections (e.g., yeast infections) and frequent bouts of the common cold.

CFS symptoms and their duration vary widely from individual to individual. Approximately 50 percent of people with CFS return to a fairly normal lifestyle within five years. The other half will still be dramatically ill even after ten years. Some people recover from the disease in two to three years, only to suffer a relapse at a later time. CFS can be cyclical, producing alternating periods of illness and relatively good health.

Who's at Risk?

CFS is thought to affect 20,000 to 30,000 Canadians.[1] Studies from the early 1980s revealed that it was mainly well-educated, affluent Caucasian women between the ages of 25 and 45 years who suffered from CFS. However, as a growing number of doctors recognize CFS as a legitimate disorder, newly gathered data shows that the illness can occur in all income, racial and age groups. Women still seem to report the condition two to four times more often than men, possibly because women are more willing to seek medical treatment for fatigue.[2]

Conventional Treatment

Medications prescribed for CFS are intended to provide relief of symptoms. They are not considered to cure the disease. Today, doctors use a combination of therapies and a gradual approach to rehabilitation in treating this disease.

Low-dose *tricyclic antidepressants* seem to have a positive effect on some people with CFS, possibly because they improve the quality of sleep. Another form of antidepressant, *SSRIs (serotonin reuptake inhibitors),* also provides treatment benefits. In some cases, *benzodiazepines,* a type of drug used to treat anxiety and sleep problems, will improve the quality of life for CFS sufferers. *NSAIDs* (nonsteroidal anti-inflammatory drugs) will help fight the aches and pains and *antihistamines* may relieve the allergy symptoms associated with the condition.

Learning to manage your fatigue will help you improve the ability to function. Behavior therapy can help you find effective ways to plan daily activities so that you can take advantage of peak energy levels. Exercise is also important in the management of CFS. Although exercise may seem to aggravate the symptoms, it is essential to maintain some muscle strength and conditioning. Throughout the course of this disease, it is important to learn to pace yourself physically, emotionally and mentally, because extra stress can make your symptoms much worse.

Managing CFS

Nutrition plays an important role in the recovery to good health. However, scientists have identified a number of vitamins and minerals that are deficient in many people with CFS. This seems to be mostly due to the illness itself, rather than a poor diet. Even marginal nutrient deficiencies can contribute to fatigue symptoms. But lacking important nutrients can also delay the healing process.

Dietary Strategies

Follow a wholesome, healthy diet. The quality of the foods eaten seems to be most important in helping to restore energy levels.

1. *Emphasize plant foods* in your daily diet. Fill your plate with grains, fruits and vegetables. If you eat animal protein foods like meat or poultry, they should take up no more than one-quarter of your plate. Try vegetarian sources of protein like beans and soy.

2. *Choose foods and oils that are rich in essential fatty acids.* Fish, nuts, seeds, flaxseed and flaxseed oil, canola oil, Omega-3 eggs, wheat germ and leafy green vegetables are examples.

3. *Choose foods rich in vitamins, minerals and protective plant compounds.* Reach for whole

grains as often as possible. Eat at least three different colored fruits and three different colored vegetables every day.

4. *Eliminate sources of refined sugar* as often as possible: cookies, cakes, pastries, frozen desserts, soft drinks, sweetened fruit juices, fruit drinks, candy, etc.

5. *Buy organic produce* or *wash fruits and vegetables* to remove pesticide residues.

6. *Limit foods with chemical additives.*

7. *Avoid caffeine* (this can worsen fatigue by interrupting sleep patterns).

8. *Drink at least 8 to 12 cups (2 to 3 liters) of water every day.*

9. *Avoid alcohol.* If you drink, limit your alcohol intake. Women should consume no more than one drink a day, or seven per week, men no more than two drinks per day, to a limit of nine drinks per week.

10. *Take a multivitamin and mineral supplement each day* to ensure you are meeting your needs for most nutrients. Buy a product that contains no artificial preservatives, colors, flavors or added sugar, starch, lactose or yeast. This should be declared in small print below the ingredients list. If you experience gastrointestinal upset when taking a multivitamin, try a "professional brand" supplement available at certain health food stores. These products contain no binding materials and are suitable for people with food sensitivities. However, they're expensive, and you have to take at least three to six capsules a day to meet your recommended intake levels. Brand names include Genestra® and Thorne Research®.

To help you follow these principles, reread Chapter 5. You'll learn what foods you should be eating more often. You'll also learn how many servings of these foods you should be striving for each day.

If you experience bloating, cramps, gas, diarrhea or skin rashes after eating, it's a good idea to be tested for food allergies. Ask your family doctor for a referral to an allergy specialist.

Essential Fatty Acids

The fat in foods or in the body are made up of individual building blocks called fatty acids. The body can make all but two fatty acids: linoleic acid and alpha-linolenic acid (ALA). Because these two fatty acids are essential to our health and well-being, they must be supplied by the diet. Linoleic acid is considered an omega-6 fatty acid. It's found in leafy vegetables, seeds, nuts, grains and vegetable oils made from corn, safflower, sunflower, soybean and sesame. Alpha-linolenic acid belongs to the omega-3 family of fats. Good food sources include canola oil, flaxseed and flaxseed oil, walnuts and walnut oil, wheat germ and soybeans.

It's thought that people with CFS don't metabolize essential fatty acids properly and that this leads to a faulty immune system. One of the body's natural antivirus agents, called interferon, requires essential fatty acids in order to exert its virus-fighting power. Some studies have determined that many CFS sufferers have lowered levels of essential fats in their body. Some researchers have reported symptom improvements in many patients treated with essential fatty acids.[3]

Your daily diet should include 3 to 6 teaspoons (15 to 30 ml) of fat or oil rich in essential fatty acids. Emphasize sources of alpha-linolenic acid, since this particular fatty acid is emerging as a very healthy part of the diet.

Vitamins and Minerals

B Vitamins

Without B vitamins, our bodies would lack energy. These eight nutrients are indispensable for yielding energy compounds from the foods we eat.

Many B vitamins serve as helpers to enzymes that release energy from fat, protein and carbohydrate. Compared with healthy people, patients with CFS often have lower levels of B vitamins in their blood.[4-7] One study also found that enzymes dependent on B vitamins were less active in people with CFS. No published studies could be found that assessed the effect of vitamin B supplements on fatigue symptoms.

Vitamin B Supplements

In Chapter 4, I discuss in detail each B vitamin, daily requirements and food sources. To ensure you are getting your daily B vitamins, it is wise to take a good-quality multivitamin and mineral supplement each day. If you're looking for more B vitamins than a regular multi gives you, choose a high-potency or super formula that contains 50 to 100 milligrams of B vitamins (or micrograms in the case of folic acid and B12). You can also take a B complex formula that gives you all the B vitamins, often combined with vitamin C.

Magnesium

Magnesium is a part of adenosine triphosphate (ATP), the active energy compound that's used by every cell in your body. It's believed that a deficiency in magnesium can lead to the decreased energy and weakness seen in CFS. Some investigations have found low levels of magnesium in the red blood cells of patients with CFS.[8,9] When these patients are regularly given magnesium by injection, they reported more energy, less pain and more balanced emotions.

Although there is no concrete evidence to support the use of extra magnesium in CFS, there is no harm done by increasing your intake of this mineral. In fact, research from the United States suggests that only 25 percent of the population is meeting its daily magnesium needs. Some of the best food sources include nuts, seeds, legumes, prunes, whole grains, leafy green vegetables, Brewer's yeast, cheddar cheese and shrimp.

Magnesium Supplements

If you decide to supplement, choose a product made from magnesium citrate, a form that's more easily absorbed by the body. No definite dose has been established for CFS. Doses of 200 to 300 milligrams have been used to reduce the muscle pain and joint tenderness associated with fibromyalgia. The daily upper limit for supplemental magnesium is 350 milligrams. Doses higher than this can cause diarrhea and stomach upset.

Herbal Remedies

The following herbs have been shown to boost the body's production of infection-fighting immune compounds. Of the three I discuss, echinacea and Panax ginseng have been shown to enhance the activity of immune cells in people with CFS.[10] Echinacea can be beneficial to help treat bothersome colds, while ginseng and aged garlic extract can be used longer term for immune stimulation.

Echinacea

Studies have found that this herb can reduce the duration of cold symptoms by as much as 50 percent. Echinacea's active ingredients enhance the body's immune system by increasing production of certain white blood cells that fight off viruses and bacteria. Three species of echinacea are found in products—*Echinacea purpurea, Echinacea angustifolia* and *Echinacea pallida*—and all have medicinal benefits.

To ensure you're getting a quality product, buy one that's standardized. Take a total of 900 milligrams of echinacea three to four times daily at the first sign of cold or flu. Limit daily use to eight consecutive weeks; there is some concern that long-term use of echinacea might depress the immune system. Do not use echinacea if you're allergic to plants in the Asteracease/Compositae family (ragweed, daisy, marigold and chrysanthemum).

Panax Ginseng

This ginseng goes by many names, including Asian, Korean and Chinese. Studies have shown the herb to have strong immune-enhancing properties. A large Italian study found that individuals taking 100 milligrams of a standardized ginseng product (G115 extract) had significantly higher levels of antibodies in response to a flu shot compared with those who did not take the herb. Killer white blood cell counts were nearly twice as high in the ginseng group after eight weeks of supplementation. These and other white blood cells are an important part of the body's defense against viruses and foreign molecules.

Buy a product with a statement of standardization or "G115" printed on the label (such as Ginsana® from Pharmaton® Natural Health Products). The typical dosage of a standardized extract is 100 or 200 milligrams once daily. Take ginseng for three weeks to three months and follow with a one- to two-week rest period before you resume taking the herb. In some people, it may cause mild stomach upset, irritability and insomnia. To avoid overstimulation, start with 100 milligrams a day and avoid taking the herb with caffeine. Ginseng should not be used during pregnancy, breastfeeding or in individuals with poorly controlled high blood pressure.

Siberian Ginseng (*Eleutherococcus senticosus*)

Unlike Panax ginseng, this herb has a much milder effect and fewer reported side effects. Pregnant and nursing women can safely take Siberian ginseng, and it is much less likely to cause overstimulation in sensitive individuals. To ensure quality, choose a product standardized for eleutherosides B and E. The usual dosage is 300 to 400 milligrams once daily for six to eight weeks, followed by a one- to two-week break.

Garlic (*Allium sativum*)

A daily intake of garlic and its accompanying sulfur compounds has been used to enhance the body's immune system and kill many types of bacteria and fungi (including the Candida organism that causes yeast infections). One-half to one clove a day is recommended.

To supplement, buy *aged* garlic extract. The aging process used to make this supplement increases the concentration of the special sulfur compounds that stimulate the immune system. In fact, animal studies have found that the amount of garlic equivalent to three aged garlic extract capsules dramatically increases activity of white blood cells (killer cells, macrophages and leukocytes). Generally, two to six capsules a day (one or two with meals) are recommended. You can also buy aged garlic in a liquid form (Kyolic® brand) that you then add to foods.

Other Natural Health Products

Fish Oil Supplements

Fish oils are concentrated in omega-3 fatty acids and play an important role in cell membrane function and immune function. Based on the finding that CFS patients have depressed essential fatty acids in their blood cells, Scottish researchers had 63 adults with CFS take either fish oil (eight 500 milligram capsules per day) or placebo capsules for three months.[11] When the study was over, 85 percent of patients taking the fish oil had a significant improvement in their symptoms. As would be expected, there was also an increase in cellular levels of essential fatty acids. Researchers from the United Kingdom tried to replicate these results among 50 patients with CFS and found no difference in symptoms between those taking fish oil and the placebo group.[12]

Despite the mixed findings, you may still decide to add fish oil capsules to your nutritional regime, especially if you don't eat oily fish. Buy a product that offers a combination of EPA and DHA. A good-quality fish oil supplement should also contain vitamin E to help stabilize the oils. The brand used in clinical studies was Efamol® Marine. Avoid fish *liver* oil capsules. Supplements made from fish liver are a concentrated source of vitamin A and D; too much of these vitamins can be toxic when taken in large amounts for long periods.

Fish oil has a blood-thinning effect. If you take anticlotting medication, consult your physician first. Follow your health care practitioner's advice for dosage.

L-Carnitine

This compound is not considered an essential nutrient because the body makes it in sufficient quantities. Carnitine helps all cells in the body generate energy, especially muscle cells. It's possible that a deficiency of this compound can cause the fatigue associated with CFS. Studies have shown that CFS patients tend to have lower levels of carnitine in their blood, and higher levels are linked with less severe symptoms.[13,14]

Researchers from Chicago took the carnitine-and-CFS hypothesis one step further. They gave 30 people with CFS either carnitine or a drug treatment for two months.[15] After a two-week rest period, the treatments were switched. Those who originally got the drug were given carnitine. The researchers found a significant improvement in those taking the carnitine supplements after eight weeks.

L-carnitine is found in meat and dairy products. As a general dietary supplement, the recommended dose is 1 to 3 grams per day. If you have been diagnosed with a carnitine deficiency, the recommended dose is 990 milligrams taken as tablets two to three times daily (people with carnitine deficiencies should be monitored by their physician to make sure their dose is appropriate).

L-carnitine is available in the United States but it is not legally available in Canada. However, some health food stores do stock it.

Avoid products that contain D-carnitine or DL-carnitine. These forms compete with L-carnitine in the body and could lead to a deficiency. The supplement is considered safe. Occasional side effects of gastrointestinal upset have been reported.

Nutrition Strategy Checklist for Chronic Fatigue Syndrome

☐ Follow a healthy diet   ☐ Magnesium
☐ Identify food allergies   ☐ Echinacea
☐ Healthy oils   ☐ Panax ginseng
☐ Fish   ☐ Garlic
☐ Multivitamin/mineral   ☐ L-carnitine
☐ B vitamins

Recommended Resources

www.cfids.org
The CFIDS (Chronic Fatigue and Immune Dysfunction Syndrome)
Association of America, Inc.
P.O. Box 220398
Charlotte, NC, USA 28222-0398
Tel: 704-365-2343 (resource line) or 1-800-442-3437 (voice mail)
Fax: 704-365-9755

www.niaid.nih.gov
National Institute of Allergy and Infectious Diseases
Office of Communications and Public Liaison
Building 31, Room 7A-50
31 Center Drive, MSC 2520
Bethesda, MD, USA 20892-2520

Cirrhosis of the Liver

Weighing in at three pounds and roughly the size of a football, the liver is the largest internal organ in the body. Every minute, one quarter of the body's blood supply flows into the liver, where it is processed and cleaned to remove all harmful substances before flowing out again. The liver performs countless other functions essential for maintaining good health. It stores energy to fuel your muscles, produces over a thousand different enzymes, manufactures bile and cholesterol, regulates hormones and processes waste products. Because the liver plays such a crucial role in supporting your bodily functions, you cannot survive if your liver stops functioning.

Cirrhosis is a term that refers to several chronic diseases that can affect the normal functioning of the liver. These diseases damage healthy liver tissue, replacing it with scar tissue. The scar tissue restricts the flow of blood and prevents the liver from performing its many essential tasks.

What Causes Cirrhosis?

In North America, the most common cause of cirrhosis is alcohol abuse. Heavy drinkers are nearly 30 times more likely to develop cirrhosis than nondrinkers. Alcoholic cirrhosis usually develops in people who have been heavy drinkers for more than ten years. The amount of alcohol necessary to damage the liver varies from person to person. Because men are more inclined than women to drink excessively, alcoholic liver disease is twice as common in men than it is in women. However, even though women drink less, they are more easily affected by alcohol and more susceptible to alcohol-related liver injury.

Not everyone who drinks excessively will develop cirrhosis. Approximately 15 percent of alcoholics acquire the condition, while others experience less serious forms of liver damage.

Even social drinkers have been known to develop cirrhosis. Frequency and regularity of alcohol intake are the greatest risk factors influencing the prognosis of this disease. In alcoholics, nutritional deficiencies caused by a poor diet may also trigger the development of cirrhosis.

Hepatitis B ranks as a major cause of cirrhosis worldwide, although it is not as common a problem in North America. In the Western world, hepatitis C is the culprit behind cirrhosis. Both of these viral diseases provoke low-grade inflammation of the liver that often continues over several decades. The long-term damage to liver tissue associated with this type of inflammation often leads to cirrhosis.

Several inherited diseases, including hemochromatosis and glycogen storage diseases, interfere with the way the liver produces and stores a variety of essential substances, such as proteins, metals and enzymes. Blocked bile ducts cause bile to back up into the liver, resulting in serious tissue damage. Environmental toxins, reactions to prescription drugs and parasitic infections are additional factors that can cause scar tissue to develop in the liver.

Liver damage associated with cirrhosis is irreversible, no matter how it is caused. Early diagnosis and treatment is essential to prevent long-term damage. It is important to have regular medical checkups because a significant portion of the liver may have stopped functioning before any signs or symptoms of cirrhosis become apparent. While there are some treatments that can delay the progression of the scar tissue and reduce complications, there is no cure for this disease.

Symptoms

Some people feel no symptoms at all for many years. Common symptoms include feeling weak, sick and nauseated, loss of appetite and weight loss. As well, the liver may feel larger and harder.

As the disease progresses, complications may develop due to loss of liver function, including

- fluid accumulation in the leg (edema) and abdomen (ascites)

- bruising and bleeding easily

- yellowing of the skin (jaundice), gallstones and itching

- impaired mental function, personality changes, coma or death caused by toxins that accumulate in the blood and brain because the liver can no longer process the blood to remove them

- high blood pressure in the veins that run from the intestine to the liver

- enlarged blood vessels (varices) in the lower end of the esophagus (varices have thin walls and are more likely to burst under high pressure, resulting in serious bleeding problems)

- bacterial infections

- kidney dysfunction and possible kidney failure

- increased sensitivity to medications and drugs

Who's at Risk?

- Individuals who drink more than two alcoholic drinks a day for more than ten years (women are more susceptible to alcohol-related liver damage than men).

- Individuals who suffer from chronic viral hepatitis types B, C, D, autoimmune hepatitis and nonalcoholic steatohepatitis.

- Individuals with prolonged obstruction of the bile ducts or diseases of the bile ducts.

- Individuals with an inherited disease such as hemochromatoisis, Wilson's disease, glycogen storage diseases and alpha-1antitrypsin deficiency.

- Individuals exposed to environmental toxins or parasitic infections.

Conventional Treatment

The treatment for cirrhosis depends on the cause of the disease and the complications that have developed. A healthy, wholesome diet is always necessary to provide the body with essential nutrients. The following are common treatments for the causes and complications of cirrhosis:

- *Alcoholic cirrhosis:* avoid alcohol to prevent further liver damage and to allow for some improvement in liver function

- *Hepatitis-related cirrhosis:* medications, such as interferon and corticosteroids, are used to treat the hepatitis

- *Edema and ascites:* low-sodium diet or diuretics (medication to remove fluid from the body)

- *Infections:* antibiotics

- *Itching:* medication

- *Toxins:* protein-restricted diet to reduce build-up of toxins in the blood and brain

- *Portal hypertension:* beta-blocker medication

- *Varices:* injection with anticlotting agents

Severe cases of liver damage require a liver transplant: the diseased liver is removed and replaced with a healthy one from an organ donor. Survival rates have improved and 80 to 90 percent of liver transplant patients now survive the surgery.

Nutritional therapies for liver disease are individualized for each person, depending on the cause of the disease and its severity. A registered dietitian who specializes in liver disease should be consulted to develop an appropriate nutritional care plan. The following guidelines are general and should be tailored to each patient's specific condition.

Managing Cirrhosis

Dietary Strategies

Dietary Calories and Protein

Weight loss is common in people with severe liver disease, so following a diet that contains adequate calories and protein is important to help prevent muscle breakdown. Individuals with liver cirrhosis should increase their intake of protein-rich foods. The recommended intake of protein for healthy people is 0.8 grams protein per kilogram of body weight. This should be almost doubled to 1.2 to 1.5 grams per kilogram of body weight for people with cirrhosis.[1,2] A registered dietitian will help you plan a diet that provides sufficient protein. A list of foods and their protein content can be found in Chapter 2.

Some evidence supports the use of vegetable protein foods (legumes, soy, unsalted nuts) in people with cirrhosis who develop mental confusion, a condition called hepatic encephalopathy.[3] It is believed that an imbalance in circulating amino acids and high levels of ammonia in the bloodstream contribute to an altered mental state. When consumed with lactulose medication to lower blood ammonia levels, diets containing mainly vegetable protein rather than animal protein resulted in improvements in mental status symptoms.

Some research suggests that people with cirrhosis fare better by eating four to seven smaller meals per day, including a good breakfast and a late-evening meal.[4] A grazing pattern of eating appears to minimize some of the muscle breakdown that accompanies cirrhosis.

In people who experience impaired fat absorption because of decreased production and secretion of bile, the digestive aid that helps absorb dietary fat, a low-fat diet is required.

Branched Chain Amino Acids (BCAAs)

Branched chain amino acids (BCAAs) are found naturally in protein foods. Based on how they are metabolized in the body, they have been shown to normalize blood amino acids and lower ammonia levels in people with hepatic encephalopathy. Studies have shown that adding BCAAs to the diet can also decrease muscle breakdown in liver cirrhosis.[5-7] The typical dose used in studies is 240 to 250 milligrams per kilogram of body weight per day. These products are found in health food and supplement stores. Special BCAA formulas can be used for hospitalized patients.

Carbohydrates

Liver disease leads to malfunctions in carbohydrate metabolism and can result in hyper (high) or hypo (low) blood sugars. Choosing carbohydrate-containing foods that get digested and converted to blood sugar slowly may help minimize symptoms of carbohydrate intolerance. Toronto researchers found that a low glycemic index diet had beneficial effects in individuals with cirrhosis.[8] A list of low glycemic index foods can be found on page 7, Chapter 1.

Sodium

Restricting the intake of sodium is necessary to alleviate fluid retention that occurs with leg or stomach swelling.[9-11] A diet containing no more than 2 grams (2000 milligrams) of sodium is usually adequate to reduce swelling. In cases of severe fluid retention, your dietitian may prescribe a lower sodium diet. The sodium content of many foods can be found on page 80, Chapter 5.

Vitamins and Minerals

Multivitamin and Mineral Supplements

Since the liver is responsible for activating vitamins into forms the body can use, nutrient deficiencies are common in people with liver disease, especially if alcoholism is the cause. Deficiencies of B vitamins occur often, particularly deficiencies of folate, B1 (thiamin), B6 and B12. A daily multivitamin and mineral pill can help correct these nutrient deficits. A B complex supplement can also be used. This supplement contains the whole family of B vitamins in greater amounts than a standard multivitamin pill.

Antioxidants

Studies reveal that liver cirrhosis is accompanied by deficiencies in vitamins C and E, beta-carotene and selenium, important antioxidants that protect cells from damage caused by free radicals.[12,13] Free radicals are unstable oxygen molecules that cause damage to virtually every cell in the body, including liver cells. Research suggests that higher levels of free radical activity may be present in people with liver cirrhosis, especially when heavy drinking is the cause.[14] Supplementation with vitamin E and selenium has been shown to improve nutrient status.[15,16] The following antioxidant nutrients should be included from the diet and supplements.

Vitamin C

The recommended dietary allowance (RDA) of this vitamin is 75 and 90 milligrams for women and men respectively (smokers need an additional 35 milligrams). Best food sources include citrus fruit, citrus juices, cantaloupe, kiwi, mango, strawberries, broccoli, Brussels sprouts, cauliflower, red pepper and tomato juice. To supplement, take a 500 or 600 milligram supplement of Ester C once daily. The daily upper limit for vitamin C is 2000 milligrams.

Vitamin E

The RDA for vitamin E is 22 international units (IU). Best food sources include wheat germ, nuts, seeds, vegetable oils, whole grains and kale. To supplement, take 200 to 800 IU of natural source vitamin E. Buy a mixed vitamin E supplement if possible. The daily upper limit is 1500 IU.

Beta-Carotene

No RDA has been established for beta-carotene as it is not considered an essential nutrient. Best food sources are orange and dark green produce, including carrots, sweet potato, winter squash, broccoli, collard greens, kale, spinach, apricots, cantaloupe, peaches, nectarines, mango and papaya. Choose a multivitamin and mineral with beta-carotene added.

Selenium

The RDA for this trace mineral for adults is 55 micrograms. Best food sources are seafood, chicken, organ meats, whole grains, nuts, onions, garlic and mushrooms. To supplement, take 200 micrograms of selenium-rich yeast per day. Check how much your multivitamin and mineral gives you before you buy a separate selenium pill. The daily upper limit is 400 micrograms.

Herbal Remedies
Milk Thistle (*Silybum marianum*)

The active ingredients of this herb (known collectively as silymarin) can support and enhance liver function.[17-20] Silymarin can prevent toxic substances from penetrating liver cells and may even help liver cells regenerate more quickly. Milk thistle also seems to act as an antioxidant, protecting liver cells from damage caused by free radicals. Buy a product that's standardized to 70 percent silymarin. The dose for liver cirrhosis is 200 milligrams, three times daily. Use milk thistle with caution if you are allergic to plants in the Asteracease/Compositae family (ragweed, daisy, marigold and chrysanthemum).

Other Natural Health Products
Grapeseed Extract

Individuals with liver cirrhosis tend to bruise and bleed easily because the liver slows or stops production of the proteins needed for blood clotting. Grapeseed extract contains natural chemicals called anthocyanins, which are thought to keep blood vessels healthy by inhibiting the action of enzymes that break down connective tissue. In Europe, grapeseed extract is widely used to treat conditions related to fragile blood capillaries.

While no studies have assessed the effectiveness of grapeseed extract in patients with cirrhosis, it is a very safe supplement and it may be beneficial. The typical dose is 50 milligrams once daily, but studies have used higher doses for a three-week period, followed by a lower maintenance dose of 40 to 80 milligrams daily.

Lecithin (Phosphatidylcholine)

Lecithin and phosphatidylcholine supplements are thought to exert their health benefits by supplying the body with choline, a member of the B vitamin family. Once ingested, choline becomes incorporated into the membranes of cells. Phosphatidylcholine supplements are used in Europe to treat alcoholic liver disorders. Studies suggest that phosphatidylcholine supplements can reduce alcohol-induced liver damage.[21]

Most lecithin supplements contain 10 to 20 percent phosphatidylcholine. Others, however, are almost pure phosphatidylcholine; they will be labeled as such. For the most part, researchers use phosphatidylcholine supplements in clinical studies. Buy a supplement labeled phosphatidylcholine. Take 1200 to 2220 milligrams per day, in divided doses.

SAMe (S-Adenosyl-Methionine)

SAMe is a compound that our body makes naturally from certain amino acids in high-protein foods like fish and meat. It is found in virtually all body tissues and fluids. The production of SAMe is closely linked with folate and vitamin B12, so deficiencies of these B vitamins can lead to depressed levels of SAMe. In the body, SAMe is used to synthesize hormones, brain neurotransmitters, proteins and cell membranes.

It's thought that SAMe acts as an essential nutrient by restoring biochemical compounds that are depleted in people with alcoholic liver disease. People with liver disease lose the ability to form SAMe, and this leads to deficiencies in choline and glutathione, an enzyme that plays a critical role in liver detoxification and antioxidant reactions.[22-25] One study conducted on patients with alcoholic liver cirrhosis found that compared with the placebo, SAMe resulted in improved survival and reduced the need for liver transplants among subjects with severe cirrhosis.[26]

To supplement, take 400 milligrams on an empty stomach, three times daily. Buy an enteric-coated product. If you have a manic-depressive illness or you take antidepressant medication, consult your physician before taking SAMe.

Nutrition Strategy Checklist for Cirrhosis

- ☐ Diet high in vegetable protein
- ☐ Eat small frequent meals
- ☐ Branched chain amino acids
- ☐ Low glycemic index carbohydrates
- ☐ Limit sodium
- ☐ High-potency multivitamin/mineral OR B complex
- ☐ Vitamin C
- ☐ Vitamin E
- ☐ Beta-carotene
- ☐ Selenium
- ☐ Milk thistle
- ☐ Grapeseed extract
- ☐ Lecithin (Phosphatidylcholine)
- ☐ SAMe

Recommended Resources

www.liverfoundation.org
American Liver Foundation
75 Marden Lane, Suite 603
New York, NY, USA 10038
Tel: 973-256-2550 or 1-800-465-4837

www.liver.ca
Canadian Liver Foundation
2235 Sheppard Avenue E
Toronto, ON, Canada M2J 5B5
Tel: 416-491-3353 or 1-800-563-5483
Fax: 416-491-4952

www.niddk.nih.gov
National Digestive Diseases Information Clearinghouse
2 Information Way
Bethesda, MD, USA 20892-3570
Tel: 301-654-3810

Colorectal Cancer

Colorectal cancer is the third most common type of cancer in the world and the second leading cause of cancer deaths in North America.[1] It targets the large intestine and the rectum. Cancer of the large intestine, called colon cancer, affects men and women equally, while rectal cancer is more common among men.

The colon and the rectum are essential components of your digestive system. When you eat, food passes from the stomach into the small intestine, where digestive juices break the food down into individual nutrients. Any waste products that remain make their way to the large intestine, where they're processed to remove excess water and other fluids. The remaining solid waste, or stool, is moved into the rectum, where it is passed out of the body in a bowel movement.

Cancer develops when the cells in the lining of the colon or rectum begin to grow out of control. These cells divide and multiply at abnormal rates, forming small clumps or growths known as polyps. When polyps first form, they are noncancerous (benign). Eventually some of the polyps can change to become cancerous (malignant). Polyps smaller than 1 centimeter (0.5 inch) rarely become malignant, but the cancer risk increases as the polyps grow in size. There's almost a 50 percent chance of cancer developing from polyps that are larger than 2 centimeters (1 inch). Several different types of polyps can grow in the intestine, but those called adenomatous polyps are most likely to cause cancer.

What Causes Colorectal Cancer?

Scientists don't know what triggers polyps to develop. A hereditary factor may be involved. Studies indicate that people with a family history of colorectal cancer are much more likely to develop malignant growths in their intestinal tract. Colon cancer may also be stimulated by familial polyposis, a rare hereditary genetic disorder that causes thousands of polyps to develop in the intestinal tract. People with familial polyposis frequently develop colon cancer before the age of 40. Other risk factors for colorectal cancer include inflammatory bowel diseases such as ulcerative colitis and Crohn's disease.

Scientists also suspect that diet and lifestyle play important roles in the development of colorectal cancer. People at highest risk tend to eat more fat, red meat and refined carbohydrates. Studies indicate that people who exercise regularly and who eat high-fiber diets, with plenty of fruits and vegetables, have a lower risk of colon cancer.[2,3]

Colorectal cancer develops very slowly, usually over a period of seven to ten years. By reacting quickly to certain warning signs, it is possible to prevent cancer from developing. There are also several screening tests that can detect the presence of polyps. Removing polyps is the best way to prevent colorectal cancer. Screening tests can also find cancer in the early stages, when treatment is more effective and a full recovery is still likely. Colorectal cancer often develops with no symptoms, which makes screening even more important.

Symptoms

There may be no symptoms in the early stages of colorectal cancer. See your doctor if you have any of these warning signs:

- a change in normal bowel habits for more than two weeks, such as constipation or diarrhea or both
- narrow, pencil-thin stools
- bright or dark red blood in or on your stools on more than one occasion
- constant abdominal pain or cramping
- frequent gas pain
- a feeling that your bowel doesn't empty completely
- weight loss for no apparent reason
- constant tiredness

These symptoms may be caused by other conditions, such as ulcers or hemorrhoids. However, changes in your stools or bowel habits should not be ignored and require immediate medical attention. People with a family history of colorectal cancer should be screened regularly for the disease.

Who's at Risk?

You are at risk for colorectal cancer if you

- are over the age of 40; risk rises significantly at ages 50 to 55
- have a family history; risk is higher if the cancer affects more than one relative
- have an inflammatory bowel disease (ulcerative colitis, Crohn's disease)
- have a genetic disease such as Gardner's syndrome, familial polyposis or hereditary nonpolyposis colorectal cancer (HNPCC)
- are of Jewish or Eastern European ancestry
- are obese[4]

- are sedentary
- smoke cigarettes

Conventional Treatment

Polyps and early stage cancers can be removed during a *colonoscopy* (insertion of specialized instruments into the rectum) or *laparoscopic surgery* (insertion of specialized instruments through tiny incisions in the abdomen). Traditional surgery, in which diseased sections of the colon are removed, is used for more advanced cases. Nearby lymph nodes may also be removed during surgery if they have been invaded by cancer. Inherited disorders, such as familial polyposis, may require removal of the entire length of the colon and rectum.

A *colostomy* may be necessary if larger areas of the colon are removed. This involves creating an opening in the abdominal wall for elimination of waste material into an external bag. A small pouch may instead be constructed from the end of the small intestine and attached to the anus to allow for normal waste elimination.

Chemotherapy and radiation therapy may be necessary after surgery to destroy any remaining cancer cells. After surgery for colorectal cancer, five-year survival rates can be as high as 90 percent if the cancer has not spread into the lymph glands. If the lymph glands are affected, the survival rate drops to 65 percent or lower.

Preventing Colorectal Cancer

Dietary Strategies

Dietary Fat

Diets high in total fat and saturated animal fat may increase the risk of colon and rectal cancer. Animal studies show that a high fat intake induces colon tumors, and studies in humans have linked a high fat intake with high rates of colon cancer.[5,6]

A high-fat diet may increase the chances of colon and rectal cancer by increasing the amount of bile acids in the intestinal tract. After a meal, bile acids are released from the gallbladder to help break down fat. Despite their action as a digestive aid, bile acids also appear to enter colon cells and initiate cancer development.

To reduce your fat intake, choose lean meats, poultry breast and foods prepared with little or no added fat. See page 18, Chapter 3, for a list of lower-fat food choices.

Meat also seems to increase the risk of colorectal cancer. Many studies have found that higher intakes of meat increase the risk of the cancer.[7-9] In a study conducted among Seventh Day Adventists, compared to non-meat eaters, those who ate red and white meat at least once per week almost doubled the risk for colon cancer.[10] Cooking meat, poultry and fish at a high temperature forms heterocyclic amines, compounds found to be cancer-causing in laboratory studies. Cancer experts recommend consuming no more than 3 ounces (90 grams) of red meat per day (if eaten at all).[11]

Omega-3 Fatty Acids

These special fats found in oily fish may reduce the risk of colon cancer by inhibiting normal cells from becoming cancerous. Fish oils may also inhibit the growth of cancerous cells. A few studies have found that fish oil supplements taken for up to six months actually improve the health of colon cells in people at high risk for colorectal cancer.[12-16] While it is premature to recommend fish oil capsules for the prevention of colon and rectal cancer, it makes sense to add fish to your weekly menu. Aim to eat oily fish at least three times per week. Salmon, trout, herring, sardines and mackerel are good choices.

Carbohydrates: Sugar and Starch

High intakes of refined starches, especially foods made with white flour, seem to increase the risk of colorectal cancer.[17-20] There is also evidence that sucrose-containing foods increase the risk. It's thought that refined starches and sugars increase the risk by elevating blood-glucose and insulin levels. Insulin, a hormone that clears glucose from the bloodstream, appears to be related to colorectal cancer.

As often as possible, avoid consuming too much table sugar, cookies, cakes, desserts, candy, chocolate, fruit drinks, soft drinks, syrup, corn syrup and jam. Refined foods such as white bread, crackers, presweetened breakfast cereals, cereal bars, granola bars, white pasta and white rice should be replaced with whole-grain products.

Dietary Fiber

It's long been thought that a diet high in fiber prevents colon and rectal cancer in a number of ways. Dietary fiber can bind bile acids before they can enter colon cells (certain bile acids are toxic to colon cells). A high fiber intake can increase stool bulk and dilute the concentration of cancer-causing substances. By speeding the rate at which waste products are removed from the colon, dietary fiber can prevent carcinogens from making contact with colon and rectal cells. Finally, bacterial fermentation of fiber in the colon produces short chain fatty acids, substances that have anticancer properties.

An analysis of 13 studies of people with colorectal cancer concluded that an intake of fiber-rich foods is associated with a lower risk for the two cancers.[21] However, two large studies revealed that when people at high risk for colon cancer (they have adenomatous polyps) were given a high-fiber diet or daily fiber supplements for a number of years, there was no reduction in the growth of polyps.[22,23] The famous Nurses' Health Study also found no difference in the risk of colorectal cancer between women with the highest and lowest fiber intakes.[24]

Whether fiber reduces the risk of developing colon cancer remains to be proven. It may be that high-fiber foods provide other anticancer compounds such as vitamins and antioxidants. However, because dietary fiber is associated with so many other health benefits, current recommendations are to consume 25 to 35 grams per day. See page 3, Chapter 1, for a list of fiber-rich foods.

Vegetables

Evidence that diets rich in vegetables protect from colorectal cancer is convincing. Many studies have found that many types of vegetables significantly reduce the risk of polyp recurrence and colorectal cancer. One large American study revealed that higher vegetable intakes were associated with a 40 percent lower risk in women and a 20 percent lower risk in men.[25] Raw vegetables, leafy green vegetables, cruciferous vegetables (broccoli, cauliflower, cabbage, turnip) and carotenoid-containing vegetables (carrots, tomatoes) seem to offer protection. A high dietary intake of the carotenoid compound lutein has been found to lower the risk of colon cancer, especially in women.[26] The major sources of lutein consumed by study participants were spinach, broccoli, lettuce, tomatoes, oranges, carrots, celery and greens.

Vegetables contain many substances that may keep the bowel healthy. Beta-carotene, lutein, B vitamins, vitamin C and other natural plant chemicals all may have anticancer properties. Vegetables are also rich in fiber. And certain vegetables such as asparagus and Jerusalem artichokes may promote the growth of health-enhancing bacteria in the intestinal tract. See page 67, Chapter 5, for a list of vegetables categorized by their predominant plant chemicals (e.g., beta-carotene, lutein).

Green Tea

Research suggests that antioxidant compounds in green tea may prevent colon cells from becoming cancerous.[27] Population studies have shown that drinking green tea is associated with lower rates of colon and rectum cancer. A study conducted in China found that the more green tea consumed, the lower the risk for colorectal cancer.[28]

While we don't yet know if drinking green tea over the long term will decrease your risk of getting colon or rectal cancer, current evidence indicates that this beverage offers protection. Try adding a cup of green tea to your daily diet—replace coffee, soft drinks and fruit drinks with green tea. It's available loose in specialty tea shops or in tea bags in grocery stores.

Alcohol

There is evidence that all types of alcoholic beverages increase the risk of colorectal cancer.[29,30] When it comes to rectal cancer in men, beer may be more harmful than other types of alcohol. It's thought that alcohol may stimulate colon cells, causing them to rapidly divide, and it may activate cancer-causing substances. Alcohol may also stimulate the transformation of polyps into cancer.[31]

Cancer experts do not recommend the consumption of alcohol. If you drink, limit yourself to no more than two drinks per day or a maximum of nine per week (men), and one drink per day or seven per week (women).

Vitamins and Minerals
Vitamins C and E

An intake of foods rich in these two nutrients has been linked with a lower risk of colorectal cancer. A study conducted among Iowa women found that those with the highest intake of vitamin E had an 84 percent lower risk of the cancer compared with women who consumed the least.[32] Vitamin E was particularly protective in women under the age of 65. One Finnish study found that vitamin E supplements offered protection from colorectal cancer in men.[33]

Both vitamin C and vitamin E are strong antioxidant nutrients, able to protect the genetic material of cells from damage caused by free radical molecules. Cells with faulty genetic material may progress to polyps and eventually cancer. Studies have revealed that the colon cells in patients with colorectal cancer have a diminished antioxidant capacity.[34]

Foods rich in vitamin C include citrus fruit, citrus juices, cantaloupe, kiwi, mango, strawberries, broccoli, Brussels sprouts, cauliflower, red pepper and tomato juice. To supplement, take 500 or 600 milligrams once daily. Keep in mind that studies have not found vitamin C supplements to lower cancer risk; only high intakes of foods containing vitamin C have been linked to a lower risk of colorectal cancer.

The best food sources of vitamin E are wheat germ, nuts, seeds, vegetable oils, whole grains and leafy greens. To supplement, take 200 to 800 international units (IU) of natural source vitamin E once daily. Preliminary research in the lab suggests that supplements labeled "mixed" vitamin E may offer additional cancer protection.

Folate

A deficiency of this B vitamin has been linked with colorectal cancer. Folate is essential for the production of a cell's genetic material, DNA (deoxyribonucleic acid), in cells. DNA is the blueprint in every cell that controls cell division and all body processes. A lack of folate may also make the harmful effect of alcohol on colon cells more pronounced. One study found that compared with an intake of 200 micrograms or less, 400 micrograms of folic acid from a multivitamin pill was related to a 31 percent lower risk of colon cancer in women.[35]

Folate-rich foods include spinach, lentils, orange juice, whole grains, fortified breakfast cereals, asparagus, artichoke, avocado and seeds. To supplement, take a multivitamin and mineral that contains 400 to 1000 micrograms of folic acid (the synthetic form of folate) or take a B complex formula.

Calcium

Several studies have linked higher calcium intakes from supplements (1200 to 2000 milligrams per day) and low-fat dairy foods with lower risks of colorectal cancer and recurrence of polyps.[36-40] It is thought that once calcium is ingested, the mineral binds with bile acids in the intestinal tract, thereby preventing their toxic effects on colon cells.

Be sure to meet your daily calcium requirements by eating three to four one-cup servings of low-fat yogurt or milk. If you don't eat dairy foods, calcium-fortified soy or rice beverages and orange juice can be substituted. For each serving your diet lacks, take a 300 milligram calcium supplement with vitamin D added. You'll find more about calcium requirements, food sources and supplements on page 43, Chapter 4.

Selenium

This trace mineral is needed to form a selenium-containing enzyme called glutathione peroxidase. As a part of glutathione peroxidase, selenium acts as an antioxidant, protecting the genetic material of cells from free radical damage. Studies show that compared with people free of colorectal cancer, individuals with the disease have lower selenium and glutathione peroxidase levels in their body.[41-43]

One large American study found that when men and women were given a 200 microgram selenium supplement or placebo pill once daily, those taking selenium experienced a 50 percent reduction in colon cancer.[44]

Selenium-rich foods include seafood, chicken, organ meats, whole grains, nuts, onions, garlic and mushrooms. To supplement, take 100 to 200 micrograms of selenium-rich yeast per day. Check how much your multivitamin and mineral pill gives you before you buy a separate selenium pill, since some multis contain as much as 100 micrograms.

Herbal Remedies

Garlic (*Allium sativum*)

A daily intake of raw and cooked garlic and its accompanying sulfur compounds is associated with a lower risk of colon and rectal cancer.[45] The Iowa Women's Health Study, which followed 42,000 women for five years, found that women who consumed 0.7 grams of garlic per day (less than one clove) had a 32 percent lower risk of colon cancer compared with those who did not consume garlic.[46]

Garlic may help prevent cancer in a number of ways. Like vitamins C and E, garlic possesses antioxidant properties, which may keep DNA healthy. The sulfur compounds in garlic may also help the liver detoxify cancer-causing substances. Garlic may have a direct toxic effect on certain types of cancer cells. And finally, studies have shown that garlic, in particular the allyl sulfides in aged garlic extract, stimulate the body's immune system.

Include one to two cloves of cooked or raw garlic in your daily diet. To supplement, buy aged garlic extract. The aging process used to make this supplement increases the concentration of the sulfur compounds that stimulate the immune system. Aged garlic is also odor free and gentler on the stomach. Generally, two to six capsules a day (one or two with meals) are recommended. You can also buy aged garlic in a liquid form (Kyolic® brand) that you add to foods.

Nutrition Strategy Checklist for Preventing Colorectal Cancer

☐ Diet low in animal fat and meat	☐ Green tea
	☐ Limit alcohol
☐ Fish	☐ Vitamin E
☐ Whole grains	☐ Folate
☐ Dietary fiber	☐ Calcium
☐ Limit sugar and sweets	☐ Selenium
☐ Vegetables	☐ Garlic

Recommended Resources

www.cancer.ca
Canadian Cancer Society
10 Alcorn Avenue, Suite 200
Toronto, ON, Canada M4V 3B1
Tel: 416-961-7223
Fax: 416-961-4189

www.ccalliance.org
Colon Cancer Alliance, Inc.
175 Ninth Avenue
New York, NY, USA 10011
Tel: 1-877-422-2030 (help-line)
Fax: 425-940-6147

www.ccac-accc.ca
Colorectal Cancer Association of Canada
Ottawa Regional Cancer Center
501 Smyth Road
Ottawa, ON, Canada K1H 8L6
Tel: 1-888-318-9442

www.cancernet.nci.nih.gov
A service provided by National Cancer
Institute (www.nci.nih.gov)
National Cancer Institute
Public Inquiries Office
Building 31, Room 10A31, 31 Center Drive,
MSC 2580
Bethesda, MD, USA 20892-2580
Tel: 301-435-3848 or 1-800-4-CANCER (1-800-422-6237) (help-line)

Common Cold

Cold is the common name for a viral infection of the upper respiratory tract, which includes the sinuses, the lining of the nose, the throat and the large airways. Most people suffer from at least one a year. Current estimates indicate that the North American population suffers more than one billion colds annually, making this pesky condition a leading cause of doctor visits and school and work absenteeism. While colds may be annoying, they are fairly harmless and usually cause nothing more than an inconvenience in our busy lives.

What Causes the Common Cold?

There are over 200 viruses that can cause a cold. Most colds are caused by rhinoviruses, but influenza and other respiratory viruses can also be the culprits. Because these viruses are so widespread and varied, conventional medicine has been unable to cure or prevent the common cold.

Cold viruses can be spread very easily. When someone coughs or sneezes or even talks, viruses are spread through the air. Inhaling the contaminated droplets allows viruses that have entered the nose to infect the nasal membranes. Cold viruses can remain infective for several hours outside the body, which means that the viruses can also be spread by direct and indirect contact. Rubbing your nose or eyes after touching an object that has been contaminated with saliva or nasal secretions (door handles, toys, used tissue) will transfer the virus. Even shaking hands with someone who has a cold can expose you to infectious secretions.

People seem to suffer from colds more often during the winter months. This is probably because the winter temperatures keep people indoors, where they are more likely to come into prolonged contact with other people suffering from cold viruses. As well, the many cold viruses survive better when humidity is low, which is usually during the colder months. It's also possible that cold weather dries out the lining of the nasal passages, making them more susceptible to infection. A cold will usually last from four to ten days and is most contagious when the first symptoms appear, approximately two to three days after the infection was contracted.

Symptoms

Symptoms of the common cold include

- sore, scratchy throat; cough
- husky voice
- sneezing; runny nose
- mild feeling of illness
- tired and achy
- headache
- watering eyes

Cold symptoms may be complicated by other illnesses that develop when the body's defenses are weakened. For instance, children often suffer from middle ear infections during or after a cold. Bacterial infections of the sinuses may also follow a bout with a cold virus. Complications such as these increase the severity of cold symptoms and may be dangerous for some people. Contact a doctor if you develop a high fever that lasts longer than two days; if you experience chest pains, wheezing, hard coughing spells or earache; if you cough up thick green, yellow or bloody sputum; if your symptoms last more than a week or if you feel more ill than usual with a cold.

Who's at Risk?

Children have colds more often than adults. Women are also at high risk, possibly because of their often close contact with children or as an effect of their menstrual cycle.

People who are fatigued, stressed or have allergies of the nose and throat are also more susceptible.

Conventional Treatment

Colds are viruses and therefore cannot be treated with antibiotics. Antibiotic treatment is prescribed only if colds are complicated by bacterial infections. To help ease symptoms of the common cold

- stay warm and comfortable
- drink fluids to help keep mucus membranes moist
- rest at home if you have a fever or severe symptoms
- take acetaminophen or ibuprofen for relief of pain or fever (Note: Children and adolescents should not take aspirin because of increased risk of Reye's syndrome, a potentially fatal condition.)
- try nasal decongestants to provide temporary relief
- take antihistamines to reduce allergic reactions that may accompany colds
- use cough suppressants for severe coughs (Coughing helps clear secretions and mucus from the airways and should be left untreated, if possible.)
- use a vaporizer to loosen secretions and ease chest tightness

Preventing and Managing the Common Cold

Although colds can't actually be prevented, good personal hygiene will help protect you, your family and your coworkers from cold viruses.

- Wash hands thoroughly and frequently.
- Cover your mouth when coughing or sneezing, preferably with a tissue.
- Clean surfaces that you touch with germ-killing disinfectant.
- Avoid rubbing your eyes and nose with dirty hands.
- Eat a nutritious diet.
- Get plenty of sleep.
- Avoid drinking alcohol.
- If possible, avoid crowded places or close contact with people with colds.

Vaccines to prevent influenza are readily available. However, because there are so many types of cold viruses, it is impossible to prevent most colds with a vaccine. Scientists are experimenting with new antiviral agents, such as interferon, a substance produced naturally by human cells. Interferon is being produced by genetic engineering and shows promise in preventing viral infections.

Dietary Strategies

Fluids

During a cold, drink at least 8 cups (2 liters) of fluid per day to prevent dehydration and constipation. Hot fluids are most effective for alleviating nasal congestion. Drink hot water, hot tea, soups and broths. Fluid also helps keep the lining of the respiratory tract moist, which can ease the symptoms of a sore throat.

Drinking plenty of fluids each day is an important way to help prevent the common cold. When you are dehydrated, tiny cracks form in your nasal membranes. These cracks allow virus-filled droplets to take up residence and promote infection. Always consume 8 to 12 glasses of fluid daily.

Chicken Soup

Research from Mount Sinai Hospital in Miami, Florida, suggests that chicken soup may help treat a cold.[1] A compound in the soup called cystine appears to have a decongestant effect. And it's thought that the spicier the soup, the better. Hot peppers contain capsacian, a natural compound that has the ability to act as a decongestant.

Probiotics

Fermented milk products such as yogurt, kefir and acidophilus milk contain lactic acid bacteria, healthy bacteria that may help prevent the common cold. Once ingested, these microbes take up residence in the gastrointestinal tract, where they exert their health benefits. A number of studies have shown that regular consumption of probiotic foods as well as probiotic supplements enhances the activity of the immune system.[2,3] Recent research suggests that a deficiency of lactic acid bacteria in the intestinal tract of children may be responsible for viral infections of the respiratory tract.[4]

Include one fermented milk product in your daily diet. To supplement, buy a product that contains 1 to 10 billion live cells per dose (capsule). Take 1 to 10 billion viable cells three times daily with food. Children's products are available on the market. These usually contain one-quarter to one-half of the adult dose (250 to 500 billion live cells).

Vitamins and Minerals

Vitamin C

So far, more than 60 studies have examined the effects of large doses of vitamin C on the common cold. While vitamin C supplements do not appear to prevent a cold, they do appear to reduce the duration and severity of symptoms. Studies have tested doses of 1000 milligrams and higher, more than ten times the recommended daily intake.[5-7] The greatest benefit is seen when a daily dose of 2000 milligrams (2 grams) or more is taken. Children, people under physical stress and people with low dietary intakes of vitamin C tend to respond best to the nutrient.

Vitamin C promotes the body's production of interferon, a natural antiviral agent that fights infection. Vitamin C also has a slight antihistaminic effect. To treat a cold, take a 1000 milligram time-released vitamin C pill twice daily. High doses of vitamin C can cause diarrhea, but this side effect resolves after continued use. You may have to build up to 2000 milligrams per day. Once your cold symptoms have subsided, return to a typical supplemental dose of 500 milligrams per day.

There is some concern that vitamin C supplements can cause kidney stones even though no studies have found this to be the case. Individuals with a history of kidney stones or kidney failure should restrict their intake to 100 milligrams per day.

Vitamin E

Vitamin E does not treat a cold, but it may play a role in preventing one. Research in healthy older adults determined that a daily vitamin E supplement taken for one month improved the responsiveness of the immune system.[8,9] Vitamin E appears to help certain white blood cells, called natural killer cells, fight infection.

Foods rich in vitamin E include wheat germ, nuts, seeds, vegetable oils, whole grains and leafy green vegetables. To supplement, take 200 to 800 international units (IU) of natural source vitamin E. Buy a "mixed" vitamin E supplement if possible. The daily upper limit is 1500 IU.

Zinc

Studies support the use of zinc lozenges to reduce the duration of cold symptoms. Compared with cold sufferers taking placebo pills, those taking zinc gluconate or zinc acetate lozenges experienced faster recovery from coughing, sore throat, runny nose and headache.[10-12] However, not all studies have found zinc lozenges to be effective.[13] It has been suggested that this may be because of the chemical form of zinc used or the addition of certain flavoring agents that may interfere with zinc's activity.[14]

When zinc lozenges are dissolved in the mouth, the zinc is released and attaches to cold viruses. By doing so, cold viruses are unable to bind to cells in the mouth and throat and cannot cause infection.

To treat a cold, take one zinc lozenge made of zinc gluconate or zinc acetate every two hours, for a total of five per day. More is *not* better, since taking high doses of zinc can cause toxic effects. Once your cold symptoms have disappeared, discontinue use of zinc lozenges.

It is important to ensure your daily diet contains zinc-rich foods, since the mineral is vital to a healthy immune system. Zinc-rich foods include oysters, seafood, red meat, poultry, yogurt, wheat bran, wheat germ, whole grains and enriched breakfast cereals. Your diet and a multivitamin and mineral supplement will provide all the zinc you need to stay healthy.

Herbal Remedies

Echinacea

Many studies in the laboratory have shown the ability of echinacea to enhance the body's production of white blood cells that fight infection. Despite the positive results in the lab, clinical trials in adults taking echinacea to treat a cold or flu have not conclusively shown that the herb is effective, perhaps because so many different brands were used. However, a recent review of 16 studies conducted with 3396 participants found that most studies report a positive effect.[15]

To ensure quality, buy a product that's standardized to contain 4 percent echinacosides (*Echinacea angustifolia*) and 0.7 percent flavonoids (*Echinacea purpurea*), two of the herb's active ingredients. Take a total of 900 milligrams three to four times daily. For fluid extracts (1:1), take 0.25 to 1.0 milliliter three times daily. For tinctures (1:5), take 1 to 2 milliliters three times daily. For teas, take 125 to 250 milliliters three to four times daily. Take until symptoms are relieved, then continue taking two to three times daily for one week. Guidelines for doses in children can be found in Chapter 7. Don't use echinacea if you are allergic to plants in the Asteracease/Compositae family (ragweed, daisy, marigold and chrysanthemum).

Garlic (*Allium sativum*)

The sulfur compounds in garlic have been shown to stimulate the body's immune system, making garlic a potential agent in the prevention of colds.[16-18] A number of studies have focused on the specific sulfur compounds in aged garlic extract, a special supplement that is aged for up to 20 months. Whether garlic actually heals a cold remains to be proven by clinical studies. However, the herb does have a long history of use in the treatment of infection.

Use one-half to one clove each day in cooking. To supplement, buy a product made with aged garlic extract. Take two to six capsules a day in divided doses. Aged garlic extract is odorless and less irritating to the gastrointestinal tract than other forms of garlic supplement (garlic oil capsules, garlic powder tablets).

Panax Ginseng

This herbal remedy may help prevent cold through its ability to stimulate the immune system. A well-controlled trial in Italy found that 100 milligrams of Panax ginseng (G115 extract) taken daily resulted in a significant decline in the frequency of colds and flus.[19]

To supplement, choose a product with a statement of standardization or "G115" printed on the label, such as Ginsana® (Pharmaton® Natural Health Products). Take 100 milligrams once daily. Take ginseng for three weeks to three months and follow with a one- to two-week rest period before you resume taking the herb. In some people, it may cause mild stomach upset, irritability and insomnia. To prevent overstimulation, avoid taking the herb with caffeine. Ginseng should not be used during pregnancy, breastfeeding or if you have poorly controlled high blood pressure.

Nutrition Strategy Checklist for Treating and Preventing Colds

☐ Hot fluids

☐ Chicken soup

☐ Probiotics

☐ Vitamin C

☐ Vitamin E

☐ Zinc lozenges

☐ Echinacea

☐ Garlic

☐ Panax ginseng

Recommended Resources

www.fda.gov/opacom/lowlit/clds&flu.html
Department of Health and Human Services
Food and Drug Administration
5600 Fishers Lane (HFI-40)
Rockville, MD, USA 20857
Tel: 1-888-463-6332

www.lung.ca/diseases/common_cold.html
The Lung Association
3 Raymond Street, Suite 300
Ottawa, ON, Canada K1R 1A3
Tel: 613-569-6411
Fax: 613-569-8860

www.niaid.nih.gov/factsheets/cold.htm
National Institutes of Health
National Institute of Allergy and Infectious Diseases
NIAID Office of Communications and Public Liaison
Building 31, Room 7A-50, 31 Center Drive,
MSC 2520
Bethesda, MD, USA 20892-2520

Congestive Heart Failure (CHF)

Congestive heart failure (CHF) is a serious medical disorder that requires monitoring by a physician. The term heart failure can be misleading, because this condition does not actually cause your heart to fail or stop beating. What it does mean is that your heart has become weakened and is no longer working well enough to meet the needs of your body.

The heart is a hollow, muscular organ that circulates blood to all parts of your body. Blood is pumped by the right side of your heart to the lungs, where it becomes loaded with oxygen, a fuel essential for maintaining your bodily functions. The oxygenated blood then returns to the heart, from where the chambers on its left side circulate the blood to your brain and other vital organs. Once your cells have absorbed the oxygen and nutrients, the blood returns to the heart and the cycle begins again.

When your heart becomes damaged and weak, its ability to pump blood is weakened. Less blood is forced into your system, causing a backup of fluid (congestion) in your lungs and other tissues. Your organs become deprived of the oxygen and vital nutrients they need for fuel, which means that they can no longer function properly. Congestive heart failure can leave you feeling tired and short of breath after even the slightest exertion.

As the damage from CHF progresses, the heart must work harder to compensate for its reduced pumping power. This extra workload causes the heart to undergo significant changes. Over time, the heart may become enlarged and stretched so that it can pump larger quantities of blood. Or the heart muscle may thicken, building extra strength to increase the force of each pump. In some cases, the heart may beat faster, attempting to compensate for its shortcomings by pumping blood more frequently. These changes weaken the heart even more by causing it to strain and overwork.

Congestive heart failure also affects the kidneys. The kidneys, which normally eliminate excess water from your body, begin to retain salt (sodium) and water, increasing the volume of blood circulating in your system. Initially, this improves the heart's performance. However, the excess fluid eventually accumulates in various parts of the body, causing swelling (edema) in your legs and feet when you are standing or in your back and abdomen when you are lying down. Weight gain is frequently a result of this increased retention of sodium and water.

What Causes Congestive Heart Failure?

Any disease that affects the heart can lead to congestive heart failure. The most common causes include

- *coronary artery disease:* fatty deposits occur that narrow the arteries that supply blood to your heart

- *heart attack*

- *high blood pressure*

- *heart valve problems:* damage to tiny valves in your heart that keep the blood flowing in the right direction

- *cardiomyopathy:* damage to the heart muscle caused by viral infections, drug and alcohol abuse

- *congenital heart disease:* the heart may be damaged at birth

- *arrhythmias:* abnormal heart rhythms may cause the heart to beat too fast

- *other medical conditions:* diabetes, extreme obesity or an overactive thyroid gland

CHF is an incurable disease. However, symptoms can be managed and progression of the disease can be controlled with medications and lifestyle changes. Unfortunately, only 20 percent of people diagnosed with this condition survive longer than eight to ten years and nearly one in five die within the first year of diagnosis.

Symptoms

CHF progresses gradually and symptoms develop slowly, which include

- shortness of breath when you exert yourself
- shortness of breath when lying down
- wheezing or coughing, accompanied by shortness of breath
- fatigue and weakness
- swelling in your legs, ankles or feet
- swollen neck veins
- rapid weight gain
- dizzy spells

Who's at Risk?

Because older people tend to suffer most often from diseases that cause congestive heart failure, they are the most susceptible to developing CHF. The risk is higher for people with poorly controlled high blood pressure, heart disease, kidney disease and diabetes. The disease affects men and women equally.

Conventional Treatment

The following lifestyle modifications can ease symptoms and help prevent CHF from becoming worse:

- *increasing daily exercise*—moderate exercise helps your heart pump more efficiently; try 20 to 40 minutes of moderate walking three to five days per week[1-4]

- *stopping smoking*—smoking damages your heart muscle and reduces the amount of oxygen in your blood
- *managing stress*—chronic stress can make your heart beat faster

The following medications may be used to treat heart failure:

- *ACE (angiotensin-converting enzyme) inhibitors* to lower blood pressure and help blood flow more easily
- *diuretics* to keep fluids from accumulating in your body by increasing urination
- *digoxin* to slow the heartbeat and increase the power of each beat
- *beta-blockers* to slow your heart rate and reduce blood pressure

Surgery may be necessary to replace faulty heart valves or repair damage caused by coronary artery disease. A heart transplant may be needed in severe cases of CHF.

Managing Congestive Heart Failure

Dietary Strategies

Individuals with severe heart failure may need to restrict daily fluids to 1000 to 2000 milliliters (1 to 2 liters) to prevent fluid retention. To monitor fluid gain, weigh yourself daily before breakfast (after urinating). A rapid weight gain of more than 3 pounds (1.3 kilograms) may indicate that you're retaining fluid and may require additional treatment. Notify your doctor if you gain weight suddenly.

Avoid alcohol and caffeine. Alcohol can reduce your heart's ability to pump effectively and can interact with heart medications.[5] As well, limit or avoid beverages and foods containing caffeine. Caffeine should be restricted because of its potential to increase the heart rate and cause abnormal heart rhythms. (See page 82, Chapter 5, for the caffeine content of selected foods.)

Eating small, frequent meals may reduce the workload of the heart and help improve your intake of calories and nutrients. Calorie needs for people with CHF are higher because of the additional workload of the heart and an increased metabolism. By eating five or six times a day, you will be more likely to meet your energy needs.

Sodium

Sodium restriction is the primary dietary intervention for treating CHF. Too much salt causes the body to retain water, making your heart work harder. This causes shortness of breath and swelling. For mild to moderate heart failure, reduce your intake to no more than 3000 milligrams (3 grams) of sodium per day. Some individuals will require further sodium restriction as recommended by their registered dietitian. To reduce sodium intake, practice the following:

- Eliminate salty processed foods (see page 79, Chapter 5).

- Read food labels to see how much sodium is present. If nutrition labels are not present, read the ingredients list, which lists items in order of the amount present. Look for the words sodium, salt or soda.

- Remove the saltshaker from the table; don't add salt when cooking.

- Avoid beverages high in salt: vegetable juice, diet pop, mineral water and hot malt beverages.

- Use herbs and spices for seasonings: pepper, garlic powder, onion powder and lemon juice.

- When dining out, ask that no salt be added to meals.

- Discuss the use of salt substitutes with your dietitian. Some brands should not be used if you are taking certain diuretic medications.

Vitamins and Minerals
Multivitamin and Mineral Supplements
Many people with advanced heart failure are undernourished and can benefit from a daily multivitamin and mineral supplement. People with CHF often have difficulty eating enough food to meet their increased energy requirements. To prevent nutrient deficiencies, take one multivitamin and mineral pill daily.

Antioxidants
It is a well-accepted assertion that damage caused by free radicals contributes to the development and progression of CHF.[6-8] Free radicals are unstable oxygen molecules generated by normal body processes. If produced in excess, they can damage virtually every cell in the body. A regular intake of dietary antioxidants (vitamins C and E, beta-carotene, selenium) helps the body keep free radical activity under control.

Whether antioxidant supplements help treat CHF remains to be seen. It is possible they may help prevent a worsening of heart failure. A few studies have shown that supplementation with vitamins C and E can reduce free radical activity in CHF.[9,10] Therefore, be sure to include the following antioxidants in your daily diet.

- *Vitamin C* Best food sources include citrus fruit, citrus juices, cantaloupe, kiwi, mango, strawberries, broccoli, Brussels sprouts, cauliflower, red pepper and tomato juice. To supplement, take 500 or 600 milligram, of Ester C once daily.

- *Vitamin E* Best food sources include wheat germ, nuts, seeds, vegetable oils, whole grains and kale. To supplement, take 200 to 800 IU of natural source vitamin E. Buy a "mixed" vitamin E supplement if possible.

- *Selenium* Best food sources are seafood, chicken, organ meats, whole grains, nuts, onions, garlic and mushrooms. To supplement, take 200 micrograms of selenium-rich yeast per day.

- *Beta-Carotene* Best food sources are orange and dark green produce, including carrots, sweet potato, winter squash, broccoli, collard greens, kale, spinach, apricots, cantaloupe, peaches, nectarines, mango and papaya. Choose a multivitamin and mineral with beta-carotene added.

Thiamin (Vitamin B1)

Long-term use of a diuretic called Lasix® (furosemide) leads to a loss of thiamin in the urine, and a deficiency of the B vitamin may worsen heart performance. Many studies have found that patients with heart failure who take these diuretics are deficient in thiamin.[11-13] Researchers have also found that a daily thiamin supplement can replenish the body's supply of the vitamin and improve the functioning of the heart.[14]

If you are taking Lasix®, your doctor should monitor your thiamin status. To treat a deficiency, take 100 milligrams of thiamin twice daily. Thiamin is very safe and rarely causes an adverse reaction.

Magnesium

This mineral is essential for the functioning of heart cell membranes, and many enzymes that catalyze reactions in the heart muscle use it. A number of medications used to treat CHF can alter magnesium levels in the body.[15] A decrease in magnesium in patients with CHF has been linked to heart arrhythmias and a poorer prognosis.[16,17] Studies have shown that supplementation of magnesium improves mineral levels in the body and reduces heart arrhythmias.[18-20]

Good food sources of magnesium include nuts and seeds (choose unsalted varieties), legumes, prunes, whole grains, leafy green vegetables, Brewer's yeast, cheddar cheese and shrimp. Your heart specialist will monitor your magnesium levels and determine if magnesium supplements are required. If you decide to take magnesium supplements to prevent a deficiency, take 200 to 250 milligrams twice daily. Buy a supplement made from magnesium gluconate, citrate, aspartate, succinate or fumarte. The body absorbs these forms of the mineral more efficiently. Magnesium gluconate is less likely to cause diarrhea than other forms of the mineral. It may take six months to see improvement with magnesium.

Potassium

Certain diuretic drugs can cause potassium to be excreted in the urine. Because potassium helps maintain normal function of the heart, your doctor may recommend potassium supplements if you take potassium-wasting diuretics such as Lasix® (furosemide) or Hydrodiuril® (hydrochlorothiazide).

Include potassium-rich foods in your daily diet—raisins, prunes, dates, dried apricots, bananas, oranges, citrus juices, strawberries, watermelon, beets, greens, spinach, tomatoes, legumes and peas are good choices.

Herbal Remedies

Hawthorn (species *Crataegus*)

The active components (flavonoids and procyanidins) in this plant act on the heart by increasing the force of contraction, lengthening the period between heartbeats, reducing oxygen use and increasing nerve transmission. The herb may also improve blood flow by dilating blood vessels.

There is a substantial amount of evidence for hawthorn's beneficial effects in congestive heart failure.[21-23] To supplement, buy a product standardized to 2 to 3 percent flavonoids or 18 to 20 percent procyanidins. Take 100 to 300 milligrams three times daily. It may take six to eight weeks for the herb to reach its full effect. Hawthorn can interact with certain heart medications; check with your pharmacist. If you are on certain heart drugs, take hawthorn only under your physician's supervision. Do not take hawthorn with digitalis.

Other Natural Health Products

Coenzyme Q10 (CoQ10)

CoQ10 works with many different enzymes in the body and so is needed for many important metabolic reactions. One very important function of CoQ10 is the production of the body's energy compounds, ATP (adenosine triphosphate). Studies have shown that CoQ10 levels are much lower in the heart cells of individuals with CHF than they are in healthy people.

Many clinical trials have shown that CoQ10 supplements (along with medication) improve the quality of life in patients with CHF.[24-28] Studies show that supplementation with CoQ10 can decrease hospitalization and significantly decrease many of the symptoms associated with heart failure. CoQ10 also acts as an antioxidant.

Choose an oil-based CoQ10 supplement. Take 50 milligrams, twice daily.

L-Propionyl-Carnitine

Carnitine is an amino acid found in all body cells, where it is used to metabolize fatty acids into energy. Carnitine helps the heart contract and produce energy more efficiently, and as a result, use less oxygen. A handful of studies have found that L-carnitine supplementation improves exercise tolerance and heart functioning in patients with CHF.[29-33]

Most studies use the form of carnitine called L-propionyl-carnitine. If you can't find it, buy L-carnitine. L-carnitine is available in the United States but is not legally available in Canada. However, some health food stores do stock it.

Take 1000 milligrams, two or three times daily. The supplement is considered to be very safe. Do not take D-carnitine or DL-carnitine, which can cause heart and muscle dysfunction.

L-Taurine

This is an amino acid that's used to make many different proteins in the body. It's found in meat, poultry, eggs, fish and dairy products. The body can also make taurine from vitamin B6 and other amino acids in food.

It's believed that taurine helps the heart beat and maintains healthy cell membranes. Studies have found that supplementation of taurine (2 grams three times daily) improved shortness of breath, edema and heart palpitations in patients with CHF.[34-35] Taurine supplements are considered to be very safe. However, be sure to buy a product made by a reputable manufacturer. This is the case for any supplement you are taking in large doses (grams).

Nutrition Strategy Checklist for Congestive Heart Failure

- ☐ Restrict fluids and sodium
- ☐ Avoid alcohol and caffeine
- ☐ Eat small frequent meals
- ☐ Multivitamin/mineral
- ☐ Vitamin C
- ☐ Vitamin E
- ☐ Thiamin (vitamin B1)
- ☐ Magnesium
- ☐ Hawthorn
- ☐ Coenzyme Q10
- ☐ L-propionyl-carnitine
- ☐ L-taurine

Recommended Resources

www.americanheart.org
American Heart Association
7272 Greenville Avenue
Dallas, Texas, USA 75231
Tel: 1-800-AHA-USA1 (1-800-242-8721)

www.heartandstroke.ca
Heart and Stroke Foundation of Canada
222 Queen Street, Suite 1402
Ottawa, ON, Canada K1P 5V9
Tel: 613-569-4361
Fax: 613-569-3278

www.nhlbi.nih.gov
National Institutes of Health
National Heart, Lung and Blood Institute
Information Center
P.O. Box 30105
Bethesda, MD, USA 20824-0105
Tel: 301-592-8573

Constipation

An increasingly sedentary lifestyle and a growing preference for a diet of refined and overprocessed food can make us more susceptible to constipation. But many people worry unnecessarily about their bowel habits, expressing concern if they don't have a bowel movement every day. Bowel habits are highly individualized and frequency can vary considerably. In healthy adults, it is quite normal for bowel movements to range in frequency from three times a day to three times a week.

A person who is suffering from acute or chronic constipation usually has fewer than three bowel movements a week and produces small, hard stools that are difficult to pass. Bloating, gas pains, cramps and sluggishness often accompany constipation. Some people may also have the feeling that their rectum is not fully emptied.

What Causes Constipation?

Acute constipation comes on suddenly and is usually triggered by medications, illness or recent changes in diet. Chronic constipation takes a longer time to develop and can last for months or years. While constipation may be uncomfortable,

it tends to be a temporary condition and rarely causes serious problems.

Under normal circumstances, your bowels function very efficiently. During the digestive process, a series of wave-like muscle contractions move food through the small intestine, where it is broken down into absorbable nutrients. The digested food then enters the large intestine, or bowel, for further processing. At this stage, fluid and electrolytes, such as sodium and potassium, are removed, and most of the water content is absorbed in the colon. Muscle contractions move the remaining semi-solid waste material into the rectum, where it collects and is passed out of the body as a bowel movement.

Constipation usually develops when the muscles of the colon contract sluggishly or too slowly, allowing waste material to linger in the bowel. As a result, the colon absorbs excessive amounts of water, leaving the stool hard, dry and difficult to pass. Often, constipation is caused by a diet that is low in fiber or fluids or by a lack of physical activity. Other factors that may result in constipation include

- medications, such as pain killers and iron supplements

- changes in routine, such as travel, stress or irregular sleeping habits

- life changes, such as pregnancy or aging

- abuse of laxatives

- ignoring the urge to have a bowel movement

- irritable bowel syndrome or other problems affecting the intestines, colon or rectum

- illness or diseases, such as multiple sclerosis, stroke, diabetes or lupus

While constipation is not a life-threatening condition, it can sometimes lead to complications. Straining and excessive pushing to pass the stool may lead to hemorrhoids or small tears around the anus (anal fissures). Too much straining may also cause a small portion of the intestinal lining to push out through the rectum; this condition is called a rectal prolapse. Less often, the hard stool may pack so tightly into the intestine and rectum that the normal contractions of the colon cannot move it out of the body. This is called a fecal impaction. In rare cases, constipation may be a sign of colorectal cancer, heart disease or kidney failure.

Symptoms

Symptoms of constipation include

- small, hard, dry stools
- difficult bowel movements
- fewer than three bowel movements a week
- abdominal cramps, gas pain, bloating
- a feeling of sluggishness

Who's at Risk?

Constipation is the most common gastrointestinal complaint in North America, affecting almost everyone at one time or another. Women, children and adults over age 65 report constipation most often. Pregnant women also tend to experience constipation. As well, people who are sedentary or bedridden or who have recently had surgery often experience constipation.

Conventional Treatment

To prevent constipation, always respond to your body's urges to have a bowel movement. If constipation persists, laxatives, stool softeners or enemas may be recommended for a short period. These include

- *bulking agents,* such as bran or psyllium, to add volume and draw fluid into the stool so that it can be passed more easily

- *stool softeners* to allow water to penetrate the stool and soften it, triggering natural contractions of the colon
- *mineral oil* to soften stool
- *glycerin suppositories* to lubricate the rectum, making it easier to pass hard, dry stool
- *magnesium salts* to pull large amounts of water into the intestine, making the stool soft and loose and stretching the intestinal walls to stimulate contractions
- *bowel stimulants* to irritate the intestine, causing it to contract and move the stool through more quickly
- *enemas* to fill the bowel with fluid, stimulating a bowel movement

Excessive use of constipation medications may lead to lazy bowel syndrome by damaging the nerve cells and interfering with the normal muscle contractions of the colon. Use laxatives only when necessary. Instead, rely on the dietary strategies listed below to promote regular bowel movements. It's also important to increase physical activity to stimulate bowel function. Aim to be active for at least 20 minutes three times per week.

Preventing and Managing Constipation

Dietary Strategies

Develop regular eating habits and try to eat on a schedule. This helps to promote bowel motility. If your busy schedule interferes with your ability to respond to your body's defecation signals, revise your schedule. Go to bed earlier in order to rise earlier, allowing time for breakfast and a bowel movement. And remember, try not to worry excessively about your bowel movements: anxiety can aggravate constipation.

Dietary Fiber

Foods contain varying amounts of insoluble fibers and soluble fibers. Foods that have a greater proportion of insoluble fibers such as wheat bran, whole grains, nuts, seeds and certain fruits and vegetables are used to treat and prevent constipation.[1-5] Once consumed, insoluble fibers make their way to the intestinal tract, where they absorb water, help form larger, softer stools and speed evacuation. Psyllium, a type of soluble fiber, also adds bulk to stools and can be used to treat constipation.

Adults are recommended to get 25 to 35 grams of fiber per day; children two years and older should be getting 5 grams plus their age in years (e.g., a seven-year-old should be consuming 5 + 7 grams for a total of 12 grams per day). Chapter 1 outlines the fiber content of selected foods.

Despite widespread promotion by Health Canada and other organizations of the importance of fiber, the average Canadian consumes only 14 grams per day.[6] Popular foods like bagels, cereal bars, pasta, pizza and fast food tend to be low in fiber. And usual serving sizes of whole grains, fruits and vegetables provide only 1 to 3 grams of fiber. To ensure an adequate intake of vitamins and minerals, increased fiber should come from a variety of foods rather than from fiber supplements.

To treat constipation, add high-fiber foods to your daily diet. Below is a list of selected foods and their fiber content.

Food	Fiber (grams)
100% bran cereal, 1/2 cup (125 ml)	10 g
Kellogg's All Bran Buds (psyllium), 1/3 cup (75 ml)	13 g
Natural wheat bran, 2 tbsp (30 ml)	2.4 g
Flaxseed, ground, 2 tbsp (30 ml)	4.5 g
Almonds, 1/4 cup (60 ml)	4.8 g

Also choose higher-fiber fruits and vegetables:

Fruit	Vegetables
High Fiber (5+ grams)	*High Fiber (5+ grams)*
Apple, with skin	Green peas, 1/2 cup (125 ml)
Blackberries, 1/2 cup (125 ml)	Snow peas, 10
Blueberries, 1 cup (250 ml)	Swiss chard, cooked, 1 cup (250 ml)
Figs, dates, 10	
Kiwi, 2	
Mango, 1 medium	
Pear, 1 medium	
Prunes, dried, 5	
Prunes, stewed, 1/2 cup (125 ml)	
Raspberries, 1/2 cup (125 ml)	
Medium Fiber (2 to 4 grams)	*Medium Fiber (2 to 4 grams)*
Orange, 1 medium	Bean sprouts, 1/2 cup (125 ml)
Raisins, 2 tbsp (30 ml)	Beans, string, 1/2 cup (125 ml)
Rhubarb, cooked, 1/2 cup (125 ml)	Broccoli, 1/2 cup (125 ml)
Strawberries, 1 cup (250 ml)	Brussels sprouts, 1/2 cup (125 ml)
Tangerine, 1 medium	Carrots, raw, 1/2 cup (125 ml)
	Eggplant, 1/2 cup (125 ml)
	Parsnips, 1/2 cup (125 ml)
	Vegetables, mixed, 1/2 cup (125 ml)

Increase your fiber intake gradually to prevent intestinal discomfort. To minimize possible side effects such as bloating and gas, spread your fiber intake over the course of the day, rather than consuming it all at once. It is normal to experience some flatulence upon starting a high-fiber diet. This usually resolves within a few weeks, once the bacteria residing in your large intestine adjust to a higher fiber intake.

Dietary fiber needs to absorb fluid in the intestinal tract in order to add bulk to stool.

Drink 8 to 12 cups (2 to 3 liters) of fluid every day. Always include 1 cup (250 ml) of fluid with high-fiber meals and snacks.

Prunes

Prunes are high in fiber (1 gram of fiber per prune) and also contain a natural laxative substance called dihydroxyphenyl isatin. Eat four dried or stewed prunes as a snack. Drink prune juice for a concentrated source of prune's natural laxative. For a morning bowel movement, drink prune juice at bedtime. If an evening bowel movement is preferred, drink prune juice at breakfast.

Psyllium

Psyllium seed husks are a bulk-forming laxative high in both insoluble and soluble fibers. Studies have found psyllium to effectively treat constipation.[7-10] The laxative properties of psyllium are due to the swelling of the husk when it comes in contact with water. Once consumed, psyllium forms a gelatinous mass and keeps the feces hydrated and soft. The increased bulk stimulates a reflex contraction of the walls of the bowel. Take 5 to 10 grams of the husks with 2 cups (500 ml) water, one to three times per day.

Probiotics

Foods and supplements that contain friendly lactic acid bacteria (e.g., acidophilus, bifidobacteria) can help prevent constipation. These bacteria normally reside in the intestinal tract, where they perform a number of tasks that keep the bowel healthy. To achieve the health benefits of these bacteria, scientists are learning that it is important to consume them regularly.[11-12]

Eat 1 cup (250 ml) of a fermented dairy product daily: yogurt, kefir or acidophilus milk. All yogurts in Canada are made with lactic acid bacteria, whether or not they are labeled as such. To supplement, take 1 to 10 billion live cells (per capsule) with one to three meals daily. See Chapter 8 for more about probiotic supplements.

Herbal Remedies

Short-term use of one of the following herbal remedies may be tried if dietary strategies have failed. Seek medical attention for unresolved constipation.

Aloe (*Aloe vera, Aloe barbadensis*)

The components in the aloe leaf that cause a laxative effect are known as anthraquinones. These molecules exert the laxative action in the large bowel when they interact with intestinal bacteria. Take a single 50 to 200 milligram capsule of aloe leaf gel and/or latex daily in the evening for a maximum of ten days. If used longer, aloe can aggravate constipation, cause dependency and deplete body potassium.

Cascara (*Rhamnus purshiani cortex*)

Cascara bark is high in cascarosides, compounds that induce the large intestine to increase its muscular contraction and result in bowel movement. Use only the dried form of cascara. Two capsules containing dried cascara can be taken up to two times per day. As a tincture, 2 to 5 milliliters per day is generally taken. Use the smallest dosage necessary.

Cascara should be taken for a maximum of ten days. *It should not be taken long term.* Long-term use or abuse of cascara may cause a loss of potassium in the body, strengthening the action of certain heart medications, with fatal consequences. Long-term use of this herb may also weaken the colon. Women who are pregnant or lactating should not use cascara without the advice of a physician. Do not use this herb if you have abdominal pain or diarrhea.

Nutrition Strategy Checklist for Constipation

- ☐ Eat on a regular schedule
- ☐ Insoluble fiber
- ☐ Fluids
- ☐ Psyllium
- ☐ Prunes
- ☐ Probiotics

Recommended Resources

www.crha-health.ab.ca
Calgary Regional Health Authority Communications
1035-7th Avenue SW
Calgary, AB, Canada T2P 3E9
Tel: 403-265-INFO (403-265-4636) or
1-800-860-2742 (Alberta only)
E-mail: publicweb@crha-health.ab.ca

www.sickkids.on.ca
Hospital for Sick Children
555 University Avenue
Toronto, ON, Canada M5G 1X8
Tel: 416-813-5817 (medical information line)

www.niddk.nih.gov
National Digestive Diseases Information Clearinghouse
2 Information Way
Bethesda, MD, USA 20892-3570
Tel: 301-654-3810

Cystic Fibrosis

Cystic fibrosis is a progressive, potentially fatal, inherited disorder that affects the glands in the body that produce sweat and mucus. The defective cystic fibrosis gene produces an abnormal protein that interferes with the ability of the body to move sodium chloride (salt) and water through the cells. This causes the exocrine glands (the glands that produce sweat, saliva, mucus and tears) to malfunction. The fluids or secretions from the exocrine glands are used as lubricants in the body and are normally quite thin and slippery. By altering the transportation of chloride and water, the defective cystic fibrosis genes cause the glands to produce secretions that are abnormally thick and sticky.

The problems caused by cystic fibrosis are most evident in the respiratory and digestive systems. The thick secretions block the passages of the lungs, clogging the airways and creating an ideal environment for infection-causing bacteria to flourish. Breathing difficulties, recurrent infections and permanent lung damage are typical symptoms of cystic fibrosis.

The sticky mucus also blocks the ducts of the pancreas, which prevents digestive enzymes from reaching the intestinal tract. As a result of this mucus build-up, the body is unable to break down and absorb adequate nutrition from food. Chronic diarrhea, abdominal pain and nutritional deficiencies are common problems associated with cystic fibrosis.

People with cystic fibrosis tend to lose excessive amounts of salt through their sweat and saliva. This salt loss can upset the mineral balance in the body and may cause abnormalities in heart rhythms or shock. Cystic fibrosis also affects the reproductive system of both men and women. Men with the disease are usually infertile and women may have difficulty conceiving or may have more complications during pregnancy.

The severity of cystic fibrosis varies from person to person and usually depends on the degree of lung damage caused by the disease. Improved treatments have postponed some of the lung damage associated with cystic fibrosis, and many people with the disorder now have a life expectancy of 30 years or longer. Research in gene therapy is promising and may eventually prevent the progression of cystic fibrosis. However, at this time there is no cure for cystic fibrosis, and the disorder inevitably leads to death, usually as a result of lung disease and heart failure.

What Causes Cystic Fibrosis?

Approximately one in every 2500 children born in North America has the disease. To be born with cystic fibrosis, a child must inherit two defective cystic fibrosis genes, one from each parent. Most people have two normal genes. However, approximately 5 percent of all Caucasians who don't show any signs of cystic fibrosis are carriers of the disease. That means they are born with one normal gene and one defective cystic fibrosis gene.

If a child's mother and father are both carriers of a defective gene, then there is a

- 25 percent chance the child will be born with cystic fibrosis

- 50 percent chance the child will not have cystic fibrosis but will be a carrier

- 25 percent chance the child will not have cystic fibrosis and will not be a carrier

Most babies are diagnosed with the disease before they are one year old. In some cases, symptoms of the disease may not become apparent until the child is a teenager or even an adult.

Symptoms

Symptoms of cystic fibrosis include

- constant cough that expels thick mucus

- recurring respiratory infections, such as pneumonia or bronchitis

- growths (polyps) in the nose due to excess fluid in the mucus lining of the nasal passages

- skin that tastes salty

- frequent, bulky, foul-smelling, greasy stools

- failure (for children) to grow, despite a large or normal appetite

- barrel-shaped chest

- clubbing of the fingers and toes and bluish skin, caused by lack of oxygen

- night blindness, rickets, anemia and bleeding disorders caused by vitamin deficiencies

- delayed puberty, slowed growth and declining physical stamina in teenagers

- collapsed lung, coughing up blood, impaired reproductive function, liver disease and heart failure in adults

Who's at Risk?

As I mentioned above, approximately one in 25 North Americans carry the defective gene responsible for cystic fibrosis. Cystic fibrosis occurs mainly in Caucasians, especially those of Northern European heritage. The disease affects both boys and girls equally. Long-term survival is better in males, in people without pancreatic problems and in people who have only digestive problems in the early stages of the disease.

Conventional Treatment

Treatment programs are usually tailored to individual needs, depending on the severity of the disease and the organs affected. Home treatments include

- clapping or tapping the chest vigorously (percussion or vibration) and postural drainage to loosen the mucus clogging the lungs (mechanical devices are available to assist with this process)

- taking pancreatic enzymes with meals to aid digestion

- taking nutritional supplements to improve general nutrition

- taking salt supplements during a fever, exercise or exposure to hot weather

Medications may be prescribed to treat various symptoms:

- antibiotics to fight bacteria causing lung infections

- a bronchodilator to prevent narrowing of the airways

- mucus-thinning drugs to make the secretions thinner and easier to cough up

- anti-inflammatory drugs to reduce lung inflammation

- routine immunizations and influenza vaccines to prevent viral infections that can damage lungs

Oxygen therapy may be required for those patients with low oxygen levels. Surgery may be necessary for specific complications of the disease.

Managing Cystic Fibrosis

Dietary Strategies

High-Calorie Diet

The impaired digestion caused by cystic fibrosis results in weight loss and may, in children, result in improper growth. When food isn't digested properly, calories and nutrients are lost. For normal growth, people with cystic fibrosis often require 50 to 100 percent more calories than they would if they were healthy. These calories should come from fat, protein and carbohydrate. A registered dietitian who specializes in cystic fibrosis can help develop a diet with adequate calories for both children and adults.

Essential Fatty Acids

Many studies have revealed that patients with cystic fibrosis are deficient in both alpha-linolenic and linoleic acid because of poor absorption of dietary fat and faulty metabolism of these fatty acids.[1] A deficiency of these essential fatty acids can contribute to the kidney complications, lung damage and liver disease seen in cystic fibrosis.[2,3]

Children and adults should consume at least 2 tablespoons (30 ml) of oil rich in essential fatty acids (your dietitian will determine how much fat is required for an optimal calorie intake). Flaxseed oil, walnut oil and canola oil are good sources. A commercial product called Udo's Choice Ultimate Oil Blend is available in health food stores. It contains a balance of both alpha-linolenic and linoleic fatty acids from organic flaxseed, sesame and sunflower seeds, wheat germ, rice germ and oat germ. Flaxseed oil, walnut oil and Udo's oil should not be used for sautéing or frying, since their essential fatty acids are easily destroyed by heat. Store these oils in the refrigerator and use in salad dressings, dips and smoothies or add to foods like pasta sauces and soups after cooking.

Essential Fatty Acid Supplements
Supplements of essential fatty acids may help correct imbalances that occur in cystic fibrosis. One study found that borage oil that contained the fatty acid gamma-linolenic acid (GLA), taken daily for four weeks, improved essential fatty acid levels in patients with the disease.[4] While supplements of borage oil and evening primrose oil, which also contains GLA, may help, it is very important to get these healthy oils from your daily diet in order to provide extra calories.

To supplement with evening primrose oil, take 1000 to 1500 milligrams twice daily. Buy a product standardized for 9 percent GLA.

Food Sensitivities

Some children continue to have diarrhea and fail to thrive despite adequate dietary treatment. These children should be evaluated for possible food allergies. Studies have found that when allergenic foods are removed from the diet, diarrhea stops and weight gain occurs.[5,6] Your doctor should consider the possibility of food allergies if improvement does not occur with standard treatment. Ask for a referral to an allergy specialist for testing.

Vitamins and Minerals

Multivitamin and Mineral Supplements

Because of impaired absorption of nutrients, people with cystic fibrosis should take a multivitamin and mineral supplement twice daily with meals. This supplement will provide many of the nutrients that are commonly depressed in people with cystic fibrosis—beta-carotene, zinc, copper and vitamins A, D, E and C. These fat-soluble vitamins, with the exception of water-soluble vitamin C, are poorly absorbed in cystic fibrosis. As a result, deficiencies are common and can have important implications for the long-term health of people with the disease.

Vitamin A

Vitamin A levels should be monitored routinely in adults with cystic fibrosis who drive cars, since a deficiency causes night blindness.[7-10] Inflammatory lung flare-ups may also increase the risk for vitamin A deficiency. The best food sources of vitamin A include liver, oily fish, milk, cheese, butter and whole eggs. Your doctor will have you undertake blood tests to determine if it is necessary for you to take vitamin A supplements.

Vitamin D

Vitamin D is necessary for bone health, and a deficiency can increase the risk of bone loss and osteoporosis, two conditions often seen in people with cystic fibrosis.[11-15] Children with low vitamin E levels, teenagers and adults with cystic fibrosis should get regular blood tests to evaluate their vitamin D status. If a deficiency exists, your doctor will recommend a daily 400 to 800 international unit (IU) vitamin D supplement. Good food sources of vitamin D include milk, oily fish, margarine and whole eggs.

Vitamin E

Vitamin E levels are often reduced in cystic fibrosis, primarily because of poor absorption.[16-19] This antioxidant vitamin plays an important role in scavenging harmful free radical molecules whose damage can reduce lung function and increase the risk of heart disease. In cystic fibrosis, levels of many antioxidant nutrients are depressed (E, C, beta-carotene) and levels of free radicals are increased by inflammatory reactions of the disease. As a result, people with cystic fibrosis may have inadequate antioxidant defenses to protect their health.

Studies of patients with the disease have found that vitamin E supplements improve vitamin E levels and prevent free radical damage to blood cholesterol.[20-22] To supplement, take water-soluble (synthetic) vitamin E, 200 to 400 IU per day. The best food sources of vitamin E include wheat germ, nuts, seeds, vegetable oils, whole grains and leafy greens.

Vitamin K

Vitamin K status may also be impaired in people with cystic fibrosis because of impaired fat absorption.[23,24] Vitamin K is essential for blood clotting and healthy bone growth. Regular blood tests will detect a vitamin K deficiency and your doctor may recommend supplements. Good food sources of this vitamin include green peas, broccoli, spinach, leafy green vegetables, Brussels sprouts, Romaine lettuce, cabbage and liver.

Beta-Carotene

Studies show that people with cystic fibrosis tend to be deficient in beta-carotene.[25-27] This nutrient is found in orange and dark green produce, including carrots, sweet potato, winter squash, broccoli, collard greens, kale, spinach, apricots, cantaloupe, peaches, nectarines, mango and papaya. Beta-carotene helps provide the body with vitamin A. This carotenoid also acts as an antioxidant and can help protect the body from oxidative stress.

To get additional beta-carotene, choose a multivitamin and mineral supplement with the nutrient added.

Vitamin C

Ensuring an optimal intake of vitamin C can help prevent some of the free radical damage that occurs in cystic fibrosis. Researchers have found that patients who did not take a multivitamin supplement had low blood vitamin C levels and evidence of increased lung inflammation.[28] In patients who received low-dose vitamin C from a multivitamin pill, vitamin C levels were normal and levels of certain compounds in the blood that are markers of inflammation were much lower.

Foods rich in vitamin C include citrus fruit and juices, cantaloupe, kiwi, mango, strawberries, broccoli, Brussels sprouts, cauliflower, red pepper and tomato juice. To supplement, take 500 or 600 milligrams, once or twice daily.

Calcium

Many adults and adolescents with cystic fibrosis have evidence of bone loss.[29,30] Low bone mass and osteoporosis are caused by a deficiency of vitamin D and poor intake of calcium. It is very important to ensure an adequate intake of calcium, since critical periods of bone growth occur throughout childhood and adolescence. To determine your calcium requirements, turn to page 43, Chapter 4.

Calcium-rich foods include milk, yogurt, cheese, fortified soy and rice beverages, fortified orange juice, tofu, salmon (with bones), kale, bok choy, broccoli and Swiss chard. To supplement, take 300 milligrams of calcium citrate

with added vitamin D, one to three times daily. Your dose will depend on how much calcium your diet provides.

Zinc

Getting more zinc may help people with cystic fibrosis fight bacterial lung infections. This mineral is needed to activate thymulin, a hormone that enhances the immune system. Zinc is also needed for proper growth and development. Research suggests that zinc metabolism is altered in cystic fibrosis and that people with the disease may have lower blood levels of the mineral.[31-35]

Zinc-rich foods include oysters, seafood, red meat, poultry, yogurt, wheat bran, wheat germ, whole grains and enriched breakfast cereals. Most adult multivitamin and mineral supplements provide 10 milligrams; children's formulas may or may not contain zinc. Take single zinc supplements only on the advice of your doctor. Too much zinc taken for long periods has toxic effects and may suppress the immune system.

Other Natural Health Products

Digestive Enzymes

In cystic fibrosis, insufficient amounts of digestive enzymes enter the intestine because the ducts from the pancreas are blocked with mucus. As a result, carbohydrates, proteins and fats are not completely broken down and nutrients cannot be absorbed into the bloodstream. Taking a digestive enzyme supplement with each meal can help the body digest food and increase nutrients available for absorption.

With supplements, the amount of digestive enzymes is expressed in activity units rather than milligrams. These units refer to the enzyme's potency. Dosage will vary, depending on the type of enzymes in the product, so be sure to follow the manufacturer's directions.

Buy a broad-based enzyme supplement that contains protease (digests proteins), amylase (digests starch) and lipase (digests fat). Buy an enteric-coated product to withstand the acidity of the stomach.

Nutrition Strategy Checklist for Cystic Fibrosis

☐ High-calorie diet   ☐ Vitamin E

☐ Healthy oils   ☐ Vitamin K

☐ Evening primrose oil   ☐ Beta-carotene

☐ Identify food allergies   ☐ Vitamin C

☐ Multivitamin/mineral   ☐ Calcium

☐ Vitamin A   ☐ Zinc

☐ Vitamin D   ☐ Digestive enzymes

Recommended Resources

www.ccff.ca
Canadian Cystic Fibrosis Foundation
2221 Yonge Street, Suite 601
Toronto, ON, Canada M4S 2B4
Tel: 416-485-9149 or 1-800-378-2233
Fax: 416-485-0960

www.cff.org
The Cystic Fibrosis Foundation
6931 Arlington Road, Suite 200
Bethesda, MD, USA 20814
Tel: 301-951-4422 or 1-800-344-4823

www.nhlbi.nih.gov/health/public/lung/other/cystfib.htm
National Institutes of Health
National Heart, Lung and Blood Institute
NHLBI Health Information Network
P.O. Box 30105
Bethesda, MD, USA 20824-0105
Tel: 301-592-8573
Fax: 301-592-8563

Depression

It is estimated that one in every four Canadians will experience a degree of depression serious enough to require treatment at some time in their lives.[1] When faced with the stresses and losses of life, the natural response is sadness and grief. Everyone experiences emotional highs and lows in life and it's very normal to suffer through a bout of the "blues" once in a while. But depressive illness goes beyond these reactions.

Depression is a prolonged emotional response that significantly interferes with the ability to cope with daily living. Without treatment, symptoms may linger for months or even years. There are three types of depression:

1. *Unipolar major depression (clinical depression)* the diagnosis for this condition is made if symptoms of deep despair persist and consistently interfere with normal functioning during a two-week period.

2. *Dysthymia* a milder form of depression, dysthymia is a chronic mood disorder that lasts for at least two years.

3. *Manic depression (bipolar illness)* less common than the other forms of depression, manic depression involves disruptive cycles of elation or euphoria, alternating with depressive episodes, irritable excitement and mania.

What Causes Depression?

The actual causes of depression are not fully understood. It's thought to result from a combination of factors that include environmental and hereditary conditions, lifestyle choices, stress levels and body chemistry. Modern brain imaging technologies reveal that specific neural circuits in the brain do not function properly during depression, impairing the performance of crucial brain chemicals called neurotransmitters. Another theory holds that depression is caused by an imbalance in the body's response to stress, which results in an overactive hormonal system. Some studies also suggest that low levels of certain brain chemicals, known as amines, may slow down the nervous system and impair brain function enough to cause depression.

In women, there is evidence that the hormonal fluctuations of menstruation and pregnancy can trigger mental disorders. That women suffer depression more often than men also may be related to the fact that women synthesize serotonin, a brain chemical that carries messages between brain cells, at a lower rate than men. Melatonin, a chemical involved in regulating certain bodily functions, is also produced at different levels in women and men. Both differences may predispose women to become depressed with a lack of sunlight, a condition known as seasonal affective disorder (SAD).

Symptoms

Symptoms of depression develop gradually, over a period of days or weeks. The severity of symptoms can vary from person to person. To be diagnosed with depression, you must be experiencing at least four of the following indicators consistently over a period of at least two weeks:

- general sluggishness or agitation
- loss of interest in daily activities
- withdrawal
- acute sadness or feeling of emptiness
- demoralization, despair, feelings of worthlessness and hopelessness
- anxiety
- frequent outbursts of anger and rage
- concentration difficulties, memory loss, unusual indecisiveness
- self-criticism, self-deprecation

- changes in eating habits
- sleep disorders (insomnia, frequent awakening)
- chronic fatigue, lack of energy
- physical discomfort, such as constipation, headaches

In dysthymia, these symptoms are present in a milder form. People with manic depression often appear elated, uncontrollably enthusiastic and intrusively friendly. But they may just as easily become irritable or hostile. As the condition progresses, mental activity speeds up and the need for sleep decreases. A manic person is easily distracted, shifting constantly from one task or project to another, and may indulge in inappropriate sexual or personal behaviors or have delusions of power and wealth.

A typical depression can last for six to nine months, and episodes may recur several times over a lifetime. Symptoms rarely go away on their own, but with professional diagnosis and treatment, depression can be managed and controlled very successfully.

Who's at Risk?

Depression can affect anyone, at any time. Some of the main risk factors associated with depression include

- *Family history* If you have an immediate family member with depression, your risk for depression is greater.
- *Traumatic life events* Early childhood events, such as the loss of a parent, sexual abuse or divorce, increase the risk of adult depression.
- *Stress* Work-related pressures, the loss of a loved one, divorce, financial problems or a move to a new location might trigger depression.

- *Marital and work status* Depression is highest among divorced, separated or widowed people. Unemployment lasting more than six months is also a factor.

- *Physical illness* Cancer, heart disease, AIDS/HIV, hormonal disorders and thyroid conditions are associated with depression.

- *Medications* Many medications, including sedatives and pain medications, produce mood disorders as a side effect.

- *Gender and age* Women suffer from depression and attempt suicide more often than men. Children, adolescents and the elderly experience stressful life events that may predispose them to depression.

- *Alcohol or drug use* Alcohol is a depressive drug and will aggravate the symptoms of depression. Mood-altering drugs tend to complicate depression and interfere with its treatment.

Conventional Treatment

Depression is one of the most common and treatable mental disorders. It is usually treated without hospitalization, using a combination of medications and psychotherapy. The earlier treatment begins, the more effective it is and the more likely it will prevent serious recurrences. However, even when treatment is successful, depression may recur. Results of any treatment should be apparent within two to three months.

Several different types of antidepressant drugs are available. They work by influencing the activity of brain neurotransmitters, primarily serotonin, norepinephrine and dopamine, and must be taken for several weeks before they begin to work. Antidepressant drugs include

- *Selective serotonin reuptake inhibitors (SSRIs)*—Prozac®, Effexor®, Paxil®, Zoloft®, Serzone®. These drugs raise serotonin levels in the brain. SSRIs have fewer side effects and are often the first choice of treatment for depression. They may cause mild nausea, diarrhea and headaches that usually subside over time. SSRIs commonly cause sexual dysfunction as a side effect.

- *Monoamine oxidase inhibitors (MAOIs)* — Manerix®. This type of drug increases the level of various brain chemicals, including amines. It is rarely used today because of its serious interactions with other medications and with foods that contain tyramine (such as red wine, aged cheeses, soy sauce and yeast extracts).

- *Tricyclic antidepressants*—Elavil®, Tofranil®, Norpramin®. These drugs are useful in treating depression, but they bring with them a host of unpleasant side effects, such as weight gain, drowsiness, dizziness and an increased heart rate. They are not usually used to treat mild to moderate depression, because the side effects are often worse than the disease.

Psychotherapy—individual and group therapy—can help to gradually change negative attitudes and feelings of hopelessness and can provide guidance in adjusting to the normal pressures of life. It is often used in conjunction with antidepressant drugs. Electroconvulsive therapy (ECT) is used for severe cases of depression. An electric current is applied to the head to induce a seizure in the brain. For reasons not completely understood, the seizure will quickly and very effectively alleviate depression.

Managing Depression

Dietary Strategies

Carbohydrates

Carbohydrate has been one of the most widely studied nutrients with respect to mood. High-carbohydrate meals have been associated with a calming, relaxing effect and even drowsiness.[2,3] Carbohydrate-rich meals allow an amino acid called tryptophan to get into the brain, which is then used to make the neurotransmitter serotonin. Many studies associate high serotonin levels with happier moods and low levels with mild depression.

If you're feeling depressed, try a high-carbohydrate meal that contains very little protein. Protein foods like chicken, meat or fish provide many different amino acids that compete with tryptophan for entry into the brain. That means that less serotonin will be produced. Good choices include pasta with tomato sauce, a toasted whole-grain bagel with jam or a bowl of whole-grain cereal with low-fat milk. High-carbohydrate beverages such as unsweetened fruit juice, sports recovery drinks and milk are good alternatives.

Omega-3 Fats

Omega-3 fatty acids, special fats that are plentiful in fish, are lower in people who are depressed. These fatty acids are important components of nerve and brain cell membranes, where they help cells communicate messages effectively. Fish contains two special omega-3 fats, DHA and EPA. It's a lack of DHA that seems to be an important factor in depression. DHA may work to ease depression by altering the structure of cell membranes in the brain, making them more responsive to the effects of serotonin. DHA may also have anti-inflammatory effects in the brain, which can also influence mood. Some research suggests that fish oil supplements can improve symptoms in patients with clinical depression.[4-6]

The best sources of omega-3 oils are cold-water fish such as salmon, trout, mackerel, herring, sardines and fresh tuna. Aim to eat fish at least three times a week. If you have clinical depression, you might try fish oil supplements. Buy a product that offers a combination of EPA and DHA. A good-quality fish oil supplement should also contain vitamin E, which is added to help stabilize the oils. Avoid fish *liver* oil capsules.

Supplements made from fish livers are a concentrated source of vitamin A and D. Too much vitamin A and D can be toxic when taken in large amounts for long periods.

The precise dose of fish oil for treating depression is not yet known. Some experts recommend getting anywhere from 5 to 15 grams of omega-3 fats three times daily. High doses of fish oil can have side effects, such as leaving an unpleasant taste in the mouth. Fish oil also has a blood-thinning effect. If you take medication that thins the blood, consult your physician first. *Fish oil supplements should never replace your medication. Always discuss any alternative or complementary treatment with your doctor first.*

Vitamins and Minerals

Vitamin B6

Even marginal deficiencies of the B vitamins have been associated with irritability, depression and mood changes. Vitamin B6 has been the focus of study in more than 900 women suffering from depression related to premenstrual syndrome (PMS). Based on the evidence available, a daily supplement of B6 seems likely to balance emotions in women suffering from PMS-related depression.[7]

The body uses B6 to form an important enzyme that's needed to convert tryptophan to serotonin in the brain. Based on the evidence available, a daily supplement of B6 appears to be effective in helping relieve depression.

The best sources of B6 are high-protein foods like meat, fish, poultry, whole grains, bananas and potatoes. To supplement, take 50 to 100 milligrams once daily. Because the B vitamins work together (there are eight B vitamins), I recommend a B complex supplement that's balanced with all the Bs. Taking only one B vitamin in high doses could upset the body's balance. Do not exceed 100 milligrams per day as too much vitamin B6 can cause irreversible nerve damage.

Folate and Vitamin B12

A number of studies have found that many depressed people are deficient in both of these B vitamins.[8-12] It has been suggested that lack of these interrelated nutrients may work in a number of ways to cause depression. Both folate and B12 are required in the body for the synthesis of a compound called S-adenosyl-methionine or SAMe (see below, and also page 139, Chapter 8). SAMe, in turn, is used by the brain to produce neurotransmitters, in particular the amines. So a lack of B12 and/or folate can interfere with this process and result in low levels of brain amines. This could cause or worsen depression.

A folate deficiency may also impair the brain's ability to synthesize many neurotransmitters, including serotonin. Low folate levels in the body are linked with a poorer response to serotonin reuptake inhibitor drugs (Prozac®, Effexor®, Paxil®, Zoloft®, Serzone®).

Best food sources of folate include spinach, artichokes, asparagus, lentils, dried peas and beans, chicken liver, orange juice and wheat germ. To supplement, choose a multivitamin and mineral formula with 0.4 to 1.0 milligram (400 to 1000 micrograms) of folic acid (folic acid is the synthetic form of folate) or choose a B complex formula. If you take single supplements of folic acid, ensure that it has B12 added.

Best food sources of vitamin B12 include all animal foods and fortified soy and rice beverages. Adults over the age of 50 should get B12 from a supplement or fortified foods since the body's ability to absorb this nutrient from food becomes less efficient as we age. Supplement choices include a multivitamin and mineral or a B complex formula. Complete vegetarians (vegans) who do not use fortified soy or rice beverages should take a single B12 supplement offering 500 to 1000 micrograms.

Herbal Remedies

St. John's Wort (*Hypericum perforatum*)

For years, this herb has been used in Europe to treat both mild depression and seasonal affective disorder. In 1997, British researchers analyzed 26 controlled studies conducted in 1700 patients and concluded that the herb was as effective as certain antidepressant drugs in treating mild to moderate depression.[13]

Experts believe that St. John's wort works by keeping brain serotonin levels high for a longer period, just like the popular antidepressant drugs Paxil®, Zoloft® and Prozac®. It seems that the power of St. John's wort lies in two active ingredients, hypericin and hyperforin. Researchers attribute most of the herb's effectiveness to hyperforin. When selecting a St. John's wort product, look for a brand that meets the following criteria:

- It should be standardized to contain 0.3 percent hypericin.

- It should contain a high amount (3 to 5 percent) of hyperforin. Movana®, manufactured in Europe and available in North America, is an advanced formula that contains hyperforin. This extract has been used in clinical studies.

The effective dosage is one 300 milligram tablet three times a day. The herb is generally well tolerated. When taken in high doses for a long period, the herb may cause sensitivity to sunlight in very light-skinned individuals. St. John's wort has the potential to interact with a number of medications. Do not take the herb if you are using any of the following drugs: indinavir, cyclosporine, theophylline, warfarin, birth control pills or digoxin. It is not recommended for use during pregnancy and breastfeeding. If you are currently taking a prescription antidepressant drug, do not take it concurrently with St. John's wort. *Always consult your physician before stopping any medication.*

Ginkgo Biloba

A few studies have found that this herb helped improve depressive symptoms, especially in older adults.[14,15] Animal research suggests that ginkgo might work by blocking an age-related loss of serotonin receptors in the brain.[16] Instead of increasing the amount of serotonin in the brain, ginkgo seems to enhance the brain's ability to respond to serotonin.

If you are taking an SSRI drug (Prozac®, Effexor®, Paxil®, Zoloft®, Serzone®) for your depression and experiencing side effects that affect your sex life, consider adding ginkgo to your nutrition regime. Californian researchers found that a standardized extract of the herb was 84 percent effective in treating sexual dysfunction associated with antidepressant therapy.[17] Women were more responsive than men, with success rates of 91 percent versus 76 percent. Components in the herb called terpene lactones and ginkgo flavone glycosides act to increase blood flow to the extremities.

The recommended dose of ginkgo is 40 to 80 milligrams taken three times daily. To reverse sexual dysfunction, take 60 milligrams twice daily. Choose a product that is standardized to contain 24 percent ginkgo flavone glycosides and 6 percent terpene lactones.

The extract used in the scientific research is sold as Ginkoba® in Canada and the United States. On rare occasions, ginkgo may cause gastrointestinal upset, headache or an allergic skin reaction in susceptible individuals.

Other Natural Health Products

Inositol

This compound is sometimes referred to as vitamin B8, though it is not an essential nutrient.

Inositol is found all body tissues, but it is concentrated in the heart and brain.

It is found in beans, nuts, seeds, whole grains and citrus fruit as a substance called phytic acid. Once consumed, intestinal bacteria release inositol from phytic acid.

Research suggests that inositol may be involved in depression, since it works with serotonin in the brain. A few small studies have found the supplement to significantly improve symptoms of depression compared with placebo treatment.[18-20] The recommended dose is 12 grams per day. No side effects have been reported. Because the recommended dosage of inositol is high (grams rather than milligrams), be sure to buy a product made by a reputable manufacturer. There is a greater risk for ill effects from contaminants when taking products in large doses, even if the contaminant is present in small amounts. See Chapter 8 for more information on inositol.

SAMe (S-Adenosyl-Methionine)

SAMe is a compound the body makes naturally from certain amino acids found in high-protein foods like fish and meat. The production of SAMe is closely linked with folate and vitamin B12, and deficiencies of these two nutrients can lead to depressed levels of SAMe in the brain and nervous system.

The results of recent well-controlled studies show that SAMe is significantly better than a placebo in treating depression, and it may even be more effective than tricyclic antidepressant medication.[21-26] In patients taking SAMe, symptoms improve in as few as four to five days. Exactly how SAMe works to treat depressive symptoms is not entirely clear. It is associated with higher levels of brain neurotransmitters. But it may also work by favorably changing the composition of cell membranes in the brain, enabling neurotransmitters and cell receptors to work more efficiently.

SAMe is approved as a prescription drug in 14 countries, and is available as a dietary supplement in the United States. To treat depression, studies use 800 to 1600 milligrams per day in divided doses. Buy an enteric-coated product. Start with one 400 milligram tablet twice daily, then work up to two tablets three times daily. Take SAMe on an empty stomach. The supplement is very well tolerated at the recommended doses, but it may cause nausea and gastrointestinal upset in doses higher than 1600 milligrams. European studies did not find any long-term problems associated with taking SAMe.

If you are currently taking medication for depression and you are thinking about trying SAMe, do not discontinue your medication without first speaking to your doctor. When taken with antidepressant drugs, SAMe may have an additive effect causing potentially dangerous side effects.

Nutrition Strategy Checklist for Depression

- ☐ Carbohydrate-rich foods
- ☐ Fish oils
- ☐ Vitamin B6
- ☐ Folate
- ☐ Vitamin B12
- ☐ St. John's wort* OR Ginkgo biloba OR Inositol
- ☐ SAMe

* Strongest evidence—start here.

Recommended Resources

www.fhs.mcmaster.ca/direct
Depression and Anxiety Information and Education Resource Centre (DIRECT)
McMaster University
100 West 5th, Box 585
Hamilton, ON, Canada L8N 3K7
Tel: 1-888-557-5051, ext. 8000

www.ndmda.org
National Depressive and Manic Depressive Association
730 N Franklin Street, Suite 501
Chicago, IL, USA 60601
Tel: 1-312-642-0049 or 1-800-826-3632

www.nim.nih.gov
National Institute of Mental Health Information Resources and Inquiries Branch
6001 Executive Boulevard, Room 8184, MSC 9663
Bethesda, MD, USA 20892-9663
Tel: 1-301-443-4513
Fax: 1-301-443-4279

www.nmha.org
National Mental Health Association
1021 Prince Street
Alexandria, VA, USA 22314-2971
Tel: 703-684-7722
1-800-969-NMHA (1-800-969-6642) (Mental Health Information Center)
TTY: 1-800-433-5959
Fax: 703-684-5968

Dermatitis and Eczema

Dermatitis and eczema are skin conditions that cause itching, blistering and inflammation. The common types of dermatitis include

- *Contact dermatitis* This condition develops when allergy-causing substances (allergens) come in contact with the skin, triggering redness, itchiness, burning sensations and blisters on the skin surface. Perfumes, cosmetics, metal jewelry, household-cleaning products, preservatives in creams and lotions and plants such as poison ivy are examples of allergens known to cause contact dermatitis. The reaction usually disappears when contact with the allergen is avoided.

- *Seborrheic dermatitis* Yellowish, oily, scaling patches appear on the scalp, face and other areas of the body where the sebaceous (oil-producing) glands are numerous. It often appears as a stubborn, itchy form of dandruff. It tends to be an inherited condition and is treated with medicated shampoos and hydrocortisone creams or lotions.

- *Neurodematitis* This condition develops when a skin irritant, such as a tight garment or an insect bite, triggers a cycle of constant rubbing or scratching. Scaly patches appear on the affected area and become thickened and leathery (lichenified) because of the persistent scratching. Treatment usually involves applying dressings over the irritated spot to prevent further scratching or rubbing, plus topical hydrocortisone creams or ointments to soothe the skin.

- *Nummular eczema* Round, coin-shaped patches of irritated skin develop on the arms, backs, lower legs and buttocks. These patches may become crusty, dry, red and leathery. It is common in older adults and children and is often triggered by stress or extremely dry or humid climates.

- *Statsis dermatitis* This condition occurs when fluid gathers in the tissues under the skin. People with varicose veins or other circulatory problems in the legs are prone to developing this condition. It causes the skin on the ankles to become fragile, discolored, thickened and itchy. Treatment focuses on correcting the condition that causes the fluid build-up. Elastic support hose or varicose vein surgery may be necessary.

Atopic Dermatitis (Eczema)

One of the most prevalent types of dermatitis is atopic dermatitis, commonly known as eczema. "Atopic" refers to a group of allergic diseases that are hereditary and often affect several members of a family. Asthma and hay fever are part of this group, as are the skin eruptions that are characteristic of atopic dermatitis.

Atopic dermatitis affects over 15 million children and adults in North America and accounts for nearly 20 percent of all patient referrals to a dermatologist. It is a chronic, recurrent condition that causes the skin to become extremely itchy, inflamed, swollen, dry and cracked. Atopic dermatitis occurs most often in children and infants. One-third of all cases appear in the first year of life and 90 percent of patients show symptoms before the age of five.[1] The disease rarely develops after the age of 30. The majority of children with atopic dermatitis will continue to experience flare-ups into adulthood.

The cause of atopic dermatitis is unclear. It is not a contagious condition and cannot be spread from one person to another. It seems to be associated with a malfunction of the immune system, triggered in response to infectious or irritating conditions. Current research also indicates that it may be linked to a defect in the conversion of linoleic acid, a fatty acid the body must get from food. Atopic dermatitis is often aggravated by a combination of hereditary and environmental factors such as

- inherited tendencies to allergies or asthma

- dry skin

- extremely high or low temperatures

- irritants such as household cleaning products, detergents, perfumes and cosmetics, wool and other rough or synthetic fabrics, cigarette smoke, dust and sand

- allergens such as pollen, dog or cat dander or foods known to trigger allergic reactions (peanuts, eggs, soy products, fish, milk and wheat)

- emotional issues, anxiety and stress

- bacterial or viral skin infections

Symptoms

The symptoms of atopic dermatitis vary from person to person and include

- dry itchy skin
- cracks behind the ears
- rashes on the cheeks, arms and legs; small red bumps (papules) may develop, becoming crusty and infected when scratched
- red and scaly skin; skin may become thick and leathery (lichenified) due to constant scratching
- extra fold of skin around eyes (atopic pleat)
- darkened skin on the eyelids due to inflammation
- sparse and patchy eyebrows and eyelashes due to rubbing

Who's at Risk?

The incidence of atopic dermatitis has increased 30 percent since 1970, possibly because of increased exposure to environmental irritants, allergens and emotional stress. The skin condition affects men and women equally and tends to run in families. Atopic dermatitis occurs most often in children and infants. It's estimated that up to 20 percent of all infants suffer from atopic dermatitis and nearly 40 percent outgrow it by adulthood.[2]

Conventional Treatment

To keep the skin healthy, it is important to develop a proper skin-care routine. Avoid hot or long showers and use mild soaps or nonsoap cleansers to avoid drying the skin. After bathing, pat skin dry gently—avoid rubbing briskly. Moisturize the skin with creams or ointments immediately after bathing or showering.

If the skin shows signs of infection such as oozing areas or crusty or pus-filled blisters, begin medical treatment immediately. Commonly prescribed treatments include the following.

- *Corticosteroid creams and ointments* may be prescribed to treat flare-ups. Oral or systemic corticosteroid medications may be necessary for more severe episodes.
- *Antibiotics* may be needed to treat skin infections.
- *Antihistamines* may be prescribed to cause drowsiness to reduce nighttime scratching.
- *Phototherapy* with ultraviolet A or B light may be helpful.
- *Immunosuppressive drugs* may be used in adults to treat attacks that are not responding to other forms of therapy.
- *Topical immunomodulators,* new drugs under development, are offering hope for an improved, steroid-free approach to management of atopic dermatitis.

Managing Atopic Dermatitis

Dietary Strategies

Food Allergies

Certain food proteins known to cause allergic reactions may be involved in the development of eczema or may exacerbate its condition. In fact, it is estimated that food allergies contribute to atopic eczema in as many as one-third of children with the skin condition.[3] Common food allergens that can cause eczema include eggs, fish, milk and wheat. It is important to be tested for food allergies by a trained doctor to avoid dietary limitations that may be unnecessary and even harmful. Studies have shown that once food allergies are confirmed by testing, elimination of these foods results in improvement of skin symptoms.[4-6]

To determine if food allergies trigger your atopic eczema, try an elimination/challenge diet as outlined below. A registered dietitian (**www.dietitians.ca**) can help you identify problematic foods and plan a healthy diet that avoids them.

1. *Elimination phase* For a period of two weeks, eliminate common food allergens— dairy products, soy foods, citrus fruits, nuts, wheat, shellfish, fish, eggs, corn and sulfite food additives.

2. *Challenge phase* After two weeks, start introducing one food every three days. Keep a food and symptom diary. Record everything you eat, amounts eaten and what time you ate the food or meal. Document any skin symptoms. If symptoms recur when a particular food is added back, you may be allergic. Consult your doctor for further food allergy testing.

Dietary Fat

People with atopic dermatitis are thought to have impaired fatty acid metabolism.[7-9] The body uses essential fatty acids in food to produce compounds called eicosanoids, which have a wide range of health effects in the body. Linoleic acid, an essential fatty acid found in vegetable oils, is converted in the body to gamma-linolenic acid (GLA), which in turn is used to make health-enhancing eicosanoids.

Some experts think that the conversion of linoleic acid to GLA is impaired in people with atopic dermatitis (see the section on evening primrose oil, below). A diet that is high in saturated fat and processed vegetable fats further slows down this conversion. Choose lean cuts of meat, poultry breast and low-fat dairy products. Avoid processed foods that contain hydrogenated vegetable oils. Choose a margarine made with nonhydrogenated oil. Use added fats and oils sparingly. Eat fish more often, since fish contains special fatty acids that the body uses to make healthy eicosanoids.

Breastfeeding

Atopic disease (dermatitis, allergies, asthma) can possibly be prevented in high-risk infants by breastfeeding. An infant is considered to be at risk if one or both parents have an atopic illness. Breast milk contains many protective compounds that can bolster an infant's developing immune system.

Finnish researchers studied 236 high-risk infants at age 1, 3, 5, 10 and 17 to determine the effect of breastfeeding on atopic disease.[10] They found that the prevalence of atopic eczema, food allergy and respiratory illness was the lowest for those who were breastfed for longer than six months and the highest in those who had little or no breastfeeding.

Vitamins and Minerals

Zinc

A deficiency of this mineral leads to a number of health problems, including a weakened immune system and atopic dermatitis.[11,12] Scandinavian researchers have found that compared with healthy children, those with allergies tend to have lower zinc levels.[13] To prevent a deficiency, include zinc-rich foods in your daily diet. Zinc is abundant in red meat, oysters, seafood, poultry, wheat bran, wheat germ, whole grains, enriched breakfast cereals and yogurt. Adult multivitamin and mineral supplements provide 10 to 20 milligrams of the mineral. Children's products may or may not contain zinc because of its potential toxicity when consumed in large amounts. If they do have zinc, very small amounts are present (e.g., 2 milligrams).

If you have been diagnosed with a zinc deficiency, take 10 to 40 milligrams of zinc once daily. Children under ten years of age should take no more than 10 milligrams of zinc. Buy a zinc supplement with 1 milligram of copper for every 10 milligrams of zinc (large amounts of zinc deplete the body's copper stores). Consumi amounts greater than 40 to 50 milligrams per day can depress the immune system and cause toxic effects. Do not exceed 40 milligrams of zinc per day.

Herbal Remedies
Evening Primrose Oil
(*Oenothera biennis*)
Linoleic acid is an essential fatty acid abundant in corn, sunflower, safflower and soybean oils. To be fully utilized by the body, linoleic acid must be converted to other substances. The first step in this process is the transformation of linoleic acid to gamma-linolenic acid (GLA). GLA is then used to produce a number of important anti-inflammatory compounds called eicosanoids. It is hypothesized that people with atopic dermatitis have difficulty converting linoleic acid to GLA and would benefit from a direct supply in the form of GLA supplements (such as evening primrose oil supplements).

While some studies have found no benefit, a number have found evening primrose oil to be effective in reducing the severity of eczema symptoms, including skin redness and roughness and especially itchiness.[14-17] The standard dose is 6 to 8 grams per day, split in two equal doses; half that for children. Buy a product standardized to contain at least 9 percent GLA. Many studies have evaluated the effect of a brand called Efamol®. Evening primrose oil in combination with fish oil may also be effective.

It can take at least four weeks before there are any noticeable effects, and full results may take up to nine months. The doses of evening primrose oil used to treat eczema are considered safe.

Herbal Creams
Topical creams of calendula, chamomile and licorice alone or in combination are often used in Europe to ease the symptoms of eczema. When used topically, these creams have anti-inflammatory properties. Researchers from Germany found the use of chamomile cream equally effective or superior to hydrocortisone creams.[18,19] Apply one of these creams to the affected areas one to four times daily.

Other Natural Health Products
Probiotics
A group of health-enhancing microbes called lactic acid bacteria may be useful in treating eczema. Researchers from Finland evaluated the effect of Lactobacillus and bifidobacteria supplemental infant formula in 27 infants with atopic eczema.[20,21] After two months of treatment, the infants receiving the probiotic formula experienced a significant improvement in their skin condition, whereas those on regular formula did not.

Lactic acid bacteria exert their health benefits in the intestinal tract. Here they may help treat eczema by enhancing the body's immune system, preventing the attachment of harmful microbes to the intestinal tract and secreting substances that destroy infection-causing bacteria.

Take 1 to 10 billion viable cells, in three or four divided doses with food. Children's products usually contain one-quarter to one-half the adult dose, or 250 to 500 billion live cells. Probiotic supplements may cause flatulence, which usually subsides as you continue treatment. There are no safety issues associated with taking these supplements.

Nutrition Strategy Checklist for Dermatitis and Eczema

☐ Identify food allergies   ☐ Evening primrose oil
☐ Limit saturated fat   ☐ Chamomile cream
☐ Fish   ☐ Probiotic supplements
☐ Zinc

Recommended Resources

www.aaaai.org
American Academy of Allergy, Asthma and Immunology
611 E Wells Street
Milwaukee, WI, USA 53202
Tel: 414-272-6071
Fax: 414-272-6070
E-mail: membership@aaaai.org

www.aad.org
American Academy of Dermatology
930 N Meacham Road
P.O. Box 4014
Schaumburg, IL, USA 60168-4014
Tel: 847-330-0230
Fax: 847-330-0050

Canadian Eczema Society for Education & Research
(no Web site available)
11 Sapling Court
Toronto, ON, Canada M9C 1K9
Tel: 416-695-8787
Fax: 416-695-2396

www.nih.gov.niams/healthinfo
National Institute of Arthritis and Musculoskeletal and Skin Diseases Information Clearinghouse
National Institutes of Health
1 AMS Circle
Bethesda, MD, USA 20892-3675
Tel: 301-495-4484 or 1-877-226-4267 (toll-free)
Fax: 301-718-6366

Diabetes Mellitus

It is estimated that as many as 120 million people live with diabetes worldwide. Although more than 800,000 new cases are identified every year, research indicates that almost one-third of the people suffering with diabetes don't even know they have it.[1]

Diabetes is a metabolic disorder that affects the way the body uses food for growth and energy. The body's main source of fuel comes from glucose, a form of sugar that is produced during the digestive process. The bloodstream carries glucose to the cells, where it is used to fuel cell growth and essential bodily functions. Glucose (blood-sugar) levels vary frequently during the day, rising and falling as you eat food or drink fluids containing sugar or other carbohydrates. To help the body maintain your blood-sugar level within a safe and normal range, the pancreas produces a hormone called insulin. Glucose cannot pass through cell membranes without the help of insulin.

Diabetes results when the body does not produce enough insulin or does not use it properly. Glucose builds up in the blood and passes out of the body as urine, causing the cells to lose their main source of fuel. There are three types of diabetes.

Type 1 diabetes develops when the immune system attacks and destroys the insulin-producing cells in the pancreas. Scientists suspect that a genetic predisposition to diabetes, combined with environmental factors such as a virus or a nutritional problem, may trigger the immune system to malfunction. Type 1 diabetes develops most often in children and young adults, but it can strike at any age. A person with this type of diabetes must take insulin daily to stay alive. Type 1 accounts for 10 percent of all diagnosed cases of diabetes.

Type 2 diabetes is the most common form of the disease, affecting nearly 95 percent of all people with diabetes. It results when the body cannot use insulin properly. In type 2 diabetes, the pancreas usually produces adequate amounts of insulin, but the body is no longer capable of using it effectively. This condition is known as insulin resistance. In type 2 diabetes, the cells of the pancreas produce less insulin, so the body is unable to overcome insulin resistance. Type 2 diabetes also occurs when the liver releases sugar into the bloodstream overnight, causing an elevated fasting blood-glucose test (a test to measure blood glucose, done before breakfast, when nothing has been eaten in the past 12 hours).

Type 2 diabetes usually develops in people over the age of 40; the older you are, the greater your risk. It is often associated with abdominal obesity and is more prevalent in certain racial and cultural groups, such as African Americans and Hispanics. Type 2 diabetes tends to develop very gradually and may not produce any obvious symptoms. Often, people don't discover they have type 2 diabetes until they experience one of the many complications that result from the disease.

Gestational diabetes develops only during pregnancy and disappears when the pregnancy is over. It affects 2 to 5 percent of all pregnant women. Women with gestational diabetes are at higher risk of developing type 2 diabetes in later life.

During its insidious progress, diabetes damages both large and small blood vessels and nerves. This usually leads to a number of associated health problems, including

- *Eye disease* People with diabetes are four times more likely to become blind. In fact, diabetes is the leading cause of adult blindness in North America. *Diabetic retinopathy* is caused by a deterioration of the blood vessels in the eyes. It affects almost everyone with type 1 diabetes and 60 percent of people with type 2 diabetes. People with diabetes are also at greater risk of developing glaucoma, cataracts and damage to the macula of the eye. Regular visits to an ophthalmologist can prevent the progression of diabetic retinopathy and preserve eyesight.

- *Kidney disease* As many as 20 to 30 percent of people with diabetes develop kidney disease within 15 years of their diagnosis. Damage to the kidneys can ultimately lead to kidney failure, requiring treatment with dialysis or organ transplant.

- *Nerve damage* Diabetes can generate nerve damage (neuropathy) that will cause numbness and tingling sensations, especially in the feet. Nerve damage can also result in insensitivity to pain or extreme sensitivity to touch. Nerves also control gastrointestinal function and the ability to achieve an erection. Neuropathy can affect all of these bodily functions.

- *Heart disease* People with diabetes are five times more likely to have a stroke and up to four times more likely to have coronary artery disease. Chronic high blood-sugar levels lead to narrowing of the arteries, high blood pressure, heart attack and stroke.

- *Infections* Poor blood supply and nerve damage caused by diabetes can lead to ulcers on the skin and slow healing of wounds. Chronic high glucose levels increase the risk of infection and interfere with the body's immune system.

- *Impotence* Because of blood vessel blockage, impotence affects between 8 and 13 percent of all men with diabetes.

- *Pregnancy complications* Women with diabetes have a higher risk of delivering babies with birth defects and often have complications in their pregnancies.

These long-term complications usually develop after more than ten years of diabetes and are related to the level of blood-sugar control and hereditary factors. Cigarette smoking, high blood pressure and high blood cholesterol and triglycerides can further increase the chances of complications. These statistics may sound bleak, but two large intervention studies have demonstrated that tight control of blood sugar can significantly reduce the risk of eye, nerve and kidney disease.[2,3] Early diagnosis of diabetes and tight control of blood sugars are essential to help delay or prevent the complications of this disease.

Symptoms

Symptoms of type 1 and type 2 diabetes include the following. However, some people with type 2 diabetes may have no symptoms at all.

- extreme thirst
- frequent urination
- unusual weight loss
- excessive hunger
- extreme fatigue or lack of energy
- blurred vision
- recurring infections, especially in the skin, gums and bladder
- cuts and bruises that are slow to heal

Who's at Risk?

- older adults; the risk of type 2 diabetes increases after the age of 45, though the disease is also being diagnosed in overweight younger adults and children of Aboriginal, Hispanic, Asian or African descent
- obese individuals, especially if extra weight is carried around the abdomen
- people who have a close relative with diabetes
- women with gestational diabetes are at risk of developing type 2 diabetes later in life
- children of mothers with gestational diabetes have a greater risk of developing diabetes as young adults
- individuals with normal or high blood triglyceride levels and low HDL (good) cholesterol levels
- individuals with impaired glucose tolerance or elevated fasting blood sugar

Conventional Treatment

Controlling blood sugar is the most important goal of treatment. Type 1 diabetes always requires daily injections of insulin administered by needle or an insulin pump. Type 2 diabetes may require oral medications to increase insulin secretion by the pancreas (drugs such as DiaBeta®, Diamicron® or GlucoNorm®) or to enhance the action of insulin (drugs such as Metformin®, Avandia®, Actose®, Prandase®). Some people with type 2 diabetes may require insulin injections or a combination of insulin and oral medications to lower their blood sugar.

Managing diabetes includes eating healthy foods on a regular schedule, exercising regularly, achieving and maintaining a healthy weight and reducing stress. Exercise improves the body's sensitivity to insulin and lowers blood sugar to the same extent as some type 2 diabetes medications.

Self-monitoring with a home blood-glucose meter (glucometer) is essential to keep a check on sugar levels and adjust diet and medication accordingly. Maintaining blood glucose at optimal levels can significantly reduce the risk of long-term complications such as eye problems, nerve damage and heart disease.

Once you are diagnosed with diabetes, proper education by registered dietitians, nurses and certified diabetes educators is crucial to learn how to manage your medication, eating habits, exercise regimen and stress levels. Diabetes education centers in hospitals offer intensive training programs for those newly diagnosed with the disease and their families.

Managing Diabetes

Dietary Strategies

The cornerstone of diabetes management is diet therapy. Dietary advice for people with diabetes follows the principles of Canada's Food Guide to Healthy Eating.[4,5] A registered dietitian is a key member of the diabetes healthcare team and will help develop a healthy diet that is tailored to your food preferences, medication and lifestyle. Research shows that following the advice of a dietitian trained in diabetes management results in significant improvements in blood-sugar control.[6]

An appropriate meal plan can help achieve and maintain optimal blood-sugar and blood-fat levels and prevent or delay the long-term complications of diabetes. Depending on the type of diabetes, your education level and whether or not medications are used, your dietitian may develop a meal plan using either Canada's Food Guide to Healthy Eating or Good Health Eating Guide Food Choice Values. Both guides provide the number of servings per day and appropriate serving sizes for food choices. They also outline which food groups and specific foods affect blood sugar the most.

Carbohydrates

Carbohydrate-containing foods such as cereals, breads, grains, legumes, fruits, vegetables and milk products are digested and converted to blood glucose. Contrary to what some people might think, diabetic diets are not low in carbohydrate. Just like healthy individuals, a person with diabetes is recommended to consume 50 to 60 percent of daily calories from carbohydrates. But in diabetes, it is important to manage the total amount and type of carbohydrate eaten at each meal and snack. A dietitian will determine the appropriate amount of carbohydrate you need to consume, and distribute it evenly throughout the day.

Both the type of carbohydrate and the amount eaten affect blood-sugar levels. Not too long ago, dietitians used the terms simple and complex to classify carbohydrates, with simple carbohydrates such as table sugar resulting in a rapid rise in blood sugar and complex carbohydrates such as starchy foods leading to a gradual

rise in glucose. However, these terms are no longer used because they do not indicate the impact that a food has on blood-glucose levels. For instance, scientists have determined that some starchy foods, such as white bread, mashed potatoes and instant rice, result in a fast rise in blood sugar.

The glycemic index is now used to express the rise in blood sugar caused by a carbohydrate food. Studies have found that incorporating foods with a low glycemic index value into the diabetic diet can improve blood-sugar control in people with type 2 diabetes by resulting in a slow, gradual rise in blood sugar.[7-9] Lentils, kidney beans, barley, whole-grain pumpernickel bread, oatmeal, 100 percent bran cereal, pasta, yogurt and soy milk are all low glycemic index foods that can help optimize blood-glucose control. Foods are listed with their corresponding glycemic index value on page 7, Chapter 1.

Some dietitians may help their patients manage blood-sugar levels through *carbohydrate counting*. You and your registered dietitian will determine the total amount of carbohydrate to be consumed at each meal and snack, then you will be taught how to determine the amounts of carbohydrates in different portions of carbohydrate foods (e.g., milk, yogurt, cereal, bread, fruit) in order to count your carbohydrate intake. As you master carbohydrate counting, you will be able to make adjustments to medication, food and exercise. This involves learning how to identify blood-sugar patterns, interpret the causes for blood-sugar fluctuations and determine appropriate strategies to achieve blood-glucose targets.

Sugars

In the past, people with diabetes were told to avoid sugar in order to control their blood-glucose levels. However, researchers have now determined that natural sugars in fruit, milk and vegetables are an acceptable part of a healthy diabetic diet.[10] Added sugars such as sucrose (table sugar), syrup, jam, honey, molasses, maltose, dextrose and fruit juice are also allowed in small quantities. When developing a personal meal plan, a dietitian can include these sugars as part of the total daily carbohydrate intake.

Dietary Fiber

People with diabetes are recommended to achieve an intake of 25 to 35 grams of fiber per day (see page 3, Chapter 1, for a list of fiber-rich foods). Good sources of soluble fiber, such as legumes, barley, oats and psyllium-enriched breakfast cereals, have been shown to improve blood-sugar control in people with type 2 diabetes and should be included in the diet.[11-13] This type of fiber slows the absorption of sugar from the digestive tract, causing a slower rise in blood glucose. A daily intake of soluble fiber combined with a low-fat diet can also lower blood cholesterol levels by 5 to 10 percent.

Dietary Fat

Like all Canadians, people with diabetes are recommended to follow a lower-fat diet. A number of studies have found that high-fat diets impair glucose tolerance, promote obesity and cause high blood cholesterol levels.[14,15] Scientists have learned that limiting the amount of saturated fat by choosing lower-fat animal foods and avoiding packaged foods made with hydrogenated vegetable oil can improve blood-sugar abnormalities. To help reduce your fat intake, refer to Chapter 3.

Adding more monounsaturated fat to the diet may help people with diabetes lower elevated blood triglyceride levels. The best sources of monounsaturated fats are olive oil, canola oil, peanut oil and avocado. Your dietitian will help you balance your daily fat and oil servings to achieve a fat intake that contains proportionately more monounsaturated fat than polyunsaturated and saturated fat.

Alcohol

A moderate intake of one drink per day to a maximum of nine per week (men) or one drink per day or seven per week (women) is acceptable for people whose diabetes is under good control. However, because alcohol can impair the liver's ability to release glucose into the bloodstream, it may cause a low blood-sugar reaction (hypoglycemia) in people who take insulin or certain oral diabetes medications, such as DiaBeta®, Diamicron® or GlucoNorm®. Symptoms of hypoglycemia include hunger, dizziness, nervousness, anxiety, shakiness, weakness, sweating, lightheadedness and confusion. Combining alcohol with exercise and a lack of food will further increase the risk of hypoglycemia. If you take medication for your diabetes, it is best to consume alcohol with a carbohydrate-containing meal to avoid a low blood-sugar reaction.

Weight Control

Approximately 80 percent of people with type 2 diabetes are overweight. Experts believe that managing body weight can prevent or delay many cases of type 2 diabetes. Carrying excess body fat around the abdomen is linked with higher levels of insulin in the blood and insulin resistance. Having an "apple" shaped, rather than a "pear" shaped, figure increases the risk of diabetes. Losing as little as 5 to 10 percent of body weight enhances the body's sensitivity to insulin and improves blood-glucose levels. Some people with type 2 diabetes who take oral hypoglycemic medications are able to decrease or discontinue medication once they have lost weight.

To determine whether you are at an acceptable weight, turn to page 439, Obesity and Weight Loss, to calculate your body mass index (BMI). Having a BMI greater than 25 indicates overweight, and a BMI greater than 27 is defined as obese. A BMI of 22 is associated with a reduced risk of diabetes. If you have been newly diagnosed with type 2 diabetes, your dietitian will develop a meal plan that promotes gradual weight loss. Weight loss is best achieved by a combination of reduction in calorie intake and increase in physical exercise. If you have type 2 diabetes that does not require medication, refer to page 442, Obesity and Weight Loss, for strategies to help you lose weight.

The following sections discuss nutrients and supplements that may be helpful in preventing diabetes complications or possibly even controlling blood sugar in people with type 2 diabetes. Keep in mind that research in these areas is limited and *in no circumstances should they be used as a sole therapy for diabetes*. The only effective ways to lower and control blood sugar are through diet, exercise and medication. If your diabetes is not well controlled, the strategies below will not help you lower your blood sugar.

Vitamins and Minerals

Antioxidants

Research has revealed that people with uncontrolled diabetes have increased levels of free radicals in the body.[16] Free radicals are unstable oxygen molecules, generated by normal body processes, that damage cells and increase the risk of many chronic diseases, including heart disease. Some researchers have found that diabetic patients have lower levels of vitamin E and beta-carotene, two antioxidant nutrients that neutralize free radicals, rendering them harmless.[17] Such decreased levels of antioxidants may increase the risk of long-term diabetes complications.

Free radical damage to LDL cholesterol can increase the risk of heart disease in diabetes. A few studies have found that a daily vitamin E supplement can lower the level of free radical byproducts and may even improve symptoms of nerve damage in diabetes.[18,19] Some evidence also suggests that vitamin C works with insulin to maintain tight blood-sugar control.[20, 21]

To help combat free radicals, incorporate foods rich in the following antioxidants into your diet:

- *Vitamin E* The recommended dietary allowance (RDA) is 22 international units (IU). Best food sources include wheat germ, nuts, seeds, vegetable oils, whole grains and kale. To supplement, take 200 to 800 IU of natural source vitamin E. Buy a "mixed" vitamin E supplement if possible. The daily upper limit is 1500 IU.

- *Beta-Carotene* No RDA has been established for beta-carotene. Best food sources are orange and dark green produce, including carrots, sweet potato, winter squash, broccoli, collard greens, kale, spinach, apricots, cantaloupe, peaches and nectarines. To supplement, choose a multivitamin and mineral with beta-carotene added.

- *Vitamin C* The RDA is 75 and 90 milligrams for women and men respectively (smokers need an additional 35 milligrams). Best food sources include citrus fruit, cantaloupe, kiwi, mango, strawberries, broccoli, Brussels sprouts, cauliflower, red pepper and tomato juice. To supplement, take 500 milligrams of Ester C once daily. The daily upper limit is 2000 milligrams.

Magnesium

A lack of magnesium may play a role in the development of insulin resistance, poor blood-sugar control and high blood pressure. A few short-term studies have found that a daily magnesium supplement improved the body's sensitivity to insulin and glucose removal from the blood.[22,23] To prevent a magnesium deficiency, be sure to include foods rich in the mineral in your daily diet—nuts, seeds, legumes, prunes, whole grains, leafy green vegetables, Brewer's yeast, cheddar cheese and shrimp are all good sources. See page

48, Chapter 4, for an extensive list of foods rich in magnesium.

If you find it a challenge to eat magnesium-rich foods on a regular basis, consider a magnesium supplement. If you take calcium pills, buy one with magnesium added (look for a 2:1 ratio of calcium to magnesium). If you do not need to take calcium supplements, take 150 to 200 milligrams of magnesium citrate once or twice daily. Taking more than 350 milligrams of supplemental magnesium may cause diarrhea, nausea and stomach cramps.

Chromium

A deficiency of this trace mineral is associated with reduced glucose tolerance.[24] Chromium is used to make glucose tolerance factor, a compound that interacts with insulin and helps maintain normal blood-sugar levels. With adequate amounts of chromium present, the body uses less insulin to do its job. Some studies suggest that chromium is lost from the body at an increased rate with aging and in the presence of type 2 diabetes.[25,26]

Many studies have looked at the effect of chromium supplements on blood-glucose control in people with type 2 diabetes, and most report a beneficial effect. One study found that 500 micrograms of chromium picinolate taken twice daily significantly improved blood-glucose control in type 2 diabetics. (This amount of chromium is well above what is considered safe.[27]) In the same study, 100 micrograms taken twice daily did not result in significant improvements. It is likely that both the amount and type of chromium are important in achieving a beneficial effect.

The best sources of chromium are Brewer's yeast, calf's liver, blackstrap molasses, wheat germ, wheat bran, whole grains, mushrooms, apples with the skin, green peas, chicken breast, refried beans and oysters. Processed foods and refined starchy foods like white bread, white rice and pasta, sugar and sweets all contain very little chromium.

If you're concerned that you're not getting enough chromium in your diet, check your multivitamin and mineral supplement to see how much it contains. Most brands supply 25 to 50 micrograms. If you choose to take a separate chromium supplement, *do not exceed 200 micrograms* per day. High doses of chromium can cause cognitive impairment, anemia and kidney damage. Supplements made from chromium picinolate are thought to be absorbed more efficiently than those made from chromium chloride or chromium nicotinate.

Herbal Remedies

American Ginseng (*Panax quinquefolius L*)

Preliminary research conducted at the University of Toronto suggests that this herb may be useful in helping people with type 2 diabetes manage their blood sugar.[28,29] Researchers gave people with type 2 diabetes 3 grams of ground American ginseng root or a placebo pill either 40 minutes before, or together with, a glucose drink. Significant reductions in blood glucose were observed in those who had been given the ginseng, whether it had been taken before or with the sugary drink.

Ginseng contains active ingredients called ginsenosides, and American ginseng contains primarily a ginsenoside called Rb-1. Most research has been conducted using a related species of the plant, Panax ginseng, which contains Rb-1, Rg-1 and Rc ginsenosides. No adverse reactions have been reported with the use of American ginseng, but Panax ginseng may cause insomnia (see page 111, Chapter 7). If you have type 2 diabetes and decide to try American ginseng, take the herb with a meal to avoid a possible low blood-sugar reaction. Because the herb may enhance the action of diabetes medication, monitor your blood-glucose levels closely if you take oral hypoglycemic agents. Be sure to inform your healthcare practitioner that you are taking ginseng.

Other Natural Health Products

Alpha-Lipoic Acid (Lipoic Acid)

Since 1950, alpha-lipoic acid has been actively studied for its potential to help control blood-sugar levels and complications of diabetes. Lipoic acid helps enzymes turn carbohydrate from foods into a usable source of energy for the body. But lipoic acid is also an antioxidant and, as such, is able to neutralize harmful compounds called free radicals. Unlike other well-known antioxidants such as vitamins C and E, lipoic acid works in both a water and fat environment, allowing it to have a broad effect. Because of its antioxidant effects in fat tissue, lipoic acid is able to enter nerve cells where it may offer protection. The body also uses lipoic acid to regenerate vitamins C and E.

European studies have found that intravenous injections of lipoic acid are effective at improving symptoms of diabetes neuropathy (nerve damage), including pain, tingling and numbness of the arms and legs.[30-32] Studies using oral supplements of lipoic acid suggest that it can improve and may help prevent diabetic neuropathy.[33] Lipoic acid also seems to help people with type 2 diabetes control their blood-sugar level. German researchers found that a daily lipoic acid supplement taken for one month improved insulin sensitivity and glucose clearance from the bloodstream in people with type 2 diabetes.[34]

To supplement, take 600 milligrams of lipoic acid three times daily on an empty stomach. Lipoic acid supplements appear to have no significant side effects. If you decide to supplement,

monitor your blood-sugar levels closely. Because of its potential to lower blood glucose, lipoic acid could have additive effects when taken together with diabetes medications, ginseng, garlic and psyllium.

Nutrition Strategy Checklist for Diabetes

☐ Diabetic diet
☐ Low-glycemic carbohydrates
☐ Soluble fiber
☐ Low saturated fat
☐ Weight control (type 2)
☐ Antioxidants: vitamin C, vitamin E
☐ Magnesium (type 2)
☐ Chromium (type 2)
☐ Alpha-lipoic acid

Recommended Resources

www.diabetes.org
American Diabetes Association
Attn: Customer Service
1701 N Beauregard Street
Alexandria, VA, USA 22311
Tel: 703-549-1500 or 1-800-DIABETES (1-800-342-2383)

www.diabetes.ca
Canadian Diabetes Association
15 Toronto Street, Suite 800
Toronto, ON, Canada M5C 2E3
Tel: 416-363-3373

www.niddk.nih.gov/health/diabetes/diabetes.htm
National Diabetes Information Clearinghouse
1 Information Way
Bethesda, MD, USA 20892-3560
Tel: 301-654-3327 or 1-800-860-8747

Diarrhea

Few people manage to get through life without experiencing at least one bout of diarrhea. In fact, most healthy adults can expect to have as many as four episodes every year.[1] Fortunately, diarrhea is usually just a temporary condition that goes away without any special treatment.

Acute diarrhea usually lasts less than three weeks and is associated with temporary conditions, such as bacterial, viral or parasitic infections. Chronic diarrhea is usually related to intestinal disorders and may persist for weeks or months at a time. Often people who travel, especially in developing countries, will experience bouts of diarrhea. This is usually caused by contaminated food or water.

One of the most serious complications of diarrhea is dehydration. Dehydration occurs when the body loses excessive amounts of water and electrolytes (sodium, potassium, chloride). Dehydration can lead to fainting and heart problems, caused by a rapid drop in blood pressure. Dehydration is particularly dangerous for young children, the elderly and people who are physically debilitated.

What Causes Diarrhea?

Diarrhea can be triggered by many different conditions, including:

- *Bacterial infections* Consuming contaminated water or food can cause diarrhea due to bacterial infections. *Salmonella* and *Escherichia coli* (*E. coli*) are two well-known culprits.

- *Viral infections* An invading virus, such as rotavirus or Norwalk virus, can irritate the lining of the intestine, interfering with fluid absorption in the digestive process.

- *Parasites* Contaminated food or water can carry parasites into the digestive system, where they can cause bloody, watery diarrhea, often accompanied by a high fever.

- *Food allergies or intolerance* Some people have difficulty digesting certain components of the food they eat, resulting in intestinal irritation and diarrhea.

- *Medications* Some medications may cause adverse reactions, including diarrhea.

- *Intestinal diseases and bowel disorders* Diarrhea is a frequent symptom of chronic medical conditions such as inflammatory bowel disease or irritable bowel syndrome.

Symptoms

Along with the possible nausea, vomiting and fever, symptoms of diarrhea are

- loose, watery stools

- urgent need to have a bowel movement at least three times a day or more

- abdominal pain, cramping and bloating

Although diarrhea is usually a temporary condition, it may sometimes be a symptom of more serious problems. Contact your doctor if you have any of the following symptoms:

- severe pain in the abdomen or rectum

- fever of 39°C (102°F) or higher

- signs of dehydration, including thirst, less frequent urination, light-headedness, dry skin and dark-colored urine

- blood in the stool

Who's at Risk?

Diarrhea is most common among people who

- have direct exposure to others suffering from gastrointestinal infections

- consume food or drinking water contaminated with bacteria, viruses or parasites

- take certain medications, especially antibiotics and magnesium-containing antacids
- suffer from food allergies or food intolerance
- suffer from chronic intestinal disorders
- are in hospital receiving feedings by nasogastric (nose to stomach) tube

Conventional Treatment

Diarrhea will usually resolve on its own without medical treatment. In most cases, drinking enough fluids to prevent dehydration is the only treatment necessary. Some over-the-counter medications may slow down the diarrhea, but they won't speed recovery. These medications are not to be used if diarrhea is caused by a bacterial or parasitic infection because they trap the organisms inside the gut, prolonging the problem. Antibiotics are usually prescribed to shorten the duration of diarrhea caused by bacterial infections. Diarrhea caused by a virus is either treated with medication or left to run its course, depending on the severity and type of virus.

Managing Diarrhea

Dietary Strategies

To prevent dehydration, drink eight to ten glasses of water or other fluids each day. Fluids that help replace lost electrolytes include broth, clear sodas, weak tea, fruit juice and sports drinks.

To treat mild diarrhea, it may be helpful to allow your intestine time to rest by temporarily following a liquid diet. Gradually add semisolid, low-fiber foods such as crackers, toast, rice, bananas, cooked carrots, boiled potatoes and chicken. For children, doctors often prescribe the BRAT diet consisting of bananas, rice, applesauce and toast.

Avoid foods and food ingredients that can make diarrhea worse, such as milk, fatty foods, grapes, figs, dates, prune juice, gassy vegetables (broccoli, cauliflower, Brussels sprouts, cabbage), nuts, sweets and sugars, chocolate, sugar-free gums, honey, soft drinks, spicy foods, caffeine and alcohol. Avoid nicotine.

Fruit Juice

Excessive consumption of fruit juice, especially apple juice and pear nectar, is often the cause of so-called "toddler's diarrhea."[2-4] In one study from the UCLA School of Medicine, elimination of these fruit juices immediately stopped diarrhea in all cases of chronic, nonspecific diarrhea.[5] These juices contain higher amounts of fructose and sorbitol, types of carbohydrate that may be poorly absorbed.

Preschoolers should drink no more than 4 ounces (1/2 cup or 125 ml) of unsweetened juice per day, and older children no more than 6 to 8 ounces (3/4 to 1 cup or 175 to 250 ml) per day. Encourage your child to drink water when thirsty. Excessive juice consumption (12 ounces per day or more) can also displace other important nutrients in the diet and cause failure to thrive in small children. In older children, too much juice has been linked with overweight.

Fermented Milk Products

To help recover from diarrhea, include one serving of yogurt or kefir in your daily diet. These foods contain live bacterial cultures that help recolonize the digestive tract with friendly, protective bacteria (probiotics). These bacteria are known collectively as lactic acid bacteria and have been shown in numerous studies to reduce the duration of antibiotic-associated diarrhea, traveler's (*E. coli*) diarrhea and viral diarrhea in both adults and children.[6-9] *Lactobacillus* and *bifidobacteria* are the most researched types of bacteria.

Lactic acid bacteria are thought to help treat diarrhea by preventing the attachment of harmful microbes to the intestinal tract, secreting substances that destroy infection-causing bacteria and enhancing the body's immune system. Fermented milk products are appropriate for people with a mild to moderate lactose (milk sugar) intolerance (see page 407, Lactose Intolerance), since they have a lower lactose content and take longer to be digested than plain milk.

Food Allergies

Research suggests that persistent diarrhea in infants and young children may indicate a food allergy to cow's milk.[10-12] Whereas many food allergy symptoms are dramatic and can be linked to eating a certain food, others are not. Some signs of sensitivity to cow's milk are chronic, less acute and more difficult for doctors to diagnose. These types of food allergies usually occur in infants between one week and three months of age. Vomiting and diarrhea are signs of a cow's milk sensitivity. A thorough examination and medical history by a pediatrician will help diagnose a food allergy (skin tests are not useful in these types of allergies). Eliminating the problematic food is the only way of dealing with the allergy.

If formula made from cow's milk is causing your infant gastrointestinal distress, switch to a soy-based formula. About 85 percent of infants will outgrow their symptoms sometime between one month and three years of age. However, older children and adults are less likely to outgrow their sensitivity.

Vitamins and Minerals

Zinc

Many studies have linked a deficiency of zinc to diarrhea.[13-16] A lack of zinc suppresses the body's immune system and increases the intestine's susceptibility to toxin-producing bacteria or viruses. It's thought that the gastrointestinal tract may be one of the first target areas where a zinc deficiency manifests itself. Zinc deficiency may also impair the gut's absorption of water and electrolytes, prolonging diarrhea.

Studies in children in developing countries have shown short-term zinc supplementation improves immunity and reduces the duration of diarrhea. While zinc malnutrition is most often seen in developing countries, cases of zinc deficiency have been reported among children and adolescents in Canada and the United States. Zinc is abundant in red meat, which is common in the North American diet. Other good sources include seafood, poultry, wheat bran, wheat germ, whole grains, enriched breakfast cereals and yogurt.

Although North Americans consume adequate amounts of zinc, there are some people who are at increased risk for a deficiency:

- Children who follow a vegan (no animal products) diet. Zinc in plant foods is less available to the body than the zinc in animal foods. Strict vegetarians may need to consume twice as much zinc-rich (plant) food than nonvegetarians in order to meet their daily requirement.

- People who do not eat enough protein. High-protein foods are the best sources of zinc.

- The elderly. Older people absorb zinc less efficiently and tend to have a poor intake of high-protein foods.

To ensure that you and your family members are meeting your daily zinc needs, refer to page 61, Chapter 4, for recommended dietary allowances and food sources. If your doctor identifies a zinc deficiency as the cause of diarrhea, take 10 to 40 milligrams of zinc once daily. Children under ten years of age should take no more than 10 milligrams of zinc. Buy a zinc supplement with 1 milligram of copper for every 10 milligrams of zinc (large amounts of zinc deplete the body's copper stores). Consuming zinc in amounts greater than 40 to 50 milligrams per day can depress the immune system and cause toxic effects; do not exceed 40 milligrams per day.

Herbal Remedies

Goldenseal (*Hydrastis canadensis*)

This native North American plant is well known for its antibiotic and anti-infective properties. One of the herb's active ingredients, berebine, exerts its antimicrobial activity in the intestine, where it prevents infectious microbes from attaching to the gut and blocks the action of toxins produced by a number of disease-causing bacteria.[17,18]

Studies have found berebine to be effective against diarrhea caused by *E. coli*, *Salmonella*, *Shigella*, and *Giardia lamblia* (giardiasis).[19-22] When combined with conventional antibiotic therapy, berebine helped adults with acute diarrhea recover faster than standard antibiotics alone.

To take goldenseal, buy a product standardized to 8 to 12 percent alkaloid content. Take 250 to 500 milligrams three times daily. Goldenseal should not be used by pregnant and breastfeeding women.

Other Natural Health Products

Probiotics

Many studies support taking lactic acid bacteria in doses higher than what can be consumed from fermented milk products. Researchers have used lactic acid bacteria pills or fortified milk products to treat diarrhea in study subjects. Many experts believe that probiotic supplements are needed to ensure that sufficient numbers of live bacteria survive the acidic contents of the stomach and reach the intestine.

Buy a product that offers 1 to 10 billion live cells per dose. The number of living organisms in each capsule refers to the strength of the product. Choose a product that is stable at room temperature and does not require refrigeration. This allows you to continue taking your supplement while traveling.

Take 1 to 10 billion viable cells, in three or four divided doses with food. If your product contains 1 billion cells per capsule, take one capsule three times daily. To reduce antibiotic-related diarrhea, take the supplement when you start your antibiotic therapy and continue taking for five days after antibiotics are stopped.

Children's products usually contain one-quarter to one-half the adult dose, or 250 to 500 billion live cells. Probiotic supplements may cause flatulence, which usually subsides as you continue treatment. There are no safety issues associated with taking these supplements.

Nutrition Strategy Checklist for Diarrhea

☐ Fluids
☐ Limit fruit juice
☐ Fermented milk products
☐ Identify food allergies
☐ Zinc
☐ Goldenseal
☐ Probiotic supplements

Recommended Resources

www.mayoclinic.com
The Mayo Foundation for Medical Education and Research provides one of the best patient education sites on the Internet. The information is reliable, thorough and clearly written.

www.niddk.nih.gov
National Digestive Diseases Information Clearinghouse
2 Information Way
Bethesda, MD, USA 20892-3570
Tel: 301-654-3810

Diverticulosis and Diverticulitis

Almost 50 percent of North Americans over the age of 60 have diverticulosis, a condition that develops when small pouches, called diverticula, form in the gastrointestinal tract. Although diverticula can appear almost anywhere in the body, they typically develop in the walls of the large intestine, particularly in the colon. As we age, the walls of our intestines gradually become weaker. Over time, the lining of the bowel can force its way out through the weakened areas, forming these tiny, sac-like bulges.

Diverticulosis rarely displays any physical symptoms. However, feces and food particles can become trapped in the pouches, resulting in diverticulitis (inflammation of the diverticula). Bleeding, infection or inflammation may develop, causing tenderness in the abdomen, crampy pain, fever and possibly nausea. Approximately 10 to 25 percent of the people with diverticulosis will go on to develop diverticulitis.

What Causes Diverticular Disease?

Scientists have linked diverticular disease to aging and low-fiber diets. With advancing age, the outer walls of the intestine become thickened, narrowing the passageway through the colon. This makes it increasingly difficult for the muscles in the intestine to move waste products through the colon. When waste products linger in the colon too long, the stool becomes hard and dry, often resulting in constipation. The muscle straining associated with constipation puts increased pressure on the intestinal walls and may force the bowel lining to bulge through any weak spots.

A diet low in fiber may be a contributing factor in constipation and may increase the pressure inside the digestive tract. The incidence of diverticulitis has steadily increased as North Americans have added more refined and processed food to their diets.

While diverticulitis is usually not a serious disease, it can lead to medical complications. Infected diverticula can cause an abscess to form on the colon. Small holes (perforations) may develop in the diverticula, allowing pus and bacteria to leak into the abdomen. Infection that spreads into the abdomen causes peritonitis, a condition that can be fatal. Immediate surgery is necessary to clean out the infection and remove the damaged areas of the colon.

Infection may also cause damaged tissue from neighboring organs to stick together, forming a fistula. Fistulas are more common in men than women and can result in serious, long-term infections. The scar tissue that often develops after an infection is another complication of diverticulitis, as it can block the intestines and prevent normal bowel movements.

Symptoms

Most people with diverticulosis don't have symptoms or discomfort. Mild cramps, bloating and constipation may develop in some cases. Symptoms of diverticulitis include

- abdominal pain that may develop quite suddenly
- tenderness on the lower left side of the abdomen
- fever, nausea, vomiting, cramps and constipation
- rectal bleeding that is caused by burst blood vessels in the diverticula

Who's at Risk?

Those at risk for diverticulosis include older adults, especially those who follow a low-fiber diet. One-half of all North Americans between the ages of 60 and 80 have diverticulosis and nearly everyone over 80 years old has the condition.[1] As many as one-quarter of people with diverticulosis go on to develop diverticulitis.

Conventional Treatment

During an attack of diverticulitis, the following may help the colon heal faster:

- a liquid diet followed for a short time to allow the bowel to rest

- bed rest

- antibiotic medications to treat infection

- surgery may be necessary to remove the diseased part of the intestine

If you have diverticulosis, it is important to avoid constipation, which can increase the risk of a diverticulitis flare-up. Respond to your body's urge for bowel movements. Exercise regularly to promote normal bowel functions. If you have diverticulosis, the nutritional strategies below can help prevent diverticulitis.

Managing Diverticulitis
Dietary Strategies

Many practitioners tell their patients to avoid certain foods that may irritate the diverticula, such as nuts, seeds, corn, popcorn, raspberries, strawberries, figs, grapes with seeds and cucumbers with seeds. The recommendation to avoid nuts and seeds appears to have originated from one single study. There is little evidence to support the link between nuts and seeds and diverticulitis. People following a low-fiber diet have more symptoms than people on a liberal diet.

Despite this, some individuals may find that certain foods cause inflammation and pain; these foods should be avoided.

Dietary Fiber

It is well accepted that a high-fiber diet prevents diverticulitis.[2,3] The role of fiber in gastrointestinal health was recognized when researchers observed much lower rates of colonic problems in South African blacks who followed a very high-fiber diet compared with North Americans who consume dramatically less fiber.

Since that time, many studies have linked higher-fiber diets to a lower incidence of diverticulosis.[4-6] A study from Harvard University followed almost 48,000 men for four years and found that, compared with men with the lowest fiber intake, those who consumed the most fiber had a 42 percent lower risk of diverticulitis.[7] Fiber from fruits and vegetables offered the most protection. In the same study, men who followed a high-fat, low-fiber diet had a 2.3-fold higher risk of the disease, and men on a high red-meat, low-fiber diet had a 3.3-fold greater chance of having diverticulitis.

Over the past 20 years, fiber supplementation has received widespread acceptance in the management of diverticulitis. Patients treated with fiber develop fewer complications and require less surgery compared with those on low-fiber diets. Insoluble fibers in whole grains, fruits and vegetables have a significant water-retaining capacity, which helps to increase stool bulk and softness and promote regularity. By speeding the removal of waste material, dietary fiber lowers pressure in the colon.

To prevent diverticulitis, gradually increase daily fiber intake to 25 to 35 grams. See page 3, Chapter 1, for a list of the fiber content of selected foods. Include some of the following high-fiber foods in your daily diet (all have 5 or more grams per serving):

Starchy Foods	Fruits	Vegetables
100% bran cereals	Apple, with skin	Green peas
All Bran Buds cereal	Blackberries	Snow peas
Corn bran cereal	Blueberries	Swiss chard
Fiber One	Figs and dates	
Oat bran	Kiwi	
Red River cereal	Mango	
Barley	Pear, raw and canned	
Rye crackers	Prunes	
Whole-wheat pasta	Raspberries	
Dried peas, beans, lentils		
Popcorn		

Almonds are also high in fiber; add a few to your daily diet.

Bulk-forming fiber supplements may be used to promote regularity. Psyllium husk powder, Metamucil® and Prodiem® may be purchased at health food stores and pharmacies.

Drink at least 8 glasses of water or other liquids daily to help fiber produce soft stools. Adults require at least 2 to 3 liters (8 to 12 cups) of fluid each day. Water, juice, milk, soups, teas and herbal teas all contribute to your fluid intake.

Fermented Milk Products

Consuming one cup (250 ml) of yogurt or kefir per day can help the body fight infection during diverticulitis and may prevent bacterial overgrowth in unaffected diverticula. These foods contain live bacterial cultures (lactic acid bacteria) that help recolonize the digestive tract with friendly, protective bacteria; they are often referred to as probiotics. Once consumed, lactic acid bacteria make their way to the colon, where they colonize and prevent the attachment of harmful microbes to the intestinal tract, secrete substances that destroy infection-causing bacteria and enhance the body's immune system.

Lactic acid bacteria are especially important if you are taking antibiotics to treat infection in the diverticula. Antibiotics destroy both the harmful and beneficial bacteria in the gut. Probiotic foods and supplements (see below) provide a means of re-establishing growth of healthy bacteria in the intestine.

Vitamins and Minerals

If an infection is present during an attack of diverticulitis, your body's immune system will need many nutrients. Vitamins A, C, and E and zinc are all important. Refer to Chapter 4 to learn the best food sources for these nutrients. A daily multivitamin and mineral supplement will help ensure that you meet your daily requirements.

Herbal Remedies

Garlic (*Allium sativum*)

This herb may be a worthwhile addition to your daily nutritional regime if an infection is present during diverticulitis. Natural sulfur compounds in garlic have been shown to enhance the activity of infection-fighting white blood cells. Laboratory studies have also shown garlic to inhibit the growth of a number of bacteria and yeast organisms.

Add one half to one clove of garlic to your meals each day. If you choose to supplement, buy a product made with aged garlic extract. Take two to six capsules a day in divided doses throughout the day. Aged garlic extract is odorless and less irritating to the gastrointestinal tract than other forms of garlic supplements (e.g., garlic oil capsules, garlic powder tablets). You'll find more information about garlic on page 106, Chapter 7.

Other Natural Health Products

Probiotics

Lactic acid bacteria are available in supplements that provide doses higher than what can be consumed from fermented milk products. Buy a product that offers 1 to 10 billion live cells per dose. The number of living organisms in each capsule refers to the strength of the product. Choose a product that is stable at room temperature and so does not require refrigeration; this will be more convenient if you are traveling or at the office.

Take 1 to 10 billion viable cells, in three or four divided doses, with food. To reduce antibiotic-related diarrhea, take the supplement when you start your antibiotic therapy and continue taking for five days after antibiotics are stopped.

Nutrition Strategy Checklist for Diverticulitis

☐ Insoluble fiber ☐ Fermented milk products
☐ Psyllium ☐ Multivitamin/mineral
☐ Fluids ☐ Probiotic supplements

Recommended Resources

www.crha-health.ab.ca
Calgary Regional Health Authority Communications
1035-7th Avenue SW
Calgary, AB, Canada T2P 3E9
Tel: 403-265-INFO (403-265-4636) or 1-800-860-2742 (Alberta only)
E-mail: publicweb@crha-health.ab.ca

www.mayoclinic.com
The Mayo Foundation for Medical Education and Research provides one of the best patient education sites on the Internet. The information is reliable, thorough and clearly written.

www.niddk.nih.gov
National Digestive Diseases Information Clearinghouse
2 Information Way
Bethesda, MD, USA 20892-3570
Tel: 301-654-3810

Ear Infections (Otitis Media)

By the time most children reach the age of three, they will have had at least one ear infection. Although ear infections can affect anyone, they are most common among children, particularly those between three months and three years of age. According to a study conducted by the Mayo Clinic, incidence of ear infections is on the rise. Between 1975 and 1990, ear infections prompted triple the number of doctor's visits for North American children under the age of two and double the number for children between ages two to five.[1]

The ear is divided into three main parts: the inner ear, middle ear and outer ear. The inner ear contains a highly sensitive hearing sense organ known as the cochlea, as well as the fluid-filled semicircular canals that control balance. The middle ear is the passageway between the eardrum and the eustachian tube. The eustachian tube conducts sound vibrations from the outer ear to the eardrum and connects the middle ear to the nose and the back of the throat. The outer ear is the area connecting the external opening of the ear to the eardrum. Earaches usually originate in the outer or middle ear.

What Causes Earache?

An earache is a symptom that may be caused by a variety of medical conditions. In most cases, earaches are the result of a bacterial or viral infection, often developing as a complication of the common cold. Allergies, mumps, tonsillitis or other illnesses that cause nasal congestion or sore throat will also trigger earache symptoms. Occasionally, ear pain may occur even though there is nothing wrong with the ear. The head is a very nerve-rich area of the body, and many of the structures in the jaw, face and neck share the same sensory nerve pathways to the brain. As a result, even a mild inflammation in the nose, sinus, teeth, throat or tonsils can refer severe pain and tenderness to the ear.

The most common cause of earache in children is a bacterial infection of the middle ear known as otitis media. Normally, the middle ear is filled with air and the eustachian tube acts like a vent to maintain a constant air pressure. During an illness, bacteria travel from the nose and throat, along the eustachian tube, to the middle ear. The bacteria inflame the lining of the eustachian tube, causing it to become swollen and filled with mucus. This blocks the flow of air into the middle ear, decreasing the pressure and allowing fluid to build up. The fluid remains trapped inside the ear and can deaden sound, resulting in hearing loss in one or both ears. The fluid accumulation also puts increased pressure on the eardrum, causing intense pain. Children are particularly susceptible to otitis media because their eustachian tubes are smaller and narrower than those of adults and are more easily blocked by inflammation.

Skin infections of the outer ear are also frequent sources of earaches. Popularly referred to as swimmer's ear, they are often caused by an accumulation of moisture in the outer ear canal. When water enters the ear during swimming or showering, the dampness creates an ideal breeding ground for bacteria. The bacteria enter the skin through tiny cuts or scratches caused by activities such as rubbing or cleaning the ears too vigorously or poking the ear with Q-tips or dirty fingernails.

Ear infections are not contagious, but the respiratory illnesses that lead to earache symptoms are infectious. Although children with earaches may suffer some temporary loss of hearing, most ear infections do not lead to permanent damage. However, infections that aren't treated can spread to the inner ear, where they can harm delicate hearing structures and cause permanent hearing loss. Children with otitis media may develop complications such as *secretory otitis media*, which is a persistent accumulation of fluid in the middle ear, *mastoiditis*, an infection of the bone behind the ear or, occasionally, *spinal meningitis*. Recurring ear infections may also affect a child's speech and language development by causing frequent, short-term hearing losses.

Most ear infections will clear up by themselves, often through a harmless rupture of the eardrum. A break in the eardrum releases the pressure and fluid in the middle ear and usually ends the painful symptoms immediately. A ruptured eardrum will normally heal over without any further difficulty, but repeated ruptures may cause serious scarring and some hearing loss.

Symptoms

- earache or feeling of pressure in the ear
- temporary hearing loss
- symptoms of the common cold, including cough or sore throat
- irritability
- dizziness
- sudden loss of appetite
- fever
- nausea or vomiting
- fluid or pus draining from the ear
- in children, pulling or tugging on the ear
- in young children, crying frequently, especially during the night

Who's at Risk?

Ear infections can develop in people of all ages, but they are most common in children, particularly those between the ages of three months and three years. Earaches are more common in boys than girls. Estimates indicate that up to 95 percent of all children in North America will have an ear infection before the age of seven.[2] Children who are more susceptible to ear infections include those who

- have brothers or sisters with a history of recurring ear infections
- have their first ear infection before they are four months old
- are in group childcare situations
- are exposed to cigarette smoke
- have frequent upper respiratory infections or allergies
- were bottle-fed rather than breastfed

Conventional Treatment

Many doctors prescribe antibiotics to treat a bacteria-caused ear infection. Symptoms will usually subside within 72 hours after the medication is started. However, there is growing controversy about using antibiotics to treat ear infections. Antibiotic treatment has the advantage of minimizing many of the complications that may develop as a result of otitis media and other infections. However, it is well documented that most ear infections will clear up without any treatment. As a result, some doctors are now recommending supervised watchful waiting for 48 to 72 hours before prescribing antibiotics, particularly in children over the age of two.[3,4] Further research is necessary to determine whether immediate treatment with antibiotics is the best approach to managing earaches.

If antibiotics are prescribed, they must be taken as directed, for the course. This will prevent recurring infections and the development of drug-resistant strains of bacteria. Other treatments that may be recommended include

- acetaminophen or ibuprofen for fever or pain relief (aspirin should not be used by children or teens)

- antihistamines for children with allergies
- decongestants to relieve feelings of pressure in the ear
- soothing ear drops to ease swimmer's ear
- a warm, moist towel or hot water bottle wrapped in a towel applied to the ear to reduce pain

Persistent ear infections lasting more than three months may be treated with a *myringotomy*, a procedure that puts a small hole in the eardrum to release the fluid. Children with persistent secretory otitis media may be treated with a *tympanotomy*, which involves inserting small plastic tubes into the blocked ear to help equalize the pressure and improve airflow.

Although most ear infections clear up without treatment, children must be seen by a doctor if they have

- an earache that becomes worse, despite treatment
- a fever that lasts more than three days or is higher than 39°C (102°F)
- fluid (blood or pus) leaking from the ear
- a headache, fever and stiff neck
- a skin rash
- rapid or difficult breathing
- hearing loss or dizziness
- periods of excessive sleepiness, irritability or unusual fussiness

Preventing and Managing Ear Infections

The following strategies will help reduce the risk of ear infections in your child:

- Breastfeed rather than bottle-feed your baby for as long as possible.
- Hold your baby in a semi-sitting position when breast- or bottle-feeding.

- Avoid exposing your child to tobacco smoke.

- Avoid exposure to people with upper respiratory tract illnesses such as cold or flu.

- Teach your child good hand-washing techniques to prevent the transfer of bacteria that may cause upper respiratory tract infections.

- Teach your child to blow his or her nose gently and not to block the flow of air during a sneeze. Blowing the nose forcefully or blocking a sneeze may cause bacteria to travel up the eustachian tubes to the ear.

Dietary Strategies
Food Allergies
Many studies provide evidence that food allergies can cause recurrent ear infections in children.[5-9] One American study found a significant association between food allergies and recurrent otitis media in 78 percent of the children studied, and that a food elimination diet led to significant improvement in 86 percent of the children identified as allergic. Researchers have found that once food allergies are diagnosed, appropriate food-elimination diets resolve symptoms and prevent recurrent infections.

It is thought that immune compounds formed in the body in response to an allergic food can block the eustachian tube by changing pressure and increasing fluid in the middle ear. If your child suffers from recurrent ear infections, discuss the possibility of food allergies with his or her pediatrician. Skin tests, RAST testing and food challenges are all methods used to identify food allergies.

If avoidance of certain foods is required based on allergy testing, consult a registered dietitian (**www.dietitians.ca**) for advice on how to ensure your child is meeting his or her nutrient needs. For more information on food allergies, see page 36, Food Allergies.

Probiotics
Fermented milk products such as yogurt, kefir and acidophilus milk contain lactic acid bacteria (Lactobacillus, bifidobacteria, Streptococcus strains) that may help prevent recurrent ear infections. Foods and supplements that contain these live bacteria are referred to as probiotics. Once ingested, lactic acid bacteria take up residence in the gastrointestinal tract, where they exert their health benefits. A number of studies have shown that regular consumption of probiotic foods as well as probiotic supplements enhances the activity of the immune system. Research also suggests that a deficiency of lactic acid bacteria in the intestinal tract of children may be responsible for viral infections of the respiratory tract.[10]

Healthy bacteria belonging to the *Streptococci* family also reside in the nose, throat and ear, where they protect the body from bacteria that cause ear infection. Studies have found that children prone to otitis media have reduced numbers of these protective bacteria. A recent study conducted among 130 children prone to ear infections found that those treated with an oral spray containing streptococci bacteria experienced a significantly reduced number of ear infections compared with those receiving the placebo treatment.[11]

Include one fermented milk product in your daily diet. Probiotic supplements are available for children with a milk allergy. Children's products are available that contain 250 to 500 billion live cells per capsule. Take one capsule one to three times daily with a meal.

Vitamins and Minerals
Vitamin C
This nutrient is well known for its ability to reduce the duration and severity of cold symptoms. Children, people under physical stress and people with low dietary intakes of vitamin C tend to respond best to the nutrient.[12,13]

Vitamin C promotes the body's production of interferon, an immune compound that helps the body fight infection. Based on its ability to enhance the immune system, vitamin C is important for a child's overall health. The best food sources are citrus fruit and juices, cantaloupe, kiwi, mango, strawberries, broccoli, Brussels sprouts, cauliflower, red pepper and tomato juice. Most children's multivitamin formulas contain 20 to 60 milligrams of vitamin C.

Vitamin E

Vitamin E may play a role in preventing ear infections. The vitamin appears to help certain white blood cells, called natural killer cells, fight infection. Vitamin E's role as an antioxidant may also help combat the inflammation involved in otitis media. Russian researchers investigated the effects of vitamin E (and vitamin C) in children with ear infections and found beneficial effects.[14] Foods rich in vitamin E include wheat germ, nuts, seeds, vegetable oils, whole grains and leafy green vegetables. Adults can supplement by taking 200 to 800 international units (IU) of natural source vitamin E. Choose a "mixed" vitamin E supplement if possible. Young children should be encouraged to get their vitamin E from nutrient-dense foods like nuts and seeds, nut butters and avocado.

Zinc

It is important to ensure that your child's daily diet contains zinc-rich foods, since this mineral is vital to a healthy immune system. Scandinavian researchers found that children susceptible to recurrent ear infections had significantly lower blood levels of zinc compared with healthy children.[15]

Zinc-rich foods include oysters, seafood, red meat, poultry, yogurt, wheat bran, wheat germ, whole grains and enriched breakfast cereals. If a blood test identifies that your child has a zinc deficiency, short-term zinc supplementation will

likely be prescribed. Children under ten years of age should take 10 milligrams of zinc with 1 milligram of copper added, once daily. Consuming amounts greater than 40 milligrams per day can depress the immune system and cause toxic effects. See Chapter 4 for more information on zinc.

Herbal Remedies
Echinacea

Many studies in the laboratory have shown the ability of echinacea to enhance the body's production of white blood cells that fight infection. Based on this, many natural health practitioners recommend echinacea to treat ear infections in children. At the time of writing, the University of Arizona, in Tucson, had initiated a study to evaluate the use of echinacea in the prevention of recurrent otitis media. The results are pending.

In view of the controversy over antibiotic use and the development of drug-resistant bacteria, there may be value in alternative therapies such as echinacea.[16,17] Buy an alcohol-free echinacea tincture for children. The adult dose of a 1:5 tincture is 1 to 2 milligrams three times daily. Doses for children are based on their body weight. For children under the age of 12, a general guideline is as follows:

- Adult dose (milligrams) × (age of child/12) = child's dose, or
- Adult dose (milligrams) × (body weight in pounds/150) = child's dose

For older children who are at acceptable percentiles for height and weight, use half the recommended adult dosage. Limit daily use to eight consecutive weeks because of concern that long-term use of echinacea might depress the immune system. Children allergic to plants in the Asteracease/Compositae family (ragweed, daisy, marigold and chrysanthemum) should not use echinacea.

Garlic *(Allium sativum)*

The sulfur compounds in garlic have been shown to stimulate the body's immune system, making garlic a potential preventative agent for recurrent ear infections. Laboratory studies have determined that garlic's sulfur compounds are able to kill the major bacteria that cause otitis media. Studies have focused on the many types of sulfur compounds found in raw garlic and specific sulfur compounds present in aged garlic extract.

Use one-half to one clove each day in cooking. To supplement, buy a product made with aged garlic extract. Take two to six capsules a day in divided doses; children should take one to three capsules per day. Aged garlic extract is odorless and less irritating to the gastrointestinal tract than other forms of garlic supplements (e.g., garlic oil capsules, garlic powder tablets).

Other Natural Health Products

Xylitol

This natural sugar found in plums, strawberries and raspberries is used as a sweetener in some sugarless gums, syrups and lozenges. Xylitol is known to inhibit the growth of two bacteria that cause ear infections (otitis media), *Streptococcus pneumoniae* and *Haemophilus influenza*. Based on this, researchers have evaluated the ability of xylitol-sweetened chewing gums, syrups and lozenges to prevent ear infections in children.

Two studies conducted with over 1200 children attending daycare found that xylitol significantly reduced the number of ear infections and the need for antibiotics.[18,19] The greatest success was found with the chewing gum and the syrup. The children chewing the gum received 8.4 grams of xylitol per day, while those taking the syrup received 10 grams per day.

Nutrition Strategy Checklist for Ear Infections

☐ Identify food allergies　☐ Zinc
☐ Fermented milk products　☐ Echinacea
☐ Probiotic supplements　☐ Garlic
☐ Vitamin C　☐ Xylitol
☐ Vitamin E

Recommended Resources

www.crha-health.ab.ca
Calgary Regional Health Authority Communications
1035-7th Avenue SW
Calgary, AB, Canada T2P 3E9
Tel: 403-265-INFO (403-265-4690) or
1-800-860-2742
E-mail: publicweb@crha-health.ab.ca

www.mayoclinic.com
Mayo Foundation for Medical Education and Research

www.merckhomeedition.com
Merck & Co., Inc.
1 Merck Drive
P.O. Box 100
Whitehouse Station, NJ, USA 08889-0100
Tel: 1-800-225-5675

www.nidcd.nih.gov
National Institute on Deafness and Other Communication Disorders
National Institutes of Health
31 Center Drive, MSC 2320
Bethesda, MD USA 20892-2320

Eating Disorders

We live in a society that's dominated by the cult of thinness. Everywhere we look, we're bombarded with the message that thin is beautiful. The waifish looks of ultra-thin models and Hollywood actors have become our ideal—establishing standards of beauty that are not only unattainable, but unhealthy as well. It's no wonder that so many North Americans, particularly women, struggle with their body image. By the time they reach adulthood, nearly half of all North American females have concerns about their weight and many have already begun the vicious cycle of dieting and weight gain. Recent studies show that girls as young as nine years are preoccupied with their weight.

Anorexia nervosa, bulimia nervosa and *binge eating disorder* are the three main types of eating disorders. Individuals who suffer from these conditions experience physical, psychological and social symptoms that eventually threaten their well-being, their overall health and even their lives. Eating disorders can be treated with long-term therapy but usually require the intervention of a variety of health professionals, including registered dietitians, physicians and mental-health specialists.

Because the treatment for each type of eating disorder is unique and involves a multidisciplinary approach, it is beyond the scope of this chapter to outline all possible nutrition recommendations. Instead, I have presented important information about each condition to help you better understand the causes, risk factors and symptoms. I also provide a list of treatment programs across Canada. If your eating disorder is not serious enough to warrant this type of intervention, seek the advice of a registered dietitian (**www.dietitians.ca**) to help you normalize your eating patterns and correct any nutritional deficiencies. This is imperative to prevent long-term health problems associated with eating disorders.

Anorexia Nervosa

This eating disorder is characterized by an extreme fear of gaining weight. People with anorexia nervosa are obsessed with being thin and have an unrealistic concept of their body image. Even though they are noticeably underweight, anorexics always believe they're fat. To achieve their goal of weight loss, they eat very little and may exercise excessively. Sometimes they will even engage in self-induced vomiting or they may misuse laxatives or diuretics as part of a binge-purge cycle. Anorexia nervosa is an extremely dangerous and potentially life-threatening condition. People suffering from this eating disorder can literally starve themselves to death.

People suffering from anorexia nervosa often ritualize food preparation and will sometimes hide food in special places, but never eat it. They get pleasure from controlling their eating and, as they begin to starve, they may even achieve a sense of euphoria from being so disciplined and successful in achieving their goals.

There is no precise cause of anorexia nervosa, but it is thought to be an illness of psychological origin. What begins as a normal desire to lose a few pounds rapidly becomes a compulsive obsession with body image. Anorexia nervosa primarily affects women, particularly young women. Often, women with anorexia nervosa have very low self-esteem. In an attempt to change their self-image, these women may take their interest in dieting and weight loss to an extreme. For these women, anorexia nervosa is a means of taking control of their lives. By taking rigid control of their eating, they are able to maintain a sense of control over some aspect of their lives. This response is frequently triggered by stress, anxiety or anger toward family members or in other personal relationships.

In many cases, women who suffer from anorexia are perfectionists and overachievers.

They are overly critical of themselves, set unreasonable standards of performance and have a compulsive need to please others. Having low self-confidence and setting unrealistic goals often result in feelings of ineffectiveness that may lead to abnormal eating behaviors.

Studies indicate that certain brain chemicals, known as neurotransmitters, are at lower levels in people with anorexia. Reduced levels of serotonin, a powerful neurotransmitter, are known to be associated with depression, and it is thought that there may be a link between anorexia and depression. Higher levels of cortisol, a brain hormone released in response to stress, and vasopressin, a brain chemical associated with obsessive-compulsive disorders, have also been identified with anorexia nervosa.

Symptoms

The warning signs of anorexia nervosa include

- a preoccupation with food and weight
- distorted vision of body image
- significant weight loss, with no evidence of related illness
- depression
- denial of hunger, despite an extreme reduction in eating
- strange eating habits: cutting food into small pieces, preferring food of specific texture or color, refusing to eat in front of others
- complaints of feeling cold because of dropping body temperatures
- appearance of long, fine hair on the body as a way of conserving body heat
- brittle hair and nails
- dry, yellow skin
- loss of sex drive
- cessation of menstrual periods

As anorexia nervosa progresses, the symptoms of starvation become increasingly evident. Eventually, every major organ in the body will be affected. The heart becomes weaker and pumps less blood through the body. Dehydration sets in and fainting spells are common. Electrolyte imbalances develop, as the body loses potassium, sodium and chloride. This results in fatigue, muscle weakness, irritability, muscle spasms and depression. In severe cases, these physical changes will cause irregular heartbeats, convulsions and death due to kidney or heart failure. Approximately one in ten women suffering from anorexia will die—a death rate that is among the highest for a psychiatric disease.

Who's at Risk?

Not surprisingly, women suffer from eating disorders far more often than men, representing nearly 90 percent of all cases. In Canada, it's estimated that 200,000 to 300,000 women between the ages of 13 and 40 suffer from anorexia nervosa. It is a condition that usually surfaces during the teenage years, when girls are between 14 and 18 years old.

In many cases, the incidence of anorexia is influenced by social environment. Girls with a peer group or family network that emphasizes physical attractiveness and thinness are more likely to acquire eating disturbances. Girls and women with low self-esteem or depressive tendencies are also very susceptible to the condition, especially if they are dealing with high levels of stress or traumatic events such as rape or abuse. There are also indications that anorexia nervosa may run in families.

In our society, there are certain professions or activities that emphasize thinness and appearance to an exceptional degree. People who participate in dancing, gymnastics, wrestling, modeling, acting and long-distance running are likely to be very aware of their weight or body image and may be particularly susceptible to developing anorexia nervosa.

Conventional Treatment

The goal of therapy for most eating disorders is to restore a normal weight, develop normal eating patterns, overcome unhealthy attitudes about body image and self-worth and provide support to family and friends who may be helping with the recovery process. Because anorexia nervosa has such a widespread influence and affects so many aspects of daily life, effective treatment requires a collaborative effort from a team of health professionals. Often, the team consists of a family physician to manage physical symptoms, a psychiatrist or psychologist to introduce behavioral modification and a nutritionist to establish a healthy diet for recovery.

The sooner anorexia nervosa is identified and treated, the better the eventual outcome. In the early stages, the disorder may be treated without hospitalization. But when weight loss is severe, hospitalization is necessary to restore weight and prevent further physical deterioration. A structured approach that involves careful observation of all eating and elimination (urinating, bowel movements and vomiting) is the first stage of treatment.

When weight is restored and symptoms are stabilized, some type of psychotherapy is required to deal with the underlying emotional issues triggering the abnormal eating patterns. Family therapy is especially helpful for younger girls and behavioral or cognitive therapy is effective in helping replace destructive attitudes with positive ones. A nutritionist will add support by providing advice on proper diet and eating regimens. In some cases, antidepressant medications may be prescribed, but they should not be used as a substitute for appropriate psychological treatment.

Unfortunately, many people with anorexia nervosa have a tendency to relapse and return to dysfunctional eating habits. Long-term therapy and regular health monitoring are essential for a successful result. A strong network of love and support from family and friends is also crucial to the recovery process.

Bulimia Nervosa

Bulimia nervosa is the most common type of eating disorder in North America. A person with this condition will eat large amounts of high-calorie food in a very short period, then use vomiting, diuretics or laxatives to eliminate the food before the body can absorb it. Fasting or excessive exercising are other methods that bulimics may use to counteract the weight gain caused by binge eating.

People suffering from bulimia will binge as often as several times a day, sometimes consuming 10,000 calories or more in a matter of minutes or hours. Comfort foods that are sweet, soft and high in calories, such as ice cream, cake or pastry, are favorite choices for bingeing. Immediately after the binge comes the purge, when some bulimics will use as many as 20 or more laxatives a day to rid their bodies of these huge quantities of food.

Like people with anorexia nervosa, bulimics are extremely afraid of becoming fat and are obsessed with body image. People with bulimia usually look quite normal and often show few signs of their condition. Their weight may fluctuate, but it usually stays within normal ranges. They may even be slightly heavy. Because bulimics are often very secretive about their abnormal behavior, the presence of bulimia can be hard to identify.

People with bulimia nervosa are very aware of their behavior and feel guilty or remorseful. Nearly half of all people with anorexia go on to develop some symptoms of bulimia.

Studies have shown that bulimics are particularly prone to impulsive behavior. They have difficulty dealing with anxiety, have little self-control and often indulge in drug or alcohol abuse or sexual promiscuity. They are also susceptible to depression, anxiety disorders and social phobias. People with bulimia have lower levels of brain neurotransmitters, such as serotonin, which may predispose them to developing these psychological disturbances.

Symptoms

In addition to the preoccupation with food and weight characteristic of most eating disorders, symptoms of bulimia may include

- evidence of binge eating, large amounts of food missing, stealing money or food

- food cravings

- frequent weight fluctuations

- evidence of purging, vomiting, abuse of laxatives or diuretics, frequent fasting or excessive exercising

- swelling of glands under the jaw, caused by vomiting

- erosion of tooth enamel and other dental problems caused by vomiting

- feelings of shame, self-reproach and guilt

- emotional changes, depression, irritability, social withdrawal

The purging behavior associated with bulimia can cause physical complications that are dangerous to long-term health. Vomiting and purging can lead to imbalances in fluids and electrolytes. When potassium levels fall too low, abnormal heart rhythms develop. Some bulimics use a medication called ipecac to induce vomiting. Overuse of this substance has been known to cause sudden death.

Who's at Risk?

Like anorexia, bulimia is primarily a woman's disorder. Nearly twice as many women suffer from bulimia as anorexia and, in Canada, estimates run as high as 600,000 women affected by this eating disorder. Bulimia tends to develop in later adolescence, often striking young women between the ages of 18 and 20. However, it can appear in earlier adolescence.

As with other eating disorders, bulimia surfaces most often in people who have low self-confidence and are insecure about their appearance. Girls reporting sexual or physical abuse are very susceptible to developing bulimia nervosa. Studies also indicate that the disorder may have a genetic element and may run in families. As well, bulimia may be triggered by elevated stress levels and often affects women who are intelligent and high achievers.

Conventional Treatment

In most cases, bulimia nervosa is treated without hospitalization. Cognitive and behavior therapies are necessary to deal with the emotional issues underlying the symptoms of this disorder. A multidisciplinary approach to treatment works best. Physicians, nutritionists and mental-health professionals will work together to address bulimia's many different facets. In particular, long-term psychotherapy is needed to help reduce destructive tendencies and develop better coping strategies. Antidepressant medication has proven to be an effective psychological intervention.

Binge Eating Disorder

Binge eating disorder (BED) is a newly recognized condition that has many similarities to bulimia nervosa. People with BED frequently eat huge quantities of food and feel that they have no control over their eating. Unlike bulimia, however, they don't purge afterwards with vomiting or laxatives.

BED is often accompanied by depression. At this time, scientists are uncertain whether depression is a symptom of BED or an underlying cause of the condition. People do report that emotions such as anger, sadness, anxiety or boredom will trigger episodes of binge eating. Studies are currently being done on neurotransmitters and other brain chemicals to determine if they are linked to binge eating disorder.

Symptoms

Symptoms of BED include

- frequently eating an abnormally large amount of food
- feeling unable to control what or how much food is eaten
- eating more rapidly than usual
- eating until uncomfortably full
- eating large amounts of food, even when not hungry
- feelings of disgust, guilt or depression after overeating
- eating alone because of embarrassment at the quantity of food being eaten

Who's at Risk?

BED occurs most often in people who are obese (with a BMI greater than 27), and becomes more prevalent as body weight increases. Obese people with BED become overweight at an earlier age than those without the disorder and may suffer more frequent bouts of losing and regaining weight. However, it is not uncommon for people with normal, healthy weight to suffer from BED. It occurs slightly more often in women than in men and tends to appear in later years, affecting an older population than does either anorexia or bulimia nervosa.

Conventional Treatment

Many of the medical problems related to obesity are also associated with binge eating disorder. Treatment may be necessary for conditions such as high cholesterol, high blood pressure, diabetes, gallbladder disease and heart disease. Other than the appropriate therapies for obesity-related disorders, there are no standard treatments for BED. As with most eating disorders, an approach that involves psychotherapy and antidepressant drugs seems to be most effective. It is essential to deal with the emotional issues of the illness in striving for a successful result. Because people with BED find it very difficult to stay on a treatment regimen and frequently return to inappropriate behavior, long-term therapy is always recommended.

Comprehensive Treatment Centers

Eating Disorders Clinic
St. Paul's Hospital
1081 Burrard Street
Vancouver, BC, Canada V6Z 1Y6
Tel: 604-682-2344

Pickhaven Centre
P.O. Box 73136
206-525 Woodview Drive SW
Calgary, AB, Canada T2W 6E0
Tel: 403-251-5228

BridgePoint Centre for Eating Disorders
P.O. Box 190
Milden, SK, Canada S0L 2L0
Tel: 306-935-2240

Westwind Eating Disorder Recovery Centre
458-14th Street
Brandon, MB, Canada R7A 4T3
Tel: 204-728-2499 or 1-888-353-3372

National Eating Disorder Information Centre
200 Elizabeth Street
College Wing 1-211
Toronto, ON, Canada M5G 2C4
Tel: 416-340-4156

Eating Disorder Unit
Douglas Hospital
6875 LaSalle Boulevard
Montreal, PQ H4H 1R3
Tel: 514-761-6131, ext. 2895

Eating Disorder Clinic
Queen Elizabeth II Health Sciences Centre
5909 Jubilee Road
Halifax, NS, Canada B3H 2E1
Tel: 902-473-6288

Recommended Resources

www.phe.queensu.ca/anab
Anorexia Nervosa and Bulimia Association
767 Bayridge Drive
P.O. Box 20058
Kingston, ON, Canada K7P 1C0
Tel: 613-547-3684

www.anad.org
National Association of Anorexia Nervosa and Associated Disorders (ANAD)
P.O. Box 7
Highland Park, IL, USA 60035
Tel: 847-831-3438
Fax: 847-433-4632

www.nedic.on.ca
National Eating Disorder Information Centre
200 Elizabeth Street
College Wing 1-211
Toronto, ON, Canada M5G 2C4
Tel: 416-340-4156
Fax: 416-340-4736

www.something-fishy.org
The Something Fishy Web Site on Eating Disorders is an extensive resource on eating disorders posted by a recovering sufferer of anorexia nervosa.

Endometriosis

Endometriosis develops in women when uterine-type cells grow outside of the uterus. These cells may travel throughout the body and attach to a number of different areas. The misplaced cells develop into nodules, lesions, implants or growths that are affected by the hormonal fluctuations of the menstrual cycle. These growths cause pelvic pain, pain during intercourse, infertility and other problems.

What Causes Endometriosis?

The uterus, a reproductive organ located within the abdominal cavity, is lined with a type of tissue called endometrium. When you have endometriosis, tissue that looks and acts like endometrium is found living outside the uterus. In most cases, the misplaced tissue is discovered growing somewhere within the abdominal cavity attached to the ovaries, bowel, bladder, fallopian tubes or cervix. Endometrial growths can vary in size and penetration of the surrounding tissue. Endometrial growths are generally not cancerous; rather, they are normal types of tissue found growing outside the normal location.

During the course of a normal menstrual cycle, the endometrial lining of the uterus gradually builds up in preparation for pregnancy. If a woman does not become pregnant, the lining breaks down, bleeds and is discharged from the body during a menstrual period. Unfortunately, the endometrial tissue living outside of the uterus responds to the hormonal cycles of menstruation in exactly the same way. But, unlike the menstrual flow from the uterus, the blood from the misplaced tissue has no place to go. This causes episodes of internal bleeding and inflammation that can result in internal scarring, severe pain and infertility.

Scientists still don't know what causes endometriosis. The most commonly held view is the *retrograde menstruation theory*. This theory suggests that menstrual tissue occasionally flows backwards through the fallopian tubes during menstruation. The tissue is discharged from the fallopian tubes into the abdomen, where it becomes implanted and develops into endometrial growths. Another theory proposes that endometrial tissue may be distributed from the uterus to other parts of the body through the lymph glands or blood vessels. In some cases, endometrial tissue may be accidentally transplanted into distant sites through surgical procedures.

Symptoms

Signs that you might have endometriosis include

- pain before and during menstruation
- severe menstrual cramps
- irregular vaginal bleeding
- pelvic pain
- painful sexual intercourse
- painful bowel movements
- pain with exercise
- painful and frequent urination
- backache
- constipation or diarrhea
- fatigue
- infertility

The symptoms of endometriosis have little to do with the extent of the endometrial growths. Some women with mild endometriosis and small growths may experience excruciating pain, while other women with large growths and severe endometriosis may have no painful symptoms at all. Symptoms usually start after the onset of menstruation and subside after menopause, when the growths tend to shrink or disappear.

Many women with endometriosis experience ongoing gastrointestinal discomfort, including diarrhea, painful bowel movements and general intestinal distress. Studies have revealed that endometriosis is associated with changes to the intestinal tract such as altered motility and bacterial overgrowth. There are four possible reasons why women with endometriosis experience bowel problems:

1. Endometrial growths develop directly on the bowel, usually the latter part of the large intestine. Most specialists carefully check the bowel for the presence of endometriosis but, because the intestine is so long, it is possible for growths to be missed.

2. Adhesions can result from the endometriosis itself, or from past surgeries. (Adhesions are fibrous bands or structures by which parts normally adhere.) These adhesions pull on the bowel and cause pain.

3. Prostaglandins may cause intestinal symptoms in women who do not have any evidence of endometriosis on their bowels. Prostaglandins are compounds produced by the body that control the smooth muscle of the uterus, bowel and blood vessels.

4. Symptoms may be caused by an overgrowth of Candida albicans (see page 195, Candidiasis), a fungus responsible for causing yeast infections in women. Women with this yeast infection often develop food sensitivities, which can contribute to gastrointestinal upset. Usually treatment of the candidiasis provides women relief of these symptoms. Unfortunately, diagnosis of yeast overgrowth is not easy to obtain, as this condition is new and controversial among the medical community.

Women with endometriosis are often told by their doctor that they have irritable bowel syndrome (IBS). Unfortunately that diagnosis is not very helpful because it does not indicate what the underlying problem is. IBS is an umbrella term used to describe gastrointestinal distress when no other diagnosis can be made. Having your doctor thoroughly investigate the cause of your bowel problems is important for effective treatment.

Who's at Risk?

More than 5.5 million North American women and girls have endometriosis.[1] The disease occurs most often in women of childbearing age, affecting 10 to 15 percent of women between the ages of 25 and 44, but teenagers can also suffer from endometriosis.[2]

The disease is believed to run in families; you are at higher risk if you have a first-degree relative (e.g., mother, sister) with endometriosis. Other risk factors include being of Caucasian descent, having your first child after the age of 30 and having an abnormal uterus.

Conventional Treatment

The choice of treatment is guided by the extent of your symptoms, your age and your plans to have a family. For mild cases, your doctor may choose to simply wait and see how the disease progresses. The only treatment may be pain relief medication such as aspirin or ibuprofen. Exercise, heat from a bath or heating pad, massage and relaxation may also help ease painful symptoms.

If a woman with endometriosis is not planning to have children, hormone suppression treatment may be recommended. This involves taking a combination of drugs to prevent ovulation and limit the amount of estrogen that stimulates the endometrial growths. By doing so, this will hopefully slow the growth of the misplaced tissue and minimize injury to surrounding organs. Drugs commonly prescribed include

- *Birth control pills* to control irregular vaginal bleeding and improve pain with a regulated, low-dose combination of estrogen and progesterone

- *Progestins* to prevent ovulation and reduce estrogen levels

- *Gonadotropin releasing hormone (GnRH) agonists* (such as Lupron® or Synarel®) to create a temporary and reversible menopause by stopping estrogen production by the ovaries. Side effects include hot flashes, mood swings, headache, vaginal dryness and some bone loss.

- *Danazol*, a synthetic testosterone, to reduce the production of estrogen from the ovaries and stop menstruation. Possible side effects include water retention, weight gain, oily skin, muscle cramps, mood changes and hot flashes. Occasionally a rash, facial hair or deepening of the voice may occur, in which case treatment with danazol should be stopped.

For cases of moderate or severe endometriosis, surgery may be necessary. As much misplaced tissue is removed as possible while preserving the woman's ability to have children by retaining the ovaries and uterus. This type of surgery usually provides only temporary relief of symptoms, since endometriosis recurs in most women.

A complete hysterectomy, which removes all reproductive organs, will be considered only for women not planning to become pregnant and those who have severe pelvic pain that is not relieved by medication. After surgery, estrogen replacement therapy may be prescribed to counteract the menopausal symptoms that will develop.

Managing Endometriosis

The nutritional approaches listed below are aimed at easing endometriosis-associated pain, improving fertility and minimizing the side effects of certain medications. While these are not cures for endometriosis, nor intended as stand-alone treatments for the condition, they can help women feel better.

Dietary Strategies

Essential Fatty Acids and Omega-3 Fats

Dietary fats are made up of building blocks called fatty acids. These fatty acids are incorporated into cell membranes, where they affect the integrity and fluidity of the membrane. The body is able to make all but two fatty acids: linoleic and alpha-linolenic acid. Because these two fatty acids are indispensable to health, they must be obtained from food and therefore are referred to as essential fatty acids (see Chapter 3). The body uses these two essential fatty acids to produce hormone-like compounds called prostaglandins (PGs), which are sometimes referred to as eicosanoids.

Prostaglandins regulate our blood pressure, blood clot formation, blood fats, immune compounds and hormones. They are produced by the lining of the uterus, by endometrial lesions and by immune compounds called macrophages. Researchers have learned that prostaglandin formation is altered in women with endometriosis. Studies have revealed that these women have significantly higher levels of prostaglandins compared with women who are free of endometriosis.[3-8] A high level of prostaglandins can alter the contractility of the uterus and fallopian tubes, resulting in painful menstrual periods and infertility. Some of these PGs can enter the bloodstream and affect smooth muscle in other parts of the body. PGs can stimulate the gastrointestinal tract, causing it to contract in an uncontrolled manner.

The body makes different types of prostaglandins. Prostaglandins can either increase inflammation or decrease it. In the case of endometriosis, two inflammatory prostaglandins called PGE and PGF appear to be involved. A diet that's high in fatty acids from animal foods and processed fat favors the production of prostaglandins that cause inflammation. A diet high in omega-3 fatty acids, such as those found in flaxseed oil, canola oil, walnuts, soybeans and fish, favors the formation of anti-inflammatory prostaglandins.

So the balance of omega-6 to omega-3 oils in the diet is very important for proper prostaglandin formation. The optimal ratio is thought to be 4:1, or four times the amount of omega-6 oils to omega-3 oils. It's estimated that we are currently following a diet that has more than 20 times more omega-6 oils than omega-3 oils. A diet with such an imbalance will lead to a greater production of inflammatory PGs.

To achieve a better balance of omega-6 oils to omega-3 oils, practice the following:

- *Reduce the amount of animal fat in your diet.* Choose lean cuts of meat and poultry (e.g., flank steak, inside round, sirloin, eye of round, extra-lean ground beef, venison, center-cut pork chops, pork tenderloin, baked ham, deli ham, skinless chicken breast, turkey breast, lean ground turkey). Choose 1 percent or skim milk, cheeses made with less than 20 percent milk fat, and yogurt with less than 2 percent milk fat.

- *Avoid foods with trans fat*, an unhealthy fat formed when manufacturers hydrogenate vegetable oils for commercial foods such as margarine and baked goods. Read ingredients lists on food packages and choose foods that contain "partially hydrogenated vegetable oils" less often.

- *Add 1 to 2 tablespoons (15 to 30 ml) of flaxseed oil to your daily diet.* This oil is one of the richest sources of omega-3 fat. Flaxseed oil is easily broken down by heat, so don't cook with it. If you want to add it to a hot dish such as pasta sauce, add it at the end of cooking. Use the oil in salad dressing and dip recipes. Store flaxseed oil in the fridge. You'll find flaxseed oil sold in the refrigerator section of your local health food store. For recipe ideas, check out **www.omegaflo.com**. If you don't want to add the oil to your diet, supplements of flaxseed oil are available. Keep in mind that it takes four capsules (4 grams) to give you a teaspoon of oil. It may be much easier—and less expensive—to use the bottled oil.

- *Eat fish at least three times a week.* Salmon, trout, sardines, herring, mackerel, swordfish and fresh tuna are good choices.

Dietary Fiber

Getting enough fiber each day is an important way to help regulate bowel habits and ease gastrointestinal symptoms of endometriosis. It's estimated that Canadians are getting 11 to 14 grams of fiber each day, only one-half of the daily recommendation. Experts agree that a daily intake of 25 to 35 grams of dietary fiber is needed to reap its health benefits. Good food choices include whole-grain breads, breakfast cereals with at least 5 grams of fiber per serving (check the nutrition panel), dried fruit, nuts and legumes. To add higher-fiber foods to your daily diet, refer to page 3, Chapter 1.

When adding fiber to your diet, gradually build up to the recommended 25 to 35 grams. Too much too soon can cause bloating, gas and diarrhea. Spread high-fiber foods out over the course of the day. And aim to drink a minimum of 8 ounces of fluid with each high-fiber meal and snack.

Probiotics

Research suggests that women with endometriosis may have bacterial or yeast overgrowth in their gastrointestinal tract, which may aggravate bloating, stomach pain, early satiety, diarrhea and/or constipation. In one study conducted at the Women's Hospital of Texas in Houston, 40 out of 50 women studied had excessive levels of bacteria.[9]

The term probiotic literally means "to promote life" and refers to living organisms that, upon ingestion in certain numbers, improve microbial balance in the intestine and exert health benefits. Such friendly bacteria are known collectively as lactic acid bacteria and include *L. acidophilus, L. bulgaricus, L. casei, S. thermophilus* and bifidobacteria. The human digestive tract contains hundreds of strains of bacteria, making up what is called the normal intestinal flora. Among the intestinal flora are lactic acid bacteria, which inhibit the growth of unfriendly, or disease-causing, bacteria by preventing their attachment to the intestine and by producing lactic acid and other antibacterial substances that suppress harmful bacteria. Plenty of studies have shown that consuming probiotic foods or supplements increases the number of lactic acid bacteria in the intestinal tract. Lactic acid bacteria have been shown to help treat diarrhea and constipation and also inhibit the growth of Candida albicans (see page 195, Candidiasis).

Lactic acid bacteria are found in fermented milk products. Include one serving of yogurt or kefir in your daily diet.

Probiotic Supplements

If you don't eat dairy products, probiotic capsules or tablets are a good alternative. In fact, many health experts believe that taking a high-quality supplement is the only way to ensure you're getting a sufficient number of friendly bacteria to the intestinal tract. Use the following guide when choosing a product:

- *Buy a product that offers 1 to 10 billion live cells per dose.* Taking more than this may result in gastrointestinal discomfort.

- For greater convenience, *choose a product that is stable at room temperature* and does not require refrigeration. This allows you to continue taking your supplement while traveling. Good manufacturers will test their products to ensure that they maintain their viability over a long period. For example, Wakunaga's probiotics supplement Kyo-Dophilus® has been tested and found to retain high bacteria counts for up to six years at room temperature.

- *Know the type and source of bacteria in the supplement.* Many experts believe that supplements made from human strains of bacteria are better adapted for growth in the human intestinal tract. When choosing a product, you might ask the pharmacist or retailer if the formula contains human or nonhuman strains.

- *Always take your supplement with food.* When eating a meal, the stomach contents become less acidic due to the presence of food. This allows live bacteria to withstand stomach acids and reach their final destination in the intestinal tract.

Prebiotics

It is possible to eat foods that promote the growth of protective lactic acid bacteria in your intestinal tract. These foods are called prebiotics and contain components called fructo-oligosaccharides (FOSs). The human intestine does not digest FOSs; instead, FOSs stay in the intestinal tract and feed the lactic acid bacteria. Good food sources include Jerusalem artichokes, asparagus, onions and garlic. But the amount we consume in our daily diet is considered too low to have any significant effect on the growth of friendly bacteria. You will likely have to visit your local farmers market and purchase a few Jerusalem artichokes. Chop one up and add it to salads and stir-fries. In the future, purified FOS may be added to commercial food products, as is already the case in Japan.

Caffeine

A study from the Harvard School of Public Health found that women with endometriosis who consumed 5 to 7 grams of caffeine per month (one to two cups of coffee per day) had almost double the risk of not conceiving compared with women who didn't drink any caffeinated beverages.[10] This study suggests that caffeine can delay conception and therefore further aggravate fertility in women with endometriosis.

Women taking a gonadotropin-releasing hormone (GnRH) drug like Lupron® (leuprolide) or Synarel® (nafarelin) should limit their consumption of caffeine. That's because these drugs cause bone loss, as does caffeine. If you can't give up your morning brew, make sure you're getting 1000 to 1500 milligrams of calcium each day.

Caffeine can also aggravate gastrointestinal symptoms. Caffeine can stimulate the intestinal tract and cause more frequent bowel movements and diarrhea.

Assess your current caffeine intake using the list of caffeine-containing beverages and foods on page 82, Chapter 5. Gradually cut back over a period of two to three weeks to minimize withdrawal symptoms such as headaches, tiredness or muscle pain. Switch to low-caffeine beverages like tea or hot chocolate or caffeine-free alternatives such as decaf coffee, herbal tea, cereal coffee, juice, milk or water.

Alcohol

When it comes to fertility, alcohol consumption is something else that should be minimized or avoided altogether. The same researchers from the Harvard School of Public Health who investigated caffeine and conception in women with endometriosis looked at the effect of alcohol.[11] They determined that women who drank one or two drinks a day had a 60 percent higher risk of infertility compared with nondrinkers. Like caffeine, alcohol can also increase bowel discomfort.

Food Sensitivities

Certain foods and spices may aggravate the bowel discomfort that is a symptom of endometriosis. To help you determine food sensitivities, keep a food and symptom diary for a two-week period. Record everything you eat, how much of the food you eat and any symptoms you feel. If you are working with a consulting dietitian, he or she will use this tool to identify food culprits.

It can be difficult to detect foods that are causing you grief because a particular food may not bother you all the time. Sometimes it isn't what you ate but how much of the food you ate, or how quickly you ate, or how many trigger foods you ate in one day or how much stress you were under at the time. Use your food diary to look for patterns, not just specific foods.

The following foods often cause intestinal problems in women with endometriosis:

- *Caffeine and alcohol*

- *Artificial sweeteners*

- *High-fat and/or high-calorie meals.* Both dietary fat and large meals have a greater stimulating effect on colon contractions.

- *Excessive sugar* from soft drinks, candy and sweets. Often, soft drinks cause problems because of the sugar, caffeine and carbonation they contain.

- *Dairy products.* Some women don't produce enough of an enzyme called lactase in the intestinal tract. Lactase breaks down the natural milk sugar, lactose. If lactose remains undigested in the intestinal tract, it will cause bloating, gas and diarrhea. Women who have moderate lactose intolerance can usually tolerate yogurt, since it has less lactose than milk. Hard cheeses have even less lactose. If you are symptomatic, try Lactaid® milk or Lacteeze® yogurt. Or buy Lactaid® pills at the pharmacy; take a pill before a meal that contains dairy. Alternatives to dairy include calcium-fortified soy and rice beverages.

- *Wheat.* In some women with endometriosis, bloating, distension and gas is caused by an intolerance to wheat-based foods such as bread, bagels, muffins, pasta, ready-to-eat breakfast cereals, crackers and baked goods made from wheat flour. If you are unsure whether wheat is causing your gas and bloating, try eliminating it from your diet for two weeks to see if your symptoms improve. Then, slowly add wheat back to your diet. Every two days, add one new wheat food. If your symptoms recur, consider alternatives to wheat such rice, rice pasta, rice crackers, quinoa, quinoa pasta, millet, potato, sweet potato, corn, rye and oats. A good health food store will have many products—breakfast cereals, pasta, crackers, cookies and breads—that are made from wheat-free grains. Some of these foods, like rice pasta and rice crackers, are available in large grocery stores.

- *Raw vegetables.* Be sure to cook your vegetables; cooked vegetables are less likely to cause gas than raw vegetables. Particularly gassy vegetables include bok choy, broccoli, Brussels sprouts, cabbage, cauliflower, kale, radishes, rutabaga, onions and raw garlic.

- *Legumes* such as kidney beans, chickpeas and black beans. A natural sugar in dried peas, beans and lentils often causes gas and bloating. To reduce potential symptoms, rinse beans before adding them to recipes and eat a smaller portion. Try Beano®, a natural enzyme available at pharmacies and health food stores that breaks down the sugar. Add a few drops on legumes.

- *Certain fruits,* such as berries, apple with the peel, melon and prunes.

- *Nuts and seeds*

- *Spices* such as chili powder, curry, ginger, garlic and hot sauce.

Vitamins and Minerals
Vitamin E
Some researchers theorize that oxygen damage caused by free radical molecules contributes to endometriosis by promoting the growth of endometrial tissue. Free radicals are highly reactive oxygen molecules that are produced by normal body processes, including the body's own immune response. It's thought that damaged red blood cells and misplaced endometrial tissue signal the recruitment and activity of immune compounds in the abdominal cavity. In the process of engulfing foreign particles and protecting the body, these activated immune compounds generate harmful free radicals, which cause oxidation.

Studies conducted in women with endometriosis have shown that compounds called lipoproteins in the fluid of the abdominal cavity do indeed have lower levels of vitamin E, an important antioxidant.[12] Antioxidants are vitamins, minerals or natural plant chemicals that protect cells in the body from damage caused by free radicals.

The best food sources of vitamin E include vegetable oils, nuts, seeds, soybeans, olives, wheat germ, whole grains and leafy green vegetables like kale. To supplement, take 200 to 800 IU of natural source vitamin E per day.

Calcium and Vitamin D
If you are taking a GnRH drug such as Lupron® (leuprolide) or Synarel® (nafarelin), your bone health is a concern. These drugs suppress estrogen production, resulting in accelerated bone loss. A review of studies of women taking GnRH drugs determined the average bone loss to be 1 percent per month or 6 percent in total.[13] If you compare that with an average bone loss of 3 percent in the first year of menopause, it seems con-

siderable. And while that may not be important when a woman is 25 years old, it may be very relevant when she is 65. Because of their negative effect on bone density, Health Canada has set a limit of six months on the use of GnRH drugs.

Ensure that you are meeting your daily requirement of 1000 to 1200 milligrams of calcium and daily adequate intake of 200 to 400 international units (IU) of vitamin D by choosing foods listed in Chapter 4. If you are not meeting your daily targets for calcium and vitamin D through diet, take a supplement. Most multivitamin and mineral supplements provide 400 IU of vitamin D. To get enough calcium, you must take a separate calcium supplement. If you consume at least three to four servings of dairy products or calcium-fortified beverages each day, you're getting approximately 900 to 1200 milligrams of calcium. For every serving you're missing and not making up with other calcium-rich foods, consider taking a 300 milligram calcium citrate supplement with added vitamin D.

Nutrition Strategy Checklist for Endometriosis

- ☐ Limit saturated fat
- ☐ Flaxseed oil
- ☐ Fish
- ☐ Dietary fiber
- ☐ Fermented milk products
- ☐ Probiotic supplements
- ☐ Limit caffeine and alcohol
- ☐ Identify food sensitivities
- ☐ Vitamin E
- ☐ Calcium
- ☐ Vitamin D

Recommended Resources

www.endometriosisassn.org
Endometriosis Association
8585 N 76th Place
Milwaukee, WI, USA 53223
Tel: 414-355-2200

www.hcgresources.com/endoindex.html
Endometriosis Awareness and Information
pages

www.mayoclinic.com
Mayo Foundation for Medical Education and Research

www.nichd.nih.gov/publications/pubs/
endomet.htm
National Institute of Child Health and Development
NICHD Clearinghouse
P.O. Box 3006
Rockville, MD, USA 20847
Tel: 1-800-370-2943
E-mail: NICHDClearinghouse@mal.nih.gov

Fibrocystic Breast Conditions

Formerly called fibrocystic breast disease, this disorder may include breast nodules, breast swelling, tenderness and pain. These symptoms are collectively referred to as fibrocystic breast conditions. Breast pain and tenderness are also called cyclic mastalagia or mastitis. A woman with fibrocystic breast conditions may experience breast pain only, lumpiness only, or both. Although these breast conditions can be painful and suspicious lumps can cause anxiety, most do not increase a woman's risk of breast cancer.

What Causes Fibrocystic Breast Conditions?

The exact cause of this disorder is not known. Breast changes usually appear during the years a woman menstruates and regress with the onset of menopause. In most cases, the small, round lumps appear in the breasts because of hormonal changes associated with menstruation. The hormones estrogen and progesterone, which control the menstrual cycle, trigger physical responses that can make breasts become lumpy, or fibrocystic, and painful. It's thought that a deficiency of progesterone and an excess of estrogen in the last 14 days of a woman's menstrual cycle are responsible for breast changes. A woman will find that her breasts become increasingly tender and painful as her body prepares for menstruation. The discomfort normally subsides once her period starts. Over time, breast lumps may develop into cysts, which fill with fluid, causing swelling and pain.

Some researchers believe that hormone-like compounds called prostaglandins are responsible for breast changes. Studies indicate that the development of lumpy breasts may also be stimulated by a diet that includes higher levels of caffeine and dietary fat. Despite these theories, most of the clues about the cause of fibrocystic breast conditions suggest that estrogen is the key.

Symptoms

One of the main symptoms of fibrocystic breast conditions is breast lumpiness. A woman may discover only one lump, but it is more common to have multiple lumps. The lumps are tender, come in different sizes and usually move freely within the breast tissue. A woman may also experience some breast pain and swelling, which will become worse just before her menstrual period.

Some women who are severely affected by this condition complain of continuous discomfort. Up to 50 percent of women with breast pain report that it interferes with their sex life and physical activity. Occasionally, a woman may develop breast cysts that require medical attention.

Who's at Risk?

Fibrocystic breast conditions can affect women from puberty to old age. However, they most often affect women between the ages of 30 and

50. Breast symptoms usually disappear with menopause, and it is quite rare to find the disorder in postmenopausal women unless they are taking hormone replacement therapy.

Conventional Treatment

Women who suffer from painful breasts at certain times during the month may find that applying cold compresses on the tender areas and wearing a well-fitting, supportive bra both day and night will relieve some of the discomfort. Your doctor may recommend pain relievers to treat the aches and pains. If fibrocystic breast conditions cause severe pain, medications such as danazol, a mild, synthetic male hormone, or tamoxifen, a drug that blocks the action of estrogen, may be used. Because these drugs can produce side effects, they should be used only for a short time.

Managing Fibrocystic Breast Conditions

At this time, there is only weak evidence pointing to dietary factors as the cause of fibrocystic breast conditions. However, certain food and food components may very well aggravate symptoms. And since a high level of estrogen, or an increased sensitivity to estrogen, seems to be the dominant theory, any dietary modification that is able to reduce the circulating level of estrogen may help lessen your symptoms.

Dietary Strategies

Dietary Fat

Reducing the amount of fat you eat, from the typical North American intake of 35 percent calories to 15 or 20 percent, may be beneficial. Although studies have not investigated the effect of a low-fat diet on fibrocystic breast conditions per se, there is indirect evidence to support this strategy. Research in women with breast dysplasia (abnormal growth of breast cells) has found a low-fat diet to have a positive effect on the density of breast tissue and the composition of breast fluid.[1]

A high-fat diet is also associated with higher levels of circulating estrogen and cholesterol, a building block of hormones. Studies reveal that when women reduce their fat intake, their levels of blood estrogen and prolactin, a hormone that may be involved in fibrocystic breast conditions, also decline. In two small studies, women with fibrocystic breast conditions who followed a 21 percent fat diet for three months experienced a significantly lower level of circulating estrogen, prolactin and cholesterol.[2,3]

To help you follow a 20 percent fat diet:

- *Choose lower-fat animal foods.* Buy lean meat, poultry breast, 1 percent or skim milk, 1 percent milk-fat yogurt and cheese made with less than 20 percent milk fat.

- *Use added fats and oils sparingly.* Replace butter on toast with sugar-reduced jam; try mustard instead of high-fat spreads on sandwiches; mix tuna with yogurt instead of mayonnaise; top a baked potato with low-fat sour cream instead of butter; order salad dressing on the side. Use oil sparingly in cooking. Invest in a few high-quality nonstick pans. Use chicken broth or apple juice to prevent sticking in stir-fry dishes.

- *Read nutrition labels on packaged foods* like crackers, frozen entrées, snack foods, cookies and cereals. A lower-fat food will have no more than 3 grams of fat per 100 calories. If you're looking for a food that has 20 percent or less fat calories, make 2 grams of fat per 100 calories your cut-off point.

Dietary Fiber

Like dietary fat, fiber may also influence a woman's circulating estrogen levels. Most of the research on fiber intake and estrogen levels has focused on breast cancer risk, but the findings may be relevant to fibrocystic breast conditions. Two studies conducted among premenopausal women suggest that diets high in wheat bran are effective in lowering circulating estrogen.[4,5] In one study, both a 10 and 20 gram wheat-bran supplement significantly lowered estrogen after four weeks. The total fiber intake of these women was between 20 and 32 grams.

Wheat bran belongs to a class of fibers known as insoluble. That means they are unable to dissolve in water. They pass through the intestinal tract intact and, in the process, are able to bind compounds, including estrogen, preventing their absorption in the bloodstream. Soluble fibers found in oatmeal, oat bran, dried beans, lentils and psyllium-enriched breakfast cereals also have this ability, even though they have not been specifically studied for their effect on estrogen levels.

Use the list of foods on page 3, Chapter 1, to gradually add higher-fiber foods to your diet. Spread fiber-rich foods out over the course of the day. Fiber needs fluid to work, so be sure to drink at least 8 ounces of fluid with each high-fiber meal and snack.

Soy Isoflavones

Research findings on soy intake and estrogen levels provide indirect evidence that this food may be beneficial in preventing fibrocystic breast conditions. Many studies have found that a diet rich in soy foods lowers the level of circulating estrogen in women.[6-9] Soybeans contain natural chemicals called isoflavones, a class of plant compounds that have weak estrogen activity in the body. One of the main isoflavones in soybeans, called genistein, is able to compete with a woman's own estrogen for binding to estrogen receptors. In so doing, soy isoflavones are able to reduce the amount of estrogen that contacts breast cells.

Aim to include one soy food in your daily diet. A list of soy foods and how to use them can be found on page 72, Chapter 5.

Caffeine

It's long been thought that caffeine plays a role in fibrocystic breast conditions. The interest in caffeine dates back to the late 1970s and early 1980s, when researchers noted higher intakes of caffeine in women with fibrocystic breast conditions. It has been hypothesized that caffeine causes an abnormally high level of energy compounds called cAMP in cells, which may lead to symptoms.

Studies over the past decade have failed to find a relationship between caffeine intake and the development of fibrocystic breast conditions. Drinking coffee may, however, make your symptoms worse. A study from Duke University in Durham, North Carolina, asked 147 women with fibrocystic breast conditions to abstain from caffeine-containing foods, beverages and medication.[10] Among those women who successfully removed caffeine from their diet for one year, 69 percent reported a decrease or absence of breast pain.

Currently, Health Canada recommends a daily maximum of 450 milligrams of caffeine. While your goal is to avoid as much caffeine as possible, use this amount as a benchmark to see how much you're consuming now. Eliminate caffeine for three months before you assess its effect on reducing your breast symptoms. A list of caffeine-containing foods and beverages can be found in page 82, Chapter 5.

Vitamins and Minerals
Vitamin E

The use of vitamin E for treating fibrocystic breast conditions dates back to the 1960s. Vitamin E has been claimed to alter blood levels of certain hormones, especially progesterone, but this has not yet been proven. A few small studies from the early 1980s did find that vitamin E was effective at reducing symptoms.[11,12] However, subsequent well-designed studies that looked at the effect of 150, 300 and 600 international units (IU) of vitamin E in larger numbers of women found no effect on breast pain or lumps. These studies lasted only two or three months, and it is possible that vitamin E might be beneficial if taken for a longer period.

While the balance of evidence does not support the use of vitamin E supplements for managing fibrocystic breast conditions, it is certainly worth a try. Take 200 to 800 IU of natural source vitamin E per day. Foods rich in vitamin E include vegetable oils, nuts, seeds, wheat germ and leafy green vegetables.

Herbal Remedies

Evening Primrose Oil
(*Oenothera biennis*)

The oil from the evening primrose plant is a rich source of a fatty acid called gamma-linoleic acid (GLA). GLA is an omega-6 fatty acid that our bodies produce from linoleic acid, an essential fatty acid found in corn, sunflower and safflower oils.

By providing the body with GLA, evening primrose oil may help ease breast pain and tenderness in two ways. GLA is a polyunsaturated fat, which means it belongs to a class of fats with a different chemical structure than saturated fats (found in meat and dairy products). As a result, they behave differently in the body. Taking evening primrose oil is thought to increase the ratio of polyunsaturated to saturated fats in the body. Some experts believe that if saturated fats dominate, your body will be overly sensitive to hormones like estrogen. That's because hormones made from saturated fat are more potent and attach more readily to receptors. What's more, a diet that's high in saturated fat is also

believed to impair the conversion of dietary linoleic acid to GLA inside the body. Interestingly, research has found abnormally high levels of saturated fatty acids in women with fibrocystic breast conditions.

Supplementing with evening primrose oil may also alter your body's production of hormone-like compounds called prostaglandins. Many prostaglandins are made in the body. Some are inflammatory and may cause breast pain, while others are considered friendly as they do not lead to inflammation. GLA produces a special class of friendly prostaglandins called PGE1. These prostaglandins are also thought to reduce the activity of prolactin, a hormone possibly involved in fibrocystic breast conditions.

Results of studies conducted in 291 women with persistent breast pain have found evening primrose oil to be beneficial in easing symptoms.[13] The effective dose is 1.5 to 2 grams taken twice daily. Take three 500 milligram pills at breakfast and repeat at dinner. Buy a supplement that is standardized to 9 percent GLA. It may take three menstrual cycles before you feel the effects of evening primrose oil and up to eight months for the supplement to reach its full effect.

Ginkgo Biloba

French researchers studied 143 women with PMS and found that ginkgo biloba significantly reduced PMS-related breast tenderness (as well as abdominal bloating and swollen hands, legs and feet).[14] The women took ginkgo on day 16 of their cycle and continued until day 5 of the next cycle, at which time they stopped. They resumed taking the herb again on day 16.

The recommended dose of ginkgo is 40 to 80 milligrams three times daily. Start on day 16 (counting from the first day of your period) and continue until the end of your next period. This means you will take ginkgo for two weeks each month. To buy a high-quality product, choose a product standardized to 24 percent ginkgo flavone glycosides. On rare occasions, ginkgo may cause gastrointestinal upset, headache or an allergic skin reaction in susceptible individuals. Ginkgo should not be taken with blood-thinning drugs such as Coumadin® (warfarin) or heparin without medical supervision. Ginkgo may enhance the blood-thinning effect of other natural health products (like vitamin E or garlic), so be sure to inform your physician and pharmacist if you are taking a number of these supplements.

Nutrition Strategy Checklist for Fibrocystic Breast Conditions

☐ Diet low in fat

☐ Dietary fiber

☐ Soy foods

☐ Avoid caffeine

☐ Vitamin E

☐ Evening primrose oil

☐ Ginkgo biloba

Recommended Resources

www.cancer.org
American Cancer Society
2420 N Coliseum Boulevard, Suite 200
Fort Wayne, IN, USA 46805
Tel: 219-471-3911

www.fwradiology.com/fibrobrst.htm
Supported by the American Cancer Society, this Web site provides an excellent overview of fibrocystic breast conditions.

www.askdrkoop.com
Founded by former US Surgeon General Dr. Everett Koop.

Fibromyalgia

Fibromyalgia (FM) is a chronic, debilitating disorder characterized by widespread, persistent pain, fatigue and tenderness in numerous muscle areas throughout the body. The pain of FM is centered in the soft tissues located around joints, internal organs and skin. Although pain symptoms are similar to those of arthritis, fibromyalgia doesn't affect the joints, nor does it cause the crippling deterioration that is so common in arthritis. Instead, it attacks the muscles and connective tissue, causing stiffness, burning or aching pain and muscle spasms that vary in intensity. Local points of tenderness develop all over the body, particularly in the neck, spine, shoulders and hips. The pain of fibromyalgia is usually accompanied by an exhausting fatigue that limits activities and has a negative effect on mental health.

What Causes Fibromyalgia?

The cause of fibromyalgia has not been established, but many experts think that it is a biological response to stress. Researchers have also identified abnormalities in brain chemical activities that may be responsible for fibromyalgia symptoms. People with fibromyalgia have lower levels of brain chemicals such as serotonin and tryptophan and higher levels of a growth hormone known as somatomedin C. These chemical imbalances have been linked to other stress-related disorders such as depression, migraines and heightened pain sensitivity.

Scientists are beginning to suspect that certain people may be susceptible to stressful conditions if they are genetically predisposed to chronic pain disorders. Post-traumatic stress disorder, an anxiety disorder that emerges after traumatic events such as sexual or physical abuse, has been known to cause changes in brain activity that can be linked to FM syndrome. Physical traumas, such as accidents, injuries or severe illness, also seem to promote the onset of fibromyalgia by affecting the central nervous system. This response is especially prevalent in injuries that involve the neck.

Another popular theory suggests that FM may be an autoimmune disease that develops when a defect in the immune system stimulates antibodies to attack the body's own tissue. Studies have indicated that inadequate or disturbed sleep patterns very often trigger immune system reactions, causing inflammation and pain. Almost all FM sufferers experience chronic sleep disturbances, and many people report that their FM pain is much worse after a night of disturbed sleep.

Symptoms

The symptoms of fibromyalgia vary from person to person. In most cases, the disorder causes burning or aching pain that begins in a specific spot and radiates outward through the body. The pain can change location and vary in severity from day to day. Weather changes, physical activity and stressful events can affect the degree of FM pain symptoms.

Most people with FM feel tired, sometimes to the point of exhaustion. Energy levels may be low, and the ability to concentrate may be impaired. Numbness and tingling in parts of your body and occasional muscle spasms are also common symptoms. Your body may feel stiff and tight after you wake up in the morning or after long periods of standing or sitting. Digestive problems, including diarrhea, constipation, abdominal pain, gas and heartburn, as well as bladder pain and frequent urination, may all be associated with FM. Women with fibromyalgia often experience pelvic pain and may have pain during menstrual periods or during sexual intercourse.

Fibromyalgia is associated with a number of other symptoms and syndromes. At least 25 per-

cent of all people who suffer from FM are prone to depression or mood disorders. Sleep disturbances are also very common. Fibromyalgia sufferers are prone to migraines and other types of headaches. Sensitivities to temperature and to environmental conditions such as light, noise and weather patterns are also common in FM.

Because of its complex nature, fibromyalgia is very difficult to diagnose and is often confused with other psychological or autoimmune disorders, such as depression, arthritis or sleep disturbances caused by other conditions.

Who's at Risk?

Fibromyalgia affects between 2 and 6 percent of the Canadian population.[1] Women are four times more likely to develop fibromyalgia than men, especially after the age of 50. Evidence suggests that fibromyalgia runs in families and is inherited through the female line. The risk of developing fibromyalgia may also increase if you are exposed to high levels of stress or suffer a physical injury or accident, especially one that involves the neck.

Conventional Treatment

Treatment of fibromyalgia usually involves a combination of therapeutic approaches. A regular program of low-impact aerobic exercise has been shown to be very effective. Yet many people with the disease avoid physical activity because it seems to aggravate pain. However, without physical activity, your muscles will become weak. As the muscles weaken, it takes less and less physical activity to produce painful symptoms. This vicious cycle of inactivity and muscle weakness can prolong and heighten the exhausting symptoms of FM. Swimming, water-exercise programs, walking and stationary biking are all good activity choices. When undertaking any physical activity, it is important to incorporate stretching at the beginning and end of the exercise.

Learning to cope with the disease is an important component to healing. Respecting the limitations of your body and recognizing circumstances that aggravate the condition are important lifestyle management skills. Reducing stress and adopting a positive approach to pain management can help establish better control over FM symptoms. Psychological therapy may be beneficial in helping to gain such life skills.

Various physical rehabilitation therapies, massage, heat applications and relaxation techniques have all been useful in managing FM symptoms. In some cases, medication may be required to treat symptoms, including

- *Tricyclic antidepressants* to improve sleep and reduce muscle pain. Only small doses are necessary to provide effective relief. Side effects such as blurred vision, drowsiness and dry mouth are often associated with these drugs.

- *Selective serotonin-reuptake inhibitors (SSRIs)* to increase the level of serotonin in the brain. They are often prescribed for people with FM who are also suffering from a major depression. Side effects can include agitation, nausea and sexual dysfunction.

- *Pain relievers* such as acetaminophen for relief of pain symptoms.

- *Estrogen therapy* for women who develop fibromyalgia during menopause to improve sleep, which helps to reduce fatigue associated with FM.

None of the treatments for fibromyalgia offer a cure for the disease. It can take months or even years to become symptom-free. Occasional relapses and recurrence of symptoms are bound to occur along the path to recovery.

Managing Fibromyalgia
Dietary Strategies

There is no evidence so far that any one dietary factor is effective in managing fibromyalgia. It is important to eat a healthy, low-fat diet that provides plenty of fiber and fresh fruits and vegetables. Dietary recommendations for fibromyalgia are similar to those for chronic fatigue syndrome, since the two conditions share many of the same clinical features. In fact, 75 percent of patients fit the diagnosis for both fibromyalgia and chronic fatigue. The following dietary guidelines should be followed:

1. *Emphasize plant foods in your daily diet.* Fill your plate with grains, fruits and vegetables. If you eat animal protein foods like meat or poultry, they should take up no more than one-quarter of your plate. Try instead vegetarian sources of protein such as beans and soy.

2. *Choose foods and oils that are rich in essential fatty acids.* Fish, nuts, seeds, flaxseed and flaxseed oil, canola oil, Omega-3 eggs, wheat germ and leafy green vegetables are examples (see below).

3. *Choose foods that are rich in vitamins, minerals and protective plant compounds.* Choose whole grains as often as possible. Eat at least three different colored fruits and three different colored vegetables every day.

4. As often as possible, *eliminate sources of refined sugar:* cookies, cakes, pastries, frozen desserts, soft drinks, sweetened fruit juices, fruit drinks, candy, etc.

5. *Buy organic produce* or *wash fruits and vegetables* to remove pesticide residues.

6. *Limit foods with chemical additives.*

7. *Avoid caffeine* (this can worsen fatigue by interrupting sleep patterns).

8. *Drink at least 8 to 12 cups (2 to 3 liters) of water every day.*

9. *Avoid alcohol*. If you drink, consume no more than one drink a day, or seven per week (women), nine per week (men).

Vitamins and Minerals

Multivitamin and Mineral Supplements

A broad-based supplement will ensure that you are meeting your daily requirements for most nutrients. Some evidence suggests that a daily multivitamin and mineral pill, when combined with a supplement of freeze-dried fruits and vegetables (Phyto-Aloe® by Mannatech™ Inc., **www.mannatech.com**) and medical treatment, may help reduce the severity of pain symptoms.[2]

Buy a product that contains no artificial preservatives, colors, flavors or added sugar, starch, lactose or yeast. This should be declared in small print below the ingredients list. If you experience gastrointestinal upset when taking a multivitamin, try a "professional brand" supplement available at certain health food stores. These products contain no binding materials and are suitable for people with food sensitivities. However, they are expensive and you will need to take more than three to six capsules a day to meet your recommended intake levels. Brand names include Genestra® and Thorne Research®.

Calcium and Vitamin D

According to a small study from the Osteoporosis Prevention and Treatment Center in Santa Monica, California, women with fibromyalgia may be at increased risk for osteoporosis.[3] Among women aged 33 to 60 years with fibromyalgia, all had lower bone densities of the spine compared with healthy women. It is especially important to be meeting your daily requirements for calcium and vitamin D to slow down bone loss. Ensure that your daily diet provides adequate amounts of calcium and vitamin D, two nutrients crucial for bone health.

The recommended dietary allowance (RDA) for calcium is 1000 to 1200 milligrams; best food sources are milk, yogurt, cheese, fortified soy and rice beverages, fortified orange juice, tofu, salmon (with bones), kale, bok choy, broccoli and Swiss chard. If you take calcium supplements, buy calcium citrate with vitamin D and magnesium added.

The daily adequate intake for vitamin D is 200 to 600 international units (IU); best food sources are fluid milk, fortified soy and rice beverages, oily fish, egg yolks, butter and margarine. Most multivitamin and mineral supplements provide 200 to 400 IU of vitamin D. See Chapter 4 for more information about calcium and vitamin D.

Magnesium

This mineral plays an important role in muscle contraction and the transmission of nerve impulses. Muscle pain is associated with magnesium deficiency and some studies have linked fibromyalgia with low body stores of magnesium, despite normal blood tests.[4,5] One study found that supplemental magnesium combined with malic acid (Super Malic®, see below) provided significant reductions in the severity of pain and tenderness.[6] You may want to consider taking Super Malic® to correct a magnesium deficiency.

The RDA for magnesium is 310 to 420 milligrams per day (see page 47, Chapter 4). The best food sources include nuts, seeds, legumes, prunes, whole grains, leafy green vegetables, Brewer's yeast, cheddar cheese and shrimp. If your daily diet falls short in magnesium, consider taking a supplement. If you do not take supplemental calcium with magnesium, separate magnesium supplements are available as magnesium citrate, aspartate, succinate, fumarte or gluconate. The body absorbs these forms of the mineral more efficiently. Taking more than 350 milligrams of magnesium in a supplement may cause diarrhea, nausea and stomach cramps.

Other Natural Health Products

Capsaicin

This natural compound, responsible for the heat of chili peppers, has a long history of use as a topical agent for pain disorders. One study suggests that capsaicin cream might help relieve fibromyalgia pain and tenderness.[7] Individuals with fibromyalgia who applied the cream to tender points four times per day for one month reported less tenderness compared with those using the placebo cream. The researchers found no difference in overall pain or sleep quality.

Capsaicin creams are available in health food stores and pharmacies. Buy a cream with 0.025 to 0.075 percent capsaicin (the greater strength may be more effective). Capsaicin cream will produce a burning sensation, which will diminish after several applications. Use a small amount to begin. When you no longer feel burning upon application, increase the amount of cream you use. Be careful not to touch your eyes or other sensitive tissues after applying capsaicin cream. Wash your hands after using the product.

5-HTP (5-Hydroxytryptophan)

This supplement is made from the seeds of *Griffonia simplicifolia*, a plant native to Africa. The body uses 5-HTP to synthesize serotonin, a brain chemical that may be depressed in people with fibromyalgia. One study conducted among 50 people with fibromyalgia found that 5-HTP taken three times daily for one month reduced pain, stiffness, anxiety and fatigue and improved sleep.[8]

The recommended dose is 100 or 200 milligrams three times daily. Once the supplement begins to work, it may be possible to reduce the dose. 5-HTP may cause mild stomach upset and allergic reactions in some individuals. More serious, though, is a report issued by the US Food and Drug Administration in 1998 about product safety. Some batches of 5-HTP were found to contain a chemical called peak X, known to cause a potentially fatal blood disorder. At this time, there are no other warnings from the FDA about using 5-HTP. Ask your retailer how he or she ensures product quality and safety.

Do not take 5-HTP if you use SSRI drugs that raise serotonin levels (e.g., Prozac®, Effexor®, Paxil®, Zoloft®, Serzone®) or other antidepressants. People with Parkinson's disease who take a medication called carbidopa should not use 5-HTP as it may cause skin changes.

Malic Acid

Malic acid is a compound produced by the body; it is also abundant in apples and apple juice. Some researchers theorize that people with fibromyalgia have difficulty producing or using malic acid and that this may impair muscle function. To date, only one small study supports this theory. Researchers from Texas gave 24 individuals with fibromyalgia a supplement called Super Malic® that combined 200 milligrams of malic acid from apples with 50 milligrams of magnesium or a placebo.[9] After six months, those taking Super Malic® experienced significant reductions in pain and tenderness compared with the placebo group. Improvements were seen after two months of taking six tablets twice daily (2400 milligrams of malic acid, 600 milligrams of magnesium).

This product is recommended as a means of treating a magnesium deficiency and should not be used indefinitely. Take Super Malic® for three months, and then taper it off to see if symptoms return. The recommended dose is 2 capsules every three hours for a total of 12 capsules per day. This amount of magnesium may cause diarrhea, in which case you should reduce the dose. Do not take this product with magnesium-containing antacids. Super Malic® may also interfere with antibiotic absorption. Be sure to inform your physician if you start using this product.

SAMe (S-Adenosyl-Methionine)

SAMe is a compound the body makes naturally from certain amino acids found in high-protein foods like fish and meat. As a supplement, it is well known as a treatment for depression. SAMe is associated with higher levels of brain neurotransmitters, and it also appears to change the composition of cell membranes in the brain, enabling neurotransmitters and cell receptors to work more efficiently.

There is some evidence to suggest that SAMe may be useful in treating fibromyalgia. A handful of studies have found SAMe effective in managing symptoms when it was given by injection. Although these findings cannot be generalized to oral supplements, one study using SAMe in pill form did find the supplement beneficial.[10] In the study, individuals with fibromyalgia who took SAMe for six weeks fared better in terms of pain, fatigue and morning stiffness than those taking the placebo. Exactly how SAMe works to help ease fibromyalgia symptoms is unclear.

Take 400 milligrams twice daily on an empty stomach. Buy an enteric-coated product.

Nutrition Strategy Checklist for Fibromyalgia

☐ Low-fat, plant-based diet

☐ Healthy oils

☐ Avoid caffeine and alcohol

☐ Multivitamin/mineral

☐ Calcium

☐ Vitamin D

☐ Magnesium

☐ Capsaicin cream

☐ 5-HTP OR SAMe

Recommended Resources

www.arthritis.ca
The Arthritis Society
393 University Avenue, Suite 1700
Toronto, ON, Canada M5G 1E6
Tel: 416-979-7228
Fax: 416-979-8366
E-mail: info@arthritis.ca

www.co-cure.org
Chronic Fatigue Syndrome and Fibromyalgia Information Exchange Forum

www.fmnetnews.com
Fibromyalgia Network
P.O. Box 31750
Tucson, AZ, USA 85751
Tel: 1-800-853-2929

www.nih.gov/niams/healthinfo/fibrofs.htm
National Institute of Arthritis and Musculoskeletal and Skin Diseases
National Institutes of Health
31 Center Drive, MSC 2320
Bethesda, MD USA 20892-2320

Food Allergies

According to a report by the US National Institute of Allergy and Infectious Diseases, one in three people state that they have a food allergy or have a family member with a suspected food allergy. Yet, in reality, only 2 to 8 percent of children have clinically proven allergic reactions to food, and that number drops to 1 to 2 percent in the adult population.[1]

The difficulty in assessing allergic reactions to food arises when people fail to distinguish between a true food allergy and a food intolerance such as lactose intolerance (see page 407, Lactose Intolerance). A food allergy, or hypersensitivity, involves the body's immune system, whereas a food intolerance is more of a metabolic problem. Some of the symptoms may be similar, but only a true food allergy can provoke potentially fatal reactions.

An allergic reaction to food develops when the immune system mistakenly responds to a food. Thinking that the food, or an ingredient in the food, is harmful, the immune system produces immunoglobulin E (IgE), a type of protective antibody. The IgE antibodies circulate in the bloodstream, ready to defend the body against this foreign invader. The next time the particular food is consumed, it interacts with the IgE antibodies, triggering the release of massive quantities of chemicals, such as histamine. The defensive actions of histamine and other chemicals provoke a wide range of allergic symptoms that can affect the skin, cardiovascular system, gastrointestinal tract or respiratory system.

What Causes Food Allergies?

Allergists believe that many food allergies in children are the result of immature immune systems. In other words, their bodies aren't developed enough to properly process certain foods. Children will sometimes outgrow a food allergy, especially those involving dairy products or eggs. However, allergic reactions to peanuts, fish and shellfish are usually considered life-long problems. The older a person is when he or she develops a food allergy, the less likely that person is to outgrow the allergy.

There is some evidence to suggest that breast-feeding infants for the first 6 to 12 months of life may help avoid milk or soy allergies, especially if the parents are allergic and the baby is likely to be more prone to allergies.[2-4] In some cases, a food eaten by a mother may enter the breast milk and may cause an allergic reaction in the child, so caution should be exercised during this time.[5] Delaying the introduction of foods that are known to cause allergies until the second or third year of life may also help to avoid or postpone the development of allergic reactions.

Foods That Cause Allergy

Although any food can trigger an allergic reaction, the most common food allergens are the following:

- cow's milk
- egg whites
- peanuts
- wheat
- soybeans
- fish
- shellfish
- tree nuts
- beans
- corn

In some cases, people with an allergy to one type of food may also be allergic to other foods that are similar in nature. This is known as cross-reactivity. For example, someone allergic to lobster may also be allergic to shrimp or crab and may have severe reactions to these foods if eaten unsuspectingly. Some pollen allergies, such as ragweed or birch tree pollen, have been associated with allergies to specific foods.

Food additives may cause adverse reactions but are not considered true allergens. Aspartame, monosodium glutamate (MSG) and yellow food coloring can sometimes cause mild and transitory reactions in people who are sensitive to them. Sulfites, food additives used in wine and as preservatives in certain processed foods, seafood, fresh or dehydrated fruit and some soft drinks have been known to cause unpredictable, and sometimes severe, reactions in people who suffer from asthma.

Symptoms

Allergic reactions range from mild to severe and may even be life threatening. The allergens in food are most often proteins that manage to survive the heat of cooking and the digestive action of stomach acids or enzymes. As these proteins pass through the body, they create a pathway of allergic reactions. As you begin to eat the food, you may experience itching in your mouth. Once the food reaches the stomach, vomiting, diarrhea or gas pains may develop. When the allergens enter the bloodstream, they may cause a drop in blood pressure or may travel to the skin, where they can cause hives or eczema. If the allergens reach the lungs, the result may be asthma or other breathing difficulties. These reactions will usually develop within a few minutes to a few hours of eating the particular food.

In rare cases, the reactions are severe enough to trigger heart malfunctions and a dramatic loss of blood pressure that can lead to shock and sudden death—a response known as anaphylaxis. For people prone to severe allergic reactions, eating even the tiniest trace of the offending food may be enough to cause anaphylaxis.

Some experts believe that certain food allergies are more delayed in their onset, though this theory is controversial. Such allergies may cause gastrointestinal symptoms, rash or headache over days or weeks, making it difficult to trace your reaction to a particular food.

Symptoms of Food Allergy

- running nose, sneezing
- itchy eyes, mouth or face
- wheezing or coughing or dry throat
- rashes or hives or eczema
- nausea, vomiting, diarrhea
- abdominal pain

Symptoms of Anaphylaxis

- rash
- swelling of the throat and mouth
- labored breathing
- sudden drop in blood pressure
- dizziness
- rapid pulse
- loss of consciousness

Who's at Risk?

Children are ten times more likely to have a food allergy than adults.[6] Children of parents (one or both parents) who have food allergies are also more susceptible, as are infants of women who smoke during pregnancy. Children with other atopic diseases, such as eczema or asthma or airborne allergies (dust, pollen), are also at high risk of developing a food allergy.

Diagnosing Food Allergies

In combination with a patient's history and his or her diet and symptom diary, a doctor may use one of the following tests to identify food allergies:

- *Skin testing* This involves scratching with a needle a small amount of the food into the skin. Swelling or redness indicates an allergy. Skin testing cannot be used in extremely allergic people who have a history of anaphylactic reactions. This testing is not reliable for delayed food allergies.

- *RAST blood test* (radioallergosorbent tests) and *ELISA blood test* (enzyme-linked immunosorbent assay) Both these tests measure the presence of food-specific IgE antibodies. They are expensive, and, unlike skin testing, results are not available immediately. Blood tests are not reliable for delayed food allergies.

- *Controlled food challenge* In this test, various foods and the suspected allergen are placed in opaque capsules, the patient is asked to swallow the capsules one at a time and is watched to see if a reaction occurs. In a true food challenge, neither the doctor nor the patient knows which capsule contains the allergen. This is considered the gold standard of allergy testing.

Conventional Treatment

Desensitization or allergy shots may be recommended for some immediate-type food allergies. Antihistamines (e.g., Benadryl®) may help reduce or prevent allergic symptoms by blocking the release of histamine by the immune system. Some topical creams and ointments may help soothe skin symptoms.

Injectable epinephrine is required to treat an anaphylactic reaction. This is a synthetic version of the naturally occurring hormone adrenaline that is injected directly into a thigh muscle or vein. It acts to constrict blood vessels, reversing throat swelling and improving breathing. Individuals with a severe allergy should wear a medic alert bracelet and carry an injectable epinephrine kit with them at all times.

Managing Food Allergies

Dietary Strategies

The Elimination/Challenge Diet

If you are having difficulty identifying which foods are causing you grief, use the elimination diet to pinpoint your trigger foods. It may be a short-term hassle, but it is worth the effort. This process should help you decide what foods to avoid and what foods you can continue to enjoy.

The purpose of this diet is to demonstrate relief of symptoms upon removal of a given food item and recurrence of symptoms upon its reintroduction (elimination/challenge testing). You might consider enlisting the help of a registered dietitian to help you follow this diet.

Because milk, soybeans, eggs, wheat, peanuts, nuts, shellfish and corn are the main culprits of the majority of food allergies, these foods are usually not included in the starting diet. Make sure that these foods are not in other foods you eat. For example, egg or milk may be in mayonnaise or salad dressings. Stay on this elimination diet for 10 to 14 days.

During this period, keep a food and symptom diary. Record everything you eat, amounts eaten and what time you ate the food or meal. Document any symptoms, the time of day you started to feel the symptom and the duration of time you felt the symptom. You might want to grade your symptoms: 1 = mild, 2 = moderate, 3 = severe. If your symptoms do not subside, eliminate additional foods until your symptoms stop.

Once your symptoms disappear, suspect foods are reintroduced to the basic diet until symptoms reappear. Do this gradually, introducing the foods one at a time. Use the following procedure for testing foods:

Day 1: Introduce the food in the morning, at or after breakfast. If you do not experience symptoms, try the food again in the afternoon or with dinner.

Day 2: Do not eat any of the test food. Follow your elimination diet. If you do not experience a reaction today, the food is considered safe and can be included in your diet.

Day 3: If no symptoms occur, try the next food on your list, according to the above schedule.

Food Avoidance

Once a food allergy is diagnosed, eliminating the food from the diet is the most effective treatment. If allergy testing or an elimination/challenge diet reveals that you need to avoid certain foods, consult a registered dietitian in your community (**www.dietitians.ca**) to plan a healthy diet that is nutritionally complete. A dietitian can teach you how to read food labels for hidden ingredients and avoid restaurant-prepared foods that may contain ingredients that trigger reactions. It is especially important for parents and caregivers to learn how to protect children from foods they are allergic to, especially if the food causes an anaphylactic reaction.

Nutrition Strategy Checklist for Food Allergies

☐ Elimination/challenge diet

☐ Avoidance of certain foods

☐ Vitamin and/or mineral supplements as required

Recommended Resources

www.foodallergy.org
The Food Allergy and Anaphylaxis Network

www.ific.health.org
International Food Information Council
1100 Connecticut Avenue NW, Suite 430
Washington, DC, USA 20036
Tel: 202-296-6540
Fax: 202-296-6547
E-mail: foodinfo@ific.org

www.niaid.nih.gov
National Institute of Allergy and Infectious Diseases
Office of Communications and Public Liaison
Building 31, Room 7A-50
31 Center Drive MSC 2520
Bethesda, MD, USA 20892-2520

www.nin.ca
National Institute of Nutrition
265 Carling Avenue, Suite 302
Ottawa, ON, Canada K1S 2E1
Tel: 613-235-3355
Fax: 613-235-7032

Gallstones

Nearly one in ten people have gallstones, but many will never experience symptoms or need medical treatment.[1] However, gallstones may travel out of the gallbladder and into the digestive system, where they create a blockage that can lead to inflammation and intense pain. If left untreat-ed, complications caused by gallstone obstructions can be serious, even fatal.

The gallbladder's main job is to store bile produced by the liver from cholesterol. Bile is necessary for digestion and assists in the absorption of dietary fat, fat-soluble vitamins and minerals such as iron and calcium. Bile flows from the liver through a series of ducts to the gallbladder, where it is stored until needed for digestion. When food enters the digestive tract, the gallbladder contracts and releases bile into the small intestine to assist with digestion and absorption.

What Causes Gallstones?

Bile contains large amounts of cholesterol, which normally remains in a liquid form. However, when bile contains more cholesterol than normal, the cholesterol changes into a sludgy substance that collects in the gallbladder. Eventually, this sludge becomes hard deposits called gallstones. Occasionally, gallstones can be formed from calcium or bile salts that accumulate in the gallbladder, but most often they are cholesterol based. Gallstones can range in size from smaller than a pinhead to as much as 3 inches (7.5 cm) in diameter.

When gallstones form in the gallbladder, the condition is known as *cholelithiasis*. These stones normally don't cause any symptoms, especially if they remain in the gallbladder. Gallstones may also be passed from the gallbladder into the bile ducts, which is a condition known as *choledocholithiasis*. The stones may then travel into the small intestine without ever causing symptoms.

If gallstones become trapped in the bile ducts, causing a blockage or obstruction, symptoms will occur. A persistent obstruction will cause inflammation of the gallbladder (*acute cholecystitis*) or the pancreas (*pancreatitis*). The blockage may also cause a back-up of bile, which can result in liver damage. In rare cases, large gallstones may erode the wall of the gallbladder and enter the intestine, where they cause an obstruction called a *gallstone ileus*.

Symptoms

Fortunately, nearly 80 percent of all gallstones cause no symptoms at all.[2] Gallstones that temporarily block the bile ducts will cause occasional, minor attacks of pain. These attacks are usually brief and infrequent, occurring weeks, months or even years apart. You may also feel bloated, full, gassy and nauseated, especially after eating fried or fatty foods. It is very easy to confuse gallstone symptoms with those of indigestion.

If the gallstones are fully obstructing the bile ducts and causing an inflammation of the gallbladder, the symptoms will become much more acute. You will feel severe, recurrent pain that is focused beneath the right lower rib cage. This is one of the most reliable symptoms of gallbladder disease and often develops between midnight and 3 a.m. The pain may last from 30 minutes to several hours and may be accompanied by nausea and vomiting. Over time, the pain can radiate to the back or right shoulder blade. As the condition worsens, your urine becomes tea- or coffee-colored. Fever, chills and jaundice may also develop.

Who's at Risk?

- *Females* Gallstones are twice as common in women as they are in men. The female sex hormone estrogen stimulates the liver to remove greater amounts of cholesterol from the blood, which then accumulates in the gallbladder. Pregnancy, oral contraceptives and hormone therapy are also associated with higher estrogen levels and increased cholesterol-containing bile.

- *Older adults* Approximately 25 to 30 percent of women and 10 to 15 percent of men develop gallstones by the age of 70.[3]

- *Family history* Individuals with family members who have had gallstones are at higher risk of developing the condition.

- *Overweight individuals* Even a small weight gain can raise the cholesterol levels in the bile and cause the gallbladder to contract and empty less frequently. As a result, the bile becomes more concentrated, creating ideal conditions for gallstones. However, you should be careful in your attempts to lose weight. Rapid weight-loss, low-calorie diets will also upset your bile chemistry and encourage gallstone development.

- *People who don't exercise regularly.*

- Individuals who eat a *high-fat, high-sugar diet.*

Conventional Treatment

People who experience occasional gallbladder pain can reduce or prevent the number of pain attacks by following a diet that limits or eliminates fatty foods.

If pain continues, despite the dietary changes, surgery may be required to remove the gallbladder. A procedure called a *cholecystectomy* involves inserting a miniaturized video camera (laparoscope) and specialized surgical instruments into your abdomen through small incisions made in the abdominal wall. The gallbladder is completely removed using video monitoring. Occasionally, conventional abdominal surgery may be necessary. The removal of your gallbladder has little effect on one's overall health and imposes no dietary restrictions. You may find that you have more frequent bowel movements and looser stools once the surgery is complete.

When surgery is inadvisable, your doctor may recommend dissolving the gallstones with oral doses of bile salts. However, this takes months to produce results and the stones may recur once you stop taking the drug. Dissolving the stones with methyl-tert-butyl ether or fragmenting them with sonic shock waves are also techniques that have been used with varying degrees of effectiveness.

Preventing and Managing Gallstones

The strategies below are intended to prevent the formation of gallstones, or reduce the risk of "silent" gallstones becoming symptomatic. While many of the recommendations are healthy for all individuals, it is important to seek medical attention if you have gallbladder pain. Using alternative therapies to postpone surgery for symptomatic gallstones can result in rupture of the gallbladder or other serious complications. If gallbladder pain is only occasional, the following strategies may help but medical supervision is necessary.

Dietary Strategies

Meal Frequency

It is important to eat meals at regular intervals throughout the day. Skipping meals or fasting causes the gallbladder to contract less, which concentrates bile and may encourage stones to form.

Saturated Fat and Cholesterol

Reducing your intake of animal fat and dietary cholesterol can change the composition of bile, making gallstone formation less likely.[4,5] One study found that a diet high in saturated fat increased the risk of gallstones in men and women threefold.[6] Choose lean cuts of meat, poultry breast, and low-fat dairy products. Avoid processed foods that contain hydrogenated vegetable oils (another form of saturated fat). Choose a margarine made with nonhydrogenated oil. Use olive, canola, walnut and flaxseed oils in cooking, since these contain mainly monounsaturated or polyunsaturated fats (they contain very little saturated fat).

Health Canada recommends consuming no more than 300 milligrams of cholesterol each day. Choosing animal foods that are lower in saturated fat will help you to reduce dietary cholesterol intake. Other cholesterol-rich foods are egg yolks, shrimp and liver (see page 22, Chapter 3, for a list of cholesterol-containing foods).

While lower-fat diets may help prevent gallstones, some fat is necessary for the proper functioning of the gallbladder. Scientists have determined that 10 grams of fat (2 1/2 teaspoons of oil) should be consumed at each meal to ensure efficient gallbladder emptying of bile.[7] Very low fat intakes can decrease gallbladder contractions, encouraging the formation of gallstones.

Weight Control

Diets based on a very low calorie intake (800 calories per day or less) that cause rapid weight loss substantially increase the risk of gallstones. Studies find that up to 25 percent of obese people on such diets develop gallstones.[8-10] Dieting causes a shift in the balance of bile acids and cholesterol in the bile, favoring a cholesterol-rich bile. Fasting, going for long periods without eating, and very low fat intakes all encourage cholesterol to accumulate in the bile.

Obesity is a risk factor for the development of gallstones, and weight loss is an important prevention strategy. Diets that promote gradual weight loss (1200 to 1800 calories per day) and that provide some fat at each meal will lessen the risk of gallstones. As well, achieving a slow, steady weight loss will reduce the risk of weight regain. See page 442, Obesity and Weight Loss, for strategies for safe weight loss. Research has found that weight cycling among women increases the risk of gallstones requiring surgery.[11]

Physical activity may play an important role in the prevention of gallstones and should be a component of a weight-loss program. Harvard researchers found that 34 percent of symptomatic gallstone cases in men could be prevented by increasing exercise to 30 minutes of aerobic exercise (brisk walking, jogging, biking, stair climbing) five times per week.[12]

Dietary Fiber

A number of studies have revealed that people who eat high-fiber diets have a lower risk of gallstones.[13-15] Once fiber reaches the intestinal tract, it binds to cholesterol and a bile acid called deoxycholic acid, causing their removal from the body. Both cholesterol and deoxycholic acid contribute to gallstone formation.

Gradually increase your fiber intake to 25 to 35 grams per day (see page 3, Chapter 1). Foods rich in soluble fiber may be the most beneficial because of their cholesterol-binding properties. Oatmeal, oat bran, psyllium-enriched breakfast cereals, legumes, citrus fruit, apples and carrots are good sources of soluble fiber. Be sure to drink at least eight glasses of fluid per day to help fiber work properly.

Simple Sugars

Diets high in refined sugars have been linked to gallstones. It's thought that simple sugars can influence the composition of bile by altering the metabolism of fat in the body. Many sweets, such as muffins, pastries, cookies and cakes, are also high in fat—another risk factor for gallstones. Minimize your consumption of table sugar, syrups, soft drinks, fruit drinks, candy and other sweets.

Caffeine

According to a Harvard University study, drinking coffee may protect you from developing symptomatic gallstones.[16] Among 46,000 men, those who consumed two to three cups of coffee per day had a 40 percent lower risk of gallstones compared with men who were not regular coffee drinkers. And the risk was slightly less for men who drank four or more cups per day.

Animal studies show that caffeine causes the gallbladder to contract, which can help flush out cholesterol-rich bile. While coffee may reduce the risk, people who already have gallstones should avoid it, since caffeine can aggravate symptoms.

Vitamins and Minerals

Vitamin C

Low vitamin C intakes may increase the risk of gallstones by causing cholesterol to concentrate in the bile. Without vitamin C, the enzyme that breaks down cholesterol into bile acids cannot work efficiently. Studies have also found that people with gallstones tend to have reduced levels of vitamin C in their blood.[17,18] Swedish researchers gave 16 gallstone patients a 500 milligram vitamin C supplement daily for two weeks before surgery and found that the vitamin did influence the composition of the bile.[19]

The daily requirement for vitamin C is 75 and 90 milligrams for women and men respectively (smokers need an additional 35 milligrams). The best food sources include citrus fruit, citrus juices, cantaloupe, kiwi, mango, strawberries, broccoli, Brussels sprouts, cauliflower, red pepper and tomato juice. To supplement, take 500 milligrams of Ester C once daily.

Calcium

Like dietary fiber, calcium binds to deoxycholic acid, the bile acid that tends to form gallstones, and causes this acid's excretion from the body. This means that deoxycholic acid cannot be reabsorbed into the bloodstream and contribute to gallstone formation. One study conducted among 860 men found that those who consumed the most calcium had a 70 percent lower risk of gallstone development compared with those who consumed the least.[20]

The recommended dietary allowance (RDA) is 1000 to 1200 milligrams (see page 43, Chapter 4). Calcium-rich foods include milk, yogurt, cheese, fortified soy and rice beverages, fortified orange juice, tofu, salmon (with bones), kale, bok choy, broccoli and Swiss chard. If you take calcium supplements, buy calcium citrate with vitamin D and magnesium added.

Herbal Remedies

Milk Thistle (*Silybum marianum*)

This herb's active ingredients, known collectively as silymarin, support and enhance liver function. One study found that the herb improved the liquidity of the bile.[21] Whether this can actually prevent the development of gallstones has not been examined.

If you decide to take milk thistle, buy a product that's standardized to 70 percent silymarin. Take 200 milligrams two or three times daily. Milk thistle is very safe in the recommended doses (see page 115, Chapter 7). Use milk thistle with caution if you are allergic to plants in the Asteracease/Compositae family (ragweed, daisy, marigold and chrysanthemum).

Nutrition Strategy Checklist for Gallstones

☐ Eat at regular intervals

☐ Limit animal fat and cholesterol

☐ Avoid very low calorie diets

☐ Exercise

☐ Dietary fiber

☐ Limit sugar

☐ Caffeine

☐ Vitamin C

☐ Calcium

☐ Milk thistle

Recommended Resources

www.gastro.org
American Gastroenterological Association
7910 Woodmont Avenue, Suite 700
Bethesda, MD, USA 20814
Tel: 301-654-2055
Fax: 301-654-5920

www.mayoclinic.com
Mayo Foundation for Medical Education and Research

www.niddk.nih.gov/health/digesst/pubs/gallstns/gallstns.htm
National Digestive Diseases Information Clearinghouse
2 Information Way
Bethesda, MD, USA 20892-3570
Tel: 301-654-3810

Glaucoma

Known as the "sneak thief of sight," glaucoma develops slowly and painlessly, giving not a hint of its presence until the optic nerve is irreversibly damaged and vision loss has occurred. Glaucoma is the second leading cause of blindness in the world. Glaucoma refers to a group of eye diseases that cause damage to the optic nerve. Usually, the damage results from increased pressure within the eye, a condition referred to as elevated *intraocular pressure* (IOP).

What Causes Glaucoma?

In a healthy eye, the front part of the eyeball (anterior chamber) is filled with a thin, clear fluid called the aqueous humor. This fluid circulates through the eye, nourishing eye tissues and maintaining the eye shape. In order to keep the fluid fresh and the internal pressure constant, the eye produces a continuous supply of aqueous humor. Once the aqueous humor has circulated through the eye tissues, it leaves the anterior chamber through a drainage angle located where the iris and cornea meet. It then flows out of the eye through drainage channels called the trabecular meshwork.

This drainage system functions to prevent a dangerous build-up of pressure within the eye. However, when the aqueous humor is prevented from draining properly, the fluid backs up into the anterior chamber, raising the internal eye pressure. This increased pressure slowly damages the optic nerve fibers, causing a gradual loss of peripheral vision and eventual blindness.

The drainage system in the eye can malfunction in a number of different ways, each one resulting in a different form of glaucoma.

- *Primary open-angle glaucoma* accounts for 90 percent of all cases. Although the drainage angle in the eye is open and functional, the fluid drains out through the trabecular meshwork much too slowly. Pressure inside the eye gradually rises as the fluid accumulates, resulting in a slow, progressive vision loss. Vision loss begins at the sides or edges of your field of vision and gradually spreads until you are completely blind. The causes are unknown.

- *Closed-angle glaucoma* occurs when the drainage angle between the iris and the cornea is narrowed or blocked. The aqueous humor can't reach the angle and is prevented from leaving the eye, causing a sudden and intense build-up of pressure. Attacks usually occur only in one eye and are extremely painful. Blockage of the drainage angle can be triggered by anything that causes the pupil of the eye to dilate. Dim lighting, emotional stress, eye drops given before an eye examination and certain medications have been known to trigger these attacks. Closed-angle glaucoma is considered to be a medical emergency because it can destroy the optic nerve very quickly and cause blindness within a few days.

- *Congenital glaucoma* occurs in children who are born with a defect in the drainage angle that slows the normal drainage of the aqueous humor.

- *Secondary glaucoma* develops as a complication of other medical conditions such as:

- eye injuries
- eye surgery
- cataracts
- eye tumors
- eye inflammation
- diabetes
- corticosteroid drugs

People with normal IOP have also been known to develop glaucoma. The cause of glaucoma is not yet fully understood. It cannot be prevented, and the damage it causes cannot be reversed. Regular, complete eye examinations are the best way to monitor changes in your eyesight. Early detection and treatment is essential to prevent blindness. Eye examinations should be scheduled every two to four years between the ages of 40 and 60 and every one to two years for individuals over 65 or those with risk factors for glaucoma.

Symptoms

Open-angle glaucoma may not cause any symptoms until irreversible damage has been done. It tends to affect both eyes, though symptoms may appear in only one eye at first. These symptoms include

- gradual vision loss beginning at the sides or edges of your field of vision
- difficulty focusing on close work
- mild headaches
- visual disturbances, such as difficulty adjusting to darkness or seeing a rainbow-colored halo around electric lights
- frequent need to change prescription glasses

Early warning signs of closed-angle glaucoma include

- recurrent blurry vision
- pain around the eyes after watching TV or leaving a darkened room

- morning headaches
- sudden and severe pain in the eye and head
- rapid loss of vision
- nausea and vomiting
- eyelid swells
- eye becomes watery and red
- pupil dilates and does not respond to bright light in a normal manner

Who's at Risk?

You are at greater risk of glaucoma if you

- are over 40 years of age
- are of African ancestry (compared with Caucasians, black people are three to four times more likely to get glaucoma, six times more likely to suffer permanent blindness and will experience the onset of the disease ten years earlier)
- have an immediate relative with glaucoma
- have diabetes
- have extreme nearsightedness, high blood pressure or heart disease
- have suffered an eye injury, inflammation and abnormally high intraocular pressure
- use oral corticosteroids for a long period

Conventional Treatment

Glaucoma is a chronic disease and must be treated for a lifetime. Treatment is more successful if it is started early and maintained regularly. Treatments vary from person to person and can include

- *Beta-blockers* in eye drops to decrease fluid production
- *Miotic medications* to constrict the pupil; as the pupil constricts, it pulls the iris away from

the drainage angle and increases fluid drainage

- *Carbonic anhydrase inhibitors* or *alpha-2-adrenergic agonists* to decrease the production of aqueous humor
- *Prostaglandins*, hormone-like substances produced by your body, to increase fluid outflow
- *Laser therapy* to cut a hole in the iris to increase drainage (glaucoma drugs will still be needed after the surgery as the effects are not permanent)
- *Conventional surgery* to create a new opening for fluid to drain out; usually done after medication and laser therapy have failed to solve the problem
- *Regular exercise* to reduce eye pressure and modify associated risk factors, such as diabetes and high blood pressure
- *Avoiding head-down or inverted positions* (common in yoga or recreational exercises) because of the risk of increasing IOP
- *Relaxation* and *biofeedback* to help control cases of open-angle glaucoma

Preventing and Managing Glaucoma

Dietary Strategies

Weight Control

Achieving and maintaining a healthy weight may help prevent or delay glaucoma. Research suggests that glaucoma is more likely to develop in individuals with a high body mass index (BMI).[1] To determine whether or not you are at an acceptable weight, turn to page 439, Obesity and Weight Loss, to calculate your BMI. A BMI greater than 25 indicates overweight, and a BMI greater than 27 is defined as obese.

People who are overweight are more susceptible to diabetes and high blood pressure, two factors that increase the risk of glaucoma. If you have hypertension, losing weight is one of the most effective ways to lower blood pressure and intraocular pressure. See page 352, High Blood Pressure, for specific nutrition recommendations.

Caffeine, Alcohol and Fluids

If you have glaucoma, avoid caffeine intake. Caffeine can elevate intraocular pressure and reduce blood flow to the retina. Sources of caffeine include coffee, tea, iced tea, chocolate, soft drinks and certain medications (see page 82, Chapter 5, for a list of the caffeine content of selected items). Switch to decaffeinated coffee and tea, herbal teas or malt beverages.

Women should drink no more than one alcoholic beverage per day and men no more than two alcoholic beverages per day (to a limit of nine per week). Moderate consumption of alcohol can raise levels of HDL (good) cholesterol, which may help protect from glaucoma. However, too much alcohol damages artery walls and increases the risk of developing high blood pressure.

Drink fluids (water, juices, milk) in small amounts throughout the day. Consuming large quantities of water over a short time can elevate intraocular pressure.

Vitamins and Minerals

B Vitamins

There is some evidence to support taking a B vitamin supplement to prevent or delay the damage caused by glaucoma. Italian researchers gave 30 glaucoma patients a nutritional supplement containing the family of B vitamins, vitamin E and DHA, a fatty acid found in oily fish.[2] After three months of treatment, there were significant improvements in the visual field.

Vitamin B12 may be particularly important in glaucoma.[3] In the body, B12 works to maintain healthy nerve function and, as such, it may protect the optical nerve fiber from damage. Vitamin B12 is found exclusively in animal foods such as meat, poultry, eggs and dairy products. Fortified soy and rice beverages also contain B12. Adults over 50 should be meeting their daily B12 requirements from fortified foods or a supplement, since the vitamin is absorbed from food less efficiently as we age.

To supplement, take a high-potency multivitamin and mineral pill or a B complex supplement. Both formulas will supply anywhere from 25 to 100 micrograms of vitamin B12 as well as all the other B vitamins.

Vitamin C

This nutrient appears to play an important role in the healing process after glaucoma surgery. Unlike surgery of other parts of the body, successful glaucoma surgery depends on the incomplete healing of the surgical wound. Laboratory tests suggest that the high level of vitamin C normally present in the aqueous humor inhibits wound healing and contributes to successful surgery outcomes.[4,5]

Vitamin C's role as an antioxidant may also serve to protect from optic nerve damage. While the main cause of glaucoma is elevated intraocular pressure, some experts believe that free radical damage contributes to glaucoma by harming the optic nerve, especially in people who have normal eye pressure.

To ensure that you meet your daily vitamin C requirements (see page 37, Chapter 4), include the following foods regularly in your diet: citrus fruit, citrus juices, cantaloupe, kiwi, mango, strawberries, broccoli, Brussels sprouts, cauliflower, red pepper and tomato juice. To supplement, take 500 milligrams of Ester C once daily.

Vitamin E

Like vitamin C, vitamin E may be important for successful glaucoma surgery. Failure of glaucoma surgery is mostly due to scar formation from fibroblasts. Preliminary research in the laboratory found that vitamin E was able to prevent scar formation in human eye tissue.[6] Vitamin E is also an antioxidant and may act to protect the optic nerve from free radical damage.

The best food sources of vitamin E include wheat germ, nuts, seeds, vegetable oils, whole grains and kale. To supplement, take 200 to 800 international units (IU) of natural source vitamin E. Choose a "mixed" vitamin E supplement if possible.

Magnesium

One type of drug used for glaucoma is a calcium channel blocker, which prevents calcium from entering cells and helps maintain healthy blood vessels. Magnesium is a natural calcium channel blocker, though much less powerful than drugs. A small study from Switzerland found that 121 milligrams of magnesium taken twice daily improved visual field and peripheral circulation in glaucoma patients.[7]

The best sources of magnesium include nuts, seeds, legumes, prunes, whole grains, leafy green vegetables, Brewer's yeast, cheddar cheese and shrimp. If you decide to supplement your diet and you don't take supplemental calcium with magnesium, buy a separate magnesium supplement made from magnesium citrate, aspartate, succinate, fumarte or gluconate. Taking more than 350 milligrams of magnesium in a supplement can cause diarrhea, nausea and stomach cramps.

Herbal Remedies

Bilberry *(Vaccinium myrtillus)*

This herbal remedy contains antioxidant compounds called anthocyanins that may help pre- serve eye health. The anthocyanins in bilberry are thought to improve blood flow in the tiny capillaries of the eye. Although no research has been conducted in people with glaucoma, a handful of well-controlled studies found that bilberry significantly improved eye health in people with diabetic eye complications.[8,9]

Buy a product standardized to 25 to 36 percent anthocyanins. Take 160 milligrams twice daily. For more information on bilberry, see Chapter 7.

Ginkgo Biloba

Ginkgo can increase blood flow to the eye and may be useful in glaucoma.[10] American researchers gave healthy individuals 40 milligrams of ginkgo three times daily for two days.[11] The herb was shown to significantly increase ocular blood flow. It also acts as an antioxidant and helps to thin the blood.

Choose a product standardized to 24 percent ginkgo flavone glycosides and 6 percent terpene lactones. The EGb 761 extract used in the scientific research is sold as Ginkoba® (Pharmaton® Natural Health Products) in Canada and the United States. Take 40 milligrams three times daily. On rare occasions, ginkgo may cause gastrointestinal upset, headache or an allergic skin reaction. Ginkgo has the potential to enhance the effects of blood-thinning medications (warfarin, aspirin). If you're on blood thinners, let your doctor know if you start taking ginkgo.

Nutrition Strategy Checklist for Glaucoma

- ☐ Weight control
- ☐ Avoid caffeine
- ☐ Limit alcohol
- ☐ Vitamin B12
- ☐ Vitamin C
- ☐ Vitamin E
- ☐ Magnesium
- ☐ Bilberry
- ☐ Ginkgo biloba

Recommended Resources

www.eyenet.org
American Academy of Ophthalmology
655 Beach Street
San Francisco, CA, USA 94109-7424
Tel: 415-561-8500

www.cnib.ca
**Canadian National Institute for the Blind
(CNIB)**
National Communications
1929 Bayview Avenue
Toronto, ON, Canada M4G 3E8
Tel: 416-480-7644
Fax: 416-480-7019

www.eyesite.ca
The Canadian Ophthalmological Society
610-1525 Carling Avenue
Ottawa, ON, Canada K1Z 8R9

www.glaucoma-foundation.org/info
Glaucoma Foundation
33 Maiden Lane
New York, NY, USA 10038
Tel: 212-285-0080 or 1-800-452-8266

www.glaucoma.org
Glaucoma Research Foundation
200 Pine Street, Suite 200
San Francisco, CA, USA 94104
Tel: 415-986-3162 or 1-800-826-6693

www.nei.nih.gov
National Eye Institute
2020 Vision Place
Bethesda, MD, USA 20892-3655
Tel: 901-496-5248

Gout

Referred to throughout history as "the disease of kings," gout was once thought to be a disorder that affected only wealthy, old men—those privileged enough to afford rich foods and plenty of alcohol. Scientists now know that diet is only a contributing factor to this chronic condition. The real culprit behind the painful symptoms of gout is uric acid, a waste product that is formed naturally in the body.

Uric acid is formed when the body breaks down purines, naturally occurring substances found in the body. Purines are also present in many foods, including organ meats, dried peas, beans, herring, mackerel and trout. As the body breaks down cells and forms new ones, the bloodstream carries uric acid to the kidneys, where it is excreted as urine.

Gout develops when the body either makes too much uric acid or does not excrete it efficiently. As the level of uric acid rises above normal, crystals form and are deposited in the joints. These needle-sharp uric acid crystals inflame the joints, causing pain, redness, swelling and tenderness. The joint most commonly affected is the big toe, but gout can also affect the ankle, knee, foot, hand, wrist and elbow.

Gout attacks occur more often in the lower limbs and, typically, only one joint is affected. With proper treatment, attacks will usually last only three to ten days. More than half of the people who have a gout attack go on to experience another attack within a year. Over time, the attacks can become more frequent, last longer and may involve more than one joint.

Gout may become chronic, damaging tendons and restricting joint movement. Uric acid crystals may also form hard lumps, called tophi, under the skin. Tophi occur most often in the fingers and toes but can also develop under the skin around the ears, the elbows and in the kidney or urinary tract. If left untreated, tophi may break through the skin and discharge masses of crystals.

What Causes Gout?

A number of different factors contribute to the development of gout. Genetics, obesity, heavy alcohol and caffeine consumption and a purine-rich diet (see below) all have a role to play. Medical conditions and certain medications, especially diuretics, may interfere with the body's ability to produce or excrete uric acid efficiently and increase the risk of gout. Surgery, heart attacks, strokes, fatigue and stress have also been known to trigger gout attacks.

Symptoms

The onset of gout is often rapid and unexpected. Attacks frequently occur during the night and become progressively worse over time. The symptoms below are often more severe in people who develop the disease before the age of 30.

- acute, ongoing pain in one joint, usually the big toe (sometimes, even the weight of a sheet is unbearable)
- hot, red swollen skin and a feeling of tightness and pressure in the affected area
- feeling of stretching or tearing in the skin
- fever, chills and a general feeling of illness

Who's at Risk?

Women have lower levels of uric acid until after menopause, at which time their uric acid levels increase to equal those of men. For this reason, gout affects men four times more often than women. Men usually have their first gout attack between the ages of 30 and 50, while women don't usually develop any symptoms until they are between 50 and 70.[1]

Other people at higher risk of gout are those who have a family member with gout, overweight people, and people who consume excessive alcohol, coffee and purine-rich foods.

Conventional Treatment

Conventional treatment of gout may include

- *nonsteroidal anti-inflammatory drugs (NSAIDs)* to reduce pain, inflammation and swelling of an acute attack
- *medications such as allopurinol* to slow the production and speed up the elimination of uric acid
- *colchicine* to treat acute gout attacks (can cause side effects, such as nausea, vomiting and diarrhea)
- *corticosteroid injections* to treat severe pain and inflammation
- *applying ice packs* to the affected joint to help decrease inflammation

Preventing and Managing Gout

Some simple lifestyle changes may prevent recurrent attacks of gout:

1. *Maintain a healthy weight.* Weight loss will lessen the pressure on affected joints and may decrease levels of uric acid.
2. *Exercise* may help strengthen your joints and keep your weight under control.
3. *Avoid foods rich in purines,* such as certain animal foods (see below).
4. *Limit the amount of alcohol you drink.* Alcohol interferes with the excretion of uric acid, leading to a build-up of uric acid.
5. *Drink lots of fluids* to dilute the levels of uric acid in your blood.

Dietary Strategies

Fluids

Drinking plenty of fluids (water) helps to dilute uric acid in the urine, which in turn can help prevent the formation of kidney stones made from uric acid. Drink 2 to 3 liters (8 to 12 cups) of fluid each day. Water, herbal teas, vegetable juice, milk, unsweetened fruit juices and soup all contribute to your daily fluid intake. Limit your consumption of fruit juice if weight loss is required. Other preventative measures you can take in your daily diet are outlined below.

Weight Control

People who are overweight are more susceptible to developing gout. People with gout who are overweight have higher blood uric acid levels and suffer from gout attacks more frequently. Studies show that losing weight can reduce gout symptoms and the number of monthly attacks.[2-5] Weight loss helps to lower elevated levels of blood triglycerides (elevated levels are common in people with gout).

To determine if you are at a healthy weight, refer to page 439, Obesity and Weight Loss, to calculate your body mass index (BMI). A BMI greater than 25 indicates overweight, and a BMI over 27 is defined as obese. If you determine your BMI is greater than 25, use the strategies outlined on page 442, Obesity and Weight Loss, to promote safe, gradual weight loss.

Avoid very-low-calorie diets or high-protein weight-loss diets (e.g., Atkins's Diet, Protein Power), since these encourage the formation of ketones, metabolic byproducts that hamper the body's ability to excrete uric acid. High-protein diets can also markedly increase the risk of kidney stones in people with gout. Eating too much protein makes the urine more acidic, which encourages the formation of uric acid crystals.

Purine-Rich Foods

Certain foods contribute to the overproduction of uric acid in the body. By limiting the intake of these foods, it is possible to keep uric acid levels low. A diet low in purine-containing foods should be combined with medication to prevent attacks of gout. Purines occur mainly in animal foods, with the exception of dairy products and eggs, which do not contain purines. Use the following guidelines to restrict purine intake:[6]

Food	Recommended	Allowed in Moderate Amounts
Beverages	Low-fat milk Tea, herbal tea Vegetable/fruit juices	Alcohol with permission of doctor; No more than two drinks/day. *Avoid* beer and alcohol-free beer.
Breads, Cereals and Grains	White bread Potatoes Pasta, rice	Whole-grain breads and cereals; oatmeal; wheat germ; wheat bran
Meats and Alternatives	Eggs, low-fat cheese	Fish, beef, lamb, veal, shellfish; legumes, nut butters; soups made with beef stock, meat gravies *Avoid* liver, kidney, sweetbreads, anchovies, sardines, herring, mackerel, trout, scallops, game.
Vegetables	All except those on moderate list	Mushrooms, green peas, spinach, asparagus, cauliflower
Miscellaneous	Herbs and spices	Baker's yeast, Brewer's yeast

Alcohol and Caffeine

Alcohol not only contains purines but also interferes with the body's excretion of uric acid.[7] Studies have found that beer-drinking in particular increases the risk because of beer's high-purine content.[8-11] Heavy drinking also increases body weight and blood triglycerides, two factors implicated in gout. Speak to your doctor about the use of alcohol; moderate, infrequent drinking will likely not increase the chances of a gout attack.

Caffeinated beverages can also increase the production of uric acid and impair its removal from the body. Sources of caffeine include coffee, tea, iced tea, chocolate, soft drinks and certain medications (see page 82, Chapter 5, for a list of the caffeine content of selected items). Switch to decaffeinated coffee and tea, herbal teas or malt beverages.

Essential Fatty Acids

Some research suggests that elevated levels of inflammatory compounds called leukotrienes may be involved in gout.[12,13] Leukotrienes belong to a family of compounds called eicosanoids. The type of fat you eat will determine what kind of eicosanoids your body produces. For instance, linoleic acid from omega-6 oils (corn, sunflower, safflower oils) is used to synthesize "unfriendly" eicosanoids that cause inflammation and pain. Omega-3 oils (canola, walnut, flaxseed oils) produce "friendly" eicosanoids that tend to decrease inflammation. Both types of eicosanoids are produced using the same pathway in the body. This means that if you eat a diet that contains primarily omega-6 oils, the unfriendly eicosanoids win out. If most of your fat is rich in omega-3 oils, more friendly, anti-inflammatory eicosanoids will be formed. Eicosanoids derived from omega-3 fats are thought to help prevent heart disease, ease symptoms of rheumatoid arthritis and influence brain function.

Aim to include 2 tablespoons (30 ml) of the following oils in your daily diet: flaxseed, walnut, canola, and/or Udo's Choice Ultimate Oil Blend (Udo's oil is available in health food stores). With the exception of canola oil, these oils should not be used for high-heat cooking. Instead, use them for salad dressings or add them to hot foods after cooking.

Fish is another source of omega-3 fat. While studies have not evaluated the effect of fish oils in people with gout, these oils do show promise in relieving rheumatoid arthritis. Fish oils have also been shown to lower blood triglyceride levels. Include fish in your diet three times per week. Fish oil supplements are also available (see page 128, Chapter 8).

Cherries and Celery Juice

Cherries have long been used as a folk remedy for gout. One study did find that eating half a pound of cherries each day reduced uric acid levels and gout attacks. Cherries contain compounds called anthocyanidins, which have anti-inflammatory properties in the body.

Celery juice is another folk remedy that is used widely in Australia. If you are experiencing a gout attack, consider drinking celery juice throughout the day.

Vitamins and Minerals

Vitamin B12

If you take the medication colchicine for gout, consider adding a B12 supplement to your daily nutrition regime. This drug is known to impair the body's ability to absorb B12. Vitamin B12 is found exclusively in animal foods such as meat, poultry, eggs and dairy products. With the exception of eggs and dairy, these foods should be limited because of their purine content. Fortified soy and rice beverages also contain B12.

To supplement, take a high-potency multivitamin and mineral pill or a B complex supplement. Both formulas will supply anywhere from 25 to 100 micrograms of vitamin B12 as well as all the other B vitamins.

Herbal Remedies
Devil's Claw (*Harpagophytum procumbens*)

Based on a few studies conducted in people with rheumatoid arthritis, devil's claw is sometimes recommended for gout. Two studies found that the herb relieved pain and increased mobility in arthritis sufferers, while two others found only slight improvement. Devil's claw may work by decreasing inflammation.[14]

The recommended dose is 750 milligrams taken three times daily. Buy an extract standardized to 3 percent iridoid glycosides. People with ulcers should not use the herb. Its safety has not been established in people with liver or kidney disease.

Nutrition Strategy Checklist for Gout

☐ Fluids
☐ Weight control
☐ Limit purine-rich foods
☐ Avoid alcohol
☐ Avoid caffeine
☐ Essential fatty acids
☐ Fish
☐ Cherries
☐ Celery juice
☐ Devil's claw

Recommended Resources

www.rheumatology.org
American College of Rheumatology
1800 Century Place, Suite 250
Atlanta, GA, USA 30345
Tel: 404-633-3777
Fax: 404-633-1870

www.arthritis.ca
The Arthritis Society
393 University Avenue, Suite 1700
Toronto, ON, Canada M5G 1E6
Tel: 416-979-7228
Fax: 416-979-8366
E-mail: info@arthritis.ca

www.nih.gov.niams/healthinfo/
National Institute of Arthritis and Musculoskeletal and Skin Diseases Information Clearinghouse
National Institutes of Health
1 AMS Circle
Bethesda, MD, USA 20892-3675
Tel: 301-495-4484 or 1-877-22-NIAMS (1-877-226-4267)
Fax: 301-718-6366

Gum Disease

Most people worry that cavities will cause tooth loss. However, very few adult teeth are lost because of cavities. Rather, gum disease is the leading cause of tooth decay. At least 90 percent of Canadians suffer from some form of gum disease, which could be avoided and controlled through good oral hygiene and regular visits to the dentist.[1] Unfortunately, less than half of all Canadians visit a dentist on a regular basis and fewer still practice daily brushing and flossing.

What Causes Gum Disease?

Gum disease in its early stages is commonly referred to as *gingivitis*. Gingivitis develops when a sticky film called plaque builds up on the teeth and irritates the gums. Plaque begins to form even within minutes after you brush your teeth. If left on the teeth for more than 72 hours, plaque hardens into tartar or calculus, a tough, discolored deposit that cannot be completely removed by brushing or flossing. As the bacteria accumulate on your teeth, they release toxins that irritate your oral tissues. The body responds by triggering inflammation, making your gums red and swollen. Tender gums that bleed easily are a common sign of gingivitis.

The advanced stage of gum disease is known as *periodontitis* or *periodontal disease*. Untreated gingivitis leads to a build-up of plaque and tartar along the gum line at the base of your teeth, an area known as the gingiva. Gradually, tartar extends below the gum line, causing the gums to pull away from the teeth. In the airless environment below the gums, bacteria flourish and pockets of infection form, slowly deepening as the disease progresses. Eventually, periodontitis can destroy the tissue and bone that keep your teeth in an upright position, causing them to loosen and fall out. Approximately 10 percent of affected adults have periodontal disease severe enough to cause tooth loss.[2]

Oral bacteria may do more than cause tooth loss. These bacteria can enter your bloodstream whenever you brush, floss or even chew. Preliminary studies have linked oral bacteria to blood clots and clogged arteries. Early results suggest that people with periodontal disease seem to be more susceptible to heart attack and stroke than those with healthy mouths. Oral bacteria may also influence blood-sugar levels in people with diabetes and may lead to pneumonia if inhaled by people with lung disease. These microbes have also been linked to osteoporosis and preterm births.

Gum disease usually develops as a result of inadequate brushing and flossing, but there are other conditions that can increase one's risk. Many women suffer from gingivitis during pregnancy, a response triggered primarily by hormonal changes. Deficiencies in certain vitamins, particularly vitamin C, are known to cause bleeding gums and mouth infections. Diabetes, Crohn's disease, leukemia, Down's syndrome and AIDS can all provoke periodontitis.

Symptoms

The warning signs of gum disease include

- red, swollen, tender gums that bleed easily
- recessed gums; gums that are pulled away from the teeth
- pus between the teeth and gums when you press your gums with a finger
- unpleasant taste in the mouth
- bad breath
- teeth that seem loose or change position
- a change in your bite or the way that dentures fit

Who's at Risk?

Some people are more susceptible than others to the bacteria that cause gum disease; this predisposition may be inherited. People who take medications that decrease saliva production (saliva helps wash plaque away from the teeth) or cause an overgrowth of gum tissue may stimulate plaque build-up. People who smoke cigarettes and drink alcohol are also at a higher risk for gum disease. People with medical conditions that reduce their immunity and make them prone to infection are also more susceptible to the disease.

Conventional Treatment

The best treatment for gum disease is prevention. Brush your teeth after every meal and floss daily to prevent build-up of harmful bacteria. Soft toothbrushes are best for removing plaque. Toothbrushes should be replaced as soon as the bristles become matted or splayed. Choose a toothpaste containing fluoride to help protect against plaque build-up. Even if you brush regularly, it's possible to miss areas. Consider using a disclosing agent (a harmless dye) to show you what areas you need to concentrate on. Regular dental visits and professional dental cleaning (scaling) are critical to remove tartar that has built up on the teeth.

Antibiotic therapy may be required to reduce the levels of oral bacteria. Surgery may be necessary in more advanced cases of periodontal disease to remove a section of the infected gum tissue and/or graft new bone to replace the bone that may be destroyed by the disease.

Preventing and Managing Gum Disease

Dietary Strategies

Omega-3 Fats

These special fatty acids found in oily fish, flaxseed oil, walnut oil and canola oil may reduce gum inflammation and may help treat bone destruction in periodontal disease. French researchers examined 105 patients, 78 of whom had periodontal disease, and found that compared with healthy individuals, those with bone loss had increased levels of omega-6 fatty acids in their blood and reduced levels of omega-3 fatty acids.[3] Another study found that fish oil supplements tended to reduce gingivitis in men who abstained from brushing their teeth for three weeks.[4]

Omega-3 fats are used to produce anti-inflammatory compounds in the body called prostaglandins. Omega-6 fats (found in corn, sunflower and safflower oils) are used to produce prostaglandins that cause inflammation and may be involved in periodontal disease. Both types of prostaglandins are produced using the same pathway in the body, so the type of fat you eat will determine which kind of prostaglandins your body produces. If you eat a diet that contains primarily omega-6 oils, the inflammatory compounds win out. If most of the fat you consume is rich in omega-3 oils, anti-inflammatory prostaglandins will be formed.

Aim to include 2 tablespoons (30 ml) of the following oils in your daily diet: flaxseed, walnut, canola, and/or Udo's Choice Ultimate Oil Blend (available in health food stores). With the exception of canola oil, these oils should not be used for high-heat cooking. Instead, use them for salad dressings or add them to hot foods after cooking.

Include fish in your diet three times per week. Fish oil supplements are also available (see page 128, Chapter 8).

Vitamins and Minerals

Vitamin C

The role of vitamin C in maintaining healthy teeth and gums is unchallenged. This vitamin helps form collagen, the supportive network on which bones and teeth are formed. It also helps maintain the integrity of blood vessels. Without adequate vitamin C, gums become inflamed and bleed easily around the teeth. And because the nutrient is important for a strong immune system, it can help reduce the risk of oral infections.

Studies find that people with periodontal disease have lower intakes of vitamin C: the less vitamin C consumed in the daily diet, the greater the risk of serious gum disease.[5-9] The recommended dietary allowance (RDA) for vitamin C is 75 and 90 milligrams for women and men respectively (smokers need an additional 35 milligrams). The best food sources include citrus fruit, citrus juices, cantaloupe, kiwi, mango, strawberries, broccoli, Brussels sprouts, cauliflower, red pepper and tomato juice. To supplement, take 500 milligrams of Ester C once or twice daily. The daily upper limit is 2000 milligrams.

Vitamin E

Scientists are beginning to explore the role of free radical damage and antioxidants in periodontal disease. Although little research has been done in this area, it is possible that vitamin E might protect from free radicals produced by white blood cells attracted to diseased gums.

The RDA for vitamin E is 22 international units (IU). The best food sources include wheat germ, nuts, seeds, vegetable oils, whole grains and kale. To supplement, take 200 to 800 IU of natural source vitamin E. Buy a "mixed" vitamin E supplement if possible. The daily upper limit is 1500 IU.

Calcium and Vitamin D

Since these two nutrients are so critical to bone health, it is not surprising that a lack of either can increase the risk of periodontal disease. Research has determined that calcium intake is associated with oral health.[10] A survey of Americans found that men and women with the lowest calcium intakes had the greatest risk of periodontal disease.[11] As dietary intake of calcium declined, the risk increased. Women with the lowest calcium consumption had a 54 percent higher risk of the disease.

It is especially important to be meeting your daily requirements for calcium and vitamin D to slow down bone loss.

The RDA for calcium is 1000 to 1200 milligrams; the best food sources are milk, yogurt, cheese, fortified soy and rice beverages, fortified orange juice, tofu, salmon (with bones), kale, bok choy, broccoli and Swiss chard. To supplement, take calcium citrate with vitamin D and magnesium added.

The daily adequate intake for vitamin D is 200 to 600 IU; best food sources include fluid milk, fortified soy and rice beverages, oily fish, egg yolks, butter and margarine. Your multivitamin and mineral supplement should provide 400 IU of vitamin D. For more information, see Chapter 4.

Other Natural Health Products

Coenzyme Q10 (CoQ10)

This supplement is known for its antioxidant ability and is thought by some experts to prevent or treat periodontal disease. Most of the studies on CoQ10 in dental health are published in a language other than English. In Japan, practitioners have used CoQ10 topically to improve periodontitis.[12] At this time, it is not clear whether oral supplements of CoQ10 can help gum disease, though it is possible that the antioxidant properties of CoQ10 may be beneficial.

CoQ10 is very safe. If you decide to supplement, buy a CoQ10 in an oil base (instead of dry-powder tablets or capsules) as these are more available to the body. Take 50 to 60 milligrams once daily. For more information on CoQ10, see page 123, Chapter 8.

Nutrition Strategy Checklist for Gum Disease

☐ Omega-3 fats   ☐ Calcium
☐ Vitamin C   ☐ Vitamin D
☐ Vitamin E   ☐ Coenzyme Q10

Recommended Resources

www.ada.org
American Dental Association
211 E Chicago Avenue
Chicago, IL, USA 60611
Tel: 312-440-2500
Fax: 312-440-2800

www.adha.org
American Dental Hygienists' Association
444 N Michigan Avenue, Suite 3400
Chicago, IL, USA 60611
Tel: 1-800-243-2342

www.cda-adc.ca/public/index.html
Canadian Dental Association
1815 Alta Vista
Ottawa, ON, Canada K1G 3Y6
Tel: 613-523-1770
Fax: 613-523-7736

www.mayoclinic.com
Mayo Foundation for Medical Education and Research

Heart Disease and High Blood Cholesterol

"Heart disease" is a general term that includes coronary heart disease, congenital heart disease (a condition you're born with), congestive heart failure and malfunctioning heart valves. This chapter discusses only coronary heart disease, a disease that affects the blood vessels that feed the heart.

What Causes Heart Disease?

Coronary heart disease is caused by atherosclerosis, a gradual process that narrows the heart's arteries and leads to a heart attack. Atherosclerosis can begin in adolescence, when fatty streaks can appear on the lining of arteries as cholesterol sticks to the arteries. The next stage of atherosclerosis is an injury to the lining of an artery. An infection or virus, high blood pressure, cigarette smoke or diabetes may cause this damage. The body attempts to heal itself, just like it would with any wound. Immune cells are attracted to the injured artery wall and accumulate. Over time, the fatty streaks enlarge and become hardened with minerals, tissue, fat and cells, forming plaques. As plaques form beneath the artery wall, they stiffen arteries and narrow the passage through them. Most people have well-developed plaques by the time they are 30 years old. If atherosclerosis progresses, it can restrict blood flow to the heart.

Blood cells called platelets respond to damaged spots on blood vessels by forming clots. A clot may stick to a plaque and gradually enlarge until it blocks blood flow to an area of the heart. That portion of the heart may die slowly and form scar tissue. But a clot can also break loose and circulate in the blood until it reaches an artery too small to pass through. When a clot that's wedged in a vessel cuts off the supply of oxygen and nutrients to a part of the heart muscle, a heart attack results.

Who's at Risk?

Risk factors for heart disease are usually classified as either modifiable or nonmodifiable. You can't change nonmodifiable factors but you can help prevent heart disease by changing modifiable risk factors.

Nonmodifiable Risk Factors

- You're over 40. As you get older, your body becomes less efficient at clearing cholesterol from the bloodstream.
- You have a family history of heart attack prior to age 60.

Modifiable Risk Factors

- You have high blood cholesterol.
- You have high blood triglycerides.
- You have low HDL cholesterol.
- You have high blood pressure.
- You smoke cigarettes. Smoking damages the lining of the arteries, increasing the likelihood of plaque formation. Inhaling cigarette smoke also produces free radicals in the body, which then damage LDL cholesterol, making it stick to the artery walls. Finally, smoking increases blood pressure and makes blood clot formation more likely.
- You have a poor diet.
- You don't exercise regularly. Regular exercise helps you maintain a healthy weight. It lowers LDL cholesterol, raises HDL cholesterol and strengthens the heart and blood vessels.

- You have diabetes. In diabetes, fatty plaques develop and progress much more rapidly.

- Your body mass index (BMI) is greater than 25 (see page 439, Obesity and Weight Loss, to determine your BMI). Carrying extra weight puts stress on your heart and circulatory system. Being overweight can also cause high blood pressure and elevated blood cholesterol. Excess weight around the waist is much more dangerous to your heart than excess lower body fat.

Cholesterol Levels

There are two kinds of cholesterol. Dietary cholesterol is found in foods, and blood cholesterol is made by your liver. For most people, the two are unrelated. That means that dietary cholesterol has little or no effect on the amount of cholesterol in their blood. Cholesterol and fat are transported in your bloodstream on carrier molecules called lipoproteins. The lipoproteins that have received the most research attention are low-density lipoproteins (LDL), high-density lipoproteins (HDL) and triglycerides. If you know your cholesterol levels, use the following reference guide to determine if your level is healthy or if it puts you at higher risk for heart disease.

Blood Lipid	Desirable	Borderline Risk	At Risk
Total cholesterol	<5.2	5.2–6.2	>6.2
LDL cholesterol	2.0–3.4		>3.4
HDL cholesterol	0.9–2.4		<0.9
Triglycerides	0.6–2.3		>2.3

Blood lipids are measured in mmol per liter.

Circulating cholesterol contributes to heart disease by becoming part of the fatty plaques that build up on artery walls. The more LDL cholesterol in the blood, the more cholesterol available to attach to artery walls. The longer you have high LDL levels, the greater the chance more cholesterol has built up in your arteries. While LDL is considered bad, oxidized LDL cholesterol is deemed even worse. When LDL cholesterol is oxidized (damaged) by free radical molecules, it is more likely to accumulate in the arteries. Dietary antioxidants may help prevent such damage to LDL cholesterol particles.

The ratio of total cholesterol to HDL cholesterol is considered a better predictor of heart disease risk than LDL or HDL values alone. This measure is referred to as your risk ratio. Here's a reference guide:

Total/HDL Cholesterol (Risk Ratio)

Risk	Measurement
Below average	<3.5
Average	3.5–5.0
Above average	5.0–10.0
Much above average	>10.0

High Blood Pressure

The higher your blood pressure is above normal, the greater your risk for heart disease. Arteries that are stiff from atherosclerosis strain as blood pulses through them. And if you have high blood pressure as well, your arteries are put under much greater stress. Stressed and strained arteries develop more lesions, and fatty plaques grow more frequently.

Blood pressure results from the pressure generated by your heart as it pushes blood through your arteries. When your heart beats, the blood pressure in your arteries rises. When the heart relaxes between beats, blood pressure falls. Blood pressure is taken as two measures: a systolic and a diastolic pressure. A healthy blood pressure in adults is 120/80 (systolic/diastolic). Doctors interpret the bottom number, the diastolic blood pressure, to determine if you have hypertension. Here are the standards used:

Diastolic Blood Pressure	Measurement
Normal	<85
High-normal	80–89
Mild hypertension	90–99
Moderate hypertension	100–109
Severe hypertension	110–119
Very severe hypertension	>120

The only way you can detect high blood pressure is by having it checked regularly. Blood pressure should be taken when you are relaxed, not stressed. High blood pressure is treated by weight loss, dietary modifications and, often, medication (see page 351, High Blood Pressure).

Homocysteine

Today, many studies are focusing on a compound called homocysteine, an amino acid the body produces during cellular metabolism. Homocysteine is normally converted with the help of B vitamins to other harmless amino acids. When this conversion doesn't occur, homocysteine can accumulate in the blood and damage vessel walls, promoting the build-up of cholesterol. Homocysteine levels can accumulate as a result of an inherited genetic defect or a deficiency of B vitamins.

Many studies have discovered that people with high homocysteine levels have a much higher risk of heart disease. At this time, homocysteine is not routinely measured by doctors as it is expensive to do so and there is no clear definition of normal or healthy levels.

Preventing Heart Disease

Many of the risk factors for heart disease are influenced by what you eat. The nutrition and herbal recommendations below can keep your blood cholesterol at a healthy level, prevent damage or oxidation to your LDL cholesterol and promote weight loss.

Dietary Strategies
Dietary Fat

One of the most important strategies for keeping total and LDL cholesterol levels within the healthy range is to reduce your fat intake to no more than 30 percent of your total daily calorie intake. If you consume 2000 calories per day, that means consuming no more than 65 grams of fat. If you follow a 1200-calorie weight-loss diet, consume no more than 40 fat grams per day. Not all types of dietary fat affect your blood cholesterol the same way. Some fats have a strong impact on the risk for heart disease, whereas others are neutral and don't affect risk.

Saturated Fat

Dietary fats are named according to their chemical structure. Saturated fats are solid at room temperature. This is the type of fat found in animal foods—meat, poultry, eggs and dairy products. Diets high in saturated fat raise the risk for heart disease by increasing the level of blood cholesterol. Saturated fat seems to inhibit the activity of LDL receptors on cells so that this type of cholesterol accumulates in the bloodstream.

Foods contain many types of saturated fats, and not all of them influence blood cholesterol levels to the same degree. For instance, the saturated fat in dairy products is more cholesterol-raising than the saturated fat in meat. What's most important is to eat less saturated fat, period. Saturated fat should account for less than 10 percent of your daily calories. Choosing lower-fat foods will help you reduce your intake of saturated fat. See page 18, Chapter 3, for a list of foods and their lower-fat options. And don't forget to pay attention to portion sizes. When you eat lean meat, your portion size should not exceed 3 ounces (90 grams), the size of a deck of cards.

Butter is a concentrated source of saturated fat. If your blood cholesterol levels are normal, there is no reason why you should avoid butter. Just use it sparingly. People with high blood cholesterol can also continue to use a little butter. Many people have made the switch to margarine because, unlike butter, margarine is made from a vegetable oil that doesn't contain saturated fat. However, if you choose margarine over butter, be sure you are choosing a healthy one (see Chapter 3).

Trans Fat

If you are unfamiliar with this term, you may have heard about hydrogenated fat instead. Hydrogenation is a chemical process that adds hydrogen atoms to liquid vegetable oils. This makes vegetable fats more solid and more useful to food manufacturers. Packaged foods like cookies, crackers and baked goods made with hydrogenated vegetable oils are more palatable and have a longer shelf life. Margarines made by hydrogenating a vegetable oil are firm like butter.

When a vegetable oil is hydrogenated, it becomes saturated *and* it forms a new type of fat called trans fat. Trans fat increases LDL cholesterol and decreases HDL cholesterol. Many researchers believe that trans fat is worse for our cholesterol levels than saturated fat. A large Harvard study found that people with the highest intake of trans fat from margarine, cookies, cake and white bread had a 50 percent higher risk of heart disease compared with those who ate the least.[1]

To help reduce your intake of trans fat, start reading food labels and ingredients lists. Look for the words "partially hydrogenated vegetable oils." Eat foods that contain these types of oils less often. As much as 40 percent of the fat in foods like french fries, fast food, doughnuts, pastries, snack foods and commercial cookies is trans fat. If you eat margarine, choose one that's made with nonhydrogenated fat. Many brands state this right on the label.

Soon prepackaged foods will list the grams of trans fat on their nutrition labels. In the fall of 2000, Health Canada announced recommendations for improved nutrition labels on foods. All prepackaged foods will have to disclose nutrition facts on the label for a greater number of nutrients, including trans fat. Once these recommendations become law (expected late 2001), food manufacturers will have two years to fully conform to the new nutrition labeling laws.

Polyunsaturated Fat

This type of dietary fat is liquid at room temperature. Omega-6 polyunsaturated fats are found in all vegetable oils, including canola, sunflower, safflower, corn, sesame and flaxseed oils. Omega-3 polyunsaturated fats are found in fish and seafood. Replacing foods that provide mostly saturated fat with those rich in polyunsaturated fats can help you lower your cholesterol level.

Omega-3 fats found in fish can do more than just help you eat less saturated fat. Omega-3 fats can lower high levels of blood triglycerides and reduce the stickiness of platelets, the cells that form blood clots in arteries. Omega-3s may also increase the flexibility of red blood cells so they can pass more readily through tiny blood vessels. Many studies have found that populations that consume fish a few times each week have lower rates of heart disease.

Most experts agree that you should eat fish three times per week. Choose oilier fish such as salmon, trout, sardines, herring, mackerel, sea bass and fresh tuna (canned tuna has very little omega-3 fat).

Monounsaturated Fat

These fats are liquid at room temperature but turn semi-solid when stored in the fridge. Monounsaturated fats found in olive, canola and peanut oils are considered to be neutral because they don't influence blood cholesterol levels on their own. Research suggests that extra-virgin olive oil helps prevent blood clots from forming and acts as an antioxidant. Extra-virgin olive oil has been processed the least and has a darker color.

Dietary Cholesterol

This wax-like fatty substance is found in meat, poultry, eggs, dairy products, fish and seafood. It's particularly plentiful in shrimp, liver and egg yolks. While high-cholesterol diets cause high blood cholesterol in animals, this is not the case in humans. Dietary cholesterol has little or no effect on most people's blood cholesterol. One reason for this is that our intestines absorb only half the cholesterol we eat. A study from Harvard University did not find any significant association between egg intake and risk of heart disease or stroke in healthy men and women.[2] Eating one egg per day will not affect your risk for heart disease.

Too much dietary cholesterol can raise levels of LDL cholesterol in some people, especially people with hereditary forms of high cholesterol. Health Canada recommends that we consume no more than 300 milligrams of cholesterol each day. Choosing animal foods that are lower in saturated fat also helps to cut down on dietary cholesterol. A list of foods and their cholesterol content can be found on page 22, Chapter 3.

Soy Foods

A large body of evidence has shown that a low-fat diet containing 25 grams of soy protein per day lowers the risk for heart disease. In 1995, researchers in Lexington, Kentucky, published a report in the *New England Journal of Medicine* of their analysis of 38 studies on soy and cholesterol.[3] The researchers determined that eating soy protein instead of animal protein significantly lowered high levels of LDL cholesterol and triglycerides. Since then, a number of other studies have confirmed soy's cholesterol-lowering ability.

A regular intake of soy may also raise HDL cholesterol, lower high blood pressure and keep blood vessels healthy. Natural compounds in soybeans seem to act as antioxidants, preventing oxygen damage to LDL cholesterol.

Soybean's heart-healthy attributes are credited to its protein and isoflavone (phytoestrogen) content. To lower elevated cholesterol levels, you need both components. Supplements containing purified isoflavones have not been shown to reduce cholesterol levels. To add 25 grams of soy protein to your low-fat diet each day, use the following guide:

Soy Food	Soy Protein (grams)
Soy beverage, 1 cup (250 ml)	9 g
Soybeans, canned, 1/2 cup (125 ml)	14 g
Soy nuts, 1/4 cup (60 ml)	14 g
Soy flour, defatted, 1/4 cup (60 ml)	13 g
Soy protein powder, isolate, 1 scoop	25 g
Tempeh, 1/2 cup (125 ml)	16 g
Tofu, firm, 1/2 cup (125 ml)	19 g
Tofu, regular, 1/2 cup (125 ml)	10 g
Veggie Burger, Yves Veggie Cuisine	11 g
Veggie Dog, small, Yves Veggie Cuisine	11 g

Soluble Fiber

Plant foods contain a mix of two types of fiber, soluble and insoluble, but they will contain more of one than the other. Soluble fiber, the type that dissolves in water, has been shown to lower high blood cholesterol levels. Studies show that adding oats and beans to your diet can lower cholesterol by up to 16 percent.[4] And eating a psyllium-enriched breakfast cereal has been shown to lower LDL cholesterol by 9 percent.[5] The best food sources of these fibers include oats and oat bran, psyllium-enriched breakfast cereals, legumes and certain fruits and vegetables.

When soluble fiber reaches the intestine, it attaches to bile, causing it to be excreted in the stool. Bile is a digestive aid that's released into the intestine after you eat. The liver makes bile from cholesterol and sends it to your gallbladder to be stored until it's needed. Since soluble fiber causes your body to excrete bile, your liver has to make more of it from cholesterol in the bloodstream.

The end result is a lower blood cholesterol level. When unabsorbed fiber reaches your colon, bacteria degrade it and form compounds called short-chain fatty acids. These fatty acids may also hamper the liver's ability to produce cholesterol.

The following foods are good sources of soluble fiber:

Breakfast Cereals	Legumes	Fruits	Vegetables
Oatmeal	Kidney beans	Orange	Carrots
Oat bran	Black beans	Grapefruit	Potatoes
Kellogg's All Bran Buds	Chickpeas	Apple	Sweet potatoes
Psyllium-enriched cereals	Lentils	Strawberries	Green peas
	Soybeans	Pears	
	Navy beans	Cantaloupe	

If you've decided to try a psyllium-rich breakfast cereal, start with a small portion. Too much too soon can cause bloating and gas. It usually takes two weeks for the bacteria that reside in the intestine to adjust to a higher fiber intake. Start by adding 1/4 to 1/2 cup (60 to 125 ml) of Kellogg's All Bran Buds to your usual breakfast cereal. Over the course of two or three weeks, increase your portion. Increase fluid intake as you consume more fiber, since fiber needs fluid to exert its effect.

Whole Grains

In addition to fiber, whole-grain foods like whole-wheat bread, whole-grain breakfast cereals and oats have other protective ingredients that might help lower the risk of heart disease.[6,7] Whole grains are important sources of vitamin E, zinc, selenium, copper, iron and manganese, as well as of special phytochemicals (from plants) called phenols. All these natural compounds have antioxidant properties and may offer protection from heart disease.

A food made from whole grains means that it contains *all* parts of the grain—the outer bran layer where most of the fiber is, the germ layer that's rich in nutrients like vitamin E and the endosperm that contains the starch. When whole grains are processed into flakes, puffs or white flour, all that's left is the starchy endosperm. Refined grains offer significantly less vitamins E and B6, magnesium, potassium, zinc and fiber. A list of whole grains can be found on page 70, Chapter 5.

Nuts

Adding a handful of nuts to your diet may also help you prevent heart disease. Populations that include nuts as a regular part of their diet have lower rates of heart disease. The large Nurses' Health Study discovered that women who ate 5 ounces of nuts each week had a 35 percent lower risk of heart attack and death from heart disease compared with women who never ate nuts or ate them less than once a month.[8]

Nuts and seeds are rich sources of vitamin E, many important minerals and essential fatty acids (alpha-linolenic acid and linoleic acid) as well as dietary fiber. Add 1/4 cup (60 ml) of nuts to your diet five times a week.

Tea

According to researchers, natural antioxidants found in green and black tea may protect your heart. One American study looked at the effect of tea, coffee and decaffeinated coffee in 340 people who had had a heart attack.[9] Compared with non-tea-drinkers, those who enjoyed at least one cup a day had a 44 percent lower risk of heart attack.

Tea leaves contain flavonoid compounds called catechins. Catechins are found in green tea, black tea and oolong tea, but not herbal teas. To incorporate tea into your diet, replace coffee and soft drinks with your favorite type of tea, be it Earl Grey, orange-spice, apricot, raspberry or black currant. In the summer, make your own iced tea from freshly brewed tea and lemons.

Alcohol

Research has shown that a moderate intake of alcohol reduces the risk of heart disease.[10] Drinking alcohol, whether it's wine, beer or liquor, raises the level of HDL cholesterol and may reduce blood clotting. There is also evidence that antioxidants in wine, especially red wine, may keep LDL cholesterol healthy. The protective effects of alcohol are most apparent in people over the age of 50 and in those with more than one risk factor for heart disease. If you're a healthy young person, a drink a day probably won't do much for your heart.

Health authorities do not advise drinking a couple of glasses of wine each day, since there are too many negative health effects associated with drinking alcohol. If you do drink alcohol, keep your intake to no more than one to two drinks a day. If you are a nondrinker, don't start now. There are many other more important nutrition strategies you can implement to reduce your odds of heart disease.

Vitamins and Minerals

B Vitamins

These nutrients can help keep blood levels of homocysteine from accumulating. In order to prevent homocysteine from rising and damaging blood vessels, the body uses folate, B6 and B12 to convert it into other harmless compounds.

Harvard researchers studied 80,000 women for 14 years and found that those who consumed the most folate and vitamin B6 had a 45 percent lower risk of heart disease compared with women who consumed the least.[11] Among those women who got plenty of B vitamins in their diet, the risk of heart disease was also lower if they regularly took a multivitamin and mineral supplement, a major source of folate and B6.

The best food sources of folate include spinach, lentils, orange juice, asparagus, artichokes and whole-grain breads and cereals. Foods rich in vitamin B6 include meat, poultry, fish, liver, legumes, nuts, seeds, whole grains, green leafy vegetables, bananas and avocados. Vitamin B12 is found in animal foods such as meat, poultry, fish, eggs and dairy products and also in fortified soy and rice beverages.

If you have difficulty eating a varied diet, take a high-quality multivitamin and mineral supplement to ensure you are meeting your B vitamin requirements (see Chapter 4). Regular multivitamin and mineral supplements offer 100 to 300 percent of your daily needs. High-potency or super multivitamin formulas or B complex supplements contain higher amounts, usually 25 to 100 milligrams of B vitamins (or micrograms in the case of folic acid, a form of folate). Some manufacturers have developed special supplements tailored to the prevention of heart disease. For example, Cardio-Logic™ by Quest Vitamins® contains B vitamins, vitamin E, Coenzyme Q10 and supportive herbs.

Vitamin C

Many studies have reported a link between high dietary intakes and high blood levels of vitamin C and a lower risk of heart disease. American researchers observed that rates of heart disease were 27 percent lower in the men and women with the highest vitamin C levels compared with those with the lowest.[12] The level of vitamin C in your bloodstream is a good indicator of the amount of vitamin C in your diet. A Portuguese study conducted among 194 adults determined that compared with those individuals with marginal vitamin C intakes, those who consumed the most vitamin C had an 80 percent lower risk of heart attack.[13]

Vitamin C may protect from heart disease by acting as an antioxidant. The vitamin is able to neutralize harmful free radical molecules that damage your LDL cholesterol. Studies also suggest vitamin C may inhibit the formation of blood clots by reducing the stickiness of platelets.

The best sources of vitamin C include citrus fruit, citrus juices, cantaloupe, kiwi, mango, strawberries, broccoli, Brussels sprouts, cauliflower, red pepper and tomato juice. To supplement, take a 500 milligram supplement of Ester C daily. There's little point in swallowing much more at one time, since your body can only use about 200 milligrams at one time. If you want to take more, split your dose over the course of the day. Some multivitamin and mineral supplements supply up to 250 milligrams.

Vitamin E

Many studies suggest that vitamin E supplements can help prevent heart attacks in healthy men and women. Two large studies from Harvard University, published in the *New England Journal of Medicine*, found that healthy men and women who took supplemental vitamin E for two years had a 40 percent lower risk of heart attack compared with nonsupplement users.[14,15]

Vitamin E is a potent antioxidant. Once consumed through the diet or a supplement, vitamin E makes its way to the liver, where it is incorporated into the lipoproteins that transport cholesterol. It is here that vitamin E works to protect these compounds from oxygen damage caused by free radicals. Vitamin E may also inhibit blood clot formation and preserve the health of blood vessels that feed the heart.

The best food sources of vitamin E include wheat germ, nuts, seeds, vegetable oils, whole grains and kale. To supplement, take 200 to 800 international units (IU) of natural source vitamin E. Buy a "mixed" vitamin E supplement if possible. Do not take vitamin E supplements if you use a blood-thinning medication such as warfarin (Coumadin®).

Lycopene

Lycopene is a cousin of beta-carotene, the antioxidant nutrient that's plentiful in carrots. Compared with beta-carotene, lycopene is twice as potent as an antioxidant. Lycopene is found in red-colored fruits and vegetables. Tomatoes are the richest source of lycopene, but you'll also find some in pink grapefruit, watermelon, guava and apricots.

Researchers have observed a relationship between the amount of lycopene in the blood and in body fat stores and the risk of heart disease. As an antioxidant, lycopene is yet another dietary defense mechanism against free radical damage to LDL cholesterol. Toronto researchers studied the effect of dietary lycopene in 19 healthy adults and found that a diet supplemented with tomato products doubled lycopene blood levels *and* significantly reduced free radical damage to LDL cholesterol.[16] Lycopene may also lower the level of LDL cholesterol by hampering its production in the liver.

While the research on the role of lycopene in heart disease is preliminary, there's no reason why you shouldn't add this antioxidant to your diet. It appears that an intake of 5 to 7 milligrams offers protection.

Food	Lycopene (milligrams)
Tomato, raw, 1 small	0.8–3.8 mg
Tomatoes, cooked, 1 cup (250 ml)	9.25 mg
Tomato sauce, 1/2 cup (125 ml)	3.1 mg
Tomato paste, 2 tbsp (30 ml)	8.0 mg
Tomato juice, 1 cup (250 ml)	23.0 mg
Ketchup, 2 tbsp (30 ml)	3.1–4.2 mg
Apricots, dried, 10 halves	0.3 mg
Grapefruit, pink, 1/2	4.2 mg
Papaya, 1 whole	6.2–16.5 mg
Watermelon, 1 slice (25 cm × 2 cm)	8.5–26.4 mg

Heat-processed tomato products provide a source of lycopene that is much more available to the body. To increase the amount of lycopene you absorb, add a little olive oil to your pasta sauce. Lycopene is a fat-soluble compound and so is better absorbed when eaten along with a little fat.

Lycopene supplements are available in health food stores and drug stores. Choose a brand that's made with the Lyc-O-Mato™ or LycoRed™ extract. This source of lycopene is derived from whole tomatoes, and it's also the source that has been used in clinical studies. Most supplements offer 5 milligrams of lycopene per tablet.

Herbal Remedies

Garlic *(Allium sativum)*

Garlic contains many different sulfur compounds, and one in particular, S-allyl cysteine (SAC), has been shown to lower LDL cholesterol by up to 10 percent.[17] SAC is present in small amounts in raw garlic, but increases in concentration when garlic ages. The scientific studies that show a cholesterol-lowering effect have used an extract of aged garlic extract (Kyolic® brand).

Studies have shown that garlic can also lower blood triglyceride levels and thin the blood by reducing the stickiness of platelets. The sulfur compounds in aged garlic extract also act as antioxidants and prevent damage to LDL cholesterol. Finally, a daily dose of aged garlic may have a modest blood-pressure-lowering effect.

Scientists agree that as little as half a clove of garlic each day will offer health benefits. Add garlic to sauces, soups, casseroles and salad dressings. Most people can take one or two cloves a day without any problems. Some people, however, experience stomach upset when they eat raw garlic. The oil-soluble compounds in garlic account for its potential to irritate the stomach and to cause odor.

Although raw garlic contains very little SAC, a recent study from Pennsylvania State University found that if you let crushed garlic sit at room temperature for ten minutes before cooking with

it, more of these beneficial sulfur compounds will be formed.

When it comes to garlic supplements, the scientific research points to aged garlic extract as the supplement of choice because of its higher concentration of SAC. Generally, two to six capsules a day (one or two with each meal) are recommended.

Nutrition Strategy Checklist for Heart Disease and High Blood Cholesterol

- ☐ Low saturated and trans fat
- ☐ Low dietary cholesterol
- ☐ Fish
- ☐ Soy protein
- ☐ Soluble fiber
- ☐ Whole grains
- ☐ Nuts
- ☐ Tea
- ☐ B vitamins
- ☐ Vitamin C
- ☐ Vitamin E
- ☐ Lycopene
- ☐ Garlic

Recommended Resources

www.heartandstroke.ca
Heart and Stroke Foundation of Canada
222 Queen Street, Suite 1402
Ottawa, ON, Canada K1P 5V9
Tel: 613-569-4361
Fax: 613-569-3278

www.americanheart.org
American Heart Association
7272 Greenville Avenue
Dallas, Texas, USA 75231
Tel: 1-800-AHA-USA1

www.nih.gov/health/syh-hbc/index.htm
National Heart, Lung, and Blood Institute Information Center
P.O. Box 30105
Bethesda, MD, USA 20824-0105
Tel: 301-592-8573 (publications) or
1-800-575-9355 (blood pressure and cholesterol information)
Fax: 301-592-8563

Hemorrhoids

Hemorrhoids, or piles, are large, swollen veins that develop in the anus and lower rectum. Very similar to varicose veins in the legs, hemorrhoids occur when the blood vessels in the anal area swell and stretch under pressure. More than half of North Americans have experienced the itching, burning and pain associated with hemorrhoids at some time in their lives.

While hemorrhoids are not dangerous or life threatening, they can be persistent, annoying and sometimes quite painful. There are two types of hemorrhoids. *Internal hemorrhoids* develop in the upper area of the anal canal. They cannot be seen and, normally, cause little discomfort. Sometimes you may detect an internal hemorrhoid by the sensation of fullness that you feel in your rectum after a bowel movement.

If you strain too much during a bowel movement, you can inadvertently push an internal hemorrhoid out through the anal opening. This is known as a protruding hemorrhoid. Once the delicate tissue of the blood vessel is exposed in this way, it can become very irritated and painful and can bleed easily. While protruding hemorrhoids will usually return to their internal position without any help, it may be necessary to gently push them back into the anal canal after a bowel movement.

External hemorrhoids are swollen, skin-covered blood vessels that occur outside the anus, which can be itchy, painful and tender. When blood pools in these veins, a blood clot may form, producing a hard, inflamed lump around the anus.

What Causes Hemorrhoids?

Human beings are particularly prone to hemorrhoids because our erect posture puts extra pressure on the tissues surrounding the anus and rectum. Conditions such as pregnancy or obesity increase this pressure and are frequent causes of hemorrhoids. Hemorrhoids can also develop as a result of straining during a bowel movement, straining during childbirth, lifting heavy objects and sitting or standing in one position for a long time. Some people are genetically predisposed to hemorrhoids, due to an inherited weakness in the walls of the anal blood vessels.

Symptoms

An internal hemorrhoid may be felt protruding out of the anus after a bowel movement, whereas an external hemorrhoid may be felt as a hard lump near the anus. Other signs of hemorrhoid include

- itching and burning in the anal area
- pain or discomfort around the anus and rectum
- rectal bleeding

Rectal bleeding may be noticed as blood on the toilet paper, blood in the toilet bowl, streaks of blood on your stool or spots of blood on your underwear. It may also be a sign of other, more serious medical conditions such as diverticular disease, colon or rectal polyps, colitis, bowel cancer or an anal fissure. Do not ignore rectal bleeding, even if you are convinced that it is a symptom of hemorrhoids. When you detect any sign of bleeding from your rectum, consult your doctor.

Who's at Risk?

Hemorrhoids are rare before the age of 30 and become more frequent after the age of 50. People prone to constipation often have hemorrhoids. Pregnant women are also susceptible to developing hemorrhoids. Poor bowel habits, such as withholding stool or reading on the toilet, are contributing factors to hemorrhoids.

Conventional Treatment

Hemorrhoids require very little treatment and will usually go away on their own within a few days. The following may help relieve the discomfort of hemorrhoids:

- cold compresses applied to the affected area
- avoidance of prolonged standing or sitting
- witch hazel or other soothing lotions to reduce itching
- over-the-counter preparations to relieve itching
- warm sitz baths taken two or three times daily
- acetaminophen to relieve pain (avoid codeine as it causes constipation)
- stool softeners or psyllium to relieve constipation

Hemorrhoids may be destroyed by:

- *Tying off* Tiny rubber bands are tied around the base of the hemorrhoid to cut off the circulation; within ten days, the hemorrhoid withers and falls off.
- *Laser therapy* A laser beam vaporizes the affected tissue.
- *Injection sclerotherapy* A shrinking agent is injected to stop bleeding.
- *Infrared photocoagulation* A burst of infrared light is used to cut off circulation to an internal hemorrhoid.
- *Cryosurgery* The affected tissue is frozen to cut off circulation.
- *Electric current* A burst of electric current is used to shrink a hemorrhoid.

Preventing and Managing Hemorrhoids

Dietary Strategies

Maintaining a healthy weight is important in the prevention and management of hemorrhoids. Excess weight can add to the pressure on your anal veins. Preventing constipation is also key.

Dietary Fiber

Constipation causes straining, which promotes the development of hemorrhoids. To treat constipation, gradually increase your daily fiber intake to 25 to 35 grams (see page 3, Chapter 1, for the fiber content of selected foods). Foods contain varying amounts of insoluble fibers and soluble fibers. Foods that have a greater proportion of insoluble fibers, such as wheat bran, whole grains, nuts, seeds and certain fruits and vegetables, are used to treat and prevent constipation. Insoluble fibers absorb water and by doing so they help form larger, softer stools and speed evacuation. Psyllium, a type of soluble fiber, also adds bulk to stools and can be used to treat constipation.

Studies have shown that adding 10 grams of fiber to the diet helps reduce bleeding from internal hemorrhoids and speeds the removal of stool from the intestinal tract.[1,2] Use the following guide to add bulk-forming fiber to your diet:

Food	Fiber (grams)
100% bran cereal, 1/2 cup (125 ml)	10.0 g
Kellogg's All Bran Buds (psyllium), 1/3 cup (75 ml)	13.0 g
Natural wheat bran, 2 tbsp (30 ml)	2.4 g
Flaxseed, ground, 2 tbsp (30 ml)	4.5 g
Almonds, 1/4 cup (60 ml)	4.8 g

Choose higher-fiber fruits and vegetables. You'll find a list of fiber-rich fruits and vegetables on page 245, Constipation. Increase your fiber intake gradually to prevent intestinal discomfort, and spread your fiber intake over the course of the day, rather than consuming it all at once.

Dietary fiber needs to absorb fluid in the intestinal tract in order to add bulk to stool. Drink 8 to 12 cups (2 to 3 liters) of fluid every day. Always include 1 cup (250 ml) of fluid with high-fiber meals and snacks.

Probiotics

Foods and supplements that contain friendly lactic acid bacteria (e.g., acidophilus, bifidobacteria) are called probiotics and can help prevent constipation. These bacteria normally reside in the intestinal tract, where they perform a number of tasks that keep the bowel healthy. Scientists are learning that probiotics must be consumed regularly to have a health benefit.

Eat 1 cup (250 ml) fermented dairy product daily: yogurt, kefir or acidophilus milk. All yogurts in Canada are made with lactic acid bacteria whether or not they are labeled as such. To supplement, take 1 to 10 billion live cells (per capsule) with one to three meals daily. See Chapter 8 for information about probiotic supplements.

Herbal Remedies

Horse Chestnut
(*Aesculus hippocastanum*)

Studies have found horse chestnut effective in treating varicose veins in the legs; it may be useful for hemorrhoids as well. This herb contains active compounds called saponins that enhance circulation through the veins. Studies have demonstrated horse chestnut's ability to constrict and promote normal tone in veins so that blood returns to the heart.

Buy a product standardized to 16 to 21 percent aescin. Take one capsule up to three times per day. The extract used in the clinical studies is sold as Venastat® (Pharmaton® Natural Health Products) in Canada and the United States. In rare instances, horse chestnut seed extract can cause stomach upset, nausea and itching. Its use is not recommended during pregnancy and breastfeeding as insufficient information is available about its safety. People with liver or kidney disease should not take horse chestnut.

Other Natural Health Products

Citrus Bioflavonoids

These compounds are found in the inner peel of citrus fruit and, when consumed, they help strengthen blood capillaries. A number of studies have shown that a special formulation of two bioflavonoids, diosmin and hesperidin, is effective in reducing the duration and severity of hemorrhoid episodes.[3-9] Another citrus bioflavonoid called oxerutins may also be useful.

Bioflavonoids are very safe and may have a range of other health benefits. The typical dose is 500 milligrams twice daily. Oxerutins have been used in doses of 500 to 1000 milligrams up to three times daily.

Grapeseed Extract and Pycnogenol™

This supplement is rich in anthocyanins, natural compounds that help keep blood vessels healthy. Grapeseed extract is thought to work by inhibiting the action of enzymes that break down connective tissue. Another anthocyanin-rich supplement is Pycnogenol™. Pycnogenol™ is the US registered trademark for an extract made from the bark of pine trees. This supplement has the same effect as grapeseed extract and can be used to prevent and/or treat the same conditions.

While no studies have evaluated its use in hemorrhoids, a handful of studies have found grapeseed extract and pycnogenol to significantly reduce symptoms of peripheral venous insufficiency, including leg pain and swelling.[10-14] Anthocyanins may also help reduce blood clots.

Based on the suggested dose for vein problems, I recommend you take 150 to 300 milligrams of grapeseed extract per day. Some experts recommend taking 150 to 300 milligrams for three weeks, followed by a maintenance dose of 40 to 80 milligrams daily. Grapeseed extract is considered extremely safe. Pycnogenol is more expensive than grapeseed extract. The usual dose is 50 milligrams once daily.

Nutrition Strategy Checklist for Hemorrhoids

- ☐ Weight control
- ☐ Dietary fiber
- ☐ Fluids
- ☐ Fermented milk products
- ☐ Probiotic supplements
- ☐ Horse chestnut
- ☐ Citrus bioflavonoids
- ☐ Grapeseed extract OR Pycnogenol

Recommended Resources

www.mayoclinic.com
Mayo Foundation for Medical Education and Research

www.niddk.nih.gov
National Digestive Diseases Information Clearinghouse
2 Information Way
Bethesda, MD, USA 20892-3570
Tel: 301-654-3810

Hepatitis (see also Cirrhosis of the Liver)

Hepatitis is an infection or inflammation of the liver. Most liver infections are caused by one of five hepatitis viruses: hepatitis A, B, C, D and E. Hepatitis attacks the liver silently, with few, if any, obvious symptoms. Often, people don't even know they have been exposed to the disease until liver damage becomes apparent many years later. Because symptoms are so frequently overlooked, hepatitis can be easily and unknowingly transmitted to others.

The liver is the largest internal organ in the body, responsible for more than 500 different functions. In addition to processing nutrients and manufacturing essential chemicals, the liver removes poisons from the blood and processes waste products. Inflammation caused by a hepatitis virus interferes with normal liver function and, in some cases, may lead to serious liver disease, cancer or liver failure. Hepatitis can be acute, which means that the virus lasts less than six months, or it can become a chronic, long-term condition. Hepatitis B and C are the viruses most likely to develop into chronic hepatitis.

The characteristics of viral hepatitis vary according to the differing viruses that cause the disease.

Hepatitis A

Hepatitis A is usually transmitted from the stool of one person to the mouth of another and is often associated with poor hygiene. Waterborne and foodborne epidemics of hepatitis A are common, especially in developing countries where sewage-polluted water and food is prevalent. The disease can also be transmitted by eating contaminated raw shellfish. Hepatitis A does not lead to chronic hepatitis.

Hepatitis B

Hepatitis B is transmitted by contact with blood or blood products. In Canada and the United States, measures are taken to ensure a safe blood supply, so transmission by blood transfusion is unlikely. The disease spreads frequently through sexual contact and the exchange of body fluids by heterosexual and homosexual partners, and may be transmitted by drug users sharing needles or by improperly sterilized implements used for tattoos, body piercing, ear piercing or acupuncture. Mothers can infect their infants, possibly through breast milk.

The hepatitis B virus is very tough; it will survive and remain infective for days on household items such as toothbrushes and razors. Approximately 10 percent of people with hepatitis B continue to carry the virus in their blood and may infect others without realizing it.[1] As many as 60 to 90 percent of children and 10 percent of adults with hepatitis B go on to develop chronic hepatitis.[2]

Hepatitis C

Like hepatitis B, hepatitis C is primarily spread by contact with blood and blood products. Transmission through blood transfusion has been virtually eliminated in North America by routine blood screening for hepatitis C virus antibodies. Transmission is most common through drug users sharing contaminated needles or through improperly sterilized implements used for tattooing, body or ear piercing or acupuncture. However, unlike hepatitis B, hepatitis C is less likely to be spread through sexual contact. The disease is one of the main causes of chronic liver disease; 60 to 70 percent of acute cases develop into chronic hepatitis.[3]

Hepatitis D

This type of hepatitis occurs only as a co-infection of hepatitis B. It is spread by contact with blood and blood products and by contact with bodily fluids. Intravenous drug users are particularly at risk of contacting hepatitis D by sharing contaminated needles. When hepatitis D occurs in combination with hepatitis B, symptoms will be more severe and the chance of the disease progressing to cirrhosis, liver cancer and liver failure is substantially increased.

Hepatitis E

Hepatitis E, similar to hepatitis A, is transferred from stool to mouth through contaminated food or water or by poor hygiene. It can be very serious in young adults and may cause fatalities if contracted by pregnant women, especially in the third trimester.

Symptoms

Acute viral hepatitis may cause no symptoms at all. Symptoms that do develop usually begin suddenly:

- flu-like feeling of illness
- nausea and vomiting, poor appetite
- low-grade fever
- fatigue
- muscle and joint pain
- liver tenderness
- darkened urine
- jaundice (yellowing of the skin and eyes)
- pale stools and general itching

The symptoms usually last only one to two weeks. Most people usually recover in four to eight weeks, even without treatment.

Who's at Risk?

Those at highest risk of contracting hepatitis include

- healthcare workers exposed to blood, blood products or body fluids
- users of illegal intravenous or intranasal drugs, such as cocaine
- individuals with multiple sexual partners
- babies born to mothers who are carriers of the hepatitis B virus
- people sharing a household with a hepatitis carrier
- people who have had blood transfusions, organ transplants or received clotting factor concentrates prior to blood screening (1992 in the United States, 1990 in Canada)
- people who travel to countries where hepatitis is common

Conventional Treatment

There is no effective treatment for viral hepatitis, so prevention is the best strategy. If you have been exposed to hepatitis, you may be given an antibody preparation (immune serum globulin) as protection against the virus, but the degree of protection offered by this treatment varies from individual to individual. Infants born to mothers who are carriers of hepatitis B are vaccinated and given hepatitis B immune globulin, which prevents chronic hepatitis in approximately 70 percent of those infants.

For hepatitis C, interferon combined with broad-spectrum antiviral agents is successful in approximately 40 percent of cases. Interferon may not be used in people who have untreated thyroid disease, low blood cell counts, an autoimmune disease or those who drink alcohol or take drugs. Other treatments for hepatitis include

- eliminating alcoholic beverages, since alcohol speeds the progression of liver disease
- avoiding medications known to cause liver disease
- maintaining a healthy lifestyle
- exercising regularly and getting plenty of rest
- taking precautions to protect others from coming in contact with your blood or body fluids; never donating blood or semen

Preventing and Managing Hepatitis

A vaccine is available to protect against hepatitis B. Three injections of the vaccine over a period of time will protect most people from this disease. To prevent infection, it is also critical to practice good hygiene at all times, especially when traveling to foreign countries. Avoid unprotected sex with multiple partners or with a partner who may have been exposed to the hepatitis virus. Don't share needles or drug paraphernalia and avoid intranasal drugs such as cocaine. When considering body piercing, ear piercing, tattooing or acupuncture, make certain that all implements are properly sterilized.

Dietary Strategies

Good nutrition, in the form of a healthy, well-balanced diet, may help liver cells damaged by the hepatitis virus regenerate. Healthy eating is an important part of treatment and protecting the liver from further damage. The guidelines in Chapter 5 should be followed.

Avoid overeating carbohydrate-rich foods, since excess amounts can cause fatty deposits in the liver. Include foods rich in soluble fiber in your daily diet. The fibers found in legumes, oats, psyllium, apples and citrus fruit bind toxic bile acids (a product of digestion) in the intestine and remove them from the body.

There is some suggestion that green tea may help protect from liver disease. Japanese researchers found that men who drank green tea, especially more than 10 cups per day, had decreased liver enzymes measured by blood tests.[4] Animal research has also found that natural compounds called flavonoids, extracted from green tea, are able to protect from chemically induced liver damage.[5]

Alcohol must be avoided to allow the liver to heal and rebuild.

Vitamins and Minerals

Vitamin E and Selenium

Scientists believe that damage caused by free radical molecules may be involved in viral hepatitis.[6,7] Free radical damage may make the liver more susceptible to viruses, and it may continue to destroy liver cells after the onset of hepatitis. Free radical damage may be due to a deficiency of antioxidants, such as vitamin E and selenium and/or an overproduction of free radicals by the body.

In the body, vitamin E and selenium work closely together to mop up harmful free radicals. Both nutrients also boost the body's immune system. Researchers from China found that daily selenium supplementation reduced the risk of liver cancer among hepatitis B carriers.[8] A German study conducted among hepatitis C patients found that vitamin E, when combined with interferon therapy, reduced the amount of virus in the liver.[9] Case reports of individuals infected with hepatitis C also document improved liver tests and recovery rates when supplemented with antioxidants.[10]

The recommended dietary allowance (RDA) for vitamin E is 22 international units (IU). Best food sources include wheat germ, nuts, seeds, vegetable oils, whole grains and kale. To supplement, take 200 to 800 IU of natural source vitamin E. Buy a "mixed" vitamin E supplement if possible. The daily upper limit is 1500 IU.

The RDA for selenium is 55 micrograms. Best food sources are seafood, chicken, organ meats, whole grains, nuts, onions, garlic and mushrooms. To supplement, take 200 micrograms of selenium-rich yeast per day. The daily upper limit is 400 micrograms.

Herbal Remedies

Milk Thistle (*Silybum marianum*)

The active ingredients of this herb, known collectively as silymarin, can support and enhance liver function. Silymarin can prevent toxic substances from penetrating liver cells and may even help liver cells regenerate more quickly. Milk thistle also seems to act as an antioxidant, protecting liver cells from damage caused by free radicals. Research conducted among patients with chronic hepatitis found that when 240 milligrams of the herb was taken twice daily, the patients showed improved results of liver function tests.[11]

Buy a product that's standardized to 70 percent silymarin. The recommended dose is 200 milligrams two or three times daily. Use milk thistle with caution if you are allergic to plants in the Asteracease/Compositae family (ragweed, daisy, marigold and chrysanthemum). For more information on milk thistle, see page 114, Chapter 7.

Other Natural Health Products

Coenzyme Q10 (CoQ10)

This antioxidant may help the body respond better to the hepatitis B vaccine. Researchers gave healthy individuals either 90 or 180 milligrams of CoQ10 daily for two weeks prior to vaccination and three months afterwards.[12] The study found that CoQ10 was able to increase production of antibodies to the hepatitis B virus, with the higher dose having a greater effect.

CoQ10 may also help combat free radical damage caused by hepatitis. Japanese researchers found a significant increase in the blood levels of oxidized CoQ10 among chronic hepatitis patients compared with healthy people.[13] This suggests that the compounds may be important in protecting liver cells.

Choose a CoQ10 supplement in an oil base (instead of dry-powder tablets or capsules), since this is more available to the body. Take 50 milligrams twice daily. When taken in daily doses of 300 milligrams or more, CoQ10 can interfere with liver enzyme blood tests.

N-Acetyl Cysteine (NAC)

N-acetyl cysteine (NAC) is a modified form of cysteine, an amino acid found in protein-rich foods. The body uses NAC to make a selenium-containing antioxidant enzyme called glutathione. As such, NAC may be important for the antioxidant action of selenium and vitamin E. Studies in HIV have investigated the possible antiviral effects of NAC, but with conflicting results.

A limited amount of research suggests that NAC may be useful in conjunction with interferon. One report found that supplementation of NAC led to improved response to interferon treatment in hepatitis C.[14] The typical dose ranges from 250 to 1800 milligrams per day. NAC is very safe when taken as recommended; however, one animal study found that very high doses caused liver damage.

Phosphatidylcholine

Phosphatidylcholine supplements are thought to exert their health benefits by supplying the body with choline, a member of the B vitamin family. Once ingested, choline becomes incorporated into the membranes of cells, where it appears to have an anti-inflammatory effect.

Research suggests that phosphatidylcholine may be beneficial for people with hepatitis C. German researchers showed that when taken with interferon therapy and continued for 24 weeks after, phosphatidylcholine improved liver function to a greater extent than interferon alone.[15]

Buy a supplement labeled phosphatidylcholine. Studies in hepatitis used 1600 to 1800 milligrams per day, in divided doses. For more information about phosphatidylcholine, see page 131, Chapter 8.

Nutrition Strategy Checklist for Hepatitis

☐ Healthy diet
☐ Soluble fiber
☐ Avoid alcohol
☐ Vitamin E
☐ Selenium
☐ Milk thistle

☐ Coenzyme Q10 (Hepatitis B)
☐ N-acetyl cysteine (Hepatitis C)
☐ Phosphatidylcholine (Hepatitis C)

Recommended Resources

www.liverfoundation.org
American Liver Foundation
75 Maiden Lane, Suite 603
New York, NY, USA 10038
Tel: 1-800-465-4837

www.liver.ca
Canadian Liver Foundation
2235 Sheppard Avenue E, Suite 1500
Toronto, ON, Canada M2J 5B5
Tel: 416-4913353 or 1-800-563-5483
Fax: 416-491-4952

www.hepatitiscsociety.com
Hepatitis C Society of Canada
3050 Confederation Parkway, Suite 301B
Mississauga, ON, Canada L5B 3Z6
Tel: 905-270-1110 or 1-800-652-HepC (1-800-652-4372)
Fax: 905-270-1277

www.hepfi.org
Hepatitis Foundation International
30 Sunrise Terrace
Cedar Grove, NJ, USA 07009-1423
Tel: 973-239-1035 or 1-800-891-0707
Fax: 973-857-5044

www.hepnet.com
**HepNet—The Hepatitis Information Network
(Canadian)**

Herpes (Cold Sores and Genital Herpes)

The herpes simplex virus (HSV) is responsible for two common and painful infections: cold sores and genital herpes. A different type of herpes virus causes each infection. Cold sores, the irritating little blisters that often appear on your lips, gums, and the outside of your mouth, nose or cheeks, are usually triggered by HSV type 1. HSV type 2 is associated with genital herpes, a highly contagious, sexually transmitted disease that causes sores to develop on the penis, in and around the vaginal opening, around the anal opening, on the buttocks or on the thighs. It is important to understand, however, that either type of herpes virus can trigger cold sores and genital lesions.

The herpes virus lurks deep within the nerve cells at the base of your spine, where it may remain inactive for months or even years at a time. Every so often, something will activate the virus, causing it to travel along the nerves to the skin, where it triggers an outbreak. Usually, the first eruption of sores is the worst, with later episodes becoming milder. HSV remains in your nerve cells for life and cannot be cured.

Most outbreaks of HSV are unpredictable. Physical or emotional stress, fatigue, fever, menstruation, illness, certain foods, dental treatment or exposure to sunlight may reactivate the virus.

The frequency of recurrent attacks can vary considerably. Some people have only one or two outbreaks in a lifetime, while others deal with several attacks in a year.

Contracting the Virus

Herpes simplex is a highly contagious virus. Both cold sores and genital herpes can be passed from one person to another through skin-to-skin contact. Cold sores are spread by contact with the open sores or the saliva of an infected person. The virus is often contracted during infancy, through exposure to an adult with a cold sore. People who are exposed to oral herpes for the first time as adults frequently suffer more severe symptoms.

Genital herpes is usually transmitted through sexual intercourse with someone who is having a herpes outbreak. The sores that appear in the genital area during an active outbreak will shed viruses that can infect a sexual partner. In some instances, a person can have an HSV 2 outbreak without any visible sores. However, the virus can still be transmitted even when blisters aren't present. Unfortunately, many cases of genital herpes are contracted when someone has intercourse with a partner who does not know that he or she is infected.

If you have genital herpes or a cold sore, you may also transmit the virus to a partner during oral sex. Because the virus is so contagious, it is possible to transfer the virus to other parts of your body by touching the open sores and then accidentally rubbing or touching your genitals, eyes, mouth or other skin surfaces. If the herpes virus spreads to your eyes, it can cause corneal blindness.

A pregnant woman with genital herpes can spread the infection to her baby as the infant passes through the birth canal. Genital herpes is very dangerous during pregnancy, as babies born with it may die, suffer from nerve damage or have serious problems affecting the brain, skin or eyes. Herpes can also cause life-threatening illness in people suffering from eczema, AIDS, cancer or a suppressed immune system.

Symptoms
Cold Sores

A painful, tingling or itching sensation (called the prodome) may precede the blisters by one or two days. Then fluid-filled blisters or painful, red sores appear on or near the mouth or lips. These blisters form in clusters, before joining together into a larger single sore. After the blisters break and ooze, a yellow crust or scab forms. The dead skin then sloughs off and the area heals without a scar. During this time, your gums may be swollen and sensitive.

The first attack may also cause swollen lymph nodes, fever and flu-like symptoms. The sores normally last seven to ten days.

Genital Herpes

The symptoms of genital herpes may develop one to three weeks after sexual contact with an infected person. Sometimes symptoms don't appear until weeks or months after contact.

An itching or burning sensation in the genital or anal area precedes the blisters. The legs, buttocks or genital area will also be painful. Gradually, small red bumps appear, which join together to form fluid-filled blisters.

These blisters break to become painful open sores. As a crust or scab forms over the scar, dead skin sloughs off and the area heals, though it may be scarred.

The first outbreak may also be accompanied by fever, headache, muscle aches, painful urination, vaginal discharge and swollen glands. Sores normally last two to three weeks.

Who's at Risk?

Cold sores are very common. Estimates indicate that 80 percent of the North American population suffer from HSV 1. The virus is easily spread within families, with infants being most susceptible to infection. Outbreaks occur most often during adolescence and tend to decrease after age 35.

As much as 25 percent of the North American population suffer from HSV 2. The genital herpes virus affects both men and women. People who have unprotected sex with an infected partner are most at risk.

Conventional Treatment
Cold Sores

Cold sores usually clear up without treatment. Antiviral medications, in ointment or oral drug form, may shorten the duration of the outbreak but won't prevent recurrent attacks. Anesthetic mouthwashes or mouthwashes containing baking soda may ease the discomfort. Do not squeeze or pinch the blister. Keep the cold sore area dry to prevent the infection from worsening.

If you have burning pain in the eye or a rash near the eye, see your doctor immediately to prevent an infection that may lead to corneal blindness.

Genital Herpes

Antiviral medications (such as acyclovir, famciclovir and valacyclovir) in ointment or oral drug form may help genital herpes sores heal faster and reduce the number of recurrent outbreaks. Wear cotton underwear; synthetic fabrics hold moisture and may make the infection worse. Soaking in a shallow tub of salty water may ease discomfort. Eating a healthy diet, managing stress and getting enough rest and exercise may reduce the number of outbreaks.

You should tell anyone whom you have had sexual intercourse with in the past two years that you have genital herpes so that they can be examined and treated to prevent the spread of further infection.

Preventing and Managing Herpes

If you have HSV 1, use sun protection on your lips and face before exposure to the sun to help prevent outbreaks. Avoid spicy foods, as they may trigger a cold sore. To prevent spread of the virus, avoid skin contact (kissing, touching, oral sex) with other people when blisters are present. And always wash your hands carefully after touching a cold sore.

To prevent the spread of HSV 2, abstain from sexual intercourse (including oral sex) during an active outbreak. Use a latex condom during all sexual contact, since you may infect your partner even when blisters are not present.

Avoid touching other parts of your body after touching a genital sore and wash your hands carefully after contact with a sore.

Dietary Strategies

A nutritious, well-balanced diet provides vitamins and minerals that are important for wound healing and a strong immune system. Focus on low-fat animal-protein foods such as poultry breast, lean meat and low-fat dairy products. Be sure to eat whole-grain starchy foods, legumes and five to ten servings of fruits and vegetables each day. Include zinc-rich foods such as yogurt, wheat bran, wheat germ and enriched breakfast cereals to support immunity. Eat fish three times a week to get health-enhancing omega-3 fats. Use vegetable oils that support a healthy immune system, such as flaxseed, walnut and canola oils.

Minimize your intake of foods that can undermine the immune system and increase your susceptibility to infection. Limit animal fats, refined sugars and alcoholic beverages. You'll find guidelines for a healthy diet in Chapter 5.

Vitamins and Minerals

Vitamin A

This vitamin is essential for a healthy immune system and for healing of the skin. Some research suggests that people with HSV may be deficient in vitamin A.[1] The best food sources of this vitamin include liver, oily fish, milk, cheese and egg yolks.

Beta-carotene in foods also contributes to your daily vitamin A intake. Eat orange and dark green produce, including carrots, sweet potato, winter squash, broccoli, collard greens, kale, spinach, apricots, cantaloupe, peaches, nectarines, mango and papaya.

Your diet and a multivitamin will provide your daily requirement of vitamin A. Most multivitamins offer 2000 to 5000 international units (IU) of vitamin A. Because high doses of vitamin A can be toxic if taken for a period, separate vitamin A supplements should be taken only under the guidance of your health care provider. Do *not* take extra vitamin A during pregnancy.

Vitamins C and E

Both these nutrients are needed for proper immune function and wound healing. One study found that vitamin C combined with flavonoids was effective in treating genital herpes.[2] (Interestingly, many of the herbs used to treat herpes in developing countries contain flavonoids.)

Vitamin C is plentiful in citrus fruit, citrus juices, cantaloupe, kiwi, mango, strawberries, broccoli, Brussels sprouts, cauliflower, red pepper and tomato juice. During a herpes outbreak, take 200 milligrams of vitamin C with 200 milligrams of bioflavonoids five times daily. To help prevent a recurrence, take 500 milligrams of Ester C (with added bioflavonoids) once daily.

Vitamin E is found in wheat germ, nuts, seeds, vegetable oils, whole grains and kale. For immune system support, take 200 to 800 IU of natural source vitamin E. Buy a "mixed" vitamin E supplement if possible.

Herbal Remedies

Aloe Vera

Researchers have found that applying aloe vera gel or cream to genital herpes reduces the time needed for lesions to heal.[3] Some evidence suggests that aloe cream is better absorbed than aloe gel and therefore may be more effective. Apply aloe vera cream (containing 0.5 percent aloe) three times daily.

Lemon Balm (*Melissa officinalis*)

As a topical cream, this herb is widely used in Europe to treat cold sores and genital herpes. It is used at the first sign of symptoms or on a regular basis to prevent an attack. Studies have found that lemon balm cream provides significant reduction of pain, the number of blisters and the size of blisters.[4-6] It is thought that active components in the plant interfere with the ability of the herpes virus to attach to cells. During an outbreak, apply lemon balm cream (70:1 extract) four times daily. To prevent a recurrence, use twice daily.

Siberian Ginseng (*Eleutherococcus senticosus*)

One study found that, compared with placebo, this mild form of ginseng reduced the frequency of herpes outbreaks by 50 percent.[7] To ensure quality, choose a product standardized for eleutherosides B and E. The usual dose is 300 to 400 milligrams once daily for six to eight weeks, followed by a one- to two-week break.

Other Natural Health Products

Lysine

Lysine is an amino acid plentiful in meat and dairy products. Supplemental doses of lysine have been found to significantly reduce the severity of symptoms of herpes outbreaks and reduce the healing time.[8,9] There's also evidence that lysine can reduce or even prevent recurrences of attacks.[10] When 1543 people were surveyed after taking lysine for six months, 84 percent said that the supplement prevented recurrence or decreased the number of outbreaks. Among people not taking lysine, 79 percent said their symptoms were intolerable, whereas only 8 percent described their symptoms as intolerable when taking lysine. Studies in the laboratory have determined that lysine inhibits the growth of HSV.

Buy a supplement of L-lysine monohydrochloride. Studies vary in the dosage used. Some have used 1200 milligrams daily for six months, or 1000 milligrams three times daily for six months. Doses less than 1000 milligrams per day have not been effective. No side effects have been reported with these amounts.

Nutrition Strategy Checklist for Herpes

- ☐ Healthy diet
- ☐ Vitamin A
- ☐ Vitamin C
- ☐ Vitamin E
- ☐ Herbal creams: Aloe vera OR Lemon balm
- ☐ Siberian ginseng
- ☐ Lysine

Recommended Resources

www.ashastd.org/stdfaqs/herpes.html
American Social Health Association
P.O. Box 13827
Research Triangle Park, NC, USA 207709
Tel: 919-361-8400
Fax: 919-361-8425

www.cafeherpe.com
Café Herpé is sponsored by Novartis Pharmaceuticals Corporation.

www.advicecenter.com
Health Advice Company

2515 E Highway 54
2200 Century Plaza
Durham, NC, USA 27713
Tel: 1-888-ADVICE8 (1-888-238-4238)

www.herpes.com
www.herpesweb.net
These Web sites are sponsored by
GlaxoWellcome.

www.niaid.nih.gov/factsheets/stdherp.htm
National Institute of Allergy and Infectious
Diseases
National Institutes of Health
Office of Communications and Public Liaison
Bethesda, MD, USA 20892

www.gov.on.ca/health/
Ontario Ministry of Health and Long-Term
Care
Tel: 416-314-5518 or 1-800-268-1153
(Ontario only)

Hiatal Hernia (Gastroesophageal Reflux Disease)

A hiatal hernia develops when part of the stomach bulges through the diaphragm into the chest. The diaphragm, the muscle used for breathing, separates the chest from the abdomen. Normally, the esophagus, or food pipe, joins the stomach by passing through a small opening in the diaphragm, called the esophageal hiatus. When the muscle tissue surrounding your hiatus becomes weak, the upper part of your stomach can herniate or push through, forming a hiatal hernia.

There are two types of hiatal hernia. The most common is a sliding hernia. This is when the stomach pushes into the chest only when you swallow. As the muscle of the esophagus contracts during a swallow, the stomach is pulled up through the hiatus opening. When the swallow is finished, the esophageal muscle relaxes and the stomach falls back into the abdomen.

A para-esophageal hernia develops less often but is more serious. In this type of hernia, the stomach bulges into the chest and remains there. It does not slide up and down with each swallow. If the para-esophageal hernia becomes large enough, it can interfere with the passage of food into the stomach and may cause food to actually become stuck in the esophagus. An accumulation of stomach acid or damage caused by trapped food may also cause ulcers to form in the herniated part of the stomach.

What Causes a Hiatal Hernia?

Anything that puts intense pressure on your abdomen may lead to a hiatal hernia. Pregnancy, obesity and lifting heavy objects are risk factors for this condition. Even severe coughing, vomiting or straining during a bowel movement may generate enough pressure to push the stomach through the hiatus opening.

Symptoms

Very often, a hiatal hernia will cause no symptoms at all, especially if it is a small one. However, in some cases, a hernia may cause heartburn or other symptoms of gastroesophageal reflux (GERD). A hiatal hernia can interfere with the action of a small band of muscle that surrounds the bottom of the esophagus, called the lower esophageal sphincter. During normal digestion, this sphincter muscle acts like a valve, opening to allow food to pass into the stomach and closing to prevent food and stomach acid from flowing back into the esophagus.

As the stomach herniates into the chest, it may push the sphincter out of place, interfering with the muscles that control the activities of the valve. If the sphincter opens and closes at the wrong times, stomach acid may back up into the esophagus, causing heartburn, belching, pain and sometimes bleeding. Discomfort may be worse after eating, when lying down or after stooping over. Sometimes pain can spread into the upper chest, back and neck, similar to the pain of a heart attack, and should be assessed by a doctor. In most cases, symptoms will clear up with dietary and lifestyle changes.

Who's at Risk?

It's estimated that 10 percent of Canadians have hiatal hernias. The prevalence climbs to 40 percent in people over the age of 50.[1] Women appear to be at greater risk for developing a hiatal hernia than men. As well, pregnant women and people who are overweight are at higher risk.

Conventional Treatment

Treatment is not necessary unless you are experiencing symptoms. Lifestyle changes may help ease heartburn symptoms that often accompany a hiatal hernia. Dietary changes (see below) as well as the following strategies are useful:

- Avoid lying down after you eat to reduce the risk of food and stomach acid entering the esophagus; avoid eating two to three hours before bedtime.

- Elevate the head of your bed 6 to 8 inches (15 to 20 cm) to prevent stomach acid from moving up into your esophagus while you sleep.

- Avoid strenuous exercise immediately after eating.

- Avoid clothing that is tight around the abdominal area.

- Avoid certain medications, such as NSAIDs, sedatives, tranquilizers and calcium channel blockers, that may cause heartburn.

- Stop smoking.

- Avoid stress, which slows down digestion, encouraging esophageal reflux; try relaxation techniques to help reduce heartburn.

Certain medications may reduce heartburn, including antacids, H-2 blockers that reduce the amount of acid produced by the stomach, and proton pump inhibitors that block acid production. In severe cases, surgery may be necessary to repair the hernia.

Preventing and Managing a Hernia

Dietary Strategies
Trigger Foods
Dietary changes will help reduce heartburn by preventing reflux and irritation of a sensitive or inflamed esophagus. Fatty foods and high-fat meals often cause symptoms because they remain in the stomach longer and increase the time the esophagus is exposed to the acidic stomach contents. Cream, ice cream, milkshakes, fatty desserts and pastries, gravies, butter, margarine, vegetable oil, fried meats, sausage, cream soups, french fries and potato chips are often poorly tolerated.

Chocolate and coffee can also cause distress. Chocolate contains methylxanthine, a compound that relaxes the esophageal sphincter and increases the likelihood of reflux. Coffee also relaxes the esophageal sphincter and stimulates acid secretion by the stomach, which can make symptoms worse. If your esophagus is not inflamed, coffee may be allowed as tolerated. Alcohol, carbonated beverages, spearmint, peppermint, spicy foods, tomatoes, citrus fruit, onions and garlic can also irritate the esophagus. Eating smaller meals and drinking fluids between meals, rather than with meals, can also help prevent reflux.

Weight Loss

People who are overweight have an increased risk of developing a sliding hernia and esophageal reflux.[2-4] Weight loss helps to lessen abdominal pressure and can eliminate symptoms of heartburn.

To determine if you are at a healthy weight, refer to page 439, Obesity and Weight Loss, to calculate your body mass index (BMI). Having a BMI greater than 25 indicates overweight and a BMI over 27 is defined as obese. If you determine that your BMI is greater than 25, use the strategies outlined on page 442 to promote safe, gradual weight loss.

Vitamins and Minerals

Vitamin B12

People on acid blocking medication are at risk for developing a vitamin B12 deficiency and so should supplement this vitamin. Vitamin B12 requires stomach acid in order to be released from food proteins so that it can be absorbed into the bloodstream. Without stomach acid, the intestine cannot absorb B12.

Because the absorption of other nutrients, such as iron and zinc, can be affected by insufficient acid, a daily high-potency multivitamin and mineral supplement is recommended. These formulas will provide 25 to 100 micrograms of B12. Separate B12 supplements are also available in 500 and 1000 microgram doses. Vitamin B12 is extremely safe.

Iron

Some people with hiatal hernia may develop an iron deficiency because of slow bleeding of the hernia.[5,6] You should take care to eat an iron-rich diet. The richest sources of iron are beef, fish, poultry, pork and lamb (see page 55, Chapter 4). These foods contain heme iron, the type that can be absorbed and utilized the most efficiently by your body. Iron in plant foods such as dried fruits, whole grains, leafy green vegetables, nuts, seeds and legumes is nonheme iron, and the body is much less efficient at absorbing it. To enhance the absorption of nonheme iron, eat them along with nonirritating vitamin-C-rich foods such as red pepper, broccoli, Brussels sprouts, cantaloupe and strawberries.

To help you meet your daily iron requirements, a multivitamin and mineral supplement is a wise idea. Most formulas provide 10 milligrams, but you can find multivitamins that provide up to 18 milligrams of the mineral.

If you are diagnosed with iron-deficiency anemia, your doctor will prescribe single iron pills. Refer to page 161, Anemia, for more information on using iron supplements safely.

Nutrition Strategy Checklist for Hiatal Hernia

☐ Avoid food triggers   ☐ Vitamin B12

☐ Small, frequent meals   ☐ Iron

☐ Weight control

Recommended Resources

www.crha-health.ab.ca
Calgary Regional Health Authority Communications
1035-7th Avenue SW
Calgary, AB, Canada T2P 3E9
Tel: 403-265-INFO (403-265-4636) or
1-800-860-2742 (Alberta only)
E-mail: publicweb@crha-health.ab.ca

www.mayoclinic.com
Mayo Foundation for Medical Education and Research

www.focusondigestion.com
Site supported by MedicineNet.com.

High Blood Pressure (Hypertension)

High blood pressure, or hypertension, is one of the "big three" risk factors for heart disease (along with high cholesterol and cigarette smoking). The higher your blood pressure is above normal, the greater your risk of coronary artery disease, congestive heart failure, renal failure and stroke. Hypertension is often called the silent killer because it develops slowly, over a number of years, and usually displays no symptoms until a vital organ is irreversibly damaged.

Your blood pressure is determined by the force or pressure generated by the heart as it pushes blood through the arteries. When the heart beats, blood pressure in your arteries rises. Between beats, blood pressure falls as your heart relaxes. Blood pressure is assessed by two measurements: systolic pressure (blood pressure when the heart is contracting) and diastolic pressure (blood pressure when the heart is relaxing). A normal resting blood pressure is 120/80. The top number is the systolic reading and the bottom number is the diastolic reading.

The higher the blood pressure level, the harder your heart is working. If your resting blood pressure is consistently 140/90 or higher, you have high blood pressure. Doctors use the following guide to determine high blood pressure:

Evaluation of Blood Pressure (mm Hg)

	Systolic Blood Pressure	Diastolic Blood Pressure
Normal	<130	<85
High-normal	130–139	80–89
Mild hypertension	140–159	90–99
Moderate hypertension	160–179	100–109
Severe hypertension	180–209	110–119
Very severe hypertension	>210	>120

Blood pressure tends to increase with age. Your blood pressure will also change throughout the day, reaching its highest levels in the morning and its lowest during the night, when you are sleeping. When you are relaxed and resting, your heart beats more slowly and your blood pressure drops. Physical activity, emotional stress and anxiety increase your heart rate and blood pressure. Because of these normal variations in blood pressure, a diagnosis of hypertension is never based on just one high reading. To be certain that the diagnosis of high blood pressure is accurate, your blood pressure is taken after resting for five minutes. It is then measured on at least two other occasions.

If high blood pressure is complicated by hardening of the arteries (atherosclerosis), the condition becomes much more serious. When arteries are hardened and stiff they strain as blood pumps through them. Because hardened arteries can't expand to accommodate the blood flow, blood pressure rises. This prolonged stress damages the arteries and causes cholesterol to accumulate on the artery walls, narrowing the arteries even further. This usually leads to a reduction in the blood flowing to the kidneys. The kidneys respond by retaining sodium to increase blood volume and blood pressure.

The higher your blood pressure and the longer it remains uncontrolled, the greater the damage it can cause. Complications from high blood pressure include aneurysm (an enlarged, bulging blood vessel), stroke, kidney disorders and vision loss. Managing your blood pressure for five years or longer can decrease the risk of heart attack by 20 percent and the risk of heart failure by 50 percent.[1]

What Causes High Blood Pressure?

In 90 percent of all cases, the cause of high blood pressure is unknown. In these cases, the condition is referred to as primary or essential hypertension. Scientists suspect that high blood pressure is caused by several changes in the heart and blood vessels brought about by an interaction of genetic, lifestyle and social factors. The role of lifestyle factors such as obesity, alcohol consumption, smoking, inactivity, poor diet and stress have been well documented.

In the remaining 10 percent of cases, the cause of high blood pressure can be identified. Causes include kidney disease, hormonal disorders such as thyroid disease, certain medications, pregnancy and use of illegal drugs. When the cause of high blood pressure is known, the condition is referred to as secondary hypertension.

Symptoms

While most people don't know they have high blood pressure until it is diagnosed, the following signs or symptoms may be present:

- headaches, dizziness and nosebleeds
- damage to the eyes, kidneys, brain and heart, causing fatigue, nausea, vomiting, shortness of breath, restlessness and blurred vision
- drowsiness or coma from swelling in the brain in severe cases

Who's at Risk?

In North America, it's estimated that one person in every five suffers from high blood pressure. The following factors may increase your risk of developing the condition:

- *older age*
- *race*—high blood pressure is more common in black people
- *gender*—men have a greater risk of high blood pressure before the age of 55 and women are at greater risk over the age of 65[2]
- *genetics*—high blood pressure can run in families
- *obesity*

Conventional Treatment

Lifestyle changes are the most effective method of preventing and controlling high blood pressure. Weight loss, regular exercise and dietary changes can significantly lower blood pressure. Quitting smoking, learning to manage stress and getting proper rest are also important strategies. The following medications are sometimes prescribed to lower blood pressure:

- *diuretics*, or water pills, to help the kidneys eliminate salt and water
- *beta-blockers* to make the heart beat less often and with less force
- *alpha-blockers* to block the effects of chemicals produced by the nervous system on the blood vessels
- *alpha-beta-blockers* to combine the benefits of both alpha-blockers and beta-blockers
- *ACE (angiotensin converting enzyme) inhibitors* to dilate arteries
- *angiotensin antagonists* to protect blood vessels from narrowing
- *calcium channel blockers (CCBs)* to prevent calcium from entering the heart muscle cells and blood vessels, keeping the blood vessels dilated and relaxed
- *vasodilators* to open blood vessels by relaxing the muscle in the blood vessel walls

Preventing and Managing High Blood Pressure

Dietary Strategies

Weight Control

People who are overweight have an increased risk of developing high blood pressure. Study after study has determined overweight to be a strong risk factor for elevated blood pressure.[3-7] Weight loss should be the first line of treatment in hypertension. Even a moderate weight loss of 5 to 10 percent of body weight will cause a drop in blood pressure. In some cases, achieving and maintaining a healthy weight can reduce or eliminate the need for blood pressure medication.

To determine if you are at a healthy weight, refer to page 439, Obesity and Weight Loss, to calculate your body mass index (BMI). A BMI over 25 indicates overweight; a BMI greater than 27 is defined as obese. If you determine your BMI is greater than 25, use the strategies outlined on page 442, Obesity and Weight Loss, for safe, gradual weight loss.

The DASH Diet

Studies are now revealing that eating whole foods is much more important than focusing on single nutrients in the prevention and treatment of hypertension. The Dietary Approaches to Stop Hypertension (DASH) diet study has determined an optimal pattern of eating that produces a potent blood-pressure-lowering effect.[8] This eight-week trial measured the effects of diet on blood pressure in 459 adults. Participants were asked to follow one of three diets: 1) a control diet that contained little fruit and vegetables (3.6 servings/day) and dairy products (0.5 servings/day), 2) a diet high in fruits and vegetables (8 to 10 servings/day) and 3) a combination diet high in fruits and vegetables with added low-fat dairy products (2 servings/day). All diets had the same levels of sodium and a maximum of two alcoholic drinks per day.

Subjects on the combination diet who had mild hypertension achieved a reduction in blood pressure similar to that obtained by drug treatment. A subsequent study using the DASH combination diet lowered blood pressure within two weeks; after two months, 70 percent of the participants achieved a normal blood pressure.[9]

This DASH diet provides food choices that are high in fiber, calcium, magnesium and potassi-um, all of which have been associated with lower blood pressure. The DASH diet is also low in refined carbohydrates and saturated fats, both of which can cause salt retention and high blood pressure.

If you have high blood pressure and would like to follow the DASH diet, use the following as your guide:

Food	Servings per Day
Whole-grain foods	7 to 8
Vegetables	4 to 5
Fruits	4 to 5
Low-fat/nonfat dairy products	2
Meat, poultry, fish	4 to 6 ounces (100 to 150 grams)
Legumes, nuts, seeds	4 to 5 per week
Added fats	3
Sweets	Treat yourself to 1 serving per week

The DASH diet and portion sizes can be found at the DASH diet homepage **www.dash. bwh.harvard.edu**.

Fish and Omega-3 Fats

Studies have shown that eating fish once a day lowers blood pressure in people with hypertension.[10,11] Two studies found that adding fish to a weight-loss diet produced a greater blood-pressure-lowering effect than weight loss alone.[12,13] Omega-3 fats found in fish are used by the body to produce anti-inflammatory compounds called eicosanoids (prostaglandins, leukotrienes, prostacylcins, thromboxanes). These compounds are thought to protect from hypertension.

The best sources of omega-3 fats are salmon, sardines, herring, mackerel, trout, sea bass and fresh tuna. Aim to include one serving of fish in your daily diet. Fish oil capsules are an alternative for people who don't like fish (see below).

Alcohol and Caffeine

An excessive intake of alcohol damages blood vessel walls and increases the risk of hypertension.[14-16] Too much caffeine can exacerbate high blood pressure, especially when combined with stress. Women should limit their intake of alcohol to no more than one drink per day (or seven per week), men no more than two drinks per day (to a limit of nine per week). A drink is considered 12 ounces (340 ml) of regular beer, 5 ounces (145 ml) of wine or 1 1/2 ounces (45 ml) of 80-proof (40 percent) distilled spirits.

Since caffeine also raises blood pressure, reduce your caffeine intake to no more than 450 milligrams per day (refer to page 82, Chapter 5).[17-19] Older adults with hypertension may be more sensitive to the effect of caffeine and should limit their intake to no more than 1 cup (6 ounces) of coffee per day.[20] Avoid caffeinated beverages, especially coffee, if you are under stress.

Vitamins and Minerals

Vitamin C

Some evidence suggests that the formation of free radicals increases in people with hypertension and that this may impair the ability of blood vessels to relax and dilate.[21] As an antioxidant, vitamin C is thought to inhibit the production of free radicals in vessel walls and preserve their health. Studies have found that vitamin C supplements help lower blood pressure in people with hypertension.[22-26]

The recommended dietary allowance (RDA) is 75 and 90 milligrams for women and men respectively (smokers need an additional 35 milligrams). Foods rich in vitamin C include citrus fruit, citrus juices, cantaloupe, kiwi, mango, strawberries, broccoli, Brussels sprouts, cauliflower, red pepper and tomato juice. To supplement, take 500 milligrams of Ester C once or twice daily. The daily upper limit is 2000 milligrams.

Calcium

This mineral is important in both preventing and treating high blood pressure. Low calcium intakes are associated with hypertension and higher intakes have been shown to lower blood pressure. In a review of 22 studies, calcium supplementation was found to modestly lower systolic blood pressure but not diastolic pressure.[27-28] Based on this evidence, the Canadian Hypertension Society does not recommend calcium supplements above the recommended daily intake to treat or prevent high blood pressure.[29]

Calcium Supplements

Calcium supplements seem to be more beneficial when high blood pressure is due to pregnancy than when the condition is due to any other cause. Supplements in the range of 1500 to 2000 milligrams per day have been shown to significantly lower blood pressure during pregnancy.

To ensure you are meeting your daily recommended intake for calcium, include calcium-rich foods in your daily diet. Low-fat milk, yogurt, fortified soy and rice beverages, fortified orange juice, tofu, salmon (with bones), kale, bok choy, broccoli, Swiss chard and almonds are all good choices.

Choose a supplement made with calcium citrate, with vitamin D and magnesium added. You'll find more information about calcium starting on page 43, Chapter 4.

Magnesium

Low levels of magnesium in the diet and the blood are believed to contribute to the development of hypertension.[30,31] Magnesium influences the excitability of the heart and the reactivity of blood vessels. While studies show that magnesium-rich diets are important in preventing high blood pressure, clinical studies using magnesium supplements to treat hypertension have been less than convincing.[32] The Canadian Hypertension Society does not recommend magnesium supplements to treat or prevent high blood pressure.

The best strategy is to eat magnesium-rich foods as outlined in the DASH diet (see above). For most people this is quite a change, since a diet of refined, processed foods contains little magnesium.

The best food sources of magnesium include nuts, seeds, legumes, lentils, prunes, whole grains, leafy green vegetables, Brewer's yeast and shrimp. See page 47, Chapter 4, for a detailed food list and recommended magnesium intakes.

Potassium

Low intakes of potassium are linked with high blood pressure.[33] Depleting potassium levels in the body elevates blood pressure in both people with normal blood pressure and people with high blood pressure. Low potassium levels cause the body to retain sodium and lose calcium. Increasing potassium intake dilates blood vessels and protects vessels from the narrowing effect of stress hormones.

Some studies have found potassium supplements to lower blood pressure in people with hypertension.[34,35] However, the greatest benefit comes from following the DASH diet, which offers a combination of potassium-, calcium- and magnesium-rich foods.

Potassium-rich foods include bananas, oranges, orange juice, potatoes, avocado, cantaloupe, peaches, tomatoes, tomato juice, lima beans, salmon, cod, chicken, meat and milk.

Sodium

Until recently, experts felt that sodium restriction alone did not help all people lower their blood pressure. It is estimated that up to 50 percent of people with essential hypertension are unable to handle sodium properly and are salt sensitive.[36] Older adults and people with diabetes tend to be salt sensitive and respond to a low-sodium diet.

It now appears that reducing sodium may be an important component of a blood-pressure-

lowering diet for most people with high blood pressure. Researchers have measured the effects of the DASH diet with varying levels of salt on the blood pressure in 412 people with hypertension.[37] Participants ate foods with high, medium and low levels of sodium for 30 days. The researchers found that blood pressure fell significantly at each lower sodium level. Reducing sodium, in combination with the DASH diet, seems to have a greater blood-pressure-lowering effect than the DASH diet alone.

The table of selected foods and their sodium content, on page 80, Chapter 5, will help you make wise choices as you reduce your intake of sodium-rich foods.

Herbal Remedies

Garlic (*Allium sativum*)

Studies have shown that garlic supplements can lower elevated blood pressure by 5 to 10 percent.[38-40] Garlic is thought to work by relaxing the smooth muscle of blood vessels and activating compounds that dilate vessels. Both Kwai® garlic powder and Kyolic® aged garlic extract supplements have shown beneficial effects. Studies using Kwai® gave 600 to 900 milligrams daily, in divided doses. With Kyolic®, a reduction in blood pressure was achieved by a large dose of 7.2 grams.

Garlic supplements in high doses may be unsafe during pregnancy. Garlic may also enhance the effects of blood-thinning medications like warfarin (Coumadin®). Since garlic can prolong bleeding time, stop taking it one week prior to scheduled surgery.

Other Natural Health Products

Coenzyme Q10 (CoQ10)

Reports from several research studies deem this antioxidant to be a moderately effective treatment for hypertension.[41,42] CoQ10 may lower blood pressure by neutralizing or suppressing the action of free radicals formed in vessel walls. The recommended dose for high blood pressure is 225 milligrams daily. CoQ10 is very safe. No significant side effects have been reported. For more information about CoQ10, refer to page 123, Chapter 8.

Fish Oil Supplements

A number of studies have found that fish oil supplements help reduce blood pressure in people with hypertension.[43-47] Fish oil does not seem to be effective, however, at treating high blood pressure associated with pregnancy. Buy a product with a combination of EPA and DHA, two omega-3 fatty acids found in fish. Look for a supplement that has vitamin E added as it helps prevent the oils from going rancid. Avoid fish *liver* oil capsules. Fish liver oil is a concentrated source of vitamin A and D, which can be toxic when taken in large amounts for long periods.

The typical dosage to lower blood pressure is 4 grams per day, often taken in divided doses. Fish oil supplements can cause belching and a fishy taste. Because fish oil has a thinning effect on the blood, you should use caution if you are taking blood-thinning medication such as aspirin, warfarin (Coumadin®) or heparin. See page 126, Chapter 8, for more information on fish oils.

Nutrition Strategy Checklist for High Blood Pressure

☐ Weight control
☐ DASH diet
☐ Omega-3 fats
☐ Limit alcohol and caffeine
☐ Vitamin C
☐ Calcium
☐ Magnesium
☐ Potassium
☐ Restrict sodium
☐ Garlic
☐ Coenzyme Q10

Recommended Resources

www.americanheart.org
American Heart Association
National Center
7272 Greenville Avenue
Dallas, TX, USA 75231
Tel: 1-800-AHA-USA1 (1-800-242-8721)

www.ash-us.org
American Society of Hypertension
515 Madison Avenue, Suite 1212
New York, NY, USA 10022
Tel: 212-644-0650
Fax: 212-644-0658

www.canadianbpcoalition.org
Canadian Coalition for High Blood Pressure Prevention and Control
c/o Dr. Robert Petrella
Centre of Activity and Aging
1490 Richmond Street N, Room 208A
London, ON, Canada N6G 2M3
Tel: 519-661-1610
Fax: 519-661-1635

www.nhlbi.nih.gov
National Institutes of Health
National Heart, Lung and Blood Institute
NHLBI Health Information Network
P.O. Box 30105
Bethesda, MD, USA 20824-0105
Tel: 301-592-8573
Fax: 301-592-8563

Hyperthyroidism (Graves' Disease)

The thyroid gland is a tiny butterfly-shaped gland that weighs only an ounce. It produces a steady supply of two major thyroid hormones, tri-iodothyronine (T3) and thyroxine (T4). When you are healthy, the pituitary gland located in your brain releases thyroid stimulating-hormone (TSH), which triggers the release of T3 and T4. These thyroid hormones travel in your bloodstream to various organs in the body and determine the speed of all your internal chemical processes. In a nutshell, thyroid hormones act to control your body's metabolic rate (the speed at which you burn calories). When T3 and T4 are at normal levels, the amount of TSH in your blood will level off.

When the thyroid gland becomes overactive it secretes too many thyroid hormones, causing your cells to work harder and your metabolism to speed up by 60 to 100 percent. This condition is known as hyperthyroidism and is characterized by a high metabolic rate.

What Causes Hyperthyroidism?

Graves' Disease

Several factors may trigger hyperthyroidism but, in North America, Graves' disease causes 90 percent of all cases. This disorder is named after the Irish physician Robert Graves, who first described it in 1835. The condition is also referred to as diffuse toxic goiter, thyrotoxicosis or Basedow's disease.

Graves' disease is an autoimmune condition. Under normal circumstances, the immune system produces antibodies that protect the body from foreign invaders, such as bacteria and viruses. In Graves' disease, the immune system malfunctions and produces a protein called thyroid-stimulating antibody that causes the thyroid gland to overproduce thyroid hormones.

Little is known about the exact causes of Graves' disease. It's thought that severe emotional stress may be a factor. Stress can increase the blood levels of cortisone and adrenaline, two hormones that help prepare the body for a stressful event. Cortisone and adrenaline may also affect the production of antibodies in the immune system. It's possible that environmental conditions may cause immune system malfunctions, triggering the problems of an overactive thyroid.

Symptoms

Hyperthyroidism causes a range of symptoms, including

- anxiousness, nervousness and irritability
- fast heartbeat
- sleeplessness
- fatigue
- heat intolerance
- high blood pressure
- profuse sweating
- shakiness and tremors
- muscle weakness, especially in upper arms and thighs
- confusion
- increased appetite
- weight loss
- frequent bowel movements
- eye changes, including puffiness and a constant stare
- sensitivity to light, increased tear formation
- fine, brittle hair
- thinning skin
- lighter or less frequent menstrual periods

In addition to the symptoms of hyperthyroidism listed above, Graves' disease is characterized by three other distinctive symptoms:

- The thyroid gland may become quite enlarged, causing a bulge in the neck. This is called a goiter.

- Sometimes people with Graves' disease develop a lumpy, reddish thickening of the skin in front of the shins. This condition is called pretibial myxedema.

- Fifty percent of people with Graves' disease will have eyes that protrude out of their sockets, due to a build-up of deposits and fluid in the orbit of the eye. As a result, the muscles that move the eye are not able to function properly, causing double or blurred vision. Eyelids may not close properly because they are swollen with fluid, exposing the eye to injury from foreign particles. Eyes will be painful, red and watery.

Thyroid hormones also have an effect on the reproductive system. Women with Graves' disease may find that their menstrual periods are decreased and younger girls may experience a delay in the onset of menstruation. For many women, an overactive thyroid gland is connected with infertility. Fortunately, once the condition has been treated successfully, fertility is usually quickly restored.

Who's at Risk?

About 75 percent of all autoimmune diseases occur in women, hitting them most often between the ages of 30 and 40.[1] In North America, hyperthyroidism (from all causes) affects approximately 2 percent of women, compared with 0.2 percent of men.[2] In Canada, Graves' disease affects approximately one in every 100 people.[3] You may be at risk of developing Graves' disease if you

- are a woman between the ages of 20 and 40

- are a woman who has given birth within the last six months

- have experienced thyroid disease before

- have been overtreated for hypothyroidism

- have other autoimmune conditions (e.g., Hashimoto's thyroiditis, diabetes mellitus, rheumatoid arthritis, lupus, pernicious anemia or vitiligo)

Diseases of the immune system tend to run in families. Graves' disease has been identified as an inherited condition, although not every member of an afflicted family will develop the disorder. Cigarette smoking and stress may also increase the risk for Graves' disease.[4]

Conventional Treatment

The treatment for hyperthyroidism varies according to the needs and symptoms of each person. In developing a treatment plan, your physician will consider your age, the severity of your illness, the symptoms you are experiencing and other medical conditions you may have.

There are three main approaches to treating the problems associated with hyperthyroidism and Graves' disease.

1. *Medication* Antithyroid drugs such as Tapazole® (methimazole) and Propyl-Thyracil® (propyl-thiouracil) are most commonly used to treat hyperthyroidism. They slow down the activity of the thyroid gland by suppressing the release of thyroid hormones. The doses of these medications are adjusted according to the level of thyroid hormone in your blood. Antithyroid drugs are usually prescribed in mild cases of hyperthyroidism and for children, young adults or the elderly with the disease.

2. *Radioactive iodine* Since antithyroid drugs do not cure hyperthyroidism, you may be treated with radioactive iodine to achieve a long-term solution. A small dose of radioactive iodine is taken by mouth and travels from your stomach to your thyroid gland, where it destroys some of the cells. Treatment is usually designed to destroy only enough thyroid cells to bring

thyroid hormone production back to a normal level. Treatment with radioactive iodine usually causes your thyroid gland to slow down to the point where it underproduces thyroid hormones, creating a condition known as hypothyroidism. Hypothyroidism is easily treated by taking a daily thyroid hormone pill called Synthroid® (levothyroxine) to restore normal blood levels.

3. *Surgery* Hyperthyroidism can be permanently cured by surgically removing the thyroid gland in a procedure called a thyroidectomy. This may be considered if you have a large goiter, if you have a negative reaction to antithyroid medication or if you are in a younger age group. Once the thyroid gland is removed, the cause of hyperthyroidism is eliminated. However, you will probably become hypothyroid and so require thyroid replacement medication for the rest of your life.

In addition to one or more of these treatments, your doctor will usually prescribe beta-blocking drugs such as Inderal® (propranolol), Tenormin® (atenolol) and Lopressor® (metoprolol). Beta-blockers do not control abnormal thyroid function but are useful in managing symptoms such as increased heart rate and nervousness until other forms of treatment can be started. These drugs block the action of the thyroid hormone circulating in your bloodstream, slowing your heart rate and reducing feelings of nervousness and irritability. They are not suitable for people who have asthma or heart failure as they may cause these conditions to worsen.

Eye Symptoms

Any eye changes you are experiencing because of Graves' disease will usually improve once the hyperthyroidism is under control. In some cases, however, the condition progresses despite all thyroid gland treatments. In these situations, strong drugs such as oral steroids (prednisone) or immunosuppressants (cyclosporin) may be used

to minimize swelling and reduce pressure on the optic nerve.

Your specialist may consider radioactive treatments and surgery to remove some bone from the eye orbit to reduce swelling and prevent nerve damage. Simple ways to help you cope with your eye changes include using eye drops and eye lubricants, sleeping with the head of your bed elevated and wearing eyeglasses with prisms to improve double vision. If you are a cigarette smoker, bear in mind that smoking makes eye symptoms worse and reduces your response to treatment.

Managing Graves' Disease

The nutritional approaches recommended below are intended to help offset side effects associated with various types of treatment for Graves' disease. In addition to keeping you well during and after your course of therapy for this disease, these strategies will improve your overall health and feeling of well-being.

Dietary Strategies
Weight Control

If you have been treated for hyperthyroidism, you are at risk for gaining weight. Research suggests that up to 50 percent of women with hyperthyroidism report weight problems after therapy.[5,6] Many women increase their food intake when they are experiencing the disease to prevent weight loss. When your thyroid hormones return to lower, normal levels, your metabolic rate slows down. This means your body will burn fewer calories each day. If you do not reduce your food intake to match your lower metabolism, you will gain weight.

If you have finished your treatment program and you now weigh more than you did before you were diagnosed with Graves' disease, examine your eating habits to determine where you are going wrong. Keep a food diary for two weeks. Writing down what you eat often highlights dietary discrepancies. On page 442, Obesity and Weight Loss, I outline many strategies to help promote weight loss.

To improve your chances of long-term success, consider working one on one with a registered dietitian. To find a nutritionist in private practice in your area, log on to **www.dietitians.ca**.

Vitamins and Minerals

Antioxidants

Research suggests that hyperthyroidism is associated with a decrease in antioxidants and an increase in oxidative stress brought on by free radical molecules.[7,8] Free radicals are highly reactive oxygen molecules that are produced by normal body processes. Dietary antioxidants such as vitamins C, E and beta-carotene quench harmful free radicals and prevent them from causing damage to body cells.

Studies that measured levels of antioxidant nutrients in the blood and thyroid tissue of women with Graves' hyperthyroidism have observed decreased levels of beta-carotene and vitamin E.[9,10] Another study looked at the effect of a daily vitamin C supplement in 24 women undergoing antithyroid drug therapy for Graves' disease.[11] At the beginning of the study, the researchers found that, compared with healthy women who served as controls, those with hyperthyroidism had higher levels of oxidized compounds and lower levels of antioxidant enzymes in their blood. After taking 1000 milligrams of vitamin C for one month, these women had significant increases in antioxidant enzymes.

While the link between antioxidants and hyperthyroidism is preliminary, there is no harm in boosting your intake of these nutrients as they have many other potential health benefits.

- *Vitamin C* The recommended dietary allowance (RDA) is 75 and 90 milligrams for women and men respectively (smokers need an additional 35 milligrams). Best food sources include citrus fruit, citrus juices, cantaloupe, kiwi, mango, strawberries, broccoli, Brussels sprouts, cauliflower, red pepper and tomato juice. To supplement, take 500 milligrams of Ester C once daily. The daily upper limit is 2000 milligrams.

- *Vitamin E* The RDA is 22 international units (IU). Best food sources include wheat germ, nuts, seeds, vegetable oils, whole grains and kale. To supplement take 200 to 800 IU of natural source vitamin E. Buy a "mixed" vitamin E supplement if possible. The daily upper limit is 1500 IU.

- *Beta-Carotene* No RDA has been established for beta-carotene. Best food sources are orange and dark green produce, including carrots, sweet potato, winter squash, broccoli, collard greens, kale, spinach, apricots, cantaloupe, peaches, nectarines, mango and papaya. Choose a multivitamin and mineral supplement with beta-carotene added.

Calcium and Vitamin D

It's well documented that hyperthyroidism causes a higher rate of bone breakdown. Some studies, but not all, have found a harmful effect of antithyroid medication on bone density. To explore further the effect of thyroid medication on bone loss, French researchers summarized the results from 41 studies in 1250 patients.[12] Their results showed that medications like Tapazole® (methimazole) and Propyl-Thyracil® (propylthiouracil) that suppress thyroid hormone secretion cause significant bone loss in the lower spine and hip in postmenopausal women.

There is also evidence that women with Graves' disease are more susceptible to calcium and vitamin D deficiency during the winter months.[13] Deficiencies of these two nutrients are linked with a higher risk of tetany following surgery for Graves' disease. Tetany is a condition of mineral imbalance in the body that results in severe muscle spasms. Mild tetany is characterized by tingling in the fingers, toes and lips. More severe forms can lead to death. Tetany occurs when the concentration of calcium in body fluids falls below normal. Low calcium levels can be caused by a lack of vitamin D. Fortunately, most forms of tetany can be successfully treated with adequate calcium and vitamin D.

To protect your bones and lower the risk of postoperative tetany, make sure you meet your daily requirements for each essential nutrient (see the RDA tables in Chapter 4).

- *Calcium* The RDA is 1000 to 1200 milligrams. Best food sources are milk, yogurt, cheese, fortified soy and rice beverages, fortified orange juice, tofu, salmon (with bones), kale, bok choy, broccoli and Swiss chard. If you take calcium supplements, buy calcium citrate with vitamin D and magnesium added.

- *Vitamin D* The daily adequate intake is 200 to 600 IU. Best food sources are fluid milk, fortified soy and rice beverages, oily fish, egg yolks, butter and margarine. Most multivitamin and mineral supplements provide 400 IU of vitamin D.

Iodine

This trace mineral is an integral part of T3 and T4, the two thyroid hormones released by the thyroid gland. When the body is faced with an ongoing lack of iodine, production of thyroid hormones declines. This leads to hypothyroidism, which produces symptoms such as weight gain and sluggishness (see page 367, Hypothyroidism).

While deficiency of iodine does not lead to Graves' hyperthyroidism, short-changing your diet of this indispensable mineral might influence your remission rate after treatment with antithyroid drugs. One American study of 69 patients who took antithyroid medication for Graves' disease suggests that the more iodine in the diet, the longer the rate of remission (the longer the disease remained dormant).[14]

The major source of iodine is the ocean—seafood and seawater are excellent sources of the mineral. As you move farther inland, the amount of iodine in foods varies and generally reflects the amount of this mineral in the soil that plants grow in or animals graze on. Land that was once under the ocean contains plenty of iodine. In Canada and the United States the soil around the Great Lakes is iodine-poor. However, in Canada and the United States the fortification of table salt with iodine has eliminated the health problems associated with iodine deficiency.

The daily recommended intake for adults is 150 micrograms of iodine. During pregnancy and breastfeeding, women need to consume an additional 70 and 140 micrograms each day, respectively. North Americans are estimated to be getting approximately 200 to 500 micrograms of iodine per day, well above the requirements. Some of this excess may be coming from a diet increasingly reliant on fast foods, since these foods add a generous amount of salt to the diet. Besides iodized salt, other food sources of iodine include seafood, bread, dairy products, plants grown in iodine-rich soil and meat and poultry from animals raised on iodine-rich soil.

If antithyroid drugs are a part of your treatment regime, make sure you include iodine-rich foods in your diet. This is particularly true if you live in an area with iodine-poor soil, you avoid fast food and salty foods and you don't add table salt to your meals. Consider bringing back the saltshaker to the table—a little is all you need.

Nutrition Strategy Checklist for Hyperthyroidism

☐ Weight control   ☐ Calcium
☐ Vitamin C   ☐ Vitamin D
☐ Vitamin E   ☐ Iodine
☐ Beta-carotene

Recommended Resources

www.ngdf.org
National Graves' Disease Foundation
2 Tsitsi Court
Brevard, NC, USA 28712
Tel: 704-877-5251
Fax: 704-877-5251
E-mail: ngdf@citcom.net

www.thyroid.ca
Thyroid Foundation of Canada
1040 Gardiners Road, Suite C
Kingston, ON, Canada K7P 1R7
Tel: 1-800-267-8822
Fax: 613-634-3483
E-mail: thyroid@io.org

www.the-thyroid-society.org
Thyroid Society for Education and Research
7515 S Main Street, Suite 545
Houston, TX, USA 77030
Tel: 1-800-THYROID (1-800-849-7643)
Fax: 713-799-9919

Hypoglycemia

Hypoglycemia develops when the glucose (sugar) levels in your blood fall below normal. Low glucose or blood sugar can cause many body organs to malfunction. The brain is the most susceptible because glucose is its main energy source.

Your body relies on glucose as its main source of fuel for daily activities. During the process of digestion, the carbohydrates (sugars and starches) that you eat every day are converted into glucose. Glucose is often referred to as blood sugar because it is absorbed by your bloodstream and carried to every cell in your body. Unused glucose is stored in your muscles and liver as glycogen. Your body draws on these sugar stores for energy when your blood sugar drops.

Whenever you eat food, the breakdown of carbohydrates into glucose causes your blood-sugar level to rise. This triggers your pancreas, an organ located in your upper abdomen, to release a hormone called insulin. Insulin helps glucose enter body cells, where it supplies the energy to fuel most bodily functions. As glucose is absorbed into the cells, your blood-sugar level gradually drops back to a normal range.

A few hours later, when most of the available glucose supply is consumed, your blood-sugar levels start to fall below normal, indicating that your body needs more fuel. Your pancreas responds to the falling glucose levels by releasing a different hormone, called glucagon. Glucagon stimulates your liver to release its stored supply of glucose into the bloodstream, where it is circulated to the cells. Once again, your blood-sugar levels rise back to normal. By relying on insulin, glucagon and several other hormones, your body is able to keep your blood-glucose levels under constant control and regulate your daily energy supply.

What Causes Hypoglycemia?

Hypoglycemia occurs when your blood-glucose levels drop too low and you no longer have enough energy to fuel your daily activities. Hypoglycemia develops most often as a complication of diabetes (see page 263, Diabetes). Many people with diabetes have to take insulin or other drugs to keep their blood-sugar level in the normal range. When people with diabetes eat too little food, exercise too strenuously, drink too much alcohol or take too much medication, they are at risk of developing hypoglycemia.

Hypoglycemia can also occur in people who don't have diabetes. If you develop low blood-sugar symptoms after eating a meal, you may have *reactive hypoglycemia*. This type of low blood-sugar reaction occurs when the pancreas releases too much insulin at once, causing your blood-sugar level to fall below normal. Symptoms usually develop within two to five hours after eating a meal. If you are prone to reactive hypoglycemia, eating too many starchy or sweet foods can aggravate the condition. That's because large portions of carbohydrate-rich foods cause your blood sugar to rise very rapidly, triggering excessive insulin production and a dramatic drop in your glucose level, leaving you feeling sweaty, anxious, hungry and shaky.

Other possible causes of hypoglycemia include

- stress and anxiety
- an unbalanced diet that is high in refined grains and/or sugars
- drinking alcohol
- early pregnancy
- prolonged fasting
- long periods of strenuous exercise
- exercising while you are on beta-blocker medication (e.g., propranolol)
- liver disease
- gastric surgery that disrupts the balance between digestion and insulin release
- hereditary intolerance of foods that contain the natural sugars fructose and galactose (rare childhood conditions)

While there are many conditions that may cause hypoglycemia, only 1 percent of hypoglycemia cases occur in people who do not have diabetes.[1] Studies indicate that it is actually quite a rare disorder.

Symptoms

When your blood-sugar level falls, your body responds by releasing a hormone called epinephrine (adrenaline) from your adrenal glands. This hormone stimulates your liver to release its stored glucose into your bloodstream. But this adrenaline rush also produces the symptoms that are characteristic of hypoglycemia, such as sweating, nervousness, rapid heartbeat, hunger, faintness and trembling.

If your blood-sugar level continues to fall, the reduced glucose supply will begin to affect your brain. Symptoms include headache, dizziness, confusion, blurred vision, difficulty concentrating, anxiety, agitation and abnormal behavior that could be mistaken for drunkenness. If your condition continues to worsen, convulsions, loss of consciousness and coma may result. Such life-threatening symptoms are usually caused by too much medication in people with diabetes.

If you have symptoms of hypoglycemia and you do not have diabetes, your doctor may conduct some simple blood tests to measure your blood-sugar and insulin levels. Ideally, this test will be done while you are experiencing an episode of hypoglycemic symptoms. The diagnosis of hypoglycemia will be confirmed if the blood test indicates that your blood-sugar levels are below normal and your symptoms improve when you consume sugar.

For years, doctors used the oral glucose tolerance test to diagnose hypoglycemia. However, its use has fallen out of favor because it can produce misleading results. It is now recognized that the signs and symptoms of hypoglycemia can occur in individuals who have blood-glucose levels within the normal range. Relying on a blood-sugar test alone is often not enough to diagnose hypoglycemia.

One of the most useful ways to determine if you suffer from hypoglycemia is to assess your symptoms. In general, when symptoms appear three to four hours after eating and disappear after you've consumed food, hypoglycemia is a likely cause.

Who's at Risk?

- People who take medication for diabetes
- People who fast or follow a low-calorie diet
- Pregnant women
- People who drink alcohol after a long period without eating food

Conventional Treatment

In most cases, the symptoms of hypoglycemia will quickly improve when you consume sugar in any form. Eating candy, sugar cubes, glucose or dextrose tablets or drinking a glass of fruit juice, milk or sugar water will immediately raise your blood-sugar levels, making you feel much better. If you do experience a low blood-sugar reaction, treat it immediately by consuming 10 to 15 grams of carbohydrate such as five Lifesavers®, half a banana, or 1/2 to 3/4 cup (125 to 175 ml) of fruit juice.

If you have diabetes or are prone to recurring episodes of hypoglycemia, you should always carry some candy or other type of sugar. DextroEnergy™ are flavored dextrose tablets that are widely available in drug stores in the diet section. Three tablets give you 9 grams of carbohydrate. In severe cases of hypoglycemia, an injection of glucagon or intravenous glucose may be necessary to restore blood-sugar levels.

Hypoglycemia that develops after gastrointestinal surgery can often be managed by eating small, frequent meals and following a high-protein, low-carbohydrate diet. A hereditary intolerance of fructose (fruit sugar) or galactose (milk sugar) is treated by eliminating the foods that cause hypoglycemic symptoms.

Managing Hypoglycemia

The section below focuses on nutritional strategies that will help you maintain a consistent blood-sugar level so that you are less vulnerable to experiencing hypoglycemia. Over the years, I have had many clients seek my help for managing their hypoglycemia. They have learned that following the proper diet is key to preventing hypoglycemia. Instead of relying on fast-acting carbohydrates to treat a low blood-sugar reaction, use the strategies below to prevent a sugar low from occurring in the first place.

Dietary Strategies
Meal Timing

One of the first and most important ways to prevent a low blood-sugar reaction is to eat regularly throughout the day. Your blood sugar will peak 45 to 90 minutes after you eat a meal. After this point, your sugar level starts its decline. If you suffer from hypoglycemia, you should *eat every three hours.* That means eating *three meals and three snacks.* Here's what a daytime meal and snack schedule might look like (note that time spans show approximate time of the meal or snack, not the duration):

Breakfast:	7:00–8:00 a.m.
Snack:	10:00–10:30 a.m.
Lunch:	12:00–1:00 p.m.
Snack:	3:00–4:00 p.m.
Dinner:	6:00–7:00 p.m.
Snack:	9:00–10:00 p.m.

Once you get into a consistent pattern of eating, you will feel much better. And if you choose the right foods at your meals and snacks, chances are you'll forget that you are vulnerable to hypoglycemic reactions.

The Glycemic Index

Carbohydrate-containing foods, such as starches, fruits, milk and sugars, eventually wind up as glucose in your bloodstream. But not all carbohydrates behave the same way when it comes to raising your blood sugar. Some carbohydrate-rich foods are digested and absorbed into the bloodstream quickly, while others are broken down and converted to glucose slowly.

Foods that are converted to blood glucose quickly (e.g., white bread) trigger your pancreas to release an excessive amount of insulin, causing your blood-glucose level to drop to a very low level. On the other hand, foods such as high-fiber breakfast cereals or yogurt are digested and absorbed more slowly, causing a gradual rise in blood sugar. This means your pancreas does not release as large an amount of insulin. As a result, your blood-sugar level won't plummet. Instead, you will experience a smooth, steady blood-sugar level, leading to more consistent energy levels.

The rate at which a food causes your blood sugar to rise can be measured and assigned a value. This measure is referred to as the glycemic index value. The glycemic index (GI) is a ranking from 0 to 100. The number tells you whether a food raises your blood glucose rapidly, moderately or slowly. Foods that are digested quickly and cause your blood sugar to rise rapidly have high glycemic index values. Foods that are digested slowly, leading to a gradual rise in blood sugar, are assigned low glycemic index values. All foods are compared with pure glucose, which is given a value of 100 (fast acting).

Choose carbohydrate foods that do *not* cause large increases in blood sugar.

- Choose low GI foods at your meals and snacks.
- Avoid eating high GI foods as snacks, since they can trigger a low blood sugar.
- Combine a high GI food with a low GI food to result in a meal with a medium GI value.

You'll find a list of foods ranked by their GI value on page 7, Chapter 1.

Soluble Fiber

Many of the foods with a low glycemic index value tend to be higher in soluble fiber. Dried peas, beans, lentils, oats, barley, psyllium husks, apples and citrus fruits are all good sources of soluble fiber and, as you will see from the GI table on page 7, Chapter 1, these foods also have a low GI. When you eat these foods, the soluble fiber forms a gel in your stomach and slows the rate of digestion and absorption. That means your blood sugar will rise at a slower rate and your pancreas won't produce excessive amounts of insulin.

If you don't feel like using the GI table to choose foods, you might just plan your meals around foods rich in soluble fiber:

Food	Good Sources of Soluble Fiber
Cereals	Kellogg's All Bran Buds, oatmeal, oat bran
Grains	Barley
Legumes	All (baked beans, bean soups, black beans, chickpeas, kidney beans, lentils, soybeans, etc.)
Fruit	Apples, cantaloupe, grapefruit, oranges, pears, strawberries
Vegetables	Carrots, green peas, sweet potato

Protein

Adding a little protein to meals slows the rate at which your stomach empties its contents into the small intestine. As a result, the carbohydrate in your meal will enter your bloodstream at a slower rate. Choose lean protein foods such as lean beef, chicken breast, turkey, pork tenderloin, center-cut pork chops, seafood and eggs. If you are a vegetarian, include vegetarian protein foods in your meals—tofu, beans, veggie ground round and tempeh. Dairy products such as milk, yogurt and cheese also contribute protein to a meal.

To help manage your blood sugar, distribute your protein throughout the day. If you need to eat 60 grams of protein each day, aim for 20 grams at each meal. You'll find a list of foods and their protein content on page 15, Chapter 2.

If you enjoy a green salad with your meal, continue doing so. But toss it with a vinaigrette dressing. Studies have found that vinegars, especially red wine vinegar, also slow the rate at which food leaves your stomach.

Caffeine and Alcohol

Caffeine is known to cause a low blood-sugar reaction, especially if it has been a few hours since you last ate. Researchers from the Yale University School of Medicine found that consuming 400 milligrams of caffeine triggered hypoglycemia when blood-sugar levels were in the low-normal range, as might occur two to three hours after a meal.[2]

If you are sensitive to caffeine, switch to low-caffeine or caffeine-free beverages. Replace coffee with decaf coffee, cereal-based beverages (e.g., Ovaltine), herbal tea, weakly brewed black tea or green tea. If you don't want to part with your daily cup of coffee, drink it with a meal so that the caffeine will be less likely to trigger a low blood-sugar reaction. Between meals, stick to vegetable juice, water, milk, herbal tea or decaf lattes.

Drinking alcoholic beverages can also impair blood-sugar control and trigger a hypoglycemic reaction in susceptible individuals. It can induce reactive hypoglycemia by interfering with glucose uptake and promoting the release of insulin from your pancreas. The drop in blood sugar that follows leads to a craving for foods, especially sweets. If you reach for sugary foods in response to this low blood sugar, you'll only aggravate your symptoms.

If you have hypoglycemia, avoid drinking alcohol on an empty stomach. Instead, enjoy your drink with a meal. The presence of food in your stomach will delay the absorption of alcohol. If you do drink, limit yourself to seven alcoholic drinks per week (women) or nine per week (men) for health protection.

Vitamins and Minerals

Chromium

Supplements of this trace mineral have been promoted to manage hypoglycemia, but unfortunately research studies are few and far between. One small study was conducted in the late 1980s with eight women who had hypoglycemia.[3] Those who took 200 micrograms of chromium for three months experienced significantly fewer low blood-sugar symptoms and had higher blood-glucose levels two to four hours after eating. Another small study conducted among 20 patients with hypoglycemia found similar results using 125 micrograms of the mineral.[4] A larger number of studies have investigated the use of chromium in individuals with type 2 diabetes.

It appears that chromium does play an important role when it comes to regulating blood glucose. Chromium is used by the body to make glucose tolerance factor (GTF), a compound that interacts with insulin and helps maintain normal blood-sugar levels. With adequate amounts of chromium present, your body uses less insulin to do its job.

The recommended intake for chromium is 25 and 35 micrograms per day for women and men. Chromium-rich foods include apples with the skin, green peas, chicken breast, refried beans, mushrooms, oysters, wheat germ and Brewer's yeast. Processed foods and refined (white) starchy foods like white bread, instant rice and white pasta, sugar and sweets contain very little chromium.

If you're concerned you're not getting enough of this mineral through your diet, check your multivitamin and mineral supplement to see how much it contains. If it's less than 50 micrograms, consider taking a separate 100 or 200 microgram supplement each day. Studies show that chromium picolinate is absorbed more easily than other forms (such as chromium chloride and chromium nicotinate). At this time, however, chromium picolinate is available in the United States but not in Canada. Chromium supplements are extremely safe.

Other Lifestyle Factors

Regular Exercise

Exercise improves many aspects of blood-sugar control. Working out enhances the body's sensitivity to insulin, improves glucose uptake by your cells and increases the concentration of chromium in your tissues.

You don't need to exercise vigorously to reap the benefits. In fact, working out too intensely may bring on hypoglycemia. If you exercise with someone, you should be able to carry on a conversation (you should be a little breathless, though). If you work out at a gym, consult with a certified personal trainer to help you find your target heart-rate zone. Staying within this range while you exercise will prevent you from overdoing it. Good activities include brisk walking, jogging, stair climbing, swimming, rowing and cycling. Aim to exercise four times per week, with each session at least 30 minutes long. If you are not exercising this much, gradually work up to it.

Plan your snacks around your exercise session. If you eat lunch at noon and exercise at 3 p.m., you'll want a snack about 30 minutes before you begin. At 2:30 p.m., eat an apple, yogurt or a sports energy bar. Depending on what time you eat dinner, you'll likely need to eat another small snack around 4:30 p.m.

Nutrition Strategy Checklist for Hypoglycemia

- ☐ Eat every three hours
- ☐ Low GI carbohydrates
- ☐ Soluble fiber
- ☐ Protein-rich foods
- ☐ Avoid caffeine
- ☐ Avoid alcohol
- ☐ Chromium
- ☐ Regular exercise

Recommended Resources

www.hypoglycemia.org
The Hypoglycemia Support Foundation, Inc.
P.O. Box 451778
Sunrise, FL, USA 33345
(This Web site is founded by an author on the subject.)

www.mayoclinic.com
Mayo Foundation for Medical Education and Research

www.niddk.nih.gov/health/diabetes/pubs/hypo/hypo/htm
National Diabetes Information Clearinghouse (NDIC)
1 Information Way
Bethesda, MD, USA 20892-3560
Tel: 301-654-3327

Hypothyroidism

Hypothyroidism develops when your thyroid gland does not produce enough thyroid hormones to meet your body's needs. An underactive thyroid gland will cause your metabolic rate to slow down, making you feel slow, sluggish and constantly tired. Thyroid deficiencies have also been known to cause infertility or miscarriages in early pregnancy.

What Causes Hypothyroidism?

The thyroid gland is a small organ with a big job. Located in your neck, just below your Adam's apple, the thyroid controls and coordinates your body's main body functions, or metabolism. It produces two thyroid hormones, triiodothyronine (T3) and thyroxine (T4), which circulate through your bloodstream and act on almost every organ in your body. These hormones maintain a healthy metabolic rate by controlling the speed at which your body burns calories for energy.

A well-functioning thyroid gland is essential to normal growth and development. If your thyroid does not produce enough thyroid hormones, all your bodily functions will slow down. You will begin to feel sluggish and tired and may develop a variety of other uncomfortable symptoms. As the condition becomes more advanced, you could experience serious health problems.

The most common type of hypothyroidism is Hashimoto's thyroiditis or chronic thyroiditis. It is an autoimmune disease caused by a malfunction of your immune system. In this case, the immune system begins to produce antithyroid antibodies that attack the thyroid gland. The damage caused by these antibodies prevents the thyroid from producing adequate levels of thyroid hormones. People with Hashimoto's thyroiditis often develop a painless thyroid lump or goiter that can be seen at the lower front of their throat.

Hypothyroidism can also be caused by

- surgery to remove the thyroid gland (usually a treatment for thyroid cancer, in some cases for overactive thyroid)

- radioactive iodine therapy (usually used to treat overactive thyroid conditions)

- X-rays, especially of the head and neck

- treatment with certain medications, such as lithium

- obesity

- pregnancy and postpartum conditions

- iodine deficiencies

- absence of a thyroid gland at birth (all babies in Canada are screened for hypothyroidism to detect this condition)

- having a genetic predisposition

Another version of the disorder, *secondary hypothyroidism*, may develop if you have an abnormality in an area of your brain called the hypothalamic-pituitary axis. The pituitary gland helps the thyroid gland regulate the production of T3 and T4 by releasing thyroid-stimulating hormone (TSH). The hypothalamus gland performs a similar function by producing thyrotropin-releasing hormone (TRH). If these two glands do not secrete enough hormones to trigger your thyroid gland to function, you may experience the hormonal deficiencies that lead to hypothyroidism.

Symptoms

The symptoms of hypothyroidism vary in severity, depending on the decrease in thyroid hormone levels and the length of time a deficiency has been present. Most of the time, the symptoms are fairly mild. In the early stages of the disorder, symptoms may not be noticeable at all and you may still feel quite well. However, research indicates that people with mild hypothyroidism go on to develop more severe thyroid problems in later years.

When you have more severe hypothyroidism, you may begin to feel slow, sluggish, tired and run down. You may also feel depressed and lose interest in daily activities. Additional symptoms include

- increased sensitivity to cold

- muscle swelling or cramps, especially in your arms and legs

- weight gain

- dry, itchy skin

- constipation

- increased menstrual flow

- tingling or numbness in your hands and feet

- coarseness or loss of hair

- memory loss and mental impairment

- infertility or miscarriages

- a slow heart rate

- dull facial expression, droopy eyelids and hoarse voice

- high blood pressure

Because hypothyroidism progresses gradually, worsening over a period of months or years, you may not even realize how unwell you feel until your thyroid condition is corrected with a hormone medication.

Who's at Risk?

Hypothyroidism affects almost 5 percent of the population—approximately 500,000 Canadians have an underactive thyroid gland.[1] Although thyroid disease can affect anyone, hypothyroidism is ten times more common in women than in men. The risk of hypothyroidism increases considerably as you age. It usually strikes after age 40 and is common in elderly women. In fact, up to 10 percent of women over the age of 65 show evidence of hypothyroidism.[2]

Hashimoto's thyroiditis has been associated with a genetic component, so your risk may be greater if you have a close female relative with a related autoimmune disease.

Some women also develop thyroid conditions during or immediately after pregnancy. Thyroiditis is especially common during the period following the birth of the baby, when it can often be confused with postpartum depression.

If you have had surgery or received radioactive iodine therapy to treat thyroid conditions such as hyperthyroidism, Graves' disease or thyroid cancer, you may be predisposed to hypothyroidism. Irradiation of the head and neck through X-rays or cancer treatment may also predispose you to thyroid problems.

In countries outside North America, one of the most common causes of hypothyroidism is iodine deficiency. This mineral is an essential component of thyroid hormones. People who do not have natural sources of iodine in their diet, such as fish and other seafood, are at high risk of developing hypothyroidism. In Canada and the United States, the problem has been virtually eliminated because iodine has been added to table salt.

Conventional Treatment

In most cases, hypothyroidism is a permanent condition that requires a lifetime of treatment. The goal of treatment is to provide the body with enough thyroid hormones to maintain an efficient metabolic rate. At present, the prescription of a thyroid supplement is the only effective treatment for this disorder. The supplement is usually a form of synthetic T4 that is taken daily as a small pill. Although the supplements contain only T4, the various organs in your body can convert the hormone into the more powerful T3 as needed.

Some thyroid supplements are made from hormones extracted from animal thyroids. These are not often prescribed today because their potency levels are not consistent. They also contain T3, which can cause heart problems, especially in older people or those with heart conditions.

Your doctor will determine your daily dosage of thyroid replacement hormones, depending on your age, sex, weight, thyroid function and other medications you are taking. Usually, you will start with a low dose and increase it gradually until your blood levels of T4 and TSH are within normal range. Hypothyroidism is an ongoing process, and your dosage may change as your thyroid function continues to deteriorate. Regular blood tests will help your doctor adjust your thyroid hormone medication to suit your needs. If you become pregnant, the dose may need to be increased. Older people need less T4, so your dosage may be lowered as you age.

Managing Hypothyroidism

Dietary Strategies

Weight Control

A deficiency of thyroid hormones leads to a general decline in the rate at which the body burns carbohydrate, protein and fat for energy. As a result, weight gain is common in hypothyroidism. And it is more difficult to lose weight if your thyroid hormone levels are not in a correct balance—but it is not impossible!

If you are suffering from hypothyroidism and are experiencing difficulty controlling your weight, examine your eating habits to determine where you are going wrong. Keep a food diary for two weeks. Writing down what you eat often highlights dietary discrepancies. Strategies for weight loss are outlined on page 442, Obesity and Weight Loss.

High Blood Cholesterol

Hypothyroidism is linked with a greater risk of early heart disease as thyroid hormones influence the level of blood cholesterol. Many studies find that patients suffering from a deficiency of thyroid hormones, whether they have overt symptoms or not, have higher levels of total cholesterol, bad LDL cholesterol and triglyceride levels.[3-7] The more severe the hypothyroidism, the higher the cholesterol levels.

Researchers have also learned that people with a sluggish thyroid gland have LDL cholesterol particles that are more readily oxidized by harmful free radical molecules.[8,9] Free radicals are reactive oxygen molecules that roam the body and damage cells. When free radicals oxidize your LDL cholesterol, this cholesterol has a greater tendency to stick to your artery walls. Your body does have ways of protecting itself from free radicals, though. Special enzymes in the body and certain nutrients in foods, such as vitamins C and E, act as antioxidants and help keep free radical activity in check.

If you have high blood cholesterol, refer to page 327, Heart Disease and High Blood Cholesterol, for nutritional strategies to prevent heart disease.

Soy Foods

You may have heard that eating soy foods can harm your thyroid gland and cause hypothyroidism. This simply isn't true. It is true that raw soybeans contain compounds that prevent the body's ability to use iodine. But heating soybeans eliminates these effects, and all soy foods, from tofu to soy nuts, are manufactured using heat.

This misinformation may have stemmed from the observation that, back in the 1950s, a small number of goiter (enlargement of the thyroid gland) cases developed in infants fed soy formula. However, since the 1950s, there have been no cases of infant goiter in babies who have been fed soy formulas. What's more, over the past five years a handful of studies have found no effect of soy foods on thyroid function or thyroid hormone levels. So rest assured, you can continue to enjoy your tofu.

Vitamins and Minerals

B Vitamins

Preliminary research suggests that people with hypothyroidism may have higher blood levels of homocysteine, a known risk factor for heart disease.[10] Homocysteine is an amino acid that everyone produces. Under normal circumstances it is converted to other harmless amino acids with the help of three B vitamins: folate, B6 and B12. When this conversion does not occur rapidly enough because of a deficiency of B vitamins or a genetic defect, homocysteine can accumulate in the blood. High levels of homocysteine can damage blood vessel walls and promote the build-up of cholesterol deposits.

Getting adequate amounts of B vitamins is an important way to keep your blood homocysteine at a healthy level. The best food sources for each B vitamin are as follows:

B Vitamin	Good Food Sources
Folate	Spinach, orange juice, lentils, wheat germ, broccoli, artichokes, asparagus, leafy greens and whole grains
Vitamin B6	Whole grains, bananas, potatoes, legumes, fish, meat and poultry
Vitamin B12	All animal foods, including meat, poultry, fish, dairy products and eggs, as well as fortified soy and rice beverages

Taking a daily multivitamin and mineral pill will ensure that you meet your requirements for all B vitamins. A standard multivitamin will provide 100 to 300 percent of the recommended dietary allowance (RDA) for each nutrient. High-potency, mega or super multivitamins have higher amounts of the B vitamins. Most B complex supplements contain 50 to 100 milligram amounts of all the B vitamins. Many brands also add vitamin C.

One word of warning if you are shopping for a high-potency B vitamin supplement. Vitamin B3, or niacin, can cause flushing when taken in amounts greater than 35 milligrams. This is a harmless reaction that causes your face, chest and arms to feel hot and tingly. The reaction usually passes within 20 to 30 minutes. To avoid this niacin flush: 1) take your supplement right after eating a meal, 2) buy a supplement with less than 35 milligrams of niacin or 3) buy a multivitamin or B complex that contains niacinamide rather than niacin (niacinamide is nonflushing).

Iodine

This trace mineral is an integral part of T3 and T4, the two thyroid hormones released by the thyroid gland. The major source of iodine is the ocean—seafood and seawater are excellent sources of the mineral. As you move farther inland, the amount of iodine in foods varies and generally reflects the amount of iodine that's in the soil plants grow in or animals graze on. Land that was once under the ocean contains plenty of iodine. In Canada and the United States, the soil around the Great Lakes is iodine-poor. However, the fortification of table salt with iodine in Canada and the United States has eliminated health problems caused by iodine deficiency.

If the body is short-changed of iodine on an ongoing basis, the production of thyroid hormones slows down and eventually hypothyroidism develops. But if you eat salty processed foods and fast foods, or you add table salt to your meals, you are not at risk for consuming too little iodine.

Too much iodine in the diet can also cause hypothyroidism. Excess iodine can result in low thyroid hormone levels by halting the activity of enzymes needed for their production. There have been cases of people who develop hypothyroidism by taking in too much iodine in the form of iodine-rich seaweed and kelp supplements on a daily basis.[11]

The daily recommended intake for iodine is 150 micrograms per day. North Americans are estimated to be consuming 200 to 600 micrograms of iodine per day—well above requirements. Some of this iodine excess may come from our growing dependence on fast and processed foods, since these foods contribute a generous amount of salt to our daily diet. Besides iodized salt, other food sources of iodine include seafood, bread, dairy products, plants grown in iodine-rich soil and meat and poultry from animals raised on iodine-rich soil.

Selenium

This trace mineral is an important component of an enzyme that produces the thyroid hormone T3. Researchers have learned that a selenium deficiency in older adults is strongly associated with lower levels of the T3 hormone.[12] The relationship between impaired selenium status and reduced thyroid hormone levels may be partially responsible for the hypothyroidism that's often diagnosed in elderly women.

The best food sources of selenium include seafood and meat. Whole-wheat bread, wheat bran, wheat germ, oats, brown rice, Brazil nuts, Swiss chard and garlic are other good sources. Dietary intake from plant foods will vary according to the selenium content of the soil in which these foods were grown.

People at greatest risk for a selenium deficiency are those who eat a vegetarian diet based on plant foods grown in low-selenium areas. But because most of us eat supermarket foods that have been transported from areas throughout Canada, the United States, Mexico or South America, selenium deficiency is uncommon.

If you're considering a supplement, check your multivitamin first. Some high-potency brands contain up to 100 micrograms of selenium. If you are using single selenium supplements, a 200 microgram dose is plenty. You might want to choose one that contains selenomethionine or selenium-rich yeast, since these organic forms of the mineral appear to be more available to the body.

The daily upper limit for selenium from foods and supplements is 400 micrograms per day. Consuming too much selenium over a period has toxic effects, including hair and nail loss, gastrointestinal upset, skin rash, garlic breath odor, fatigue, irritability and nervous-system abnormalities.

Iron Supplements

If you are taking levothyroxine (Synthroid®) and are also being treated for an iron deficiency, take your medication and your iron pill two to three hours apart, rather than at the same time. Studies have found that iron supplements can reduce the body's absorption of levothyroxine.[13,14] It is possible that impaired absorption of your medication could make you hypothyroid and increase your medication requirements.

If you are taking iron supplements to correct an iron deficiency, your doctor will monitor your thyroid hormone levels closely. Iron pills should be taken only if your doctor has diagnosed you with iron deficiency. If you are taking them on your own accord, be sure to let your physician know.

Nutrition Strategy Checklist for Hypothyroidism

☐ Weight control   ☐ Iodine

☐ Manage blood   ☐ Selenium
   cholesterol

☐ B vitamins

Recommended Resources

www.thyroid.ca
Thyroid Foundation of Canada
1040 Gardiners Road, Suite C
Kingston, ON, Canada K7P 1R7
Tel: 1-800-267-8822
Fax: 613-634-3483
E-mail: thyroid@io.org

www.the-thyroid-society.org
Thyroid Society for Education and Research
7515 S Main Street, Suite 545
Houston, TX, USA 77030
Tel: 1-800-THYROID (1-800-849-7643)
Fax: 713-799-9919

Impotence (Erectile Dysfunction)

For most men, impotence, or erectile dysfunction, can be a great source of embarrassment, anxiety and fear. Defined as the inability to achieve or sustain an erection adequate for sexual intercourse, impotence can damage a man's self-image, ruin his sexual life and cause significant emotional pain in his personal relationships.

Almost all men experience occasional episodes of erectile dysfunction. As men age, their sexual abilities change. Erections may take longer to achieve and may be slightly softer. More direct stimulation may be needed to produce an erection, orgasms may be less intense and recovery time between erections may be longer. These changes are a natural part of the aging process and not a cause for concern. While a man's sexual responses may slow down over time, impotence is not an inevitable part of growing older.

Producing and sustaining an erection is a complex process. A precise sequence of events must take place, beginning with the sensory and mental stimulation provoked by sight, sound, touch, smell and thought. This state of sexual arousal triggers the brain to communicate with the nervous system, increasing blood flow to the penis. Surrounding muscles, tissues, arteries and veins respond to the message of sexual excitation by relaxing and expanding. This process allows the penis to engorge with blood. If this delicately balanced sequence of events is interrupted at any point, impotence can be the result.

What Causes Impotence?

Once thought to be primarily a psychological problem, impotence is often caused by a physical or medical condition. The most common cause of erectile dysfunction is damage to the arteries, tissues and muscles in the area of the penis.

Diseases that may be responsible for the damage include diabetes, multiple sclerosis, atherosclerosis, vascular diseases and kidney disease.

Prostate surgery or other surgical procedures can harm nerves and arteries near the penis. Impotence can also develop as a result of injuries to the penis, prostate gland, spinal cord or bladder, especially if they damage surrounding muscles, nerves and tissue. Medications such as antihistamines, antidepressants, tranquilizers and high blood pressure drugs list impotence as a side effect. Obesity and an inadequate production of testosterone or other male hormones may also contribute to erectile dysfunction. Chronic alcoholism, substance abuse and smoking often increase the risk of impotence by lowering sexual drive or by interfering with the blood flow necessary to achieve an erection.

While most cases of erectile dysfunction have an underlying medical cause, approximately 10 to 20 percent develop as a result of psychological factors.[1] Men who fail to achieve an erection because of a physical condition may find that anxiety only makes the situation worse. What may begin as an occasional physical problem can easily turn into an ongoing psychological issue. Other factors associated with impotence include stress, fatigue, guilt, depression, low self-esteem and loss of interest in a partner.

Symptoms

Signs of impotence include

- total inability to achieve an erection

- inconsistent or sporadic inability to achieve an erection

- inability to maintain an erection

Who's at Risk?

It is estimated that over 30 million men in the United States suffer from erectile dysfunction.[2]

Impotence can affect men at any age after puberty, but the incidence increases with age. Some 52 percent of men between the ages of 40 and 70 suffer from some type of erectile difficulty, with 5 in every 100 men experiencing impotence after age 40.[3,4] Diseases account for over 70 percent of all cases of impotence. In fact, 35 to 50 percent of men with diabetes have erectile dysfunction.[5] Psychological factors account for up to 20 percent of all cases of impotence.

Conventional Treatment

Treatment is necessary if erectile dysfunction lasts longer than two months or is a recurring problem. Treatment may vary according to the cause and severity of the problem. Treatments include

- *Viagra® (sildenafil)* to relax the smooth muscles in the penis during sexual stimulation, increasing blood flow necessary to achieve an erection

- *Prostaglandin E (alprostadil)* to relax smooth muscle in the penis, increasing blood flow necessary to achieve an erection

- *Testosterone replacement therapy* used in men with hormone deficiency

- *Binding devices* to slow the outflow of blood from the penis to achieve and sustain an erection

- *Vacuum devices* to create a vacuum pressure that draws blood into arteries in the penis

- *Vascular surgery* to improve blood flow to the penis (used when blood flow has been affected by an injury or a vascular blockage)

- *Penile implants* to place inflatable devices or rods into the sides of the penis to create a permanent erection; usually used after other approaches have been unsuccessful

- *Psychological counseling* to help deal with impotence problems caused by anxiety, stress or other psychological factors; most successful when both partners receive counseling

- *Behavioral sex therapy*

The following lifestyle changes may help prevent occasional episodes of erectile dysfunction:

- Quit smoking. The Massachusetts Male Aging Study found that smoking cigarettes almost doubles the likelihood of moderate or complete erectile dysfunction. Cigar smoking and secondhand smoke also increased the risk.[6]

- Limit use of alcohol or other drugs.

- Exercise regularly and eat a balanced diet.

- Reduce stress and anxiety.

- Get adequate sleep.

- Improve communication with your partner. Work on the relationship rather than the sexual intercourse.

- Create a relaxed, private and comfortable environment for intercourse.

- See your doctor for regular check-ups.

Managing Impotence
Dietary Strategies
Weight Control

A study of American men found that being overweight was associated with impotence. Researchers from the New England Research Institutes collected information from 1700 men living in Boston between 1987 and 1989.[7] When they followed up with these men ten years later, they learned that men who were overweight in 1987 to 1989 had a higher risk of erectile dysfunction regardless of any weight loss that occurred over the decade. The same study found that men who exercised regularly had the lowest risk of becoming impotent compared with sedentary men, who had the highest risk.

Research suggests that erectile dysfunction is associated with having a body mass index of 28 or greater.[8] Body mass index is a ratio used to determine if your weight is putting your health at risk. To calculate your body mass index, turn to page 439, Obesity and Weight Loss.

Dietary Fat

Since achieving and maintaining an erection involves the arteries in the penis, it is logical that a high-fat diet might increase the risk of erectile dysfunction by damaging blood vessel walls. The Massachusetts Male Aging Study also found that dietary fat and cholesterol were linked with erectile dysfunction.

To eat less fat, start by cutting back on animal fats, or saturated fat, the type of fat that raises blood cholesterol.

Food	Lower-Fat Choices or Substitutes
Milk	Skim, 1% milk fat (MF)
Yogurt	Products with less than 2% MF
Cheese	Products with less than 20% MF
Cottage cheese	Products with 1% MF
Sour cream	Products with 7% or less MF
Cream	Evaporated 2% or evaporated skim milk
Red meat	Flank steak, inside round, sirloin, eye of round, extra-lean ground beef, venison
Pork	Center-cut pork chops, pork tenderloin, pork leg (inside round, roast), baked ham, deli ham, back bacon
Poultry	Skinless chicken breast, turkey breast, lean ground turkey or chicken
Eggs	Egg whites (two whites replaces one egg). You can buy these beside the fresh eggs at your grocery store.

To learn more about dietary fat and how much you should be eating, refer to Chapter 3.

Vitamins and Minerals
Vitamin E

Although no studies have looked at the link between vitamin E and erectile dysfunction, vitamin E is a nutrient that can protect from artery damage. Vitamin E is a potent antioxidant, and as such, it prevents bad LDL cholesterol from becoming damaged by unstable oxygen molecules called free radicals. LDL cholesterol particles damaged by free radicals are much more likely to stick to artery walls. To prevent impotence, it's important to keep the arteries in the penis healthy.

The recommended dietary allowance (RDA) for vitamin E is 22 international units (IU). The best food sources include wheat germ, nuts, seeds, vegetable oils, whole grains and kale. To supplement, take 200 to 400 IU of natural source vitamin E. The daily upper limit is 1500 IU.

Zinc

This mineral is essential for growth, sexual development and sperm production. A zinc deficiency may lead to low testosterone levels and, as a result, may contribute to impotence. Certain medications can deplete the body of zinc and may cause sexual dysfunction. A South African study found that compared with healthy men, those who were taking a diuretic drug called hydrochlorothiazide for high blood pressure had lower zinc levels and a higher incidence of sexual dysfunction.[9] When these men were given supplemental zinc, symptoms of sexual dysfunction improved in some, but not all of the men.

Men require 11 milligrams of zinc per day. The best food sources include oysters, dark turkey meat, lentils, ricotta cheese, tofu, yogurt, lean beef, wheat germ, spinach, broccoli, green beans and tomato juice. If using a supplement, choose one that offers 15 to 30 milligrams of zinc (many multivitamin and mineral formulas offer this amount). Make sure your zinc supplement has 1 milligram of copper for every 10 milligrams of zinc, since supplemental zinc depletes the body's stores of copper. Do not exceed 40 milligrams per day; too much zinc has toxic effects.

Herbal Remedies

Ginkgo Biloba

Some research suggests that the active ingredients in this herb can improve blood flow to the extremities. In one study of 60 men with impotence caused by poor blood circulation, 50 percent experienced improvement after taking ginkgo for six months.[10] Another study from the University of California, in San Francisco, found ginkgo to be effective at relieving sexual dysfunction caused by certain antidepressant drugs known as serotonin reuptake inhibitors (e.g., Prozac®, Effexor®, Paxil®, Zoloft®, Serzone®).[11]

Choose a product that is standardized to 24 percent ginkgo flavone glycosides and 6 percent terpene lactones. The extract used in much of the scientific research is sold as Ginkoba® (Pharmaton® Natural Health Products) in Canada and the United States.

The recommended starting dose to reverse sexual dysfunction is 120 milligrams daily. Take 40 milligrams three times daily or 60 milligrams twice daily with meals. If needed, the dose of ginkgo can be increased with monitoring by your doctor as higher doses have a blood-thinning effect. On rare occasions, ginkgo may cause gastrointestinal upset, headache or an allergic skin reaction.

Panax Ginseng

This herb goes by many names, including Asian, Korean and Chinese ginseng. One study of 90 Korean men found that Korean ginseng was more effective in treating impotence than both the placebo treatment and the drug treatment.[12]

Buy a product standardized to contain 4 to 7 percent ginsenosides or with a statement of standardization of "G115" printed on the label. Ginsana® (Pharmaton® Natural Health Products) contains the G115 extract that has been used in many clinical studies. The typical dosage is 100 or 200 milligrams once daily. Take ginseng for three weeks to three months and follow with a one- to two-week rest period before you resume taking the herb.

In some people, ginseng may cause mild stomach upset, irritability and insomnia. To avoid overstimulation, start with 100 milligrams a day and avoid taking the herb with caffeine. Ginseng should not be used if you have poorly controlled high blood pressure.

Maca (*Lepidium meyenii*)

Also known as Peruvian ginseng, maca has been used for more than 2000 years to enhance libido, fertility and energy levels. Although little research has been done on the effectiveness of maca for erectile dysfunction, the findings to date look promising. A recent animal study found that maca significantly improved sexual functioning. Dr. David Saul from Toronto, Ontario, recently completed an observational study in which 29 men with erectile dysfunction were given 500 milligrams of maca twice daily. Within two to four weeks, 72 percent reported improvement in sexual functioning and 48 percent were able to have successful intercourse again without resorting to Viagra®.[13]

The herb is thought to work by improving testosterone levels and improving blood flow to the penis. The recommended dose is 1500 to 6000 milligrams daily, in two or three divided doses. No side effects have been reported.

Herbs to Avoid

Two herbs in particular should be avoided by men with erectile difficulties or dysfunction.

Licorice may reduce testosterone levels in men and may therefore interfere with libido and impotence.

Yohimbe, a herb from the bark of an evergreen tree native to Africa, may be effective when used to treat impotence, but it has a number of dangerous side effects, including tremor, insomnia, anxiety, high blood pressure, increased heart rate, nausea and vomiting.

Other Natural Health Products

DHEA (Dehydroepiandrosterone)

DHEA is a hormone produced by the adrenal glands, two small glands that sit above the kidneys. The body uses DHEA as a building block to make estrogen and testosterone. DHEA production in the body declines with age. Austrian researchers have found DHEA levels to be lower in men with erectile dysfunction compared with healthy volunteers.[14] Recently, a study involving 40 men with erectile dysfunction revealed that a daily 50 milligram supplement of DHEA taken for six months was associated with improved sexual performance.[15]

The dose used to treat erectile dysfunction is 50 milligrams per day. Supplemental DHEA is neither a nutrient nor a natural product. It is a hormone manufactured from compounds found in soybeans. It is sold as a dietary supplement in the United States, but at this time it is not allowed for sale in Canada.

DHEA is considered safe when taken for the short term. It is possibly unsafe used long term in amounts that raise DHEA levels above normal, as it might increase the risk of prostate cancer. Even at low doses, side effects can occur. DHEA has been shown to lower the level of good HDL cholesterol and cause acne and hair loss. DHEA may also increase or decrease the body's sensitivity to insulin, the hormone that regulates blood sugar.

If you have diabetes, have your doctor monitor your blood-glucose levels closely.

L-Arginine

This amino acid is a building block for protein. It's found in dairy products, meat, poultry, fish, nuts and chocolate. Along with its many other functions in the body, arginine is used to make nitric oxide, a compound that relaxes blood vessels. Nitric oxide is considered an important factor in achieving an erection. A well-controlled Israeli study involving 50 men with erectile dysfunction found that high-dose arginine taken for six weeks resulted in significant improvement in sexual function.[16]

The dose used to treat erectile dysfunction is 5 grams per day. Although L-arginine is considered safe, side effects can include abdominal pain and bloating. Allergic reactions have also occurred in a small number of people.

If you have stomach ulcers or take a medication that irritates the stomach (e.g., a nonsteroidal anti-inflammatory such as naproxen), use caution with this supplement, since L-arginine may cause the body to produce more stomach acid. L-arginine can also alter potassium levels in your body. If you're taking medications such as potassium-sparing diuretics or ACE inhibitors, use the supplement only under medical supervision.

Nutrition Strategy Checklist for Impotence

☐ Weight control
☐ Low fat
☐ Vitamin E
☐ Zinc
☐ Ginkgo biloba OR Ginseng OR Maca
☐ DHEA
☐ L-arginine
☐ Quit smoking

Recommended Resources

www.mayoclinic.com
Mayo Foundation for Medical Education and Research

www.niddk.nih.gov/
National Kidney and Urologic Diseases Information Clearinghouse
The National Institute of Diabetes and Digestive and Kidney Diseases
Office of Communications and Public Liaison
NIDDK, NIH, 31 Center Drive, MSC 2560
Bethesda, MD, USA 20892-2560
Tel: 1-800-622-9010

www.impotence.org
Sponsored by the Sexual Health Council of the American Foundation for Urologic Disease, Inc.

Infertility

Defined as the inability to conceive after one year of frequent, unprotected intercourse, infertility affects approximately one in six couples. Throughout North America, infertility is on the rise, possibly because of the increase in sexually transmitted diseases and the decision of a growing number of women to delay having children until later in life.

Once thought to be solely a woman's problem, failure to conceive can be caused by reproductive difficulties in both men and women. Thirty percent of all cases of infertility originate with the woman, 30 percent originate with the man, 30 percent are the result of combined factors and the remaining cases are unexplained.[1] For women, infertility is often associated with ovarian disorders, and for men, it is usually linked to problems with sperm production.

What Causes Infertility?

Conception

A woman's lifetime supply of over 7 million eggs, or ova, is created during her growth in the womb. After birth, as she grows and matures, millions of these eggs disintegrate, leaving only about 300,000 eggs available for fertilization by the time she reaches puberty. A woman becomes fertile once her menstrual cycle begins, usually between the ages of 9 and 16. From this point onward, an egg will ripen inside her ovaries once every month until she reaches menopause.

Stimulated by a sequence of hormones, the egg matures inside a tiny, sac-like structure called a follicle and is released into the fallopian tube. For conception to take place, a sperm must fertilize the egg as it travels from the ovaries and through the fallopian tubes to reach the uterus.

A man produces sperm in his testicles on a continuous basis throughout his lifetime. Sperm are shaped like tadpoles, carrying genetic material in their "heads" and capable of moving by lashing their "tails" in a swimming motion. During intercourse, a man will ejaculate millions of these sperm into a woman's vagina. Ideally, the sperm will fertilize the egg within 24 hours of ovulation, because both the sperm and egg deteriorate fairly quickly. To reach the egg, the sperm must travel through the acidic environment of the vagina into the uterus and up to the fallopian tubes. Although millions of sperm make this difficult journey, only one will penetrate the tough outer membrane of the egg.

Once the first sperm has entered the egg, a chemical reaction takes place, making the egg impenetrable to other sperm. The genetic material in the head of the sperm then combines with the genetic material contained within the egg, completing the process of conception. The fertilized egg travels down through the fallopian tubes into the uterus, where it implants on the thickened lining of the uterus wall, called the endometrium. The woman's uterus will nurture this tiny collection of cells for nine months as it grows and develops into a fully formed fetus.

Female Infertility

At any stage along the way, from the development of a woman's eggs to the journey of a fertilized egg into her uterus, the female reproductive process can go astray. Approximately one-third of female infertility is caused by a failure to ovulate, a condition known as anovulation. Unless ovulation takes place, no egg is available for the sperm to fertilize. A balance of hormones is necessary for ovulation to occur successfully. Two small glands located in the brain, the hypothalamus and the pituitary gland, regulate most of these hormonal responses.

The hypothalamus secretes gonadotropin-releasing hormone (GnRH), which stimulates the pituitary gland to relay hormonal messages to the ovaries. In response to these messages, the ovaries nurture an egg to maturity and release it into the fallopian tubes, ready to be fertilized. Emotional stress, extreme exercise, dieting, poor nutrition, low body fat, anorexia, medications and environmental toxins can interfere with the performance of the hypothalamus, preventing it from sending the correct signals to the pituitary gland and disrupting conception.

The pituitary gland produces two hormones, follicle-stimulating hormone (FSH) and luteinizing hormone (LH), that stimulate the follicles in the ovaries to grow and release mature eggs. These hormones also tell the ovaries to produce estrogen and progesterone. The pituitary gland may malfunction because of a tumor, an injury, surgical complications or various medical disorders. A defective pituitary gland can over- or underproduce FSH and LH, resulting in ovulation failure.

The pituitary gland also produces prolactin, a hormone involved in the production of breast milk. Prolactin has the effect of suppressing ovulation, acting as a natural form of birth control during pregnancy and breastfeeding. The pituitary gland may secrete too much prolactin, due to severe kidney disease, adrenal gland disorders, hypothyroidism and the effect of certain medications.

Other glands also affect hormones involved in conception. For instance, the thyroid gland establishes your metabolic rate by circulating hormones to control the speed and efficiency of bodily functions. A thyroid gland that is overactive (hyperthyroid) or underactive (hypothyroid) can interfere with the body's ability to use hormones and cause infertility.

Every woman has small amounts of male sex hormones, called androgens, circulating through her bloodstream. These hormones are secreted by the adrenal glands and are necessary for normal sexual development. If the adrenal glands malfunction, elevated levels of male hormones can suppress ovulation.

A variety of ovarian disorders, including cysts, tumors, infections and medical conditions, can also cause infertility. For some women, their ovaries simply fail to function. Because of surgery, injury, radiation or chromosomal problems, their ovaries run out of eggs too early, sending them into premature menopause. In rare instances, women are born without ovaries or without a normal supply of eggs, making ovulation impossible.

Several disorders of the uterus can also hamper conception. During a normal reproductive process, progesterone and luteinizing hormone stimulate the uterine lining to thicken into a nourishing bed for the fertilized egg. If the uterus is unable to respond to these hormones, the egg cannot implant properly. The result is usually a spontaneous abortion or miscarriage. Some women find it difficult to carry a fetus to full term because their uterus is structurally abnormal. Others discover that they are infertile because they were born without a uterus.

Sexually transmitted diseases such as gonorrhea, chlamydia and pelvic inflammatory disease affect the reproductive tract and are another cause of infertility. These infections can go undetected for long periods and, if left untreated, can scar the uterus, block the fallopian tubes and cause the formation of pelvic adhesions.

Many women fail to realize that diet, nutrition and lifestyle can also influence fertility. Excessive exercise, low-calorie diets, eating disorders, obesity, certain medications and elevated stress levels are all factors that will interfere with the reproductive process. Fortunately, these are among the easiest fertility problems to correct.

Male Infertility

Men are considered to be infertile when they don't produce enough sperm or when their sperm are of poor quality. Each time a man ejaculates, he releases approximately 50 million sperm in each milliliter of seminal fluid. If his sperm count drops below 20 million sperm per milliliter of ejaculate, his fertility will be impaired. The quality of the sperm is also important. Normal sperm have oval heads and long tails. Poor-quality sperm have large heads and deformed tails. These abnormalities interfere with the motility of the sperm, making them unable to swim to the egg in a vigorous, forward motion.

Problems with sperm production can result from

- medical illnesses, including mumps and sexually transmitted diseases
- injury to the testicles, an undescended testicle, or testicular cancer
- certain drugs, including recreational drugs such as marijuana

- cigarette smoking or drinking alcohol
- antibodies that are produced by the immune system to attack or disable the sperm
- vasectomy (surgical sterilization)
- overheating the sperm by wearing tight clothes, taking too many long baths or using saunas
- environmental toxins
- defects in the sperm-producing cells

Combined Infertility Factors

One of the main reasons behind the increased rate of infertility in North America is age. Many couples are waiting until they are well into their 30s or 40s before attempting to have children. However, the quality and numbers of both sperm and eggs deteriorate as men and women grow older.

Sometimes infertility arises because the man's sperm is incompatible with the woman's cervical mucus. Normally, the cervix secretes a thick mucus to protect the vagina from foreign invaders, such as bacteria. During ovulation, chemical changes take place to thin the mucus consistency, allowing the sperm to enter the reproductive tract. For some couples, the chemistry between the sperm and the cervix just isn't right. The mucus remains thick, creating an environment that can block or damage the sperm, preventing conception.

Approximately 10 percent of all infertile couples discover that their infertility has no apparent cause. Both partners appear to be normal, healthy and able to reproduce. However, they simply cannot conceive together.

Symptoms

The main symptom of infertility is the inability to conceive a child after one year of unprotected, frequent intercourse. Each specific medical disorder, hormonal disruption or anatomical abnormality produces additional symptoms in the woman that may indicate infertility. These symptoms may include

- history of recent weight loss or gain
- irregular menstrual periods
- absent menstrual periods (amenorrhea)
- prolonged or heavy periods
- spotting between periods
- abnormal vaginal discharge
- discomfort in the lower abdomen
- pain during sexual intercourse

Who's at Risk?

One in six couples experience infertility problems. You may be at increased risk of developing fertility problems if you

- are over 30 years old
- have irregular or absent periods
- have a history or have a partner with a history of sexually transmitted diseases (STDs), pelvic infections or genital infections
- are a woman with excessive hair growth on your face and body (hirsutism)
- have a history of using an intrauterine device (IUD) for birth control
- have had a surgical sterilization reversed or if your partner has undergone this procedure
- have had abdominal surgery or your partner has undergone this type of surgery
- have endometriosis
- have a history of emotional stress

Conventional Treatment

For the majority of couples, giving nature enough time is usually the only treatment required for successful conception. Most healthy couples under 35 years of age have a 25 percent chance of becoming pregnant in the first month of trying to conceive. That rate rises to 60 percent after three to six months and reaches 85 percent after one year.

In many cases, mistimed intercourse is the only reason for infertility. For a woman, detecting the changes in your body that signal the beginning of ovulation is often the first step toward solving your fertility problems. Keeping a record of your basal temperature will help determine your most fertile days. (There is a slight rise in the body's basal temperature when ovulation occurs. Recording your temperature each morning will help pinpoint this crucial time in your menstrual cycle.) A urine test, indicating the presence of luteinizing hormones, is another method of establishing ovulation. By planning intercourse to maximize the chances of a mature egg meeting a viable sperm, you increase the possibility of conception considerably.

Since the primary cause of infertility is anovulation, the major objective of most fertility treatments is to stimulate ovulation. The fertility drug clomiphene citrate (Clomid®) is often used to trigger ovulation by affecting the release of luteinizing hormone. Some women benefit from supplements of the hormones FSH, LH or GnRH to restore a normal menstrual cycle and stimulate egg production.

In some instances, surgery may be necessary to repair damaged reproductive organs caused by infections or endometriosis. Surgery is also helpful in correcting certain uterine abnormalities and removing polyps and fibroids.

Assisted reproductive technologies (ART), such as in vitro fertilization, are proving to be very successful in treating a wide variety of infertility problems. During this process, fertility drugs are prescribed to stimulate the ovaries to produce many eggs. When they mature, several eggs are retrieved from the ovaries and fertilized in a laboratory. Three to five embryos are then implanted in your uterus, in the hope of establishing a successful pregnancy. In vitro fertilization is used most frequently for women who have fallopian tube damage, endometriosis, antisperm antibodies and unexplained infertility.

Enhancing Female Fertility

Dietary Strategies

Weight Control

A woman's body weight can affect her chances of becoming pregnant. If a woman is obese, fat cells can produce enough estrogen to interfere with her ability to conceive. High estrogen levels tell the brain to stop stimulating the development of follicles and, as result, ovulation doesn't occur. Studies show that losing weight can lead to ovulation and pregnancy.

Weighing too little is not healthy either. Menstruation occurs at a critical level of "fatness." If you lose too much weight, or you are already thin, your body fat diminishes and hormone levels are affected. This, in turn, can lead to the inability to ovulate.

To find out if you are at a healthy weight, refer to page 439, Obesity and Weight Loss. If you are overweight and have polycystic ovary syndrome (PCOS), follow the recommendations given in the section on PCOS. If you are underweight, read the guidelines in Chapter 5. Incorporating some of these suggestions will help you ensure you are getting enough calories and nutrients in your daily diet. If you recognize that your low body weight is caused by an eating disorder, read page 284, Eating Disorders, for information on how to begin your recovery process.

Vitamins and Minerals

Vitamin B12

There is some evidence that anemia due to a deficiency of vitamin B12 can cause infertility in women.[2] Two case reports revealed that when women with this nutrient deficiency who were having trouble conceiving were given supplemental B12, pregnancy occurred.[3] How a lack of B12 affects a woman's chances of conceiving is not understood.

Ensure you are meeting your needs for this vitamin. Vitamin B12 is found in animal foods such as meat, poultry, fish, eggs and dairy products and also in fortified soy and rice beverages. If you eat very few or no animal foods, take a high-quality multivitamin and mineral supplement to ensure you are meeting your B vitamin requirements (see Chapter 4 for more information on this vitamin). Regular multivitamin and mineral supplements offer 100 to 300 percent of your daily needs. High-potency or super multivitamin formulas or B complex supplements contain higher amounts, usually 50 to 100 micrograms of B12.

Herbal Remedies

Chasteberry (*Vitex angus-castus*)

If irregular menstrual periods caused by an imbalance of hormones are interfering with your ability to become pregnant, you might consider taking chasteberry. The herb is believed to increase the pituitary gland's production of luteinizing hormone (LH). LH in turn boosts the secretion of progesterone during the last 14 days of the menstrual cycle. Chasteberry also lowers excessive levels of prolactin.

In one German study, chasteberry was successful in treating 10 out of 15 women suffering from amenorrhea.[4] Women taking the herb began having regular periods after six months of treatment. Blood tests revealed an increase in levels of LH and progesterone. A few other European studies suggest that when taken daily, chasteberry can restore progesterone and prolactin levels to normal and result in pregnancy.

Buy a product that is standardized to 0.5 percent agnuside and 0.6 percent aucubin, two of the plant's active ingredients. The recommended dose is 175 to 225 milligrams once daily. Research and clinical experience suggest that it takes five to seven months to restore regular menstrual periods. In women who have not had a period for more than two years, it can take up to 18 months to have an effect. If you become pregnant, stop taking chasteberry as it may stimulate the uterus.

Enhancing Male Fertility

Vitamins and Minerals

Antioxidants

It appears that certain vitamins and minerals affect the health and motility of sperm. Most research attention has been paid to the antioxidant nutrients, in particular vitamin E, vitamin C and selenium. It is believed that free radicals, dangerous oxygen molecules found in the body, damage sperm. Cigarette smoking, among other things, causes the formation of free radical compounds that can damage sperm. Antioxidants are able to neutralize these harmful chemicals, rendering them inactive in the body.

Two studies have found that vitamin E supplements, taken in doses of 100 and 200 international units (IU), improved sperm activity of infertile men and increased the rate of pregnancy in their partners. Preliminary research suggests that vitamin C may improve sperm count and sperm motility.[5,6] Studies have also found that compared with fertile men, infertile men have significantly lower levels of selenium in their semen, suggesting that selenium plays a role in sperm development.[7,8] These studies are far from conclusive, but even if dietary antioxidants don't improve male fertility, they are still important nutrients to be consuming in the diet.

- *Vitamin C* The recommended dietary allowance (RDA) is 90 milligrams (smokers need 125 milligrams). Best food sources include citrus fruit, citrus juices, cantaloupe, kiwi, mango, strawberries, broccoli, Brussels sprouts, cauliflower, red pepper and tomato juice. To supplement, take 500 milligrams of Ester C once daily. The daily upper limit is 2000 milligrams.

- *Vitamin E* The RDA is 22 international units (IU). Best food sources include wheat germ, nuts, seeds, vegetable oils, whole grains and kale. To supplement, take 200 to 400 IU of natural source vitamin E. Buy a "mixed" vitamin E supplement if possible. The daily upper limit is 1500 IU.

- *Selenium* The RDA is 55 micrograms. Best food sources are fish, seafood, chicken, organ meats, whole grains, nuts, onions, garlic and mushrooms. To supplement, take 200 micrograms per day. Check how much your multivitamin and mineral formula gives you before you buy a separate selenium pill. The daily upper limit is 400 micrograms.

Vitamin B12

This vitamin may also affect male fertility. There is some evidence to suggest that a B12 deficiency may lead to lower sperm counts. One study looked at the effects of B12 supplements among infertile men. Supplementing the diet with extra B12 helped only those men with low sperm counts and impaired sperm motility.[9] Taking a multivitamin and mineral supplement and including animal foods in the diet are simple ways to prevent a B12 deficiency.

Zinc

This mineral is essential for growth, sexual development and sperm production. Many studies have found a link between infertility in men and a low zinc concentration in seminal fluid. A zinc deficiency may also lead to low testosterone levels. One small study conducted in men with low testosterone levels found that zinc supplements increased sperm count and the rate of pregnancy in their partners.[10]

Zinc-rich foods include oysters, dark turkey meat, lentils, ricotta cheese, tofu, yogurt, lean beef, wheat germ, spinach, broccoli, green beans and tomato juice. If supplements are used, take from 15 to 30 milligrams (many multivitamin and mineral formulas offer 15 milligrams). A zinc supplement should have 1 milligram of copper for every 10 milligrams of zinc. Do not exceed 40 milligrams of zinc per day.

L-Carnitine

This compound is not an essential nutrient because the body makes it in sufficient quantities. Carnitine helps the body generate energy by transporting fat into cells. Most of the body's carnitine is located in muscles and the heart, but some is also found in sperm and seminal fluid. A number of studies have found a positive relationship between sperm count and motility and their concentration of L-carnitine. The higher the concentration of L-carnitine, the higher the sperm count. Researchers have also found that infertile men have much lower levels of L-carnitine in their semen compared with fertile men.[11] One Italian study revealed that 3 grams per day of supplemental L-carnitine taken for three months increased sperm count and sperm motility in 37 out of 47 men.[12]

L-carnitine is found in meat and dairy products. To get 3 grams a day, though, you will need to take supplements. To supplement, take 1 to 3 grams per day. L-carnitine is available in the United States but is not legally available in Canada. However, some health food stores do stock it. Avoid products that contain D-carnitine or DL-carnitine as they compete with L-carnitine in the body and may lead to a deficiency. Occasional side effects of gastrointestinal upset have been reported.

Nutrition Strategy Checklist for Infertility

Females:
- [ ] Weight control
- [ ] Vitamin B12
- [ ] Chasteberry

Males:
- [ ] Vitamin C
- [ ] Vitamin E
- [ ] Selenium
- [ ] Vitamin B12
- [ ] Zinc
- [ ] L-carnitine

Recommended Resources

www.asrm.org/patients/mainpati.html
American Society for Reproductive Medicine
1209 Montgomery Highway
Birmingham, AL, USA 35216-2809
Tel: 205-978-5000
Fax: 205-978-5005

www.iaac.ca
Infertility Awareness Association of Canada, Inc. (IAAC)
406 1 Nicholas Street
Ottawa, ON, Canada K1N 7B7
Tel: 613-244-7222
Fax: 613-244-8908

www.infertilitynetwork.org
Infertility Network
160 Pickering Street
Toronto, ON, Canada M4E 3J7
Tel: 416-691-3611
Fax: 416-690-8015

www.inciid.org
The International Council on Infertility Information Dissemination, Inc.
P.O. Box 6836
Arlington, VA, USA 22206
Tel: 703-379-9178

www.mayoclinic.com
Mayo Foundation for Medical Education and Research

Inflammatory Bowel Disease: Ulcerative Colitis and Crohn's Disease

Inflammatory bowel disease is a term used to describe two chronic conditions that affect the digestive tract: ulcerative colitis and Crohn's disease. These disorders cause the intestine to become inflamed, bleed easily and form sores or scars.

Ulcerative colitis (also called colitis, ileitis or proctitis) usually affects only the colon (large bowel) and rectum. Occasionally, it may affect the lower part of the small intestine, called the ileum. Inflammation always starts in the rectum and may extend into the rest of colon. Inflammation occurs only in the top layers of the bowel tissue and is continuous—there are no areas of normal tissue. Ulcers form in infected areas, which may cause bleeding and become infected.

Crohn's disease can affect any part of the digestive tract, from the mouth to the anus, and inflammation is seen in all layers of the bowel tissue. Unlike ulcerative colitis, the inflammation of Crohn's disease occurs in patches, with areas of healthy tissue in between.

While these disorders differ in some ways, they do share common characteristics. Both are unpredictable. People may experience multiple attacks, followed by weeks or years of quiet periods, or remissions. Abdominal pain, cramping, fatigue and diarrhea are typical symptoms of both Crohn's disease and ulcerative colitis.

What Causes Inflammatory Bowel Disease?

The cause of inflammatory bowel disease remains unknown. Some scientists think that it may develop as a result of a virus or bacterial infection that triggers the immune system, causing inflammation of the intestine. Food sensitivities, high-fat and high-sugar diets are also under investigation. Because inflammatory bowel disease tends to run in families, it's possible that a gene may be responsible for increased susceptibility to the disease.

Symptoms

The symptoms of inflammatory bowel disease can vary considerably in severity. Some people have only mild attacks that can be managed with dietary modifications and drugs. Others experience severe symptoms, requiring treatment with intravenous nutrition, stronger drugs, hospitalization and surgery.

Ulcerative Colitis

- diarrhea, which may be violent and urgent
- frequent bowel movements, as many as six to ten a day
- stool may be watery, bloody and filled with pus and mucus
- painful rectal spasms
- abdominal pain and cramping
- mild fever
- fatigue
- loss of appetite
- anemia
- weight loss and malnutrition
- rectal bleeding

Crohn's Disease

- diarrhea, sometimes bloody
- abdominal pain and cramping
- mild fever

- fatigue
- nausea, vomiting and bloating
- sores around the anus
- painful or swollen joints (common in children)
- slow growth and delayed puberty in children
- anemia
- a lump or swelling in the abdomen, often on the right side

Who's at Risk?

Inflammatory bowel disease affects both men and women equally. It can strike any age, race or ethnic group; however, people of Jewish or European descent are five times more likely to develop the disease. Most people develop inflammatory bowel disease before the age of 30, with symptoms usually developing between the ages of 14 and 30. Both Crohn's disease and ulcerative colitis run in families. In fact, up to 20 percent of those affected have a close relative with the disease.[1]

Conventional Treatment

In most cases, ulcerative colitis can be controlled with medication and may be cured completely through surgical removal of the colon. Crohn's disease cannot be cured with either drugs or surgery, but these and other treatments make the disease more manageable and relieve some of the discomfort. The following treatments may be used to manage inflammatory bowel disease:

- anti-inflammatory drugs such as tablets, enemas or suppositories
- corticosteroids to reduce inflammation
- immune system suppressors to reduce the immune system response, possibly preventing further damage to digestive tissues

- antibiotics to help heal fistulas and abscesses, complications of ulcerative colitis
- bulking agents to relieve diarrhea
- laxatives to treat constipation that may develop from a narrowing of the intestine
- pain relievers to manage pain and discomfort
- iron supplements to treat anemia
- vitamin and mineral supplements to treat nutritional deficiencies caused by impaired absorption
- exercise to relieve stress and help achieve normal bowel movements
- surgery to remove damaged portions of the digestive tract, close fistulas or remove scar tissue

Managing Inflammatory Bowel Disease

Dietary Strategies
During a Flare-Up
When symptoms of inflammatory bowel disease flare up, bowel rest and a low-fiber, low-fat diet can help minimize discomfort and speed healing. Medication may also be necessary. If the flare-up does not require hospitalization, liquid supplement drinks such as Ensure®, Boost® or Essentials® provide energy, protein, vitamins and minerals in an easy-to-digest form. These products are readily available in drug stores.

Many people find they cannot tolerate milk products when the disease is active.[2-4] Lactase, the enzyme necessary to digest the milk sugar lactose, is located on the lining of the small intestine. In Crohn's disease, damage to the intestinal lining causes a loss of lactase. As a result, lactose remains undigested in the intestinal tract, causing abdominal pain, bloating, gas and diarrhea. In people with ulcerative colitis, lactose intolerance is due more to age and ethnicity than the disease itself. You should avoid dairy products and lactose-containing foods during such a flare-up (see page 407, Lactose Intolerance).

Your diet therapy during the healing process will be based on your own specific food intolerances, the portion of your gastrointestinal tract affected and the severity of the flare-up. A deficiency of certain vitamins and/or minerals may occur if you have severe or long-standing disease activity. The intestine's absorption of iron, calcium, selenium, B vitamins, zinc, magnesium and vitamins A, D and E can all be affected by inflammatory bowel disease. As well, many people find that they experience digestive problems with corn, soy foods, chocolate, fats and fatty foods and artificial sweeteners.[5] A registered dietitian who specializes in inflammatory bowel disease can advise you on dietary modifications. If you do not already have a dietitian, ask your gastroenterologist to provide a referral.

During Remission

When inflammatory bowel disease is under control or in remission, a high-fiber diet will help stimulate bowel motility and improve the muscle tone of the intestinal walls, especially in the colon. Fiber also binds to compounds that may irritate the colon, causing their removal from the body.[6] Gradually increase your fiber intake to 25 to 35 grams per day. A list of fiber-rich foods can be found on page 3, Chapter 1. To help fiber work in the body, drink 2 to 3 liters of water a day. Drinking plenty of fluids is especially important for people with ulcerative colitis who take the medication sulfasalazine (Asacol®) to help prevent kidney stones.

Food intolerances often do not persist during remission.[7] Avoiding foods can limit the nutritional quality of your diet and may contribute to nutrient deficiencies.

It is also important to limit your intake of animal fat and include sources of omega-3 fats in your daily diet. These special types of fat are plentiful in oily fish; they are also present in flaxseed oil, walnut oil, canola oil, Omega-3 eggs and soybeans. The body uses fat to produce eicosanoids, powerful hormone-like compounds that regulate our blood, immune system and hormones. A diet high in animal fat and lacking omega-3s favors the production of inflammatory eicosanoids that are thought to be involved in Crohn's disease and ulcerative colitis. Research suggests that omega-3 fats, especially those in fish, may be beneficial in inflammatory bowel disease.[8] Aim to eat fish three times weekly. Good choices include salmon, sardines, trout, herring, mackerel and fresh tuna. To reduce animal-fat intake, choose lean meats, poultry breast and foods prepared with little or no added fat. Refer to 18, Chapter 3, for a list of lower-fat food suggestions.

Vitamins and Minerals
Antioxidants

When the intestinal cells are inflamed, they are capable of producing free radicals, molecules that can cause further damage to the intestinal lining. Studies have found that people with active inflammatory bowel disease often have lower levels of dietary antioxidants such as vitamins A, E and C and beta-carotene.[9-14] The body's antioxidant stores can become depleted from impaired absorption of nutrients in the intestine. Research suggests that people with Crohn's disease who have had part of the small intestine removed are more prone to a selenium deficiency.[15] Without a sufficient supply of antioxidants, the intestine is vulnerable to further damage. To ensure an optimal intake of dietary antioxidants, include the following foods in your daily diet:

- *Vitamin C* The recommended dietary allowance (RDA) is 75 and 90 milligrams for women and men respectively (smokers need an additional 35 milligrams). Best food sources include citrus fruit, citrus juices, cantaloupe, kiwi, mango, strawberries, broccoli, Brussels sprouts, cauliflower, red pepper and tomato juice. To supplement, take 500 milligrams of Ester C once daily. The daily upper limit is 2000 milligrams.

- *Vitamin E* Found in wheat germ, nuts, seeds, vegetable oils, whole grains and kale. To supplement, take 200 to 800 IU of natural source vitamin E. Buy a "mixed" vitamin E supplement if possible. The daily upper limit is 1500 IU.

- *Selenium* Food sources include seafood, chicken, organ meats, whole grains, nuts, onions, garlic and mushrooms. To supplement, take 200 micrograms of selenium-rich yeast per day. Check how much your multivitamin and mineral formula gives you before you buy a separate selenium pill. The daily upper limit is 400 micrograms.

- *Beta-Carotene* Found in orange and dark-green produce, including carrots, sweet potato, winter squash, broccoli, collard greens, kale, spinach, apricots, cantaloupe, peaches, nectarines, mango and papaya. Choose a multivitamin and mineral with beta-carotene added.

Folate

A deficiency of the B vitamin folate is often found in people with long-standing ulcerative colitis. A lack of folate can lead to DNA damage and increase the risk of colon cancer.[16] In fact, 5 percent of people with ulcerative colitis develop colon cancer. The risk increases if the disease has affected the entire colon and has lasted more than eight to ten years.[17] Studies suggest that folate supplements may reduce the risk of abnormal growth of colon cells.[18,19] In one study, patients with ulcerative colitis who took 1 milligram of folate had a 66 percent lower risk for colon cancer compared with nonsupplement

users. Folate absorption may also be impaired in people with Crohn's disease.

Folate-rich foods include spinach, lentils, orange juice, whole grains, fortified breakfast cereals, asparagus, artichoke, avocado and seeds. Folate is the B vitamin in its natural form in foods. Folic acid is the synthetic vitamin found in supplements or fortified foods like breakfast cereal. To ensure you are meeting your daily requirements for folate, take a daily multivitamin and mineral supplement or B complex formula that has 0.4 to 1.0 milligram (400 to 1000 micrograms) of folic acid.

Vitamin B12

People with Crohn's disease who have had a portion of their ileum, the lower part of the small intestine, removed are at risk for B12 deficiency, since this vitamin is absorbed through the ileum into the bloodstream.[20] Depending on the length of intestine removed, B12 supplements or injections may be required. Your doctor should monitor levels of vitamin B12 in your blood.

B12 is found in all animal foods: meat, poultry, fish, eggs and dairy products. Fortified soy and rice beverages have vitamin B12 added to them. To boost your intake of B12, take a high-potency multivitamin and mineral pill or a B complex supplement. Both formulas will supply anywhere from 25 to 100 micrograms of B12. Supplements of B12 that are dissolved under the tongue and absorbed through the mouth have been shown to be as effective as injections in replenishing B12 stores.[21]

Calcium and Vitamin D

People with inflammatory bowel disease who are undergoing corticosteroid drug therapy must pay special attention to their daily calcium and vitamin D intake. Corticosteroids cause bone loss and their use is associated with the development of low bone density and osteoporosis in Crohn's disease and ulcerative colitis.[22-25]

To protect your bones, make sure you meet your daily requirements for each essential nutrient. Calcium supplements are recommended for people who have milk intolerance (refer to Chapter 4 for more information about calcium supplements).

- *Calcium* The recommended dietary allowance (RDA) is 1000 to 1200 milligrams; best food sources are milk, Lactaid® milk, yogurt, cheese, fortified soy and rice beverages, fortified orange juice, tofu, salmon (with bones), kale, bok choy, broccoli and Swiss chard. If you take calcium supplements, buy calcium citrate with vitamin D and magnesium added.

- *Vitamin D* The daily adequate intake is 200 to 600 international units (IU); best food sources are fluid milk, fortified soy and rice beverages, oily fish, egg yolks, butter and margarine. Most multivitamin and mineral supplements provide 200 to 400 IU of vitamin D.

Magnesium

A deficiency of this mineral may occur in people with inflammatory bowel disease because of impaired absorption, a decreased intake from foods and increased losses from the body. Include in your daily diet magnesium-rich foods such as nuts, seeds, legumes, prunes, whole grains, leafy green vegetables, Brewer's yeast, cheddar cheese and shrimp.

If you decide to supplement your diet and you don't take supplemental calcium with magnesium, buy a separate magnesium supplement made from magnesium citrate, aspartate, succinate, fumarte or gluconate. The body absorbs these forms of the mineral more efficiently. Taking more than 350 milligrams of supplemental magnesium can cause diarrhea, nausea and stomach cramps.

Other Natural Health Products

Evening Primrose Oil (*Oenothera biennis*)

This supplement is a rich source of a fatty acid called gamma-linolenic acid that the body uses to synthesize noninflammatory eicosanoids. Research suggests that this remedy may be of some benefit to people with ulcerative colitis. One study found that patients taking evening primrose oil had significantly improved stool consistency compared with those taking fish oil capsules or placebo pills.[26]

The recommended dose is 3 to 4 grams per day, split in two doses. Buy a supplement that is standardized to contain 9 percent GLA. Evening primrose oil is considered very safe. For more information about evening primrose, see page 103, Chapter 7.

Fish Oil Supplements

Researchers have found that fish oils have an anti-inflammatory effect in people with Crohn's disease and ulcerative colitis. Studies have found that supplementing the diet with fish oil can help prevent a relapse of Crohn's disease and may even reduce the dose of corticosteroid medication that's needed to keep the disease in remission.[27-29]

Fish oil supplements are a concentrated source of the two omega-3 fatty acids DHA (docosahexanaenoic acid) and EPA (eicosapentanoic acid). These acids inhibit the body's production of inflammatory compounds called leukotrienes. The typical dosage is 2 to 9 grams of fish oil per day, often taken in divided doses. Fish oil supplements can cause belching and a fishy taste, and high doses can cause nausea and diarrhea. Because fish oil thins the blood, caution should be used if you are taking blood-thinning medication such as aspirin, warfarin (Coumadin®) or heparin.

Probiotics

Foods such as yogurt and nutritional supplements that contain certain live bacteria known to enhance health are called probiotics. The lactobacilli, bifidobacteria and streptococci strains of bacteria have been shown to exert health benefits in the bowel. Once consumed, these bacteria make their way to the intestinal tract, where they take up residence and protect the body from disease-causing microbes. Preliminary research conducted in animals and ulcerative colitis sufferers has found promising results with probiotic supplements. Studies suggest that probiotics can help keep ulcerative colitis in remission, and may prevent a relapse of pouchitis, inflammation of the part of the colon that remains after surgery.[30-34]

To supplement, buy a product that offers 1 to 10 billion live cells per dose. Take 1 to 10 billion live cells daily, in three or four divided doses, with food. Choose a product that is stable at room temperature and does not require refrigeration. This allows you to continue taking your supplement while traveling.

Nutrition Strategy Checklist for Inflammatory Bowel Disease

- ☐ Dietary fiber (during remission)
- ☐ Diet low in animal fat
- ☐ Omega-3 fats
- ☐ Antioxidants
- ☐ Folate (ulcerative colitis)
- ☐ Vitamin B12 (Crohn's disease)
- ☐ Calcium
- ☐ Vitamin D
- ☐ Magnesium
- ☐ Evening primrose oil (ulcerative colitis) OR Fish oil
- ☐ Probiotics

Recommended Resources

www.ccfa.org
Crohn's and Colitis Foundation of America, Inc.
386 Park Avenue S, 17th Floor
New York, NY, USA 10016-8804
Tel: 212-685-3440 or 1-800-932-2423

www.ccfa.ca
Crohn's and Colitis Foundation of Canada
301-21 St. Clair Avenue E
Toronto, ON, Canada M4T 1L9
Tel: 416-920-5035 or 1-800-387-1479
Fax: 416-929-0364

www.niddk.nih.gov
National Institute of Diabetes, Digestive and Kidney Diseases (NIDDK)
Office of Communications and Public Liaison
NIDDK, NIH, 31 Center Drive, MSC 2560
Bethesda, MD, USA 20892-2560
Tel: 1-800-622-9010

Insomnia

Sleep is a basic human need. When we sleep, our minds and bodies rest and restore vital energy. Most people need between seven and eight hours of restful sleep each night to maintain good health and to feel mentally alert during the day. A lack of sleep can result in decreased productivity, increased motor vehicle and job-related accidents and higher rates of mental and physical illness. Insomnia, the inability to sleep, is a term that refers to a number of different sleep disruptions and disturbances, including

- difficulty falling asleep
- waking up early in the morning and being unable to return to sleep

- waking up frequently during the night or having difficulty staying asleep

- waking up after a full night's sleep and not feeling rested

What Causes Insomnia?

Chronic insomnia occurs when sleep habits are disturbed regularly for more than three weeks. Usually, insomnia is a symptom of a medical condition or emotional disorder. It is often associated with psychiatric disturbances and is common in people with depression and anxiety disorders. Alzheimer's disease and other forms of dementia can also disturb sleep and cause repeated nighttime awakening. People suffering from arthritis, kidney or thyroid disease, asthma, restless leg syndrome, sleep apnea and gastrointestinal disorders will frequently experience pain and discomfort severe enough to interfere with normal sleep patterns. As well, medications used to treat these and other health conditions may trigger insomnia as an unwanted side effect.

Our sleep patterns also change as we age. Sleep efficiency is known to decrease from a high of 95 percent in adolescence to less than 80 percent in old age.[1] Consequently, older people have more difficulty falling asleep or staying asleep and often find that sleep is not as refreshing as it used to be. Many lifestyle and environmental factors can also lead to chronic insomnia, such as

- drinking excessive amounts of alcohol or taking recreational drugs

- drinking coffee or caffeinated beverages before bedtime

- smoking cigarettes before bedtime

- taking long naps in the daytime or evening

- engaging in shift work that disrupts the day/night (or sleep/wake) cycle or travel that results in jet lag

- experiencing chronic tension or stress

- sleeping in a noisy environment

- sleeping in a room that is too warm or too cold

Who's at Risk?

Nearly one-third of all Canadians suffer from insomnia.[2] Although people of all ages can experience insomnia, it seems that women experience it more frequently than men and are more willing to seek treatment. Insomnia is also common among the elderly. Studies indicate that people coping with stressful situations, such as divorce or unemployment, or who have medical or emotional conditions, are much more prone to insomnia.

Conventional Treatment

The treatment of insomnia depends, of course, on its underlying cause. Making simple lifestyle changes is often the best way to treat insomnia. Here are some recommendations for improving sleep habits:

- *Exercise* Regular, moderate-intensity exercise is known to improve sleep quality. Take a brisk walk, do some gardening or join an exercise class. Avoid exercise in the late evening before bedtime because it may overstimulate the body.

- *Change your diet* Avoid big meals late at night and limit the use of alcohol and tobacco. Foods high in sugar or caffeine should also be restricted. Avoiding spicy or high-fat foods in the evening may improve sleep. Limiting fluid intake may reduce the need to go to the bathroom during the night, allowing for a more restful sleep.

- *Control your sleep environment* Keep your bedroom dark and quiet and make sure it is not too warm or cold. Use your bedroom as a place to sleep; don't use it for watching television, eating, exercising, working or other activities associated with wakefulness.

- *Establish a regular bedtime routine* Go to bed at the same time each night, and try to get up at the same time in the morning. Following a regular evening routine of brushing your teeth, washing your face and setting your alarm will help set the mood for sleep. Avoid daytime naps that might interfere with nighttime sleep.

- *Relax* Stress and worry can trigger insomnia. Relax at bedtime by taking a warm bath, enjoying a cup of herbal tea or reading until sleepy. Try to avoid worrying about daytime problems. Some people find that alternative therapies, such as biofeedback, muscle relaxation, behavioral therapy or psychotherapy, help them achieve a more restful sleep.

If your insomnia can't be managed using these techniques, medications may be prescribed. Sleeping aids include sedatives, barbiturates and tranquilizers. All carry a risk for overdose, addiction, tolerance and withdrawal symptoms. Use hypnotic drugs only a few times a week and only for a short time (two to four weeks) to avoid future problems. Hypnotic drugs should be discontinued gradually to avoid rebound insomnia, the return of sleep problems after abruptly stopping medications.

Managing Insomnia

Dietary Strategies

Caffeine

Caffeine stimulates the central nervous system and increases the metabolic rate. Researchers have found that older adults suffering from insomnia report higher caffeine intakes. One study reported increased sleep problems in people consuming more than 240 milligrams of caffeine versus abstainers.[3-5] While one or two cups of coffee in the morning can give you that gentle lift you were hoping for, the fourth or fifth cup can overstimulate your body and cause insomnia. The daily upper limit for caffeine, 450 milligrams, is based on studies that have investigated the effect of caffeine on blood pressure and other health conditions, not your ability to sleep soundly. Studies have shown that less caffeine (one or two small cups of coffee) consumed in the morning can affect the quality of sleep that same night.[6,7] Caffeine blocks the action of adenosine, a natural sleep-inducing brain chemical.

Aim for no more than 200 milligrams of caffeine a day, and preferably none. Refer to page 82, Chapter 5, for a list of caffeine-containing beverages and foods. Avoid caffeine in the afternoon. Replace caffeinated beverages with caffeine-free or decaffeinated beverages such as herbal tea, mineral water, fruit and vegetable juice or decaf coffee.

Alcohol

Alcohol worsens insomnia and breathing disturbances during sleep.[8] Once absorbed into the bloodstream, alcohol is metabolized at a set rate by the liver. If you drink more alcohol than your liver can keep up with (more than one drink an hour), alcohol arrives in the brain, where it interferes with brain chemicals called neurotransmitters. Alcohol has been shown to impair the REM portion of sleep, the time when your body is in its restorative phase.

Alcohol also dehydrates you, which can make you feel fatigued the following day. It does so by depressing the brain's ability to produce a hormone called antidiuretic. This causes the body to lose water through the kidneys.

To lessen alcohol's effect on your sleep, avoid drinking before going to bed, and only drink alcohol with a meal or snack. When alcohol is consumed on an empty stomach, about 20 percent is absorbed directly across the walls of the stomach, reaching the brain within a minute.

When the stomach is full of food, alcohol has a lesser chance of touching the walls and passing through, so the effect on the brain is delayed.

Don't drink more than one alcoholic beverage per hour. Alternate one alcoholic drink with a nonalcoholic drink or a glass of water. One drink is equivalent to 5 ounces of wine, 12 ounces of beer, 10 ounces of wine cooler or 1.5 ounces of liquor.

Carbohydrate Before Bed
A carbohydrate-rich snack, such as a glass of milk, a small bowl of cereal or a slice of toast, provides the brain with an amino acid called tryptophan. The brain uses tryptophan as a building block to manufacture a neurotransmitter called serotonin. Serotonin has been shown to facilitate sleep, improve mood, diminish pain and even reduce appetite.

Vitamins and Minerals
Vitamin B12
Many studies have found that vitamin B12 promotes sleep in people who suffer from sleep disorders. In a randomized double-blind study, Japanese researchers determined that a daily dose of 1.5 to 3 milligrams of the vitamin restored normal sleep patterns in such patients.[9] German researchers have also found that sleep quality, concentration and "feeling refreshed" were significantly correlated with the blood level of vitamin B12 in healthy men and women.[10]

B12 may promote sleep by working with melatonin, a natural hormone in the body. Melatonin is involved in maintaining the body's internal clock, which regulates the secretion of various hormones. In so doing, melatonin helps control sleep and wakefulness. Secretion of this hormone is stimulated by darkness and suppressed by light. Vitamin B12 appears to directly influence the action of melatonin, and the vitamin may prevent disturbances in melatonin release.

Vitamin B12 is found exclusively in animal foods; meat, poultry, eggs, fish and dairy products are all good sources. Fortified soy and rice beverages also have vitamin B12. To get additional B12, take a multivitamin and mineral, a B complex formula or a single supplement of the vitamin (these come in 500 or 1000 microgram doses). For sleep disorders that are due to a deficiency of vitamin B12 (have your doctor measure your B12 stores), a dose of 500 to 1000 micrograms three times daily can be used. If you take vitamin C pills, don't take them with your vitamin B12 supplement as large amounts of vitamin C can destroy B12.

Vitamin B12 is considered safe and nontoxic, even in large amounts. However, there have been some reports of B12 supplements causing diarrhea, itching, swelling, hives and, rarely, anaphylactic reactions.

Herbal Remedies
Valerian (*Valeriana officinalis*)
This native North American plant acts like a mild sedative on the central nervous system. Studies show that valerian root makes getting to sleep easier and increases deep sleep. Valerian promotes sleep by interacting with certain brain receptors called GABA receptors and benzodiazepine receptors. Compared with drugs like Valium and Xanax, valerian binds very weakly to these receptors. And unlike conventional sleeping pills, the herb does not lead to dependence or addiction.

In one double-blind study from Germany, 44 percent of those taking valerian root reported perfect sleep, and 89 percent reported improved sleep compared with those taking the placebo pill.[11] Another small study found that individuals with mild insomnia who took 450 milligrams of valerian experienced a significant decrease in sleep problems.[12] The same researchers studied 128 individuals and found that compared with the placebo, 400 milligrams of valerian produced a significant improvement in sleep quality in people who considered themselves poor sleepers.[13]

Buy a product that's been standardized to 0.5 percent essential oils or 0.8 percent valerenic acid. Take 400 to 900 milligrams in capsule or tablet form, 30 minutes to one hour before bedtime. If you wake up feeling groggy, reduce the dose. The herb works better when it's used over a period of time; it may take two to four weeks to notice an improvement in sleep.

Valerian is not recommended for use during pregnancy or breastfeeding, since it has not been studied in these conditions. Long-term use may result in sleeping-pill-like withdrawal symptoms when the herb is discontinued.

Nutrition Strategy Checklist for Insomnia

☐ Avoid caffeine
☐ Avoid alcohol
☐ Carbohydrate bedtime snack
☐ Vitamin B12
☐ Valerian

Recommended Resources

www.nhlbi.nih.gov/health/public/sleep/insomnia.htm
National Institutes of Health
National Heart, Lung and Blood Institute
Information Center
NHLBI Health Information Network
P.O. Box 30105
Bethesda, MD, USA 20824-0105
Tel: 301-592-8573
Fax: 301-592-8563

www.sleepfoundation.org
National Sleep Foundation
1522 K Street NW, Suite 500
Washington, DC, USA 20005
Fax: 202-347-3472

www.swdca.org
Sleep/Wake Disorders Canada
3080 Yonge Street, Suite 5055
Toronto, ON, Canada M4N 3N1
Tel: 416-483-9654
Fax: 416-483-7081
E-mail: swdc@globalserve.net

Interstitial Cystitis

Interstitial cystitis is a chronic inflammatory condition that affects mainly women. It causes recurring discomfort or pain in the bladder and pelvic area and a frequent or urgent need to urinate. Although the symptoms are often very similar to those of a urinary tract infection, interstitial cystitis is not a true urinary tract infection and is resistant to conventional antibiotic therapy.

What Causes Interstitial Cystitis?

The bladder is an important part of the urinary tract that's connected to the kidneys by two small tubes called ureters. The kidneys produce urine and, as urine accumulates, it flows through the ureters into the bladder, which acts as a storage tank for the fluid waste. Gradually, the bladder expands to hold a larger quantity of urine. When maximum bladder capacity is reached, urine is released into another tube, the urethra, where it flows out of the body in a process called urination.

In interstitial cystitis, small areas on the walls of the bladder become irritated by constant inflammation. This causes the bladder wall to become scarred and stiff, impairing its normal function. The inflammation can also cause the bladder to spasm, which can reduce its capacity to store urine, causing an urgent need to urinate. As the irritation becomes more pronounced, small spots of pinpoint bleeding, called glomerulatins, develop on the bladder walls. In rare cases, ulcers appear behind the bladder lining.

The exact cause of this disabling disorder remains a mystery. One theory suggests that interstitial cystitis is the result of a defective defense barrier in the bladder lining. This would allow toxins or infective agents in the urine to leak through the lining and irritate the bladder wall. It's also possible that some type of infectious bacteria may be living in the bladder cells, yet urine tests have failed to identify any bacteria in patients with interstitial cystitis. Some researchers believe that interstitial cystitis is an autoimmune disorder and that the chronic inflammation is the body's response to an earlier bladder infection.

Symptoms

Fortunately, interstitial cystitis is not a progressive disease and symptoms do not usually become worse over time. Symptoms may go into remission for extended periods, only to recur months or years later. The most common symptoms of interstitial cystitis include

- *Frequent urination* People with interstitial cystitis feel the urge to urinate more often, both during the day and at night. In mild cases, this may be the only symptom of the disorder.

- *Urgent urination* Another symptom is the pressure to urinate immediately; this sensation may be accompanied by pain and bladder spasms.

- *Pain* People with the condition may feel mild to severe discomfort in the lower abdomen or vaginal area. Interstitial cystitis makes sexual intercourse quite painful for women and sex drive may be reduced as a result.

- *Other disorders* Muscle and joint pain, gastrointestinal discomfort, allergies and migraine headaches may also occur in some people with interstitial cystitis. There appears

to be some unknown connection between the condition and other chronic disease and pain disorders, such as fibromyalgia, lupus, endometriosis and irritable bowel syndrome.

Who's at Risk?

Although very little is known about the risk factors of interstitial cystitis, research indicates that it is much more prevalent than was previously reported. While the condition affects postmenopausal women most frequently, it is becoming evident that interstitial cystitis can attack people at any age. It can affect men and children, as well as women.

Conventional Treatment

At this time there is no cure for interstitial cystitis. Nor is there a single treatment that works effectively in all people who have the disease. The earlier a diagnosis is made, the better one's chances are of responding to medical treatment, which is aimed mainly at relieving symptoms.

One of the more recent and effective treatments is the oral drug Elmiron® (pentosan polysulfate sodium). This medication seems to repair damage to the bladder wall's defense barrier. Side effects of Elmiron® may include upset stomach, diarrhea and hair loss, which disappear when the medication is discontinued.

Pain medications such as aspirin and ibuprofen are often helpful in treating the discomfort. Antidepressants and antihistamines are sometimes prescribed to ease chronic pain and psychological stress associated with the condition. If pain is quite severe, narcotic drugs may be necessary to control symptoms.

Another treatment that can be effective is a bladder installation, or bladder wash. A solution of dimethyl sulfoxide (DMSO) is passed into the bladder, where it is held for 15 minutes before being expelled. The DSMO washes are done regularly for six to eight weeks, usually in the doctor's office. They are thought to be effective because they reach the bladder tissue more directly, reducing inflammation and pain.

If all treatment methods have failed and pain is severe, surgery may be considered. Unfortunately, the results of surgery can be unpredictable, and many people continue to have symptoms even after the surgery.

Several alternative treatments have proven to ease the chronic pain of interstitial cystitis. Transcutaneous electrical nerve stimulators (TENS) use mild electrical pulses to relieve daily discomfort. The electrical pulses generated may work by increasing blood flow to the bladder, strengthening the pelvic muscles that control the bladder or triggering substances that block pain. Self-help techniques such as exercise, bladder retraining, biofeedback and stress reduction may reduce the severity and frequency of symptom flare-ups.

Managing Interstitial Cystitis

Dietary Strategies

Food Triggers

Many people with interstitial cystitis develop painful symptoms after eating certain foods. Eliminating these foods from the diet can help control symptoms and flare-ups. No two interstitial cystitis sufferers are alike when it comes to food sensitivities. Food avoidance lists are compiled by doctors based on patient case histories. They should be used as a general guideline to help you pinpoint your triggers. Below is a list of foods that have been reported to trigger pain in people with interstitial cystitis. Many of these foods are acidic and can irritate the bladder.

Food List for People with Interstitial Cystitis

Preservatives and Additives
Avoid: benzol alcohol, citric acid, monosodium glutamate (MSG), aspartame (NutraSweet®), saccharin, artificial colors

Fruit
Avoid: apples, citrus fruit, figs, cranberries, cantaloupe, strawberries, pineapple, peaches, nectarines, plums, prunes, rhubarb

Okay: melons (not cantaloupe), pears

Vegetables
Avoid: asparagus, beets, eggplant, mushrooms, pickles, tomatoes, tomato-based sauces, raw onion, spinach, parsley, beet greens, peppers, corn, sauerkraut, sweet potatoes, dandelion greens, artichokes, turnip greens, Swiss chard, purselane

Okay: other vegetables, home-grown tomatoes (tend to be less acidic)

Meats and Fish
Avoid: aged, canned, cured, processed or smoked meats and fish, anchovies, caviar, chicken livers, corned beef and meats that contain nitrates or nitrites

Okay: Other meats, fish and poultry

Dairy Products
Avoid: aged and natural cheeses, sour cream, yogurt, goat's milk

Okay: cottage cheese, frozen yogurt, milk

Grain Foods
Avoid: yeast-based products such as leavened bread, wheat, corn, rye, oats and barley.
Grain products are usually not well tolerated; try them in small quantities.

Okay: rice, potatoes, rice pasta, pasta

Legumes
Avoid: lentils, lima beans, fava beans, soybeans, tofu

Okay: all other beans

Nuts and Seeds
Avoid: most nuts

Okay: almonds, cashews and pine nuts

Eggs
may aggravate symptoms

Herbs, Spices and Condiments
Avoid: BBQ sauce, cocktail sauce, mayonnaise, miso, spicy foods, ketchup, salsa, hot sauce, relish, soy sauce, salad dressing, vinegar, Worcestershire sauce

Okay: Garlic and other seasonings

Beverages
Avoid: alcohol (especially beer and wine), carbonated drinks, tea, coffee, cranberry juice

Okay: bottled water, decaffeinated coffee or tea, some herbal teas

Other
Avoid: caffeine (chocolate, especially dark chocolate, certain medications), junk foods, tobacco, diet pills, all vitamins that contain starch fillers

Painful symptoms often occur up to four hours after eating, making it relatively easy to pinpoint problem foods. But sometimes symptoms don't appear until the following day. In these cases, identifying foods that trigger your condition can be challenging and frustrating.

Elimination/Challenge Diet
The steps below outline an elimination diet for identifying food sensitivities.

1. *Elimination phase* For a period of two weeks, eat only foods identified above as Okay, unless you already know that one of these foods causes you bladder or pelvic pain.

   At the same time, keep a *food and symptom diary*. Record everything you eat, amounts eaten and what time you ate the food or meal. Document any symptoms, the time of day you started to feel the symptom and the duration of time you felt the symptom. You might want to grade your symptoms: 1 = mild, 2 = moderate, 3 = severe.

2. *Challenge phase* After two weeks, start introducing foods from the Avoid section. Do this gradually, introducing them one at a time. I recommend the following procedure for testing foods:

   Day 1: Introduce the food in the morning, at or after breakfast. If you do not experience symptoms, try that food again in the afternoon or with dinner.

   Day 2: Do not eat any of the test food. Follow your elimination diet, eating only foods considered okay. If you do not experience a reaction today, the food is considered safe and can be included in your diet.

   Day 3: If no symptoms occurred, try the next food on your list, according to the above schedule.

   You may find that you can tolerate some foods if you eat them once every few days, but not if they are consumed every day. You may also learn that some troublesome foods are better tolerated if eaten in small portions.

   Some people with interstitial cystitis have food allergies that contribute to their symptoms.[1] Allergies to wheat, corn, rye, oats and barley are common. If you suspect you have a food allergy, speak to your family doctor about allergy testing. The elimination diet outlined above will also help determine allergenic foods.

Low-Acid Foods

Many of the foods in the Avoid section of the food list above are acidic and can cause bladder pain and urinary urgency in people with interstitial cystitis. If your list of troublesome foods leaves you little to eat, you might want to try a dietary supplement called Prelief® (by AkPharma, in the United States). This supplement reduces the acid in foods and beverages so that they don't have to be excluded from your diet. Two studies of more than 200 interstitial cystitis sufferers found that Prelief® reduced the pain and discomfort associated with consuming foods such as pizza, tomatoes, spicy foods, coffee, fruit juices, alcohol and chocolate.[2,3]

The supplement is made of calcium glycerophosphate. It's available in tablet form to be taken upon eating, or as granules that can be mixed right into foods. The supplement is not available in Canada, but can be ordered directly from the manufacturer by calling 1-800-994-4711 or visiting www.akpharma.com. It's important to use the correct amount of Prelief® to reduce the amount of acid in certain foods. The company offers a pocket guide, free of charge, to help you do this.

If eating a certain food brings on bladder symptoms, you can neutralize the acid in your urine by drinking a glass of water mixed with 1 teaspoon (5 ml) of baking soda. Practicing this as a precautionary measure when you're dining out may also help prevent bladder irritation. To prevent a flare-up after eating, drink plenty of water to help dilute the urine.

Herbal Remedies

Uva Ursi (*Arctostaphylos uva-ursi*)

Studies suggest that when taken on a short-term basis, this herb may be effective for inflammatory conditions of the urinary tract, including interstitial cystitis.[4] When taken orally, uva ursi has antiseptic and astringent effects in the urinary tract, and may reduce inflammation. The leaf of the plant contains arbutin, tannins and hydroquinone, all of which may be responsible for its effect. It is thought that products that reduce the acidity of the urine (like Prelief® or baking soda) may actually enhance the antibacterial properties of uva ursi.

If buying a supplement, choose one standardized to contain 20 percent arbutin. The dosage of standardized uva ursi capsules should be adjusted to provide 400 to 800 mg of arbutin daily. As a fluid extract (1:1), take 1.5 to 4 milliliters three times daily. To take as a tea, steep 3 grams of the dried leaf in 150 milliliters of cold water for 12 to 24 hours and then strain. Take one cup of tea four times a day. Prepare the tea with cold water to minimize the tannin content (too many tannins can cause stomach upset; prepare tea in cold water to prevent excess tannins). Do not use the herb longer than one week without medical supervision. Tannins can irritate the stomach and limit the herb's duration of use. Hydroquinone can have toxic effects if taken in larger amounts for an extended period. *Limit your use of the herb to five times a year.* Do not take uva ursi if you are pregnant or breastfeeding, as the herb can increase the speed of labor in pregnant women and there is very little information available about its use during lactation. Do not use uva ursi if you have a kidney disorder.

Other Natural Health Products

L-Arginine

Supplementing your diet with the amino acid L-arginine can help lessen symptoms of interstitial cystitis. L-arginine is used to make an enzyme necessary for the formation of nitric oxide, a compound that relaxes the smooth muscle of the bladder. Research suggests that patients with interstitial cystitis have reduced levels of nitric oxide in their urine.[5] Women with a larger bladder capacity and/or a history of recurrent urinary infections may respond more favorably to this amino acid.

A handful of studies have found that 1500 to 2400 milligrams of L-arginine taken orally can significantly reduce voiding discomfort, urinary frequency, lower abdominal pain and pelvic pain in as little as five weeks of treatment.[6-9]

L-arginine is considered a nonessential amino acid, meaning we don't have to consume it from food because the body is able to make it on its own. Although we get this amino acid from our diet, a supplement is required to achieve an intake of 1500 milligrams per day. Pregnant and breastfeeding women should not use L-arginine as it has not been studied in these conditions.

Nutrition Strategy Checklist for Interstitial Cystitis

☐ Identify food triggers
☐ Low-acid foods
☐ Prelief®
☐ Uva ursi
☐ L-arginine

Recommended Resources

www.ichelp.org
Interstitial Cystitis Association
51 Monroe Street, Suite 1402
Rockville, MD, USA 20850
Tel: 301-610-5300
Fax: 301-610-5308
E-mail: icamail@ichelp.org

www.ic-network.com
The Interstitial Cystitis Network
5636 Del Monte Court
Santa Rosa, CA, USA 95409
Tel: 707-538-9442
Fax: 707-538-9444

www.niddk.nih.gov/health/urolog/pubs/cystitis/cystitis.htm
National Kidney and Urologic Diseases Information Clearinghouse (NIDDK)

3 Information Way
Bethesda, MD, USA 20892-3580
Tel: 301-654-4415 or 1-800-891-5390
Fax: 301-907-8906
E-mail: nkudic@info.niddk.nih.gov

Irritable Bowel Syndrome (IBS)

Irritable bowel syndrome (IBS) is a relatively common disorder of the gastrointestinal tract that often develops during periods of stress or emotional conflict. IBS causes changes in bowel habits that result in constipation, diarrhea, gassy pain and bloating. IBS does not cause any permanent harm to the gastrointestinal tract. Nor does it lead to serious diseases, such as cancer. In most cases, IBS symptoms can be managed with simple changes to lifestyle and diet.

What Causes Irritable Bowel Syndrome?

So far, researchers have not identified the exact cause of IBS. Abnormal bowel motility, psychological stress and food intolerances have all been implicated. Although the symptoms can be painful and persistent, there is usually no evidence of disease, injury or structural damage to the gastrointestinal tract in people with IBS. In fact, most people with IBS appear quite healthy. Because the function of the bowel is disturbed for no apparent reason, IBS is referred to as a functional disorder.

People with IBS appear to have very sensitive colons. Even the mildest stimulation can cause the colon muscle to overreact, triggering cramps and spasms. Irritants such as drugs, hormones, certain foods and stress can aggravate the condition and intensify bowel spasms. For some people, these muscle spasms delay the passage of food through the intestine, causing constipation.

In others, the muscle spasms cause urgent diarrhea by forcing food through the intestine much too quickly.

Symptoms

Gastrointestinal discomfort that persists for at least three months may indicate IBS. Symptoms include

- crampy abdominal pain, usually exacerbated by a meal and relieved by a bowel movement
- painful constipation or diarrhea
- periods of alternating constipation and diarrhea
- passing mucus with a bowel movement
- bloating, gas and nausea
- headaches, fatigue, depression and anxiety

Who's at Risk?

It's estimated that as many as one in five North Americans suffers from this distressing condition. Women are affected three times more often than men.[1] IBS symptoms may increase during a woman's menstrual period. The disorder usually begins in late adolescence or early adulthood, and rarely appears for the first time after the age of 50.[2] IBS often surfaces during times of emotional stress.

Conventional Treatment

The treatment for IBS varies from person to person. Since emotional stress is often a trigger for the condition, learning how to cope with stress is an important way to help prevent a flare-up. Learning relaxation techniques, exercising regularly and stress-management counseling may all be helpful.

Dietary modifications (see below) can lessen IBS symptoms and prevent a flare-up. Occasionally, medications are prescribed to relieve IBS symptoms, including

- fiber supplements or laxatives to treat constipation
- drugs to control muscle spasms in the colon
- drugs to slow the passage of food through the digestive system
- tranquilizers or antidepressants
- alosetron to slow intestinal movement and reduce nerve problems (used in women)

Managing Irritable Bowel Syndrome
Dietary Strategies

One strategy that is relatively easy to implement is to *eat slowly*. Poorly chewed foods are more difficult to digest and may lead to impaired absorption and intestinal discomfort. Eating too quickly can also lead to swallowed air and gas. Chew foods thoroughly: aim to take 20 minutes to finish a meal.

Food Intolerances

Foods may trigger or worsen the symptoms of IBS. Many people with IBS, especially those who suffer from diarrhea, report adverse reactions to certain foods and improvement once these foods are removed from their diet.[3-7] To avoid unnecessary food restrictions, keep a food and symptom diary for two to four weeks to help pinpoint problem foods. A registered dietitian (**www.dietitians.ca**) can help you identify trigger foods and make changes to your diet.

While dietary intolerance varies from person to person, the following foods may cause distress:

- *Lactose-containing foods* such as milk, yogurt and soft cheeses. These foods often cause symptoms in individuals with IBS.[8-11] When the milk sugar lactose cannot be properly absorbed in the intestine, the result can be abdominal pain, bloating, gas and diarrhea. Lactose-free milk and yogurt (e.g., Lacteeze®, Lactaid®) are available, and taking lactase pills with a meal that contains milk will also help if you have a lactose intolerance. Many people with a mild or moderate lactose intolerance can eat yogurt and cheese without experiencing any discomfort, since these foods contain much less lactose than milk. Refer to page 407, Lactose Intolerance, for lactose-reduced diet guidelines.

- *Fructose- and sorbitol-containing foods* such as fruit drinks, fruit juices, dried fruit, hard candies, cough drops, throat lozenges and dietetic cookies and wafers. Colonic bacteria will ferment the sugar fructose when it is in the colon, causing gas and bloating. Sorbitol is a sugar alcohol used to sweeten foods. Sorbitol is not absorbed as readily as sugar, which means that when you eat such foods, some sorbitol reaches the colon and may exacerbate IBS symptoms.[12-17]

- *Gas-producing foods* such as dried peas and beans, lentils, bell peppers, cucumber, onions, chives, garlic, broccoli, cauliflower, cabbage, turnip, melon, pickles, eggs, carbonated beverages and chewing gum.

- *Alcoholic beverages and caffeine* (coffee, tea, colas, chocolate, certain medications; see page 82, Chapter 5, for sources of caffeine).

Dietary Fat

Meals that are high in fat and/or calories can bring on symptoms of IBS. A low-fat diet can normalize bowel function by reducing contractions in the colon that occur in response to a meal. Avoid fatty foods such as whole milk, cream, cheese, butter, margarine and fatty cuts of meat (rib eye steak, spareribs, sausage, salami). Use smaller portions of healthy fats such as avocado, peanut butter and vegetable oils.

Eating large volumes of food at one time can cause abdominal distension and discomfort. It is better to eat small, frequent meals than three large ones. Avoid skipping meals, since this is likely to trigger overeating at the next meal.

Dietary Fiber

A high-fiber diet adds bulk to stool, reduces pressure in the colon, promotes normal bowel motility and can relieve constipation in IBS.[18-21] Gradually increase your fiber intake to 25 to 35 grams per day by choosing more whole-grain breads and cereals, vegetables and fruit. It is important to add higher-fiber foods to your diet slowly to avoid an aggravation of abdominal pain and bloating. For instance, if you are adding a bran cereal to your diet, do so in 1/4 cup (60 ml) increments. Over the course of six to eight weeks, work up to 3/4 to 1 cup (175 to 250 ml). It takes a few weeks for the body to adjust to a higher-fiber intake. Insoluble fiber in wheat bran (Kellogg's All Bran, Post 100% Bran, Fibre One) is often better tolerated than soluble fiber in psyllium (Kellogg's All Bran Buds).

Avoid refined grain products such as white bread, white rice and pasta and breakfast cereals with less than 4 grams of fiber per serving. And be sure to drink plenty of fluids when eating a high-fiber meal or snack; fiber needs fluid in order to exert its beneficial effects in the bowel. Drink 8 to 12 glasses of water each day. Fiber-rich foods can be found on page 3, Chapter 1. Refer also to page 243, Constipation.

Herbal Remedies
Peppermint (*Menthae piperitate aetheroleum*)

This herbal remedy is widely used to ease the symptoms of IBS. A number of studies have found it to significantly reduce pain, distension, stool frequency and flatulence in IBS sufferers.[22,23] The volatile oils in peppermint are known to directly affect the smooth muscle of the digestive tract and reduce spasms. Compounds called flavonoids in peppermint stimulate the secretion of bile, aiding in the digestive process.

To ease bowel spasm, the recommended dose is one to two capsules (0.2 to 0.4 ml) three times daily, taken 15 to 30 minutes before meals. Peppermint oil can cause heartburn, so be sure to buy an enteric-coated product.

Peppermint tea may help ease digestion and can be consumed with and between meals. Steep 1 tablespoon (15 ml) of dried peppermint leaf in 2/3 cup (160 ml) boiling water for 10 minutes and then strain.

Do not use peppermint oil or peppermint tea to treat infant colic as it can cause jaundice and a choking sensation.

Psyllium and Flaxseed

The seeds from both of these plants may help treat constipation in people with IBS.[24] Flaxseeds and psyllium seeds are bulk-forming laxatives high in both insoluble and soluble fibers. The laxative properties of psyllium and flax are due to the swelling of the fibers when they come in contact with water. Once consumed, they form a gelatinous mass that keeps the feces hydrated and soft. The increased bulk stimulates a reflex contraction of the walls of the bowel and prompts evacuation.

- *Psyllium seed husks* Mix 1 to 2 tablespoons (15 to 30 ml) into 2 cups (500 ml) water; take one to three times per day.

- *Ground flaxseed* Take 2 tablespoons (30 ml) once daily. Mix into hot cereal, yogurt, applesauce or smoothies. Add ground flaxseed when preparing baked goods and casseroles.

Other Natural Health Products

Probiotics

Foods and supplements that contain lactic acid bacteria are called probiotics, which means "to promote life." These health-friendly bacteria are known collectively as lactic acid bacteria. The most widely studied are the *Lactobacillus* and *bifidobacteria* species. Researchers have found that a daily supplement of Lactobacillus plantarum for one month significantly reduced pain, bloating and flatulence in IBS sufferers.[25]

Once consumed, these bacteria make their way to the intestinal tract, where they take up residence and prevent the attachment of harmful bacteria and yeasts. It is thought that people with IBS may have an imbalance in their intestinal bacteria (called the intestinal flora), which can lead to gastrointestinal symptoms. Changing the intestinal flora by taking probiotic supplements may ease or prevent IBS.

To supplement, buy a product that offers 1 to 10 billion live cells per dose. Take 1 to 10 billion viable cells, three or four times daily with food. Choose a product that is stable at room temperature and does not require refrigeration. This allows you to continue taking your supplement while traveling. Refer to page 137, Chapter 8, for further information on probiotics.

Nutrition Strategy Checklist for IBS

☐ Eat slowly; chew thoroughly	☐ Psyllium
	☐ Flaxseed
☐ Identify food intolerances	☐ Peppermint
	☐ Probiotics
☐ Low fat	
☐ Dietary fiber	

Recommended Resources

www.acg.gi.org
American College of Gastroenterology
4900 B South 31st Street
Arlington, VA, USA 22206-1656
Tel: 703-820-7400
Fax: 703-931-4520

www.iffgd.org
**International Foundation for Functional
Gastrointestinal Disorders (IFFGD)**
P.O. Box 170864
Milwaukee, WI, USA 53217
Tel: 1-888-964-2001

www.ibsgroup.org (online self-help)
The Irritable Bowel Syndrome Self Help Group

www.niddk.nig.gov
**National Institute of Diabetes, Digestive and
Kidney Diseases (NIDDK)**
Office of Communications and Public Liaison
NIDDK, NIH, 31 Center Drive, MSC 2560
Bethesda, MD, USA 20892-2560
Tel: 1-800-622-9010

**www.med,unc.edu/wrkunits/2depts/medicine/
fgidc/welcome.htm**
**University of North Carolina Center for
Functional GI and Motility Disorders**
CB #7080, 778 Burnett-Womack Building
Chapel Hill, NC, USA 27599-7080
Tel: 919-966-0144
Fax: 919-966-8929

Kidney Stones

Kidneys play a critical role in health by helping to eliminate waste products that are created by the process of digestion and the breakdown of muscle tissue. These waste materials are carried through the bloodstream to the kidneys, where impurities are cleaned out of the blood and converted into urine. Every day, your kidneys process nearly 200 quarts of fluid, removing approximately 2 quarts of waste and excess water. Without this cleansing process, toxic wastes would build up and cause extensive damage to your body.

What Causes Kidney Stones?

Sometimes, substances in the urine can cause crystals to form that then build up on the inner surfaces of the kidneys. These solid masses are called stones. Normally, the urine contains compounds that prevent crystals from forming, but these chemical inhibitors don't seem to work effectively for everyone.

Kidney stones can vary considerably in size. Some are as small as a grain of sand, others can grow to be the size of a golf ball. Tiny stones are usually passed out of the body along with your urine, causing little or no pain. However, when larger stones are washed out of the kidney, they may become stuck in the bladder or another part of the urinary tract. These stones block the flow of urine and can cause excruciating pain.

There are four main types of kidney stones:

1. *Calcium oxalate* and *calcium phosphate* stones are the most common types. These two chemicals are a part of the normal diet and contribute to bone and muscle tissues.

2. *Struvite* stones usually form after a urinary tract infection.

3. *Uric acid* stones can occur when there is too much acid in the urine.

4. *Cysteine* stones are quite rare and are usually caused by an inherited disease.

The exact cause of kidney stones remains unknown. A genetic predisposition, diet and lifestyle factors appear to play a role. Recently, scientists have identified tiny bacteria called nanobacteria inside kidney stones that are thought to trigger stone formation.

Symptoms

- extreme pain in the small of the back or lower abdomen—the pain may come and go, lasting for minutes or hours at a time

- blood in the urine
- nausea and vomiting
- fever and chills
- burning during urination
- an urge to urinate frequently
- cloudy or foul-smelling urine

Who's at Risk?

It is estimated that one out of ten Canadians will have a kidney stone at some point in his or her life.[1] Those more susceptible to stone formation include

- men—men suffer from kidney stones three to four times more often than women[2]
- people with a family history of kidney disease
- middle-aged adults
- people who live in hot climates and don't drink enough fluids
- people who have recurrent urinary tract infections, kidney disorders and metabolic disorders

Conventional Treatment

Most kidney stones pass out of the body on their own. Your doctors will prescribe pain medication as needed and suggest you drink plenty of water to help move the stone through the system. The passed stone is usually saved for testing and analysis. This helps your doctor determine the type of crystals that are forming and suggest appropriate treatment to prevent a recurrence. If a stone will not pass by itself, treatment options include:

- *Extracorporeal shockwave lithotripsy (ESWL)* Shock waves are sent through the body to break the large stone into smaller stones that will pass through the urinary tract system with the urine.

- *Percutaneous nephrolithotomy* A small incision is made in your back, creating a narrow tunnel under the skin to the stone in the kidney. Using a special instrument, the doctor can shatter or remove the stone.

- *Ureteroscope* The doctor inserts an instrument, shaped like a long wire, with a miniature camera attached, into the urinary tract. This allows the doctor to see the stone and shatter it or remove it.

- *Open or incisional surgery* This is conventional surgery to remove kidney stones, but because of the newer technologies available, very few kidney stones are now removed this way.

Preventing and Managing Kidney Stones

Dietary Strategies

In as many as 50 percent of cases, kidney stones will recur.[3] If you have kidney stones, the following dietary modifications can minimize crystal formation and help prevent a future attack.

Fluids

Drinking fluids—water or other beverages—helps flush away substances that can cause crystals to form in the kidneys. When the urine is less dilute because you are not drinking enough fluids, it becomes more concentrated with chemicals that can crystallize into stones. *Drink 12 cups (3 liters) of water in divided doses throughout the day.* In hot weather, drink an additional 2 to 4 cups (0.5 to 1 liter) to make up for fluid lost through sweating.

Depending on what kind of kidney stones you have, the type of fluid you drink may increase or decrease the chances of stone formation. (This may also be true for people with a family history of kidney disease who are at risk for stones.) Hard tap water and some bottled waters contain higher amounts of calcium and sodium (see below), two minerals that may increase the risk of stone formation. Whether or not you need to drink soft tap water or low mineral-content bottled water remains controversial. While one small study found soft water preferable to hard water, others suggest that mineral waters with a higher calcium content may protect from calcium oxalate stones by reducing the amount of oxalate in the urine.[4,5] The most important strategy is to be drinking more water in general. If you are concerned, ask your doctor or dietitian, who can advise you on your choice of water based on the type of stones you have.

Certain beverages may lower the risk of kidney stone recurrences. Coffee, decaffeinated coffee, tea, beer and wine have been shown to prevent stone formation, presumably by increasing the flow of a more dilute urine.[6,7] Grapefruit juice and apple juice increased the risk of stones for reasons unknown.[8] One study found that lemonade made from 4 ounces of reconstituted lemon juice may be beneficial for some people with calcium kidney stones.[9]

Oxalate-Rich Foods

Oxalate, or oxalic acid, is a compound found naturally in plant foods that can crystallize with calcium in the urine. If you have calcium oxalate kidney stones, restricting your intake of foods that contain oxalate is advisable, especially if a urine test reveals you excrete high amounts of oxalate.[10] Although oxalate is present in many foods, it is not always available to the body and therefore may not contribute much oxalate to the urine. Research has found eight foods to increase oxalate excretion: spinach, rhubarb, beets, nuts, chocolate, tea, wheat bran and strawberries.[11]

The following foods contain moderate or high amounts of oxalate and should be limited:[12]

Type of Food	Limit
Beverages	Draft beer, chocolate beverage mixes, cocoa, instant tea, instant coffee
Breads & Cereals	Grits (white corn), wheat bran, wheat germ, whole-wheat flour
Fruits	Berries, Concord grapes, red currants, damson plums, lemon, lime, orange peel, rhubarb, tangerines
Vegetables	Beets, celery, eggplant, endive, escarole, leeks, parsley, spinach, summer squash, sweet potatoes, Swiss chard, wax beans
Legumes	Dried peas, beans and lentils, baked beans with tomato sauce, nuts, nut butters, peanut butter, tofu
Desserts	Fruitcake, desserts containing fruits listed above
Other	Chocolate, cocoa, carob powder

Calcium-Rich Foods

If you have calcium-containing kidney stones, it is not necessary to limit your intake of calcium-rich foods. In fact, restricting dietary calcium is not recommended.[13-16] Studies have found that eating calcium-rich foods is associated with a lower risk of stone formation in men and women.[17,18] One study even found that drinking two servings of milk or a calcium-fortified orange juice per day did not increase the risk of calcium kidney stones in susceptible individuals.[19]

Researchers have learned that consuming enough calcium helps to decrease the amount of oxalate that is excreted in the urine.[20,21] Calcium in foods binds to oxalate in the intestine, preventing its absorption. Many calcium-rich foods also contain potassium and magnesium, two nutrients that might help prevent kidney stones.

A low calcium intake may not only increase the risk of kidney stones, but is also detrimental to bone health. Ensure that you are meeting your daily calcium requirements of 1000 to 1200 milligrams. Some people with calcium kidney stones may absorb too much calcium from their intestine. Specific tests will reveal this, and your doctor may advise that you limit your calcium intake to 800 milligrams daily. This means consuming no more than two milk-product servings per day (e.g., 1 cup [250 ml] milk, yogurt or calcium-fortified beverage or 45 grams of cheese). Refer to page 43, Chapter 4, for the calcium content of selected foods.

Dietary Protein

Overeating protein foods like meat, poultry, eggs and dairy products can increase the amount of calcium excreted in the urine. A handful of studies have shown that a moderately low-protein diet reduces the amount of calcium, sodium, phosphates and uric acid in the urine, components known to cause kidney stones.[22,23]

If you have calcium kidney stones, limit your protein intake to between 0.8 and 1.0 gram per kilogram of body weight per day (see page 15, Chapter 2). Substitute animal protein with legumes and soy foods more often, since vegetable proteins may reduce the risk of kidney stones.[24]

Sodium

A high-salt diet causes more calcium to be excreted in the urine and makes the urine more acidic, two factors that increase the likelihood of calcium salts crystallizing to form kidney stones. If your calcium kidney stones are caused because you excrete too much calcium in your urine, limit your sodium intake to no more than 2400 milligrams per day.

To help cut back on sodium, avoid the salt-shaker at the table, minimize the use of salt in cooking and buy commercial food products that are low in added salt. The sodium content of various foods can be found on page 80, Chapter 5.

Vitamins and Minerals

Vitamin C

When vitamin C is consumed in high doses, some is converted to oxalate in the body. Indeed, studies have shown oxalate excretion to increase with vitamin C supplementation.[25,26] For this reason, people with recurrent calcium oxalate kidney stones are often advised to consume no more than 100 milligrams of vitamin C per day.

However, recent studies suggest that restricting vitamin C intake may be unwarranted. A large Harvard study conducted among 85,500 women revealed that vitamin C intake was not associated with the risk of kidney stones.[27] Another American study did not find any link between levels of vitamin C in the blood and kidney stone formation and development among adult men and women.[28]

If your doctor has determined that you have high levels of oxalate in your urine, focus on meeting your vitamin C needs through foods (refer to page 38, Chapter 4, for a list of vitamin-C-rich foods). Because it is still not known if vitamin C supplements actually cause kidney stones to recur, take vitamin C supplements only under the advice of your doctor or dietitian.

Vitamin B6

The same Harvard study mentioned above found that higher doses of vitamin B6 (40 milligrams per day or more) reduced the risk of kidney stones in women. Vitamin B6 decreases the amount of oxalate produced in the body and therefore reduces the amount available for stone formation in the urine.

If you have calcium oxalate stones caused by high oxalate excretion in your urine, consider taking a B complex supplement with 50 milligrams of B6. Avoid products that have large doses of vitamin C added. You can also buy separate B6 supplements. Do not take more than 100 milligrams of B6 per day. Supplementing with too much B6 for an extended period has toxic effects, including irreversible nerve damage.

Calcium Supplements

If you have calcium kidney stones, you may be wise to avoid calcium supplements. Instead, aim to meet your calcium needs through foods such as milk, yogurt and calcium-fortified beverages. A large Harvard study found that women who took calcium supplements had a higher risk of stone formation compared with those who did not use supplements.[29] However, the women in the study took their calcium supplements apart from a meal, or with a meal low in oxalate content, which may affect how much oxalate ends up in the urine. A much smaller study did not find an increased risk of kidney stones in post-menopausal women who took 750 milligrams of calcium carbonate daily.[30]

Because calcium reduces the absorption of oxalate, both the type of calcium supplement you take and the timing of ingestion may be important factors in the formation of kidney stones.

Nutrition Strategy Checklist for Kidney Stones

☐ Fluids   ☐ Low sodium

☐ Low oxalate-rich foods   ☐ Vitamin C

☐ Calcium-rich foods   ☐ Vitamin B6

☐ Vegetable proteins

Recommended Resources

www.kidney.ca
The Kidney Foundation of Canada
300-5165 Sherbrooke Street W
Montreal, PQ, Canada H4A 1T6
Tel: 514-369-4806 or 1-800-361-7494
Fax: 514-369-2472

www.niddk.nih.gov
National Kidney and Urologic Diseases Information Clearinghouse
(A service of The National Institute of Diabetes and Digestive and Kidney Diseases)
Office of Communications and Public Liaison
NIDDK, NIH 31 Center Drive, MSC 2560
Bethesda, MD, USA 20892-2560
Tel: 1-800-622-9010

www.kidney.org
National Kidney Foundation
30 E 33rd Street
New York, NY, USA 10016
Tel: 1-800-622-9010

Lactose Intolerance

Food intolerance is much more common than food allergy. An intolerance usually develops when the body can't properly digest a certain type of food because the digestive system lacks certain enzymes necessary to break down food into nutrients. Other causes of food intolerance include

- digestive disorders, such as celiac disease or irritable bowel syndrome

- injuries to the small intestine

- an excess of acid in the stomach

- foods contaminated by a toxin

- certain types of bacteria growing in the intestine

- recurring stress or psychological disorders

Lactose intolerance is the best-known type of food intolerance. The fact that 70 percent of the world's population has difficulty digesting lactose, the natural sugar found in milk, has led some researchers to hypothesize that lactose intolerance is in fact normal and tolerance is the abnormal condition.

What Causes Lactose Intolerance?

Lactose is found in dairy products, including milk, yogurt and cheese. Before it can be absorbed into the bloodstream, lactose must first be broken down into smaller sugar units by an enzyme called lactase, located on the lining of the small intestine. When the lactase enzyme is deficient, undigested lactose remains in the intestine. Fluid is drawn into the intestine by the high concentration of sugar, causing diarrhea. The unabsorbed lactose is also fermented by bacteria, producing excess gas, bloating and abdominal cramps. Although the symptoms may be similar, lactose intolerance is very different from a true milk allergy.

Nearly 75 percent of all adults lack sufficient quantities of the lactase enzyme to digest milk or other dairy products properly.[1] Most infants are born with adequate levels of lactase, but these levels seem to decline after the age of two. In the majority of cases, symptoms of lactose intolerance develop before the age of 20 and intensify over time.

The inability to digest lactose can also occur as a result of an illness or a disease that injures the intestinal lining, such as celiac disease and inflammatory bowel disease, parasitic infections and antibiotic therapy. In these cases, the intolerance is often temporary and will disappear when bowel health returns to normal, usually a few days to several months.

Symptoms

Common complaints include nausea, cramps, bloating, gas pain and diarrhea. These occur 30 minutes to two hours after eating a food containing lactose. The severity of the symptoms will depend on the amount of lactose you can tolerate. Some people have mild or moderate lactose intolerance and can handle some lactose, whereas others who have a severe intolerance must avoid all lactose-containing foods and products.

Who's at Risk?

Lactose intolerance is more common among Asians, African-Americans, Hispanics, First Nations Americans and people of Jewish descent. Many individuals of these ethnic origins lose the ability to produce the enzyme lactase at about five years of age. Only 5 to 15 percent of Caucasians suffer from this highly prevalent digestive problem.[2]

Managing Lactose Intolerance

Dietary Strategies

Lactose-Controlled Diet

If you experience adverse reactions to lactose, a lactose-restricted diet will prevent or reduce symptoms of bloating, flatulence, cramps, nausea and diarrhea. Living without lactose does not necessarily mean following a dairy-free diet. In fact, research suggests that people with lactose intolerance who include milk and other lactose-containing foods in their diet may actually improve their tolerance to lactose.[3] Most people with mild or moderate lactose intolerance can consume milk in small portions (125 to 175 ml).[4] Yogurt is generally well tolerated because it has less lactose than milk, the live bacteria in yogurt having digested some of the lactose. Yogurt is also emptied from the stomach more slowly than milk. This gives the enzyme lactase more time to break down lactose.

In general, eating solid foods with lactose-containing beverages improves lactose digestion because they slow the rate at which food enters the small intestine.[5] Consuming lactose-containing foods with foods rich in soluble fiber (oats, beans, psyllium-enriched breakfast cereals) may also ease symptoms of intolerance.[6]

Below is a list of foods according to their lactose content. Depending on the severity of your symptoms, you may need to avoid some or all of these foods.

High Lactose	Moderate Lactose	Low Lactose	Lactose-Free Alternatives
Milk, whole, 2%, 1%, skim	Cream	Cream cheese	Soy beverages
Buttermilk	Sour cream	Blue cheese	Rice beverages
Evaporated milk	Ricotta cheese	Brie cheese	Lactaid® milk
Condensed milk	Goat's milk	Cheddar cheese	Lacteeze® yogurt
Ice milk	Feta cheese	Parmesan cheese	
Whipping cream	Cottage cheese	Swiss cheese	
Yogurt	Ice cream	Butter	

Lactose is found primarily in dairy products, but it may also be present as an ingredient or component of various food products. Read labels carefully to identify sources of lactose. Lactose is found in milk, milk solids, sweet or sour cream, whey, lactose, curds, cheese flavors and nonfat milk powder. Possible food sources of lactose include breads, candy, cookies, sport energy bars, cold cuts, hot dogs, processed meats, commercial sauces and gravies, dessert mixes, some ready-to-eat breakfast cereals, frostings, salad dressings and sugar substitutes. People with severe lactose intolerance must avoid lactose in medications. Ask your pharmacist for a list of lactose-free equivalents.

Lactase-Treated Products and Lactase Supplements
Lactose-reduced dairy products are readily available in the dairy section of supermarkets. Products such as Lactaid® milk and Lacteeze® yogurt have been pretreated with lactase enzyme and are very low in lactose.

You may also choose to reduce the lactose content of dairy products yourself by using commercial lactase enzyme drops such as Lactaid® (McNeil Consumer Healthcare, Inc.). Because the lactose content of dairy products can vary, you may have to adjust the number of drops you add to the food. Lactaid® is also available in capsules and should be taken upon your first bite of a lactose-containing food. Lactaid® enzyme supplements are available in drug stores.

Vitamins and Minerals
Calcium and Vitamin D
If you avoid milk and other dairy products, your intake of calcium and vitamin D may be inadequate. Use fortified soy or rice beverages in place of milk, since these provide the same amount of calcium and vitamin D as an equivalent amount of milk. When you purchase a soy or rice beverage, check the label to make sure the product is fortified; not all brands have added vitamins. Three cups (750 ml) of a fortified soy or rice beverage will provide roughly 900 milligrams of calcium and 300 IU of vitamin D.

Other sources of calcium appropriate for a lactose-reduced diet are yogurt, calcium-fortified orange juice, leafy green vegetables, almonds and tofu. Keep in mind, however, that these foods lack vitamin D. See Chapter 4 for lists of foods rich in calcium and vitamin D.

If you do not use fortified soy or rice beverages, take a calcium supplement with vitamin D added. Calcium citrate supplements supply 300 milligrams of calcium; calcium carbonate pills offer 500 milligrams. Both will provide 100 to 200 international units (IU) of vitamin D. If you take a medication that blocks or reduces stomach acid, choose calcium citrate, since the body absorbs this form of the mineral more efficiently. Depending on the amount of calcium in your diet, you may need to take a calcium pill two to three times a day.

Riboflavin (Vitamin B2)

Milk provides much of our daily intake of this B vitamin, so important for energy metabolism, vision and healthy skin. If you drink fortified soy or rice beverages each day, your riboflavin requirements will be met. Other sources of the vitamin include breakfast cereals, whole grains and meat.

If you are concerned that you are not getting enough riboflavin in your daily diet, take a multivitamin and mineral supplement each day. B complex formulas also provide plenty of riboflavin (25 to 100 milligrams, depending on the formula). Separate riboflavin supplements are also available in 25, 50, 100, 500 and 1200 milligram doses. You'll find these in health food and supplement stores.

Nutrition Strategy Checklist for Lactose Intolerance

☐ Lactose-restricted diet   ☐ Vitamin D
☐ Lactaid® products   ☐ Vitamin B2
☐ Calcium

Recommended Resources

www.ificinfo.health.org
International Food Information Council
1100 Connecticut Avenue NW, Suite 430
Washington, DC, USA 20036

www.niddk.nih.gov
National Digestive Diseases Information Clearinghouse

2 Information Way
Bethesda, MD, USA 20892-3570
Tel: 301-654-3810

www.nin.ca
National Institute of Nutrition
265 Carling Avenue, Suite 302
Ottawa, ON, Canada K1S 2E1
Tel: 613-235-3355
Fax: 613-235-7032

Lung Cancer

Lung cancer is one of the most preventable types of cancers. And yet, in Canada, it is the leading cause of cancer death for both men and women.[1] Nearly 90 percent of all lung cancers develop as a direct result of cigarette smoking.[2] The more cigarettes you smoke, the higher your risk of developing this devastating disease. Studies have indicated that even secondhand cigarette smoke can be dangerous to your respiratory system.

Lung cancer develops when mutated or abnormal cells grow out of control, dividing and multiplying much more rapidly than normal cells. When the abnormal cells accumulate faster than the body can use them, they begin to clump together to form a tumor. The cancerous cells will often spread outward from the main tumor, invading and destroying normal tissue and traveling to other parts of the body, a process called metastases.

More than 90 percent of all lung cancers begin in the bronchi, the large airways that supply the lungs. Lung cancer can take several different forms, but there are four primary types.

1. *Squamous cell cancer* forms in the cells lining the airways. It represents 40 to 45 percent of all lung cancers and is most common in men.

2. *Large-cell cancer* starts in the outer edges of the lungs and accounts for 5 to 10 percent of lung cancers.

3. *Small-cell cancer* is very aggressive, spreads rapidly and occurs most often in smokers. It accounts for 15 to 20 percent of lung cancers.

4. *Adenocarcinoma* forms in the mucus-producing cells in the lung and is most common in women and nonsmokers. It accounts for 25 to 35 percent of lung cancers.

Cancerous cells in the lungs can quickly invade a large number of blood vessels and lymph nodes. These systems can carry the cancer cells to nearby or distant organs and to tissues almost anywhere in the body. This is particularly true of small-cell cancer, which spreads aggressively and often causes death within a matter of months.

What Causes Lung Cancer?

Toxic substances in the environment such as radon gas, asbestos, coke-oven emissions, arsenic, chromate and chromium, nickel and polycyclic aromatic hydrocarbons cause a small percentage of lung cancers. Other types of industrial emissions, air pollution and motor vehicle emissions have also been linked with lung cancer. But by far the biggest danger to lung health is cigarette smoking.

When you inhale smoke from cigarettes or other forms of tobacco, you damage the ability of the lungs to protect themselves from injury. As smoke travels through the bronchi to the lungs, the mucus coating that lines the airways thickens to protect the delicate lung tissue. Cancer-causing substances then become trapped in the thick mucus. The smoke also destroys the tiny mechanisms that normally clean these substances out of the bronchi. Although eventually dislodged by coughing, the toxins remain in the airways long enough to be absorbed by the cells. The harmful chemicals gradually alter the normal body cells, beginning a process that eventually leads to cancer.

Secondhand smoke is proving to be almost as dangerous as active smoking. Secondhand smoke now ranks as the third most preventable cause of death, overshadowed only by active smoking and alcohol use. Exposure to secondhand smoke significantly increases the risk of lung cancer for nonsmokers. Smokers continue to put others at risk, making secondhand smoke one of the major environmental health problems in today's society.

Although overall use of tobacco is declining in Canada, nearly one-third of Canadians over the age of 15 still smoke.[3] Preliminary studies indicate that women who smoke may be more vulnerable to the cancer-causing agents in tobacco and may have a higher risk of developing lung cancer than men who smoke. Equally worrisome is a growing interest in smoking among youth. When smoking starts in adolescence, the risk of developing lung cancer at an early age increases substantially.

The best way to prevent lung cancer is to never start smoking. However, if you do smoke, it is never too late to quit. The moment you stop smoking, your lung cancer risk begins to slowly decline. After 10 years, your risk may be lowered by as much as 30 percent and, after 30 years of not smoking, your risk drops to 10 percent.[4]

Symptoms

There are often no signs of lung cancer until the disease reaches an advanced stage. The following symptoms may be present once the disease is advanced.

- chronic cough
- coughing up mucus and traces of blood
- fever
- chest pain

- shortness of breath
- wheezing
- repeated bouts of pneumonia
- persistent hoarseness in your voice
- weight loss, loss of appetite
- weakness
- difficulty swallowing

Who's at Risk?

People at high risk for lung cancer are

- cigarette smokers; female smokers may be at greater risk than male smokers
- people who are regularly exposed to second-hand smoke
- people who are exposed to workplace or household toxins such as industrial emissions, asbestos and radon gas

Lungs that have been damaged by cigarette smoke are more vulnerable to injury from other types of inhaled pollutants. Risk for lung cancer is also influenced by the length of time that you have smoked, the number of cigarettes you smoke and how deeply you inhale the smoke.

Conventional Treatment

Treatment for lung cancer varies, depending on the size, location and type of cancer and on your general health. Early detection is important to improve prognosis. The following treatments may be recommended:

- quitting smoking and trying not to be with other people who smoke
- supplemental oxygen to relieve shortness of breath
- corticosteroids to relieve symptoms of fever, coughing and shortness of breath

- regular exercise, a healthy diet and reducing stress to maintain your strength and vigor
- chemotherapy alone or chemotherapy in combination with radiation therapy for small-cell lung cancer
- surgery, for types of lung cancer other than small-cell, especially in the early stages
- radiation therapy or a combination of chemotherapy and radiation therapy for advanced lung cancer
- narcotics to control pain in the final stages of the disease

Preventing Lung Cancer

Dietary Strategies

Alcohol

The relationship between alcohol intake and lung cancer has been examined in a number of studies. Because alcohol drinking is strongly associated with smoking, many studies have controlled for cigarette smoking and still have found an increased risk.[5-8] Studies have shown that drinking two drinks per day (40 ounces per month) has been associated with a higher risk for lung cancer.

Alcohol may act as a solvent for cancer-causing agents in cigarette smoke. Alcohol has been shown to induce changes in the lining of the lung that might increase the susceptibility to cancer-causing substances. Alcohol may also impair the ability of liver enzymes to metabolize tobacco carcinogens, resulting in increased activation of these compounds. Finally, alcohol may bind to DNA, the genetic material of cells, enhancing the damage caused by cigarette smoke.

Cancer experts do not recommend the consumption of alcohol. Men should limit themselves to no more than two drinks per day (to a maximum of nine per week), and women should have no more than one drink per day.

Dietary Fat and Cholesterol

A number of studies suggest that a high intake of fat, especially saturated fat, and dietary cholesterol increases the risk of lung cancer in smokers and nonsmokers.[9-15] It is thought that cancer-causing substances in cigarette smoke are more easily activated by a high-fat diet. A high-fat diet may also promote the development of lung cancer by influencing cell membranes, the immune system and circulating levels of hormones. Specific foods found to increase the risk include fried foods, fatty meat, dairy products and rich desserts.

To reduce your intake of saturated fat and cholesterol, choose lower-fat animal foods, such as lean meat, poultry breast and milk and yogurt with 1 percent or less milk fat. Use added saturated fat such as butter or cream cheese sparingly. Avoid margarines and packaged foods made with hydrogenated vegetable oil, another source of saturated fat. You'll find a list of sources of saturated fat and cholesterol in Chapter 3.

Substituting vegetable oils for animal fats such as butter may help prevent lung cancer in women. American researchers found that women who had the highest intake of vegetable fat had a 30 to 40 percent lower risk of lung cancer compared with those who were consuming more animal fat.[16]

There is some evidence to suggest that omega-3 fats in fish may protect from lung cancer, especially in men who smoke or in those who have high intakes of animal fat.[17] Animal research has also demonstrated anticancer properties of fish-oil diets fed to mice with lung cancer.[18] Aim to include fish in your diet three times per week. Eating more fish also means you'll be consuming fewer animal-based meals, which are higher in saturated fat.

Vegetables and Fruit

There is substantial evidence for the protective effect of a high intake of vegetables and fruit on lung cancer. A high consumption of all types of vegetables and fruit, especially *green vegetables*, *cruciferous vegetables* (e.g., broccoli, bok choy, cabbage, cauliflower), *carrots* and *tomatoes*, has been shown to lower the risk of lung cancer.[19-26] Scientists believe that a high intake of carotenoid compounds (beta-carotene, lycopene and lutein), vitamins C and E and cruciferous chemicals called isothiocyanates are responsible for the protective effects of vegetables and fruits.

Studies that have examined vegetables as a whole (rather than measuring intake of certain kinds) have found that the highest consumers have a 40 to 90 percent lower risk of lung cancer compared with the lowest consumers. When fruit is examined as a whole, the highest consumers have a 30 to 70 percent lower risk. The evidence is most abundant and consistent for green vegetables and carrots. A high intake of green vegetables appears to lower the risk by 40 to 70 percent, and carrots by 40 to 90 percent. In one large study from Harvard University, women who consumed five or more carrots per week had a 60 percent lower risk of lung cancer compared with women who never ate carrots.[27]

Eating a diet plentiful in fruits and vegetables is one of the most important strategies to lower the risk of lung cancer, second only to quitting smoking. Be sure to eat at least five to ten servings of vegetables and fruit each day. Choose different colored vegetables and different colored fruit to get a wide range of vitamins, minerals and protective plant chemicals. Eat one orange and one dark green vegetable every day to increase your beta-carotene intake.

Beta-Carotene	Lycopene	Lutein	Cruciferous Chemicals
Carrots	Tomatoes	Spinach	Bok Choy
Sweet potato	Canned	Beet greens	Broccoli
Winter Squash	tomatoes	Collard greens	Cabbage
Broccoli	Tomato juice	Kale	Cauliflower
Brussels	Tomato sauce	Red pepper	Collards
sprouts	Pink & red	Romaine	Kale
Spinach	grapefruit	lettuce	Radish

Beta-Carotene	Lycopene	Lutein	Cruciferous Chemicals
Rapini	Guava	Okra	Rutabaga
Apricots	Watermelon	Zucchini	Turnip
Cantaloupe		Grapes	
Mango		Kiwi fruit	
Papaya		Orange juice	
Peaches			
Nectarines			

Refer to page 68, Chapter 5, for tips on how to incorporate more vegetables and fruit into your daily diet.

Flavonoids

Eating more flavonoid-rich foods may lower your chances of developing lung cancer. Plant foods contain hundreds of different flavonoids. These natural chemicals act as antioxidants and inhibit the action of liver enzymes that activate cancer-causing substances.

Two large studies found that men and women who ate the most *apples, onions* and *white grapefruit* had a significantly lower risk of lung cancer compared with those who consumed the least.[28,29] Apples and onions contain a flavonoid called quercetin and white grapefruit contains one called naringin.

Green Tea

Populations that drink green tea have lower rates of cancer, including lung cancer. And a number of laboratory studies have determined that extracts of green tea have anticancer properties.[30-33] The natural chemicals in green tea have been shown to protect the genetic material of lung cells from free radicals and inhibit the growth of lung tumors in mice. However, the concentrations of green tea required to produce these effects are much higher than can be consumed in the diet.

A large clinical trial is underway in the United States to determine the effect on cancer of drinking ten or more cups of green tea per day.[34] In the meantime, there is no harm in adding green tea to your daily diet.

Vitamins and Minerals
Folate

This B vitamin is essential for the formation of DNA, the genetic material of all cells. Research suggests that higher intakes of folate from the diet may lower the risk of lung cancer.[35] One study from Tufts University in Boston found that higher blood levels of the B vitamin were associated with better survival rates in patients who had surgery for small-cell lung cancer.[36]

Vegetables and fruit are the major sources of folate, and this might account, in part, for their protective effect. To increase your intake of folate, reach for spinach, lentils, orange juice, whole grains, fortified breakfast cereals, asparagus, artichoke, avocado and seeds. A multivitamin and mineral supplement can help you meet your daily requirements (refer to page 31, Chapter 4).

Antioxidants

Numerous studies have found that a high intake of antioxidants, especially beta-carotene, from fruits and vegetables protects from lung cancer.[37,38] It is thought that dietary antioxidants (vitamins C and E, beta-carotene and selenium) may protect lung cells from free radical damage. Some studies have even found that lung cancer is associated with a lower level of certain antioxidants in the blood.[39-42]

But when researchers examine the effect of antioxidant supplements on lung cancer risk, they are disappointed. Studies have found that supplements of vitamins C and E and beta-carotene did not protect from the disease.[43-45] In fact, two of these trials found an increased risk of lung cancer among beta-carotene users who smoked. Therefore, *avoid taking beta-carotene supplements, especially if you smoke*. At this time, there is no evidence that the small amount of beta-carotene in a multivitamin supplement is harmful.

There is no evidence yet that antioxidant supplements will protect from lung cancer. An overwhelming amount of evidence points to the protective effects of antioxidants when they are consumed as food. When it comes to cancer prevention, nutrients from supplements may have biological properties different from those consumed in foods. Aim to get more antioxidants in your daily diet.

- *Vitamin C* The recommended dietary allowance (RDA) is 75 and 90 milligrams for women and men respectively (smokers need an additional 35 milligrams). Best food sources include citrus fruit, citrus juices, cantaloupe, kiwi, mango, strawberries, broccoli, Brussels sprouts, cauliflower, red pepper and tomato juice.

- *Vitamin E* The RDA is 22 international units (IU). Best food sources include wheat germ, nuts, seeds, vegetable oils, whole grains and kale.

- *Selenium* The RDA is 55 micrograms. Best food sources are seafood, chicken, organ meats, whole grains, nuts, onions, garlic and mushrooms.

- *Beta-Carotene* No RDA has been established. Best food sources are orange and dark green produce, including carrots, sweet potato, winter squash, broccoli, collard greens, kale, spinach, apricots, cantaloupe, peaches, nectarines, mango and papaya.

Nutrition Strategy Checklist for Preventing Lung Cancer

☐ Quit smoking
☐ Limit or avoid alcohol
☐ Low animal fat
☐ Fish
☐ Vegetables (especially green vegetables and carrots) and fruit
☐ Flavonoid-rich foods
☐ Green tea
☐ Folate-rich foods
☐ Antioxidant-rich foods

Recommended Resources

www.cancer.ca
Canadian Cancer Society
10 Alcorn Avenue, Suite 200
Toronto, ON, Canada M4V 3B1
Tel: 416-961-7223
Fax: 416-961-4189

cancernet.nci.nih.gov
(A service provided by the National Cancer Institute)
Public Inquiries Office
Building 31, Room 10A31
31 Center Drive, MSC 2580
Bethesda, MD, USA 20892-2580
Tel: 301-435-3848 or 1-800-4-CANCER (1-800-422-6237) (help-line)

www.mayoclinic.com
Mayo Foundation for Medical Education and Research

Lupus

Lupus is an autoimmune disease that targets women during their childbearing years. An autoimmune disease develops when the body begins to harm its own healthy cells and tissues. Normally, your immune system protects your body from germs, viruses and bacteria by producing antibodies to fight these dangerous invaders. In lupus, the immune system malfunctions and begins to produce antibodies that attack its own body parts. This causes inflammation and tissue damage that results in a wide variety of disabling symptoms.

The most common and serious type of lupus is *systemic lupus erythematosus (SLE)*. This form of lupus has been identified as a systemic disease because it can target any tissue in the body, including the skin, muscles, blood, joints, lungs, heart, kidneys or brain. SLE affects each person differently and symptoms vary depending on which tissues and bodily organs become inflamed. The disease is chronic and is characterized by recurring periods of illness, called flares, that alternate with periods of wellness or remission.

Other types of lupus include

- *Discoid lupus erythematosus (DLE)* primarily affects the skin, causing a red, scaly rash to appear on your face, scalp, ears, arms and/or chest. Extreme sun sensitivity is a common symptom of this disease.

- *Subacute cutaneous lupus (SCLE)* causes rashes and sun sensitivity. However, the rashes develop only on the arms and upper body, and the disease rarely affects other organs.

- *Drug-induced lupus erythematosus* is very similar to SLE and the symptoms usually disappear when the medication is discontinued.

- *Neonatal lupus* affects infants born to women with immune disorders such as SLE.

What Causes Lupus?

Current research indicates that lupus does not have a single cause but, rather, is triggered by a combination of genetic, environmental and hormonal factors. High levels of estrogen may accelerate the progress of the disease. Lupus also seems to run in families, which may indicate that there is a hereditary basis for the illness.

Symptoms

Lupus affects each person in a different way. The symptoms of lupus can range from fairly mild to severe, disabling or even fatal. Generally, lupus develops slowly, with symptoms appearing over a period of weeks, months or years. Initially, the disease is quite active and symptoms will steadily increase in severity, often requiring medical attention and treatment. This phase is known as a flare. After a flare, lupus will frequently move into a chronic phase, in which symptoms are less severe, though they don't disappear entirely. Women with lupus may also experience periods of remission, when the disease is not active and symptoms subside.

The following symptoms may be early warning signs of SLE:

- fatigue—often extreme and overwhelming

- weight changes—an unexpected weight loss of more than 11 kilograms (5 pounds) may be a sign of SLE activity; a sudden weight gain may be caused by swelling associated with SLE damage to heart and kidney tissue

- fever

- swollen glands—a sudden, unexplained swelling of the lymph glands might be an immune system response triggered by SLE

There are also a number of specific symptoms that indicate the presence of lupus. Although the list of lupus symptoms below is extensive, it is rare for anyone to experience more than a few of these abnormalities.

- *Photosensitivity* At least 50 percent of people with lupus develop an abnormal skin reaction to sunlight, causing a rash on exposed skin.

- *Butterfly rash (Malar rash)* A red rash appears on the cheeks and over the nose of nearly 50 percent of all people with SLE.

- *Mucosal ulcers* Small sores often appear on the mucous lining of the mouth or nose.

- *Arthritis* Almost all women with SLE develop arthritis eventually. The arthritis associated with lupus does not usually cause crippling or deformities in the joints.
- *Pleuritis or pericarditis* Inflammation of the lining of the lungs (pleuritis) or inflammation of the lining of the heart (pericarditis) affects nearly half of all people with SLE and causes chest pain and painful breathing.
- *Kidney damage*
- *Seizures* Damage to the central nervous system caused by SLE can produce problems such as epileptic seizures, delusions, hallucinations and behavioral changes.
- *Blood cell disorders* The immune system may produce antibodies that will attack the red blood cells, causing a type of anemia. It can also reduce the number of white blood cells and may interfere with blood clotting.
- *Discoid rash* This is a raised, red, scaly rash that appears on the chest, arms, face, scalp or ears of approximately one-quarter of people with lupus. The rash will worsen if exposed to sunlight.

Who's at Risk?

Lupus strikes women between the ages of 15 and 45 most often. Women who have a relative with some type of autoimmune disease are also at greater risk of developing lupus.

Conventional Treatment

The treatment for lupus varies from person to person, depending on the severity of the disease and the type of symptoms involved. Because there is no cure for lupus, the goal of treatment is to bring the disease under control so that patients can lead a relatively normal life. Women with a mild case of lupus may not require any medical treatment. If the disease is more advanced, a variety of treatment options is available.

The most important factor in managing lupus is avoiding circumstances that trigger flares, such as excessive fatigue and high levels of stress. Following a healthy diet, quitting smoking and engaging in regular exercise can help keep the disease under control. As well, it is important that you learn to recognize the warning signs of a flare, such as increased fatigue, pain, rash, stomach upset, headache and dizziness.

In some cases, medications are used to manage the symptoms of lupus. One of the primary drugs used to treat lupus is a corticosteroid called prednisone. Because corticosteroids act rapidly to suppress inflammation in your tissues, they are usually prescribed when symptoms are severe or life-threatening. Corticosteroids are potent drugs with serious side effects such as high blood pressure, osteoporosis, weight gain, acne and stomach ulcers.

Nonsteroidal anti-inflammatory drugs (NSAIDs) are helpful in decreasing the inflammation that causes joint pain, fever and swelling. The arthritis pain often associated with SLE can usually be controlled with a mild pain-relief medication such as acetaminophen. Some people also find that their lupus symptoms respond well to antimalarial drugs. These drugs work to suppress some of the immune responses that cause joint pain, fatigue, skin rashes and lung inflammation. If the nervous system or kidneys are affected, immunosuppressive drugs may be prescribed to restrain an overactive immune system.

Managing Lupus
Dietary Strategies

It is important to eat a healthy, low-fat diet that provides plenty of fiber and fresh fruits and vegetables. These foods contain protective vitamins, minerals and antioxidants that can keep you healthy. The following dietary guidelines should be followed:

1. Emphasize plant foods in your daily diet. Fill your plate with grains, fruits and vegetables. If you eat animal-protein foods like meat or poultry, make sure they take up no more than one-quarter of your plate. Try vegetarian sources of protein like beans and soy.

2. Choose foods and oils rich in essential fatty acids. Fish, nuts, seeds, flaxseed and flaxseed oil, canola oil, Omega-3 eggs, wheat germ and leafy green vegetables are good choices.

3. Choose foods rich in vitamins, minerals and protective plant compounds. Choose whole grains as often as possible. Eat at least three different colored fruits and three different colored vegetables every day.

4. As often as possible, eliminate sources of refined sugar: cookies, cakes, pastries, frozen desserts, soft drinks, sweetened fruit juices, fruit drinks and candy.

5. Buy organic produce or wash fruits and vegetables to remove pesticide residues.

6. Limit foods that contain chemical additives.

7. Limit or avoid caffeine (caffeine can worsen fatigue by interrupting sleep patterns).

8. Drink at least 8 to 12 cups (2 to 3 liters) of water every day.

9. Avoid alcohol. If you drink, consume no more than one drink a day, or seven per week.

Alfalfa

Alfalfa seeds contain an amino acid called L-canavanine that has been shown to provoke lupus in animals.[1,2] There have also been reports that alfalfa can worsen symptoms or cause a flare in women with lupus. Avoid eating alfalfa sprouts and do not use any herbal supplements that contain alfalfa.

Flaxseed

The seed of the flax grain contains plant estrogens called lignans and the essential fatty acid, alpha-linolenic acid. Research indicates that flaxseed may inhibit the action of platelet activating factor, a substance involved in SLE kidney disease. One small study found that women with lupus who consumed 30 grams of flaxseed each day experienced improved kidney function, less inflammation and reduced blood cholesterol levels.[3] Add 1 to 2 tablespoons (15 to 30 ml) of ground flaxseed to yogurt, breakfast smoothies, applesauce, hot cereal and baked goods.

Vitamins and Minerals

Vitamin E

Some experts believe that free radical damage may play a role in the development of lupus. Studies have shown that lupus is associated with an increased level of oxidized blood fats and lower levels of circulating vitamin E.[4,5] Treatment with corticosteroid medication can further increase free radical injury. Preliminary animal research has found that supplemental vitamin E can slow the progress of lupus.[6] A study of 54 women with lupus who were taking prednisone found that vitamin E did inhibit free radical damage to blood fats.[7]

The recommended dietary allowance for vitamin E is 22 international units (IU). The best food sources include wheat germ, nuts, seeds, vegetable oils, whole grains and kale. To supplement, take 200 to 800 IU of natural source vitamin E. The daily upper limit is 1500 IU.

Calcium and Vitamin D

Women with systemic lupus undergoing corticosteroid drug therapy must pay special attention to their daily calcium and vitamin D intake. Corticosteroid drugs cause bone loss, and their use is associated with the development of low bone density. Researchers have also noted that, compared with healthy women, those with SLE had lower blood levels of vitamin D, which may also play a role in the inflammation of the disease.[8] To protect your bones, make sure you meet your daily requirements for each essential nutrient.

- *Calcium* The recommended dietary allowance (RDA) is 1000 to 1200 milligrams; best food sources are milk, yogurt, cheese, fortified soy and rice beverages, fortified orange juice, tofu, salmon (with bones), kale, bok choy, broccoli and Swiss chard. If you take calcium supplements, buy calcium citrate with vitamin D and magnesium added. Refer to Chapter 4 for more information about calcium supplements.

- *Vitamin D* The daily adequate intake is 200 to 600 IU; best food sources are fluid milk, fortified soy and rice beverages, oily fish, egg yolks, butter and margarine. Most multivitamin and mineral supplements provide 200 to 400 IU of vitamin D.

Other Natural Health Products

DHEA (Dehydroepiandrosterone)

DHEA is a hormone produced by the adrenal glands, two small triangular-shaped glands that sit above the kidneys. Once the adrenal glands secrete DHEA, it's used as a building block to make estrogen and testosterone. DHEA supplementation seems to change circulating levels of estrogen and progesterone. In women, DHEA increases blood levels of male sex hormones called androgens without increasing blood levels of estrogens. The effects of DHEA on circulating hormone levels may be responsible for its health benefits.

A handful of studies have found DHEA supplements to improve symptoms of lupus, reduce flares, and reduce the dosage of corticosteroid medication needed to manage the disease.[9-13] DHEA is not a nutrient or a natural product. It is a hormone manufactured from compounds found in soybeans. It is sold as a dietary supplement in the United States, but at this time it is not allowed for sale in Canada.

The recommended dose for lupus is 200 milligrams per day as an adjunct to conventional medication. DHEA is considered safe when taken for the short term; however, it may cause acne. DHEA has been shown to lower the level of good HDL cholesterol, raising concerns about long-term use. Because DHEA is converted to estrogen and testosterone, women with an estrogen-sensitive disease (breast cancer, uterine cancer, endometriosis) should avoid using this supplement.

Fish Oil Supplements

Researchers have found that fish oils have anti-inflammatory effects in women with lupus. Studies have found that women with lupus who take fish oil supplements experience symptom improvement, longer periods of remission and a lowering of blood triglyceride levels.[14-18] Some researchers even suggest that fish oil may reduce free radical damage and help regulate the body's production of antioxidant enzymes.[19]

Fish oil capsules are a concentrated source of two omega-3 fatty acids, DHA (docosahexanaenoic acid) and EPA (eicosapentanoic acid). These acids inhibit the body's production of inflammatory compounds called leukotrienes.

The typical dosage is 2 to 9 grams of fish oil per day, often taken in divided doses. Buy a product that offers both EPA and DHA. Fish oil supplements can cause belching and a fishy taste. High doses can cause nausea and diarrhea. Because fish oil has a blood-thinning effect, use caution if you are taking blood-thinning medication such as aspirin, warfarin (Coumadin®) or heparin.

Nutrition Strategy Checklist for Lupus

- [ ] Healthy, low-fat diet
- [ ] Avoid alfalfa
- [ ] Flaxseed
- [ ] Vitamin E
- [ ] Calcium
- [ ] Vitamin D
- [ ] DHEA
- [ ] Fish oil supplements

Recommended Resources

www.arthritis.ca
The Arthritis Society
393 University Avenue, Suite 1700
Toronto, ON, Canada M5G 1E6
Tel: 416-979-7228
Fax: 416-979-8366
E-mail: info@arthritis.ca

www.lupuscanada.org
Lupus Canada
Box 64034
5512-4 Street NW
Calgary AB, Canada T2K 6J1
Tel: 403-274-5599 or 1-800-661-1468
Fax: 403-274-5599
E-mail: info@lupuscanada.org

www.lupus.org
Lupus Foundation of America, Inc.
1300 Piccard Drive, Suite 200
Rockville, MD, USA 20850-4303
Tel: 301-670-9292 or 1-800-558-0121
Fax: 301-670-9486

Macular Degeneration

This chronic eye disease associated with aging is the leading cause of blindness in Canada and accounts for one-third of all cases of vision loss.[1] Macular degeneration gradually destroys your central vision, resulting in a progressive loss of visual sharpness and detail, which makes driving or reading very difficult.

The damage caused by macular degeneration interferes with the ability of the eye to process light. As light enters the eye, it passes through the cornea and is focused by the lens onto the retina. The retina sits at the back of the eye and contains over 137 photosensitive cells. These cells, called rods and cones, are essential for black-and-white vision and for detecting movement, color and pattern. Most of the cells required for perceiving color and fine detail are located in the center of the retina, in an area known as the macula.

There are two types of macular degeneration. Dry macular degeneration develops when the tissues of the macula gradually thin out as you get older. The light-sensitive cells clustered in the macula slowly break down, blurring central vision and making it difficult to see details. The deterioration of these cells also affects color vision, causing objects to appear hazy or washed out. Ninety percent of people with macular degeneration have the dry type of this disease.[2]

Wet macular degeneration develops when abnormal blood vessels grow under the macula. These blood vessels may leak fluid and blood, causing damage to the sensitive retinal cells. Eventually, scar tissue may form on the retina, creating a central blind spot. Wet macular degeneration is more of a threat to your vision than the dry type. Studies indicate that it is responsible for 90 percent of all cases of blindness associated with this disease. Fortunately, only 10 percent of people with macular degeneration suffer from the wet form of the disease.[3]

What Causes Macular Degeneration?

Although the exact cause of macular degeneration is still unknown, it is thought to be part of the normal aging process. Oxidative damage caused by free radicals has been implicated in the development of the disease. Scientists have also identified certain factors that may hasten the development of macular degeneration, including genetic predisposition, cigarette smoking, long-term exposure to ultraviolet light and low blood levels of antioxidant nutrients. The disease may also develop as a complication of other medical conditions, such as infections, high blood pressure, arteriosclerosis, diabetes, myopia (near-sightedness) and eye injuries that lead to retinal detachment.

Because the brain has a unique capability to fill in the vision gaps during the early stages of macular deterioration, many people don't realize that they have a vision problem until the disease is fairly advanced. The damage caused by macular degeneration can't be reversed, but early detection can help reduce the risk of vision loss.

Symptoms

Symptoms of dry macular degeneration may develop quite slowly or very rapidly. There is usually no pain associated with the disease. Blurred vision is the most common early sign; peripheral or side vision remains normal. Gradually, details become hazy and less clear when you look straight ahead. Colors appear dim and gray. Dark, empty areas or a blind spot can also appear in the center of your vision.

If you have wet macular degeneration, straight objects, such as telephone poles, appear wavy. A dark, empty area or small blind spot may appear in the center of your vision. Wet macular degeneration usually develops in both eyes, though not always at the same time.

Who's at Risk?

- Caucasians over 50 years old
- Individuals with a family history of macular degeneration

- Women are more susceptible than men
- People with light colored eyes
- People who smoke cigarettes
- People who have long-term exposure to sunlight and environmental pollution

Conventional Treatment

No treatment currently exists for dry macular degeneration. To treat wet macular degeneration, a laser may be used to seal off blood vessels in the early stages of the disease. This can prevent further damage to the retinal cells. However, only 20 percent of people with the disease are good candidates for laser surgery, and the surgery is successful only half of the time. New treatments involving more specialized forms of laser surgery are also becoming available. These are most effective at closing leaking blood vessels during the first three months of vision loss.

Although you can't avoid the consequences of normal aging, there are certain things you can do to help prevent macular degeneration or slow the progress of the disease. Eating a low-fat, antioxidant-rich diet (see below), quitting smoking, wearing sunglasses to block out ultraviolet light, controlling your blood pressure and diabetes and having regular eye examinations to detect early changes in your vision are all important strategies to protect your eyesight.

Managing Macular Degeneration

Dietary Strategies

Dietary Fat

Studies have found that people with a high intake of saturated fat and cholesterol have a much higher risk of macular degeneration.[4,5] Diets high in fatty animal foods increase the risk of heart disease and obesity, two conditions that may increase the risk of macular degeneration. Choose lower-fat animal foods such as lean meat, poultry breast and milk and yogurt with 1 percent or less milk fat. Use added saturated fat such as butter or cream cheese sparingly. Avoid margarines and packaged foods made with hydrogenated vegetable oil, another source of saturated fat. For details on how to reduce your fat intake, see Chapter 3.

The same researchers have found that eating fish more than once a week, compared with less than once per month, was associated with a 50 percent reduced risk of late macular degeneration.[6] Fish contains omega-3 fat, a special type of polyunsaturated fat that may keep arteries healthy and reduce the stickiness of the blood. Aim to include fish in your diet three times per week. Eating more fish also means consuming less animal-based meals higher in saturated fat.

Lutein-Rich Foods

Lutein, a yellow compound made by plants, is a member of the xanthophylls family, a subclass of carotenoids. When consumed, lutein is concentrated in the macula of the eye, the small part of the retina that's responsible for fine, detailed vision. In the macula, lutein acts as a filter, protecting structures of the eye from the damaging effects of the sun's ultraviolet light. Lutein contributes to the density, or thickness, of the macula: the denser the macula, the better they can absorb incoming light. Lutein also acts as an antioxidant, protecting the retina from free radical damage.

Scientists have found that a high dietary intake of carotenoids, especially lutein, is associated with a 43 percent lower risk of age-related macular degeneration.[7] A handful of studies have shown that adding lutein-rich foods or a lutein supplement (see below) to the daily diet can increase the density of the macula, in some studies in as little as three months.[8-11] In one study from the Veterans Administration Medical Center in Chicago, lutein in the form of half a cup (125 ml) of sautéed spinach or a supplement, taken four to seven times per week, improved visual function in men with age-related macular degeneration.[12]

Research suggests that a daily lutein intake of 6 to 10 milligrams, the equivalent of five to seven servings of vegetables and fruit, may protect the eyes from macular degeneration. One of the best dietary sources of lutein is egg yolk because it is readily available to the body. But substantial amounts can also be found in a wide variety of vegetables and fruit, including spinach, kiwi, grapes, orange juice, zucchini, broccoli, kale and Swiss chard.

Lutein Content of Selected Foods[13]

Food	Lutein (milligrams)
Beet greens, cooked, 1/2 cup (125 ml)	5.5 mg
Broccoli, cooked, 1/2 cup (125 ml)	1.5 mg
Brussels sprouts, cooked, 1/2 cup (125 ml)	1.0 mg
Celery, 1 stalk	2.3 mg
Collard greens, cooked, 1/2 cup (125 ml)	13.9 mg
Corn, yellow, cooked, 1/2 cup (125 ml)	0.7 mg
Endive, 1/2 cup (125 ml)	1.0 mg
Kale, cooked, 1/2 cup (125 ml)	14.2 mg
Lettuce, leaf, 1 cup (250 ml)	1.0 mg
Lettuce, romaine, 1 cup (250 ml)	3.2 mg
Mustard greens, cooked, 1/2 cup (125 ml)	6.9 mg
Okra, 8 pods	5.8 mg
Peas, green, cooked, 1/2 cup (125 ml)	1.4 mg
Pumpkin, cooked, 1/2 cup (125 ml)	1.8 mg
Red pepper, 1/2 cup (125 ml)	5.1 mg
Spinach, cooked, 1/2 cup (125 ml)	11.3 mg
Spinach, raw, 1 cup (250 ml)	3.1 mg
Squash, summer, cooked, 1/2 cup (125 ml)	1.1 mg
Swiss chard, cooked, 1/2 cup (125 ml)	9.7 mg
Watercress, 1 cup (250 ml)	4.3 mg

Lutein is a fat-soluble compound, so you will absorb more of it if you add a small amount of vegetable oil to your green salad or vegetable stir-fry.

Alcohol

There is no evidence that moderate drinking reduces the risk of developing macular degeneration, even though red wine is often touted for its antioxidant compounds. Studies actually suggest that alcohol may increase the risk of the disease. Two studies found that men who drank beer regularly had a higher risk of macular degeneration.[14,15]

Harvard researchers also found that drinking at least 30 grams of alcohol per day modestly increases the risk of early dry macular degeneration in women.[16] The researchers did not find that any specific type of alcohol protected the eyes.

Men should aim to drink no more than two drinks per day, to a limit of nine per week, and women should drink no more than one per day or seven per week. If you are at increased risk for macular degeneration, or you have the disease, avoid beer.

Vitamins and Minerals

Antioxidants

The retina of the eye is particularly vulnerable to oxidative damage from free radicals because of its high consumption of oxygen, its high content of polyunsaturated fats and its exposure to visible light. Research suggests that dietary antioxidants such as vitamins C and E, beta-carotene, lycopene and selenium may offer protection from macular degeneration.

A number of studies show that both higher blood levels and higher intakes of these nutrients are associated with a lower risk of macular degeneration.[17-22] An American study found that vitamin E supplementation resulted in a slightly reduced risk of the disease.[23] It may be that com-

binations of antioxidants are most protective. Researchers from the Veterans Medical Center in Chicago gave 32 patients with dry macular degeneration a broad-spectrum antioxidant supplement that contained vitamins C and E, selenium and beta-carotene, twice daily.[24] After 18 months, those taking the supplement had stable vision and their disease was less advanced.

- *Vitamin C* The recommended dietary allowance (RDA) is 75 and 90 milligrams for women and men respectively (smokers need an additional 35 milligrams). Best food sources include citrus fruit, citrus juices, cantaloupe, kiwi, mango, strawberries, broccoli, Brussels sprouts, cauliflower, red pepper and tomato juice. To supplement, take 500 milligrams of Ester C once or twice daily. The daily upper limit is 2000 milligrams.

- *Vitamin E* The RDA is 22 international units (IU). Best food sources include wheat germ, nuts, seeds, vegetable oils, whole grains and kale. To supplement, take 200 to 800 IU of natural source vitamin E. Buy a "mixed" vitamin E supplement if possible. The daily upper limit is 1500 IU.

- *Selenium* The RDA is 55 micrograms. Best food sources are seafood, chicken, organ meats, whole grains, nuts, onions, garlic and mushrooms. To supplement, take 200 micrograms of selenium-rich yeast per day. Check how much your multivitamin and mineral formula gives you before you buy a separate selenium pill. The daily upper limit is 400 micrograms.

- *Beta-Carotene* No RDA has been established. Best food sources are orange and dark green produce, including carrots, sweet potato, winter squash, broccoli, collard greens, kale, spinach, apricots, cantaloupe, peaches, nectarines, mango and papaya. Choose a multivitamin and mineral with beta-carotene added.

- *Lycopene* No RDA has been established. Best food sources are heat-processed tomato products such as tomato juice, tomato paste, pasta sauce and canned tomatoes. Lycopene is also found in a form less available to the body in fresh tomatoes, pink grapefruit, watermelon, guava and apricots.

If you decide to take a combined antioxidant supplement rather than a separate pill for each nutrient, look for a product that provides 500 to 750 milligrams of vitamin C, 200 IU of vitamin E, 50 to 100 micrograms of selenium and 20,000 IU of beta-carotene.

Zinc

This mineral may also protect from macular degeneration, though its role is not clear. It may act as an antioxidant or it may protect the macular pigment in some other way. Studies have found that higher blood levels and higher dietary intakes of zinc are linked with a lower risk of macular degeneration.[25] Findings from studies using high, potentially toxic doses of zinc supplements have been contradictory.[26,27]

The evidence does suggest, however, that meeting your daily zinc requirement from food for many years may prevent macular degeneration later in life. Zinc-rich foods include oysters, seafood, red meat, poultry, yogurt, wheat bran, wheat germ, whole grains and enriched breakfast cereals. Most multivitamin and mineral supplements provide 10 to 15 milligrams of zinc. Refer to page 61, Chapter 4, for information on zinc requirements.

Herbal Remedies

Bilberry (*Vaccinium myrtillus*)

This herb contains anthocyanins, a compound that belongs to the flavonoids family. Anthocyanins help form strong connective tissue and blood capillaries. The anthocyanins in bilberry are thought to improve blood flow in the tiny capillaries of the eye. A small body of evidence suggests that the herb may be useful in preventing macular degeneration.[28,29]

Buy a product standardized to 25 to 36 percent anthocyanins. Take 160 milligrams twice daily. Use for one to six months is usually recommended for improvement in visual disorders. No adverse effects have been reported with bilberry use.

Ginkgo Biloba

Ginkgo is thought to increase blood flow to the eye, thin the blood and act as an antioxidant to protect membranes in the eye from free radical damage. While the research is limited, a few studies have found the herb to have a beneficial effect in macular degeneration.[30-32] The recommended dose is 40 milligrams three times daily. The clinical studies evaluated the effectiveness of a special ginkgo extract called EGb 761, sold as Ginkoba® in Canada and the United States. Side effects may include stomach upset and headache.

Ginkgo acts to thin the blood and may increase the risk of bleeding if combined with blood-thinning drugs such as warfarin (Coumadin®), heparin and aspirin. Ginkgo may also cause bleeding problems if taken with garlic and high-dose vitamin E.

Other Natural Health Products

Grapeseed Extract

Grapeseed extract is a byproduct of wine manufacturing and is a rich source of anthocyanins. Like bilberry, this antioxidant is thought to keep eye capillaries healthy. The recommended supplemental dose for antioxidant protection is 50 milligrams once daily. No adverse effects have been reported with grapeseed extract use.

Lutein

If you are concerned you are not getting enough lutein-rich vegetables and fruit in your daily diet, use a lutein supplement. Choose a product made with FloraGlo™, a high-quality lutein extract made from marigold petals that has been used in clinical studies. Take 6 to 10 milligrams once daily with a meal.

Lycopene

If you don't eat tomato products on a regular basis, you may want to consider taking a lycopene supplement for its antioxidant protection (see Antioxidants, above). Choose a brand made with the Lyc-O-Mato™ or LycoRed™ extract. Take 5 milligrams per day.

Nutrition Strategy Checklist for Macular Degeneration

- ☐ Limit saturated fat
- ☐ Lutein
- ☐ Limit alcohol
- ☐ Vitamin C
- ☐ Vitamin E
- ☐ Beta-carotene
- ☐ Lycopene
- ☐ Zinc
- ☐ Bilberry OR Ginkgo biloba
- ☐ Grapeseed extract

Recommended Resources

www.macula.org
Association for Macular Diseases
210 E 64th Street
New York, NY, USA 10021
Tel: 212-605-3719

www.eyesite.ca
Canadian Ophthalmological Society
610-1525 Carling Avenue
Ottawa, ON, Canada K1Z 8R9
Tel: 613-729-6779 or 1-800-267-5763
Fax: 613-729-7209
E-mail: cos@eyesite.ca

www.eyesight.org
Macular Degeneration Foundation
P.O. Box 9752
San Jose, CA, USA 95157
Tel: 408-260-1335 or 1-888-633-3937
E-mail: eyesight@eyesight.org

www.nei.nih.gov
National Eye Institute, NIH, HHS
Building 31, Room 6A32, 31 Center Drive, MSC 2510
Bethesda, MD, USA 20892-2510
Tel: 301-496-5248
Fax: 301-402-1065

www.preventblindness.org
Prevent Blindness America
500 E Remington Road
Schaumburg, IL, USA 60173
Tel: 847-843-2020 or 1-800-331-2020 (hot-line)

Migraine Headaches

One in five Canadians suffers from migraine, a type of headache that results from inflammation of the blood vessels and nerves surrounding the brain.[1] The exact causes of migraine headaches are not known, but they seem to be set off by changes in brain activity. Very often, specific substances, actions or stimuli in your body or environment may trigger migraines.

Research indicates that a migraine involves both the nerves and the blood vessels that feed the brain. Scientists have recorded a spreading pattern of electrical activity within the brains of people with migraines, which may be responsible for some of the classic migraine symptoms. Many people also experience a decrease in blood flow to various parts of the brain, again connected with the onset of migraine. More recently, there has been some evidence that serotonin, a powerful chemical that has the ability to constrict blood vessels, may help stimulate the migraine mechanism.

Symptoms

There are two common types of migraine, each having slightly different symptoms:

1. *Migraine with aura.* This is referred to as a classic migraine. The aura is a set of neurological symptoms that occur approximately 10 to 30 minutes before the headache starts. During the aura phase, you may experience visual disturbances, such as flashing lights or geometric patterns in front of your eyes, or you may even suffer a brief vision loss. It is not uncommon to feel dizzy and confused or to have some facial tingling and muscle weakness as the aura progresses. Migraines with auras affect only 10 to 20 percent of migraine sufferers.

2. *Migraine without aura.* This is known as a common migraine, and it affects many more people than the classic migraine. You may have mood swings, feel depressed and fatigued or lose your appetite just before the migraine strikes.

The Canadian Headache Society has recommended a detailed set of criteria for assessing migraine symptoms. It is reasonable to assume you suffer from migraines if your headaches have some of the following characteristics:

- a sequence of at least five attacks that last between 2 and 72 hours
- pain located on one side of your head, sometimes spreading to both sides
- pain that is pulsating or throbbing
- pain that prohibits or limits daily activity
- pain that is aggravated by physical activity
- nausea or vomiting during headache attacks
- sensitivity to light, noise or smell during headache attacks

Most migraines don't conform to a typical pattern. Some people suffer a migraine only once in a while; others are incapacitated by attacks as often as three times a week. The intensity of pain can vary from reasonably mild to completely debilitating. Migraines also vary in length from a brief, 15-minute episode to an attack that can last a week. On average, the duration of a migraine ranges between 2 and 72 hours.

Who's at Risk?

Migraine is a universal condition that affects approximately 6 percent of men and 15 to 18 percent of women.[2] Although migraines can strike children and adolescents, they most often affect women between 25 and 55 years of age. As many as 50 to 70 percent of all migraine sufferers have a family history of the disease, indicating that these headaches may be hereditary.[3]

Migraine Triggers

In some cases, certain stimuli or triggers may provoke migraines. Although triggers don't actually cause a migraine, they do seem to influence the activities in the brain that stimulate the disease. Often, migraine sufferers are sensitive to the combined effect of more than one trigger.

There are many common migraine triggers, and it is important to determine which ones affect you. Keeping a migraine headache diary is a good way to identify the circumstances that set off your migraines.

1. *Diet* Certain foods and food additives are well-known migraine triggers. Alcoholic beverages (especially red wine), foods treated with monosodium glutamate (MSG), foods containing tyramine (aged cheeses, soy sauce) or aspartame (NutraSweet®) and foods preserved with nitrates and nitrites all may provoke migraines. Chocolate, caffeine and dairy products are other known culprits.

2. *Lifestyle* Changes in your behavior or your surroundings can encourage migraines. If you alter your eating or sleeping habits, experience

high levels of stress or smoke cigarettes, you may find yourself struggling with more frequent migraines.

3. *Environment* Some people find that bright lights or loud noises will bring on a migraine. Weather or temperature changes and physical exertion are common triggers, and even changing time zones may affect your headache frequency. Strong odors, perfume, high altitudes and computer screens are other recognized triggers.

4. *Female hormones* Women may be more susceptible to migraines because of the estrogen cycles associated with menstruation. Migraines become more prevalent in females after puberty, reaching a peak at age 40, and then declining in frequency as women age. But almost two-thirds of women who suffer migraines will experience a worsening of their headaches during their period. Up to 15 percent of women will get migraines only during their period. *Menstrual migraines* are typically without aura and last longer than other migraines. They are also more difficult to treat. To prevent them, it is extremely important for women to avoid migraine triggers during the premenstrual week.

5. *Oral contraceptives and estrogen therapy* These also seem to make migraines worse. Speak to your doctor about alternative contraceptive methods if birth control pills contribute to your migraines.

6. *Pregnancy* Migraines are more common in early pregnancy but usually improve by the second trimester. In a small group of women, pregnancy migraines will worsen throughout their pregnancies. During pregnancy, women should pay special attention to avoiding dietary and environmental triggers, sticking to regular sleeping and eating schedules, getting regular exercise and managing stress (as should all women with migraines).

Conventional Treatment
Migraine Relief Medications

These medications target the pain of an attack and should be taken as soon as you sense a headache beginning. General analgesics (painkillers) and NSAIDs (nonsteroidal anti-inflammatory drugs) are frequently used to relieve the discomfort of mild and moderate migraine attacks. One of the most effective is sumatriptan (Imitrex®), a drug that specifically targets the receptors for serotonin. Some combination medications may also be useful in cases where other drug therapies are not effective. Because migraines are usually accompanied by extreme nausea, you doctor may also prescribe antinausea drugs.

Overuse of these drugs may cause rebound headaches. Rebound headaches are not migraines but medication-induced and may quickly become chronic.

Severe migraine attacks that result in incapacitating pain may be treated with opiates, which are very powerful painkillers. However, they are also highly addictive and so usually prescribed only in extreme cases.

Migraine Prevention Therapies

As with migraine relief medications, these drugs will work with varying success. The main types of prevention medications are

- *Beta-blockers* These work to stabilize serotonin levels and reduce the dilation of blood vessels.
- *Ergot drugs* These affect serotonin levels and blood vessel dilation.
- *Calcium channel blockers* These modulate neurotransmitters.

- *Antidepressants* These have a positive effect on serotonin levels. However, they may have serious interactions with other medications.

Alternative Treatments

A growing body of evidence indicates that alternative therapies have a positive effect on the symptoms and frequency of migraine attacks. Resting in a quiet, dark room and applying ice or pressure often helps relieve pain. Other therapies that have shown some success in alleviating migraine are

- relaxation therapy
- biofeedback
- acupuncture
- stress-management training
- psychotherapy
- hypnosis
- physiotherapy, osteopathy and chiropractic

Managing Migraines

Dietary Strategies

Food Triggers

A number of foods have been reported to trigger a migraine attack.[4-6] One study found that when people who suffer migraines eliminate these foods from their diet, about one-third experience fewer headaches and up to 10 percent become headache-free.[7] The following are the most common foods to trigger a migraine, or make one worse:

Milk	Wine
Chocolate	Coffee, tea
Hot dogs	Garlic
Cheese, especially aged cheese	Eggs
Fish	

The following foods and food additives have also been reported to bring on a headache:

Alcoholic beverages	Lima beans
Artificial sweeteners	Lentils
Citrus fruits	Nuts
Corn	Overripe bananas
Foods with MSG	Peanuts, peanut butter

Foods with nitrites/nitrates (processed meats, smoked fish, some imported cheeses, beets, celery, collards, eggplant, lettuce, radishes, spinach, turnip greens)

Red wine	Shellfish
Soybeans	Tomato

Some migraine sufferers have actual food allergies. It's thought that certain immune compounds formed in response to an offending food can trigger a migraine headache. If you find that certain foods are triggering migraines, it might be worthwhile to have your doctor refer you to an allergy specialist for food testing.

Elimination and Challenge Diet
A registered dietitian who specializes in food sensitivities (**www.dietitians.ca**) can plan an elimination/challenge diet for you, a useful tool used to identify food triggers. You can also do this on your own. Begin by keeping a food and headache diary. List all foods, beverages, medications and dietary supplements you take. Women should also note the date of their menstrual period, since hormones may also precipitate a migraine. Keep this diary for at least two weeks or long enough to cover at least three migraine attacks. Once you've completed this exercise, look for patterns. Did you eat the same food before each migraine? Did your migraines hit you after a night of drinking wine?

Once you have identified possible culprits, eliminate them from your diet for four weeks, or longer if you experience migraines less frequently. If you are migraine-free during this period, it's very likely that you've found your triggers. The next step is to make sure these foods are the actual culprits. Test each food one by one by adding it to your diet. Wait three days before testing the next food on your list. Keep in mind that this exercise may not give you clear-cut results. A combination of events may be required to bring on a migraine. For instance, you may get a migraine only when you eat the food at a specific time in your menstrual cycle. Or, the combination of stress and a food trigger may be required to cause a migraine.

Vitamins and Minerals
Riboflavin (Vitamin B2)
You might consider adding more riboflavin to your diet (or in the form of a supplement) to help prevent migraine. Your body needs riboflavin to facilitate the release of energy from all body cells. Studies reveal that migraine sufferers have less efficient energy metabolism in their brain cells. It's thought that migraine might be prevented by increasing riboflavin intake and therefore the potential of brain cells to generate energy. In a well-controlled study conducted among 55 patients with migraine, a daily 400 milligram supplement of this B vitamin reduced the frequency of headache attacks in a manner similar to certain drugs used for this condition.[8]

The recommended dietary allowance for riboflavin is 1.1 to 1.3 milligrams per day. Riboflavin is found in many foods, including milk, meat, eggs, nuts, enriched flour and green vegetables. If you take a multivitamin or B complex supplement you'll get even more riboflavin, as much as 100 milligrams.

To prevent a migraine, take 400 milligrams of B2 once daily. B2 supplements are available in 25, 50, 100, 500 and 1200 milligram doses. It may take up to three months to notice an improvement in your headache frequency. Riboflavin supplements are nontoxic and very well tolerated.

Magnesium
Evidence shows that during a migraine headache up to 50 percent of people have low magnesium levels in their brain and red blood cells.[9-11] It's thought that a deficiency of magnesium in the brain can cause nerve cells to get overly excited, triggering a migraine attack. (A few medications can deplete magnesium stores, including estrogen, estrogen-containing birth control pills and certain diuretics.)

German researchers gave 81 migraine sufferers either 600 milligrams of magnesium or a placebo pill once daily for three months.[12] In the second month of the study, the frequency of migraine attacks was reduced to 42 percent in the magnesium group compared with only 16 percent in the placebo group. As well, both the duration of a migraine and drug use significantly decreased among those people who took magnesium supplements.

The best sources of magnesium are whole foods, including whole grains, nuts, seeds, legumes, prunes, figs, leafy green vegetables, Brewer's yeast, cheddar cheese and shrimp.

To prevent a migraine, take 600 milligrams of magnesium per day, in divided doses. Buy a magnesium citrate supplement as the body absorbs this form more readily. Taking more than 350 milligrams of supplemental magnesium per day may cause diarrhea.

Herbal Remedies
Feverfew (*Tanacetum parthenium*)
Since the 1970s, this herbal remedy has been the focus of a number of studies in people with migraines. In one study, 76 people who experienced migraines were given either whole feverfew leaf or placebo for four months. The treatments were then reversed for another four-month period.[13] Without knowing which treatment they received, 59 percent of the people taking feverfew identified the feverfew period as more effective compared with 24 percent of those who chose the placebo period. Feverfew reduced the number of classic migraines by 32 percent and common migraines by 21 percent.

Feverfew is thought to reduce the frequency and intensity of migraines by preventing the release of substances, called prostaglandins, which dilate blood vessels and cause inflammation.

The recommended dose is 80 to 100 milligrams daily of *powdered feverfew leaf.* You can also try taking the herb at the onset of a migraine to ease the symptoms. Feverfew rarely causes side effects other than mild gastrointestinal upset. The herb may cause an allergic reaction in people sensitive to members of the Asteracease/Compositae plant family: ragweed, daisy, marigold and chrysanthemum.

Nutrition Strategy Checklist for Migraine

- ☐ Identify food triggers
- ☐ Vitamin B2
- ☐ Magnesium
- ☐ Feverfew

Recommended Resources

www.achenet.org
American Council for Headache Education
19 Mantua Road
Mt. Royal, NJ, USA 08061
Tel: 609-423-0258 or 1-800-255-2243
Fax: 609-423-0082
E-mail: achehq@ache.smarthub.com

www.migraine.ca
The Migraine Association of Canada
365 Bloor Street E, Suite 1912
Toronto, ON, Canada M4W 3L4
Tel: 416-920-4916 or 1-800-663-3557
Information line: 416-920-4917
Fax: 416-920-3677
E-mail: support@migraine.ca

www.headaches.org
National Headache Foundation
428 W St. James Place, 2nd Floor
Chicago, IL, USA 60614-2750

Tel: 1-888-NHF-5552 (1-800-643-5552)
Fax: 773-525-7357

Motion Sickness and Vertigo

Motion sickness is that unpleasant feeling of nausea and dizziness that can occur when you're sitting in a speeding car or rocking boat, on a jerky amusement-park ride, or on some other moving vehicle. While motion sickness is not usually a serious problem, some people suffer so much that they are incapacitated for several days after a trip in a car, airplane or boat. Individuals who are particularly sensitive may even experience nausea and dizziness in an elevator or when sitting on a swing.

Motion sickness frequently causes vertigo, a condition that gives you a false sensation of moving or spinning. Vertigo is often accompanied by nausea and loss of balance. Both vertigo and motion sickness are associated with your sense of balance and equilibrium.

What Causes Motion Sickness and Vertigo?

Your sense of balance is maintained by an interaction involving four different parts of the nervous system. The inner ears, eyes, skin pressure receptors and muscle and joint sensory receptors all send messages to the brain. By interpreting these messages, the brain determines where your body is in relation to the world around it. The signals from these four message centers let the brain know if you are turning, bending, standing still or moving in a particular direction.

The symptoms of motion sickness and vertigo develop when the brain receives conflicting signals from the inner ears, eyes and various sensory receptors. For example, if you read a book in a moving car, your eyes will only see the pages of the book, but your inner ears and your sensory receptors will detect the movement of the car. This conflicting input confuses the brain, upsets your equilibrium and triggers motion sickness.

Motion sickness may also develop as a result of excessive stimulation of the fluid-filled semicircular canals inside the inner ear, which are normally accustomed to horizontal movements. Unfamiliar vertical motion of an airplane, elevator or amusement ride can disturb the fluid and receptors inside these sensitive canals. Your brain perceives these disturbances as a loss of balance, causing nausea and dizziness. Emotional upset, anxiety, nervousness or poor ventilation inside a moving vehicle can also provoke episodes of motion sickness.

In some cases, vertigo develops as a result of specific medical conditions that affect the inner ear, including

- abnormalities in the ear
- viral or bacterial infections of the inner ear
- circulatory problems that reduce the flow of blood to the brain or to the inner ear
- injury to the skull
- allergy
- neurological diseases
- certain medications

Symptoms

Typical symptoms of motion sickness and vertigo include

- dizziness
- headache
- facial pallor
- cold sweating
- nausea
- vomiting

Who's at Risk?

Anyone can experience motion sickness if the motion is turbulent enough and continues for long enough, but some people are more sensitive to it than others. Children are more vulnerable to motion sickness than are adults. Infants are very resistant to motion sickness, but after infancy susceptibility increases, peaking at ages 10 to 12, after which it starts to decrease.[1] Females are more prone to motion sickness than males, possibly because of hormonal influences.[2]

Conventional Treatment

Motion sickness is easier to prevent than to treat. The following strategies can help reduce the likelihood of motion sickness:

- Don't read while traveling.
- Don't sit in a seat facing backwards.
- Keep your line of vision as straight ahead as possible.
- Avoid strong odors, tobacco smoke, spicy food, heavy meals or excessive alcohol before you travel.
- Travel in well-ventilated vehicles, wherever possible; keep windows open slightly in a car or stop frequently for walks in the fresh air.
- Sit or stand where motion is less apparent, such as the front seat of a car, over the wings of an airplane and at the center of a ship (preferably on deck).

If you suffer from severe motion sickness, you may need to take anti–motion sickness medication to control symptoms. Scopolamine® (hyoscine) is the most effective drug for motion sickness and can be applied as a skin patch, which works for several days. However, this drug may cause some drowsiness. Children under the age of ten should not use it. Antihistamines are used most often for children.

Managing Motion Sickness and Vertigo

Dietary Strategies

Carbohydrates

Some research suggests that people with unexplained vertigo may have difficulties processing sugar (glucose) in the bloodstream. One small study found that more than 80 percent of the patients had abnormal levels of the glucose-clearing hormone, insulin, and abnormal glucose tolerance tests.[3] A low-carbohydrate diet improved symptoms in 90 percent of cases.

If your doctor identifies, based on glucose-tolerance tests, that you have a carbohydrate intolerance, try following a lower-carbohydrate diet, especially when you travel. Limit portions of grains, pasta, rice and potato to fill only one-quarter of your plate. The remainder of your meal should consist of vegetables and lean protein foods such as poultry breast, lean meat and fish. You may even try avoiding starchy side dishes with your meal and increasing your portion of vegetables. Low-carbohydrate breakfast suggestions include cottage cheese and berries or cantaloupe or a vegetable omelet with sliced tomato. Low-carbohydrate snacks include nuts, low-carbohydrate energy bars, low-fat cheese and vegetable sticks.

Food Triggers

American researchers studied the relationship of diet to airsickness in pilots and identified possible food triggers.[4] In females, eating high-sodium foods such as preserved meats, potato chips and corn chips as well as thiamin-rich foods like pork, beef, eggs or fish was significantly associated with airsickness. In male pilots, there was a connection between airsickness and high-protein foods such as dairy products and meat.

The researchers also found that eating more frequent meals of rich foods the day before travel was linked with a greater risk of airsickness. To prevent motion sickness, try eating two or three light, low-sodium meals the day before air travel.

Herbal Remedies

Ginger (*Zingiber officinale*)

A number of studies have found powdered gingerroot effective in treating motion sickness and vertigo. One study found that when taken 25 minutes before subjects were tested in a motor-driven rotary chair, ginger was superior to placebo and drug treatment in 36 adults susceptible to motion sickness.[5] Another study found that ginger reduced the severity of motion sickness symptoms in naval cadets unaccustomed to sailing on heavy seas.[6] The same researchers also examined the effect of ginger on vertigo, and found the herb reduced vertigo symptoms significantly more than the placebo treatment.[7]

Scientists believe that the active components in ginger, gingerol and shogal, ease feelings of motion sickness by increasing the motility of the gastrointestinal tract.[8] Gingerol compounds may also improve appetite and digestion by their ability to reduce gastric secretions and increase the release of important digestive aids. There is some speculation that ginger may also work by influencing the central nervous system.

The recommended dose of powdered gingerroot for motion sickness is 500 to 1000 milligrams per day. This is equivalent to 2 to 4 grams of fresh or candied gingerroot. Consume ginger one hour before exposure to motion.

Ginger may cause mild intestinal upset. The herb has a slight blood-thinning effect and may possibly interact with blood-thinning medications like warfarin (Coumadin®), although no studies have reported this effect. Since ginger may increase bleeding time, it should not be taken before scheduled surgery.

Ginger is a menstrual stimulant and has the potential to induce abortion when taken in doses greater than 250 milligrams, four times daily. The use of ginger during pregnancy is controversial and, if used, should be taken for a short period only and limited to 1000 milligrams per day.

Ginkgo Biloba

A few studies have found this herb effective in reducing motion sickness and vertigo. One study involving 67 people with vertigo found that 47 percent of those taking ginkgo completely recovered after three months of treatment compared with only 18 percent of people taking the placebo pill.[9] An Italian study found that ginkgo improved the symptoms of vertigo and dizziness after one month of treatment.[10] The study suggests that ginkgo may work by influencing sensory receptors in the eye. The herb also increases blood flow to the brain.

The recommended dose for treating vertigo is 80 milligrams taken twice daily. Clinical studies have evaluated the effectiveness of a special ginkgo extract called EGb 761, sold as Ginkoba® in Canada and the United States. Side effects may include stomach upset and headache in some individuals.

Ginkgo acts to thin the blood and may increase the risk of bleeding if combined with blood-thinning drugs such as Coumadin® (warfarin), heparin and aspirin. Ginkgo may also cause bleeding problems if taken with garlic and high-dose vitamin E.

Nutrition Strategy Checklist for Motion Sickness

☐ Low carbohydrate diet

☐ Identify food triggers

☐ Low-fat, low-sodium meals

☐ Ginger OR Ginkgo biloba

Recommended Resources

www.entnet.org
American Academy of Otolaryngology—Head and Neck Surgery
One Prince Street
Alexandria, VA, USA 22314-3357
Tel: 703-836-4444

www.my.webmd.com
WebMD Corporation
669 River Drive, Center 2
Elmwood Park, NJ, USA 07407
Tel: 201-703-3400
Fax: 201-703-3401

Multiple Sclerosis (MS)

Multiple sclerosis (MS) is a chronic and unpredictable disease that affects the brain and spinal cord, key communication centers that control most body movements by sending messages, in the form of electrical impulses, along nerve fibers to all parts of the body. Each of these nerve fibers is protected by a fatty sheath or covering, called myelin. Myelin insulates the nerve fibers, ensuring that the electrical impulses travel quickly and efficiently along the nerve pathways of the central nervous system.

Multiple sclerosis attacks the myelin sheath around the nerves, destroying it in sections or patches and replacing it with scar tissue. The scar tissue interrupts the electrical impulses as they travel along the nerve fibers, blocking the natural flow of communication throughout the central nervous system. MS can affect every part of your body, eventually interfering with your muscle coordination, vision, emotional responses and intellectual abilities.

There are several different types of multiple sclerosis, each characterized by different patterns of attack:

- *Relapsing-remitting* This is the most common type of MS; approximately 85 percent of people with MS begin with this form of the disease. Flare-ups occur once or twice every one to three years, usually followed by periods of remission. Symptoms may become worse after each attack.

- *Secondary-progressive* More than half of those people with relapsing-remitting MS move into this stage of continuous deterioration after a number of years. The disease progresses steadily into increasing levels of disability.

- *Benign MS* Up to 25 percent of people with relapsing-remitting MS have this type. The disease has long periods of remission with few attacks and produces little disability.

- *Primary-progressive* This type is relatively rare, affecting 10 to 15 percent of people with MS. The disease grows continuously worse from time of diagnosis, with no clearly identifiable periods of attack or remission.

- *Progressive-relapsing* Also relatively rare, this type affects less than 5 percent of people with MS. It is similar to primary-progressive in that the disease grows steadily worse, but it is aggravated by sudden attacks and episodes of worsening symptoms. There are no periods of remission.

- *Malignant MS* Quite rare, this disease progresses rapidly, and disability usually develops within five years of diagnosis.

What Causes Multiple Sclerosis?

Most researchers believe that MS is an autoimmune disease. The immune system normally produces antibodies to protect the body from disease, fighting off foreign invaders such as harmful bacteria and viruses. Scientists suspect that a common virus may somehow trigger the immune system to malfunction and develop antibodies against the cells that produce myelin, causing inflammation and damage to the myelin sheath.

Research also seems to indicate that heredity has a role to play in multiple sclerosis. There is evidence that a combination of genes may make certain people more susceptible to MS than others. Approximately 15 percent of people with MS have a close relative who is also affected by the disease.

Environmental conditions may also be a factor in multiple sclerosis. MS is five times more common in people who have spent the first 15 years of their lives in a temperate climate such as that in Canada and the northern United States. People who live in a tropical climate have a much lower risk of MS, and people who live near the equator almost never develop the disease. There may be a relationship between low levels of sunshine, vitamin D deficiency and MS. Exposure to sun stimulates the production of vitamin D, which is important for regulating your immune system. If you are genetically susceptible to MS, a lack of vitamin D may trigger the immune system to malfunction.

Symptoms

Although the disease tends to progress slowly over time, its symptoms are unpredictable and vary from person to person. Some people have very few attacks and suffer minimal damage to the myelin sheath. Others have severe attacks that leave them with serious and permanent disabilities. Most people with MS find that the disease seems to come and go, with alternating periods of relatively good health (remission) and debilitating flare-ups.

Damage to the myelin sheath produces a wide variety of symptoms, depending on which part of the central nervous system is affected. Symptoms may improve during periods of remission. Symptoms include

- numbness, weakness, tingling sensations or paralysis in various parts of the body
- extreme fatigue
- blurred or double vision
- loss of balance or coordination, unsteady gait, tremor
- stiffness in muscles, painful muscle spasms
- dizziness or spinning sensation that lasts for a few days
- loss of control over urinary or bowel functions
- sensitivity to heat
- pain on one side of the face
- difficulty in speaking or slurred speech, difficulty swallowing
- difficulty with sexual functions
- problems with short-term memory, concentration, judgment or reasoning

Who's at Risk?

An estimated 50,000 Canadians have MS.[1] As I mentioned above, Canada and other countries with a temperate climate are high-risk areas for the disease. MS usually affects men and women between the ages of 20 and 40; however, women develop the disease twice as often as men.[2]

The risk of MS increases if you have a close relative with the disease, since it seems to run in families. Studies estimate that relatives of people with MS are eight times more likely to develop the condition.[3] People of northern European descent, especially those of Scandinavian heritage, may be genetically predisposed to MS.

Conventional Treatment

Although there is no cure for MS, it is no longer considered to be a fatal disease. Medical advances and improvements in the treatment of symptoms now ensure that most people with MS live a normal or near-normal life span. Treatment with medication focuses mainly on relieving symptoms.

- *Corticosteroids* These drugs reduce inflammation in nerve tissue and shorten duration of flare-ups. Side effects of prolonged use include osteoporosis and hypertension.
- *Beta interferons* These are synthetic copies of proteins that occur naturally in your body. They are used most often for relapsing-remitting MS to help fight viral infection and regulate the immune system. These medications are prescribed cautiously because long-term effects are unknown.
- *Glatiramer acetate* This type of drug is used for those with relapsing-remitting MS to block the immune system attack on myelin.
- *Muscle relaxants* These are used to relieve muscle spasms.

Other medications, such as pain relievers and antidepressants, may help relieve common symptoms of MS. Physical and occupational therapy to strengthen muscles and to learn how to use specialized devices to assist in daily tasks helps to preserve independence. Counseling also helps those suffering from MS, and their families, cope with the emotional and physical stress of the disease.

Certain lifestyle changes may help prevent attacks or reduce the severity of symptoms.

- Get adequate rest to help combat the fatigue associated with MS.
- Exercise regularly to improve strength, muscle tone, balance and coordination, as well as to improve mental attitude.
- Eat a well-balanced diet (see below) to keep your immune system strong.
- Avoid hot tubs, since soaking too long in hot water weakens muscles.

- Have regular massages to improve muscle tone and improve circulation.

- Avoid emotional and physical stress whenever possible.

Managing Multiple Sclerosis

Dietary Strategies

A low-fat, high-fiber diet that contains plenty of whole grains, fruits and vegetables will help you manage your MS. Not only do these foods provide nutrients that may help reduce symptoms of the disease, but they can also help prevent the nutrient deficiencies and constipation that often accompany MS. Although weight gain can occur in many people with MS, nutritional wasting is also prevalent.

Fatigue, physical disability and depression can influence food intake and lead to dependence on low-nutrient convenience foods, increased intake of comfort foods, loss of interest in food and a lack of energy to eat a full meal at one sitting. As calorie intake declines, it is very important that the quality of the diet remain high to provide an optimal intake of all nutrients. You'll find a healthy eating guide in Chapter 5.

Saturated Fat

Animal fat may be directly involved in the development of MS by influencing the immune system. A number of studies have linked high intakes of saturated fat with MS.[4-7] American researchers have found that individuals with MS who followed a low-fat diet (no more than 20 grams of fat per day) showed significantly less deterioration compared with those who consumed higher-fat diets.[8] The greatest benefit was seen in women and in those with minimum disability at the start of the study.

To reduce your intake of saturated fat, choose lean cuts of meat, poultry breast, skim milk and yogurt with 1 percent or less milk fat. Use little or no added saturated fats such as butter, hard margarines and cream cheese. To achieve an intake of 20 grams of fat per day, you will need to follow a plant-based diet that contains little or no animal food. Choose vegetarian protein foods most often—they contain substantially less saturated fat. Legumes and soy foods are good choices. Eat fish more often than meat and poultry. The type of fat found in fish may actually help ease symptoms of MS (see more on fish oil supplements, below).

Polyunsaturated Fat: Linoleic Acid

Polyunsaturated fatty acids are required for growth, development and maintenance of cell membranes, including those of the central nervous system. Polyunsaturated fats are important components of the myelin sheath and are used to produce noninflammatory immune compounds.

Omega-6 polyunsaturated oils such as sunflower, safflower, corn and soybean oils provide the body with an essential fatty acid called linoleic acid. Supplementing the diet with omega-6 oils appears to slow the progression of MS and reduce the severity and duration of exacerbations. Two large two-year studies found that diets supplemented with linoleic acid from sunflower seed oil produced a significant reduction in the severity and duration of relapse in MS patients who were treated early in the course of their illness.[9,10]

Since the characteristics of the MS patients studied in each trial differed, it is premature to say that omega-6 oils are an effective treatment for MS. However, there is no harm in adding these healthy oils to your diet. The dosage used in the studies ranged from 17 to 20 grams of linoleic acid, the equivalent of 1 ounce of sunflower oil. Some researchers believe that it may take at least two years for linoleic acid to exert its effect on the myelin sheath.

Vitamins and Minerals

Antioxidants

Brain and nervous system cells are prone to free radical damage because of their relatively low content of antioxidant enzymes and high levels of polyunsaturated fats (polyunsaturated fats are easily oxidized by free radicals). Some scientists hypothesize that such free radical damage can promote the progression of MS. Some studies have found that patients with MS have lower levels of antioxidants in their blood and higher levels of oxidized compounds.[11-13]

While no well-controlled trials have investigated the effects of antioxidant supplements and disease activity, it is prudent to include antioxidant-rich foods in your daily diet.

- *Vitamin C* The recommended dietary allowance (RDA) is 75 and 90 milligrams for women and men respectively (smokers need an additional 35 milligrams). Best food sources include citrus fruit, citrus juices, cantaloupe, kiwi, mango, strawberries, broccoli, Brussels sprouts, cauliflower, red pepper and tomato juice. To supplement, take 500 milligrams of Ester C once or twice daily. The daily upper limit is 2000 milligrams.

- *Vitamin E* The RDA is 22 international units (IU). Best food sources include wheat germ, nuts, seeds, vegetable oils, whole grains and kale. To supplement, take 200 to 800 IU of natural source vitamin E. Buy a "mixed" vitamin E supplement if possible. The daily upper limit is 1500 IU.

- *Selenium* The RDA is 55 micrograms. Best food sources are seafood, chicken, organ meats, whole grains, nuts, onions, garlic and mushrooms. Check how much your multivitamin and mineral provides before buying a separate selenium pill. The daily upper limit is 400 micrograms.

- *Beta-Carotene* No RDA has been established. Best food sources are orange and dark green produce, including carrots, sweet potato, winter squash, broccoli, collard greens, kale, spinach, apricots, cantaloupe, peaches, nectarines, mango and papaya. Avoid taking beta-carotene supplements if you smoke as they may increase the risk of cancer.

Vitamin B12

Several studies have documented a deficiency of B12 in people with MS.[14-16] Since the nutrient is required for the formation of myelin and for healthy immune function, a B12 deficiency may make you more vulnerable to viral or immune system factors that may cause the disease. A deficiency may also impair recovery from MS.

One preliminary study suggests that very high doses of B12 taken for six months may improve certain test results; however, improvements in disability were not seen.[17] Since B12 is critical for nerve function, it is important to include good food sources in your daily diet. The vitamin is found naturally in animal foods such as meat, poultry, fish, eggs and dairy products. Fortified soy and rice beverages also supply B12. A multivitamin and mineral supplement will provide additional B12.

If you are a strict vegetarian and you don't drink fortified soy or rice beverages, take 500 to 1000 micrograms of B12 from a supplement.

If you are taking a high-dose B12 supplement to correct a deficiency, don't take it with a vitamin C pill. Large amounts of vitamin C can destroy B12. Take your vitamin C supplement one hour after taking B12.

Vitamin D

Some researchers believe that a vitamin D deficiency associated with a lack of sunshine may influence the immune system in such a way as to cause MS. The active form of vitamin D (D3) has been shown to completely prevent experimental MS in mice, a model used by researchers to study human MS.[18] Vitamin D3 has also been shown to prevent the progression of the disease in animal research.

Preliminary findings from a Pennsylvania State University study show that MS patients who took a daily vitamin D supplement for six months had higher blood levels of the vitamin and changes in blood chemistry that indicated positive effects on their disease.[19] Blood levels of a compound called TGF-beta were increased, and this is associated with the remission and suppression of the immune response that produces MS symptoms. People with MS have also been shown to have significantly reduced bone density and more frequent bone fractures, in part related to low levels of vitamin D in the body.[20,21]

The adequate dietary intake for vitamin D is 200 to 600 IU, depending on your age (see page 39, Chapter 4). The best food sources include fluid milk, fortified soy and rice beverages, oily fish, egg yolks, butter and margarine. Most multivitamin and mineral supplements provide 400 IU of vitamin D.

The dose of vitamin D given to patients in the Pennsylvania State University study was 1000 IU per day. The daily upper limit for vitamin D is 2000 IU. In the case of vitamin D, more is not better. High-dose vitamin D supplements can be toxic and should be taken only under the supervision of a doctor.

Other Natural Health Products

Fish Oil Supplements

Omega-3 fatty acids in fish oil provide the body with EPA (eicosapentaenoic acids) and DHA (docosahexaenoic acid), two fatty acids that may be beneficial in MS. EPA and DHA suppress the body's production of inflammatory cytokines, immune compounds involved in MS. Studies have revealed that people with MS have lower blood levels of omega-3 fats compared with people free of the disease.[22,23] Norwegian researchers found that fish oil supplements taken with vitamins for two years by newly diagnosed MS patients produced a significant reduction in exacerbation and disability ratings.[24] Despite this positive finding, randomized, double-blind, placebo-controlled trials are lacking.

The dosage used in the study was 1 gram per day. Fish oil supplements can cause belching and a fishy taste. High doses can cause nausea and diarrhea. Because fish oil has a blood-thinning effect, use caution if you are taking blood-thinning medication such as aspirin, warfarin (Coumadin®) or heparin.

L-Threonine

The body uses this naturally occurring amino acid found in protein-rich foods to synthesize glycine, an important component of the spinal cord. Some evidence suggests that this naturally occurring amino acid may be able to reduce muscle spasticity often associated with MS. Two studies found that supplemental threonine reduced signs of spasticity on clinical examination.[25,26]

The first study used a dose of 6 grams per day, the other 7.5 grams per day. No side effects were noted, in contrast to the side effects of sedation and increased muscle weakness associated with drug therapy for MS-associated muscle spasm.

Nutrition Strategy Checklist for Multiple Sclerosis

☐ Low animal fat   ☐ Beta-carotene
☐ Omega-6 oils   ☐ Vitamin B12
☐ Vitamin C   ☐ Vitamin D
☐ Vitamin E   ☐ Fish oil supplements
☐ Selenium   ☐ L-threonine

Recommended Resources

www.msfocus.org
Multiple Sclerosis Foundation
6350 N Andrews Avenue
Fort Lauderdale, FL, USA 33309-2130
Tel: 1-800-441-7055
Fax: 954-351-0630

www.mssociety.ca
Multiple Sclerosis Society of Canada
250 Bloor Street E, Suite 1000
Toronto, ON, Canada M4W 3P9
Tel: 416-922-6065
Fax: 416-922-7538

www.nationalmssociety.org
The National Multiple Sclerosis Society
733 Third Avenue
New York, NY, USA 10017
Tel: 1-800-344-4867

Obesity and Weight Loss

Canadians are getting heavier, even though we are eating less fat than we did 30 years ago. It's estimated that 30 percent of Canadian adults are overweight, which is defined as having a body mass index of 27 or greater (see below).[1] More worrisome is the growing number of Canadian children between the ages of 7 and 13 who are becoming progressively overweight and obese. In 1996, 29 percent of boys and 24 percent of girls were overweight, figures that have almost doubled since 1981.[2]

What Causes Obesity?

Obesity is an excessive accumulation of body fat. You become overweight or obese when you consume more calories than your body can burn as energy. There is general agreement among doctors and scientists that men who have more than 25 percent body fat and women who have more than 30 percent body fat are diagnosed as obese.

Scientists still do not fully understand the causes of obesity. Social, behavioral, cultural, psychological, physiological and genetic factors all play a role in the process of weight gain. In North America, obesity stems primarily from an increasingly sedentary lifestyle and a growing dependence on high-fat, high-sugar foods.

Statistics clearly show that being overweight, especially if excess weight is carried around the abdomen, significantly increases the risk of serious health problems such as heart disease and stroke, type 2 diabetes, osteoarthritis, sleep apnea, gout and gallbladder disease.

Assessing Your Weight

The most widely accepted methods used to assess your weight and body fat are body mass index (BMI), waist-to-hip ratio (WHR) and body fat measurements.

Body Mass Index (BMI)

This method is used by researchers, nutritionists and doctors to assess whether your weight is putting your health at risk. The measurement is based on a mathematical formula that includes both height and weight.

Calculate Your Body Mass Index (BMI)

Divide your weight in pounds by 2.2 = weight in kilograms (kg)	_____
Multiply your height in inches by 2.54 = height in centimeters (cm)	_____
Divide your height (cm) by 100 = height in meters	_____
Square your height in meters	_____
Your BMI = weight (in kg) ÷ height (in meters squared)	_____

Long-term studies show that the overall risk of developing chronic disease is generally related to your BMI as follows:

BMI under 20	at risk for health problems related to malnutrition
BMI 20–25	risk is very low; healthy range
BMI 25–29.9	overweight; your risk is starting to increase; caution zone
BMI 30 or greater	obese; high risk

Keep in mind that there are other factors besides weight that can increase the risk of disease. Poor diet, alcohol, a lack of exercise, smoking and high blood pressure are other important risk factors.

Waist-to-Hip Ratio (WHR)

This measures where fat is accumulated on the body. An accumulation of fat around the abdomen is closely related to increased health risks. Calculate your WHR as follows:

1. Using a tape measure, find the circumference of your waist at its narrowest point when your stomach is relaxed.

   Waist = _____ inches

2. Measure the circumference of your hips at their widest point.

   Hips = _____ inches

3. Divide your waist measurement by your hip measurement.

   Waist ÷ hip = _____

A healthy WHR is 0.8 or less. That means you're not carrying excess weight around your abdomen.

Body Fat Measurements

Some health clubs and commercial weight-loss programs estimate body fat using calipers on folds of skin or by sending harmless electrical impulses through the body. These techniques may provide inaccurate results if performed by untrained individuals.

Who's at Risk?

- people with a family history of obesity

- people of certain ancestry, including First Nation Canadians, Hispanics and African-Americans

- people who eat a high-fat, high-sugar diet

- people who do not get regular exercise at their job or in their leisure time

Symptoms

When excess fat is accumulated below the diaphragm and in the chest wall, it may put pressure on the lungs, causing shortness of breath and other breathing difficulties. Difficulty breathing may interfere with sleep, leading to daytime sleepiness and sleep apnea. Overweight and obesity can also worsen a hiatus hernia and cause heartburn and gastrointestinal distress. Excess weight can cause low back pain and other orthopedic problems, particularly in the hips, knees and ankles.

Skin disorders are common in obesity because of increased perspiration and skin folding, which encourage bacterial and fungal growth. Swelling in the feet and ankles is a frequent problem for overweight people. Psychological problems are also common in obesity, including poor self-image, poor motivation and depression.

Conventional Treatment

Safe and *gradual* weight loss is the only effective solution for obesity. Even a modest loss of 10 to 20 pounds can lower blood pressure and cholesterol and reduce the risk of developing serious health problems. The ideal treatment for obesity is a multifaceted program that includes a calorie-reduced diet, physical activity and behavior therapy. Learning how to make healthy food choices and manage emotions that influence food choices are important components of a successful weight-loss program.

In some cases, prescription drugs may be used to augment diet and exercise therapy.

There are two types of medications for obesity. Medications that affect levels of brain chemicals include Tenuate Dospan® (diethylpropion), Sonorex® and Mazanor® (mazindol), Meridia® (sibutramine) and Prozac®. The second type, Xenical® (orlistat), is a medication that affects the absorption of food. Once consumed, it attaches to enzymes in the gut that break down fat and reduces the amount of fat that can be absorbed. While some medications may improve blood pressure and blood fat levels and decrease insulin resistance (the body's inability to use blood sugar) over the short term, long-term studies are needed to determine if weight loss from weight-loss medications can improve health. All medications have side effects and risks, which should be discussed with your doctor.

A more drastic treatment is a program that uses a *very low calorie diet* (VLCD)—commercially prepared formulas of 800 calories or less that replace all food intake. VLCDs are used for moderately obese people who want to lose weight quickly. They are safe when medically supervised. However, these programs are expensive and people tend to regain weight after going off the diet.

Surgery is reserved only for severely obese individuals (those with a BMI greater than 40) with existing physical or medical complications of obesity. Weight-loss surgery is performed in hospital or a medical clinic (be sure it has a demonstrated record of efficacy and safety). Surgeries such as gastric banding and gastric stapling create a small pouch at the top of the stomach where the food enters from the esophagus. This restricts the amount of food that can be eaten at a meal. A gastric bypass operation involves reducing the size of the stomach and making a bypass of food from the stomach farther down in the bowel.

Weight-loss surgeries are not without risk. Ten to 20 percent of patients require follow-up operations to correct complications. More than one-third of obese patients who have gastric surgery develop gallstones, and nearly 30 percent of patients who have weight-loss surgery develop nutritional deficiencies such as anemia, osteoporosis and metabolic bone disease. These deficiencies can be avoided if vitamin and mineral intakes are maintained.

Choosing a Weight-Loss Program

Ideally, weight loss should occur at a fairly slow and steady pace as rapid weight loss can cause muscle loss and nutrient deficiencies. Weight that is lost rapidly is also difficult to keep off. Losing weight successfully and permanently requires making permanent changes to your eating and exercise habits.

When researching programs in your community, ask these questions:

- Is there a nutrition education component? Will you learn healthy-eating skills?

- Does the program exclude any one food group?

- Does the program rely on a food or meal supplement?

- Does the program rely on specially purchased foods?

- Does the program promote and emphasize exercise?

- Does the program incorporate behavioral therapy and/or stress management techniques?

- Does the program address social support systems?

- Does the program offer one-on-one and/or group sessions?

- Does the program emphasize weight maintenance?

- What are the qualifications of the counselors?

The most difficult part of losing weight is keeping it off by maintaining long-term changes to diet and activity patterns. There is concern among experts that repeated loss and regain of body weight, known as yo-yo dieting or weight cycling, is harmful to your health. The dietary strategies listed below will help you get started on a safe weight-loss plan.

Managing Weight Loss

Dietary Strategies

- *Set a realistic goal.* You don't have to rely on the bathroom scale when setting a goal. You may prefer to choose a size of clothing, improvements in physical fitness or improvements in blood cholesterol or blood pressure readings. If you do decide to use the scale as your measure of success, choose a realistic 5-pound weight range that you want to stay within.

- *Begin with the right mindset.* Think long-term lifestyle change instead of short-term quick fix. Having the right mindset means being comfortable with slow and steady weight loss. No weight-loss program should cause you to lose much more than 2 to 3 pounds per week.

- *Get social support.* If you need help from a spouse, family member, coworker or friend, ask for it. It often helps to have a workout partner, especially when you're beginning an exercise program. If your husband pulls out potato chips every night after dinner, ask him to be mindful of your attempt to change your eating habits. If you want positive reinforcement from someone, let that person know.

- *Consider an exercise program* if you're not already active. Calories are burned during exercise, and by building up muscle, exercise helps your body burn more calories at rest. To help you lose body fat, aim to get four cardiovascular workouts each week (brisk walking,

jogging, stair climbing, swimming, cross-country skiing, aerobics classes). Gradually build up to a minimum of 30 minutes each session. When you're ready, add in weight training two or three times a week. Studies have found that adding a weight workout to a weight-loss program speeds up weight loss.

- *Visit a consulting dietitian* (see **www.dietitians.ca**). A registered dietitian can develop a nutritious diet designed to help you lose weight based on your lifestyle. Weekly visits offer support, encouragement and nutrition education.

- *Eat at regular intervals throughout the day.* Eating a meal or snack every four to five hours will help boost your metabolism, improve your energy level and help maintain a consistent blood-sugar level. Eating regularly prevents hunger and helps eliminate mindless snacking and overeating at the next meal.

- *Don't eat dinner late.* Ideally, sit down to dinner no later than 8 p.m. Remember that as the evening approaches, the body's metabolism naturally slows down. Dinnertime is actually when your body needs the smallest meal (despite this being when most of us eat the bulk of our day's calories). If you get home late, tell yourself that you've missed dinner. Just because you walk in the door doesn't mean you have to have dinner. Have a light snack instead—yogurt, a piece of fruit or a bowl of soup.

- *If your meals are more than five hours apart, plan for a snack.* Between-meal snacks are important to help keep your energy levels up and prevent snacking on sweets (or some other unhealthy food). Depending on the meal, your blood sugar will drop three to four hours later. Since your blood sugar is the only source of fuel for your brain, a post-meal dip can make you feel sluggish and tired. And often this is when people go in search of a "pick-me-up." So plan for this energy boost.

But here's my rule: *No snacking on starchy foods* like bagels, pretzels, low-fat cookies, low-fat crackers or fat-free muffins. Because these foods are quickly converted to blood glucose (remember, they're high glycemic index foods), they're more likely to lead to further hunger and sweet cravings. Better snacks include yogurt, milk, homemade smoothies and whole fruit. Choosing these snacks will also help you get more fiber and calcium into your diet.

- *Moderate your portions of starchy foods.* When you have pasta, no bread. If you have a meal with rice or potato, no bread. Bread adds extra calories to your day. Even though bread on its own is low in fat, it still has calories and these add up. For example, one large bagel is equivalent to four or five slices of bread! If you find you have a tendency to overeat foods like pasta, rice or potatoes, consider skipping the starch at dinner. Instead, enjoy grilled fish, chicken or lean meat with plenty of vegetables.

- *Choose low glycemic index carbohydrate foods more often.* These foods tend to be higher in soluble fiber. As a result, they take longer to digest and keep you feeling full longer. A list of low glycemic index foods can be found on page 7, Chapter 1.

- *Treat yourself once a week.* Enjoy your favorite treat once a week, whether it's ice cream, a rich pastry, chicken wings or french fries. Make this weekly treat part of your plan and don't feel guilty for having it. Keep in mind that any changes you make to lose weight have to be sustainable. It's not realistic to give up sweets forever.

- *Get rid of excess sugar.* A little jam on toast or a teaspoon of sugar in coffee will not affect your weight. But drinks like regular (rather than diet) soft drinks, fruit drinks and fruit juice add extra calories to your diet.

- *Limit alcohol intake to no more than seven to nine drinks per week* (see Chapter 5). Alcohol calories in beer, wine or liquor add up. Alcohol also tends to lower one's willpower, making it more difficult to stick to a healthy meal plan.

- *Deal with momentary lapses.* The key to long-term weight maintenance is nipping small weight gains in the bud. If you want to stay trim, you've got to catch that 5-pound gain before it becomes 10 pounds. Monitor your weight on a regular weekly basis. Have a plan of action to take off any extra pounds you've gained. You might keep a food diary for a few weeks to help you identify how you gained the weight, and add an extra workout to your week for a month or give up sweets until the pounds are off.

Vitamins and Minerals

Multivitamin and Mineral Supplements

A low-calorie diet (less than 1500 calories per day) may be lacking folate, vitamin D, calcium, iron and zinc. A multivitamin and mineral supplement offers you a little extra nutritional insurance. It provides the recommended daily amounts for vitamins and minerals, with the exception of calcium, iron and vitamin E. Take one daily with a meal. See page 78, Chapter 5, for tips on choosing a multivitamin formula.

Calcium

This important mineral is often missing in a diet designed for weight loss. Unfortunately, it is often lacking in higher-calorie diets, too. If you are consuming less than three daily servings of milk, yogurt and/or calcium-fortified beverages, take a 300 milligram supplement of calcium citrate with vitamin D added for each serving you are lacking. A list of calcium-rich foods and supplement sources can be found on page 43, Chapter 4.

Iron

A daily multivitamin and mineral supplement will help you meet your iron needs. But it is also important to eat iron-rich foods such as lean red meat, seafood, poultry, eggs, legumes, whole grains, enriched breakfast cereals, dried apricots, raisins and blackstrap molasses. To enhance your body's absorption of iron from plant foods, include a source of vitamin C with your meals; 1/2 cup (125 ml) of citrus juice, red pepper, broccoli, strawberries or tomato juice are a few good choices. Avoid drinking tea with iron-rich meals as tannin compounds in the beverage interfere with iron absorption. Also don't combine an iron-rich meal with large quantities of milk or yogurt, since calcium interferes with iron absorption.

Chromium

This essential mineral is involved in the regulation of carbohydrate and fat metabolism. Chromium has been reported to increase muscle mass and decrease body fat, which could lead to weight loss. While the majority of studies have not found chromium to be effective in weight loss, a few studies do support its use. In one study researchers found that chromium supplements taken for three months resulted in a significantly greater loss of body fat among overweight adults.[3] Another study found that when chromium was taken in combination with regular exercise, weight loss occurred.[4]

Good food sources of chromium include apples with the skin, green peas, chicken breast, refried beans, mushrooms, oysters, wheat germ and Brewer's yeast. Processed and refined starchy foods such as white bread, rice and pasta, sugar and sweets contain very little chromium.

Studies have evaluated chromium picinolate, a type of chromium thought to be absorbed better than other forms of the mineral. The dosage used in weight-loss studies, 200 to 400 micrograms per day, is much higher than the recommended dietary intake. Doses of 600 micrograms can cause cognitive impairment, anemia and kidney damage. People with diabetes should consult their doctor before starting on chromium as it may lower blood-sugar levels.

Herbal Remedies

Herbal remedies for weight loss are popular items in pharmacies and supplement stores. Most formulas contain a few different herbs combined with nutrients. Whether these products will help you lose weight permanently remains to be seen. No clinical studies have evaluated their long-term success. These products should be used to *assist* you in your weight-loss effort of healthy eating and exercise. Before purchasing a herbal remedy it's important to know what's safe and what's not, as well as what might be effective and what is not.

Ephedra *(Ma huang)*

This plant contains an active ingredient called ephedrine, which stimulates the central nervous system, speeds the heart rate and increases blood pressure. When combined with other stimulant ingredients such as caffeine, it has been shown to increase metabolism.

Taking ephedra in high doses with other stimulants causes serious side effects. In the United States, there have been over 800 reported adverse reactions and 22 deaths due to ephedra abuse. In Canada, the herb is allowed for sale only in products that contain a combination of herbs. The recommended dose cannot exceed 11 milligrams. Although this dose is considered safe, it can cause insomnia and anxiety in some people. Ephedra use can also lead to dependency. Because of its negative side effects, some companies have reformulated their weight-loss products by removing ephedra and replacing it with a safer herbal extract called Advantra Z™.

Bitter Orange (*Citrus aurantium*)

Advantra Z™ is a patented extract of bitter orange that has been shown to work as effectively as ephedra but without the negative effects on the heart or nervous system. The herb stimulates certain receptors in the body, which elicit the breakdown of fat and increase the body's metabolic rate.

A 1999 study evaluated the combined effect of Citrus aurantium, caffeine and St. John's wort on weight loss in 20 overweight adults.[5] All subjects exercised three times a week and followed an 1800-calorie diet. At the end of the six-week period, those who took the herbal supplement had lost significantly more weight and body fat than those who took the placebo. The herb did not affect heart rate and blood pressure.

You'll find the standardized extract of Citrus aurantium in a few products, including Quest® Vitamin's TrimFit™, Twin Lab's Diet Fuel™ and Interactive Nutrition's Metabolean®.

Hydroxycitric Acid (HCA) (*Garcinia cambogia*)

In laboratory studies, this herbal extract has inhibited the action of a cellular enzyme and increased the breakdown of fat. Three published studies have evaluated the effect of HCA in humans, with disappointing results.[6-8] All studies found that people who took HCA burned body fat no differently from people taking the placebo. The larger of the three studies measured weight and fat loss in 135 overweight men and women who took either 1500 milligrams of HCA or a placebo. Both groups exercised and followed a high-fiber, low-calorie diet. After 12 weeks, there was no significant difference between the two groups. At this time there is no evidence that weight-loss products containing hydroxycitric acid (e.g., Citrimax™) are effective.

Other Natural Health Products

Conjugated Linoleic Acid (CLA)

This naturally occurring fatty acid is found in dairy products and meat. Because the body does not manufacture CLA itself, the only way to get it is through foods or supplements. CLA is thought to facilitate weight loss by inhibiting the action of a lipoprotein lipase, an enzyme that breaks down dietary fat so that it can be absorbed by the body. CLA is also thought to increase the activity of the enzyme responsible for breaking down body-fat stores.

Research presented at the Research Conference of the American Chemical Society in August 2000 found that CLA supplements helped people lose weight and keep the extra pounds off. In one study, Norwegian researchers studied 60 overweight individuals. Half were given CLA and the others took a placebo pill.[9] After three months, the CLA users lost more weight than those in the placebo group.

Preliminary evidence suggests that CLA may help prevent weight gain as fat. Researchers from the University of Wisconsin followed 80 overweight people for six months.[10] Subjects received either daily CLA supplements or a placebo pill. All dieted and exercised and most lost weight. After the study was over, the people who were not taking the CLA regained weight in the typical pattern—75 percent of their weight gain was fat. The people in the CLA group put weight back on very differently—half as muscle and only half as fat.

The recommended dose is 1 gram (1000 milligrams) taken three times daily with a meal. Buy a supplement made with Tonalin™ CLA or Clarinol™, brands of CLA that are manufactured to high-quality standards and have been used in clinical research.

5-HTP (5-Hydroxytryptophan)

This supplement is made from the seeds of an African plant. The body uses 5-HTP to synthesize serotonin, a brain chemical that may be involved in satiety and weight control. Two small studies found that supplemental 5-HTP promoted reduced food intake and weight loss in obese adults.[11,12]

The recommended dose is 100 to 300 milligrams three times daily. 5-HTP may cause mild stomach upset and allergic reactions. More serious, though, is a report issued by the US Food and Drug Administration (FDA) in 1998 concerning product safety. Some batches of 5-HTP were found to contain a chemical called peak X, known to cause a potentially fatal blood disorder. At this time, there are no other warnings from the FDA about using 5-HTP. Ask your retailer how he or she ensures product quality and safety.

Do not take 5-HTP if you use SSRI drugs that raise serotonin levels (e.g., Prozac®, Effexor®, Paxil®, Zoloft®, Serzone®) or other antidepressants. People with Parkinson's disease who take a medication called carbidopa should not use 5-HTP as it may cause skin changes.

Nutrition Strategy Checklist for Obesity

☐ Low-calorie diet
☐ Multivitamin/mineral
☐ Calcium
☐ Iron
☐ Chromium
☐ Bitter orange (Avantra Z™)
☐ CLA
☐ 5-HTP

Recommended Resources

www.obesite.chaire.ulaval.ca
Donald B. Brown Research Chair on Obesity
Ferdinand-Vandry Building, Room 3101J
Medicine Faculty, Université Laval
Ste-Foy, PQ, Canada G1K 7P4
Tel: 418-656-2131, ext. 8571
Fax: 418-656-7898

www.ific.org
International Food Information Council
1100 Connecticut Avenue NW, Suite 430
Washington, DC, USA 20036
Tel: 202-296-6540
Fax: 202-296-6547
E-mail: foodinfo@ific.org

www.nhbli.nih.gov
National Digestive Diseases Information Clearinghouse
2 Information Way
Bethesda, MD, USA 20892-3570
Tel: 301-654-3810

www.nlhlbi.nih.gov
National Institutes of Health
National Heart, Lung, and Blood Institute
1 AMS Circle
Bethesda, MD, USA 20892-3675
Tel: 301-495-4484 or 1-877-22-NIAMS (1-877-226-4267)
Fax: 301-718-6366

www.nin.ca
National Institute of Nutrition
265 Carling Avenue, Suite 302
Ottawa, ON, Canada K1S 2E1
Tel: 613-235-3355
Fax: 613-235-7032

Osteoarthritis

Osteoarthritis has plagued humans since the earliest days of history. Today, osteoarthritis is the most common form of arthritis and a leading cause of occupational disability. Affecting one in every ten Canadians, osteoarthritis is most prevalent in older people.[1] While not everyone with osteoarthritis has symptoms, those who do find themselves struggling with a pattern of relentless pain and stiffness that can completely destroy their quality of life.

What Causes Osteoarthritis?

Also known as degenerative joint disease, osteoarthritis is thought to be the result of wear and tear of the joints. Inside each joint is a tough, slippery tissue, called cartilage, which covers the ends of bones. Healthy cartilage allows the bones to glide smoothly over one another when we move. It also acts as a shock absorber to protect the joints from the stresses and strains of daily activities. Over time, repeated use and unusual stresses cause the cartilage to crack and wear away. Small bits of cartilage break off, finding their way into the spaces in the joints, where they irritate the muscle tissue and interfere with joint movement. Once the protective layering of cartilage disintegrates, the bones rub painfully against each other, further restricting movement. The bones may even thicken and grow spurs along the edges of the joint.

As the damage grows more extensive, osteoarthritis causes swelling, stiffness and pain. Eventually, the joint may become enlarged and may even freeze in a bent position. The pain associated with osteoarthritis does not come from the destruction of the cartilage, since cartilage has no nerves and can't sense pain. It is the nerve cells of the muscles, tendons, ligaments and bones that signal pain as they are forced to work in unaccustomed ways.

Osteoarthritis usually targets weight-bearing joints, such as the hips, knees, feet and spine. Although the finger joints and joints at the base of the thumb are not weight bearing, they are also common sites for arthritis.

Scientists think that genetics may play a role in osteoarthritis. One theory is that this type of arthritis might be caused by abnormalities in the cells that manufacture cartilage. Another theory suggests that the disease is actually a disorder of the bone rather than of the cartilage. Failure of the bone to respond to impact may lead to damage of the overlying cartilage.

Osteoarthritis may also develop from known causes such as infection, deformity, injury or diseases such as diabetes and high blood pressure. People working in certain occupational groups, such as movers and workers in manufacturing plants, may be more susceptible to osteoarthritis; for instance, if their job involves repetitive, heavy physical work. High-intensity, high-impact sports may have a similar damaging effect on the joints. Being overweight also contributes to osteoarthritis. The excess weight puts additional stress on the knees and hips and may also be associated with metabolic abnormalities that may affect the cartilage.

Symptoms

Damage from osteoarthritis progresses slowly and affects only one or two joints in the early stages of the disease. Once symptoms begin, the disease will continue to progress, gradually limiting the motion of the joint and leading to severe disability in many cases. Symptoms of osteoarthritis may include

- pain in the joint that may be made worse by exercise

- stiffness in the joint after sleep or periods of inactivity

- swelling in the joint, particularly after use

- reduced range of motion in the joint
- crackle or grind in the joint when moved
- pain when the joint is touched
- bony lumps in the joints of the fingers or the base of the thumb

Who's at Risk?

Osteoarthritis is more likely to develop in people over age 45. Women have a higher tendency to develop osteoarthritis in older age groups and to develop more severe symptoms than men. Also at greater risk are people who

- have a family history of joint disease
- are obese
- work in occupations that involve repeated, heavy physical work
- engage in high-intensity, high-impact sports
- have rheumatoid arthritis and gout
- have medical conditions, such as diabetes and high blood pressure

Conventional Treatment

Treatment is intended to control pain and improve joint care. Regular exercise will increase flexibility, decrease pain, improve your overall health and help you maintain a healthy weight. Be sure to schedule rest in order to avoid overexercising joints and to relieve some of the pressure on them. Other treatments to control pain include

- heat—applying moist heat relaxes aching muscles and reduces pain
- cold—applying cold helps reduce swelling and lessen pain
- water therapy—therapy in a heated pool or whirlpool might ease symptoms

- medications—NSAIDs (nonsteroidal anti-inflammatory drugs), COX-2 inhibitors, acetaminophen, mild narcotic painkillers, corticosteroid injections, topical pain relievers and hyaluronic acid all may be used

Surgery may be necessary to relieve pain and disability by removing pieces of cartilage from the joint, resurfacing or smoothing out bones, repositioning bones or replacing joints with artificial joints.

Physical therapy or massage may help ease stiffness and pain in joints. Acupuncture may also offer some pain relief.

Managing Osteoarthritis

Dietary Strategies
Weight Control
To help protect your joints from further damage, it is very important to control your weight. Studies have found that higher levels of body fat and obesity are significantly related to osteoarthritis pain.[2,3] Some researchers believe that losing body fat is more important than losing body weight when it comes to relieving joint pain.

To determine if you are at a healthy weight, refer to page 439, Obesity and Weight Loss, to calculate your body mass index (BMI). Having a BMI over 25 indicates overweight and a BMI greater than 27 is defined as obese. If you determine that your BMI is greater than 25, use the strategies outlined on page 442, Obesity and Weight Loss, to promote safe, gradual weight loss.

Vitamins and Minerals
Vitamin C
Since free radical damage may be involved in the progression of osteoarthritis, researchers have hypothesized that higher intakes of antioxidant

nutrients might be associated with lower rates of the disease. The best evidence to date supports the use of vitamin C.

One large study conducted among 640 patients with knee osteoarthritis found that those who consumed the most vitamin C in their diet had a threefold reduced risk for the disease progressing compared with people who consumed the least.[4] High intake of vitamin C appeared to protect against cartilage loss. Those with the highest vitamin C intake also had a 70 percent lower risk of developing knee pain.

Vitamin C acts as an antioxidant and also supports collagen synthesis, both of which may be important in slowing the progression of osteoarthritis. The best food sources are citrus fruit, strawberries, kiwi, cantaloupe, broccoli, bell peppers, Brussels sprouts, cabbage, tomatoes and potatoes (refer to page 38, Chapter 4, for the vitamin C content of selected foods). To supplement, take 500 milligrams of Ester C once or twice daily.

Vitamin D
Low intakes and low blood levels of vitamin D may impair the response of bone to osteoarthritis, making progression of the disease more likely. In a study of 556 patients with knee osteoarthritis, the risk of disease progression increased threefold in those who had lower vitamin D intakes and reduced blood levels of the nutrient.[5] Reduced vitamin D levels were associated with cartilage loss. Another study also found that low blood vitamin D was associated with a narrowing of the joint space in elderly women with hip osteoarthritis.[6]

The daily adequate intake is 200 to 600 international units (IU) depending on your age (see page 39, Chapter 4). The best food sources of vitamin D include fluid milk, fortified soy and rice beverages, oily fish, egg yolks, butter and margarine. Most multivitamin and mineral supplements provide 200 to 400 IU of vitamin D.

Herbal Remedies
Capsaicin Cream
Capsaicin, responsible for the heat of chili peppers, has a long history of use as a topical agent for pain disorders. A few studies have found that capsaicin cream is effective in providing osteoarthritis pain relief.[7,8] When applied to the skin, capsaicin depletes substance P, a compound that transmits feelings of pain from the nerves to the spinal cord.

Capsaicin creams are available with or without a prescription. Zostrix®, Capzasin-P® and Capsin® are all available over the counter. Buy a cream with 0.025 to 0.075 percent capsaicin (the greater strength may be more effective). Capsaicin cream will produce a burning sensation, which will diminish after several applications. Use a small amount to begin with. When you no longer feel burning upon application, increase the amount of cream you use. Be careful not to touch your eyes or other sensitive tissues after applying capsaicin cream. Wash your hands after using the product.

Other Natural Health Products
Chondroitin Sulfate
This compound belongs to a family of compounds called glucosaminoglycans that are a normal part of cartilage. Studies show that supplemental chondroitin sulfate can reduce the painful symptoms of hip and knee osteoarthritis and improve walking distance.[9-13] When compared with nonsteroidal anti-inflammatory drugs (NSAIDs), chondroitin sulfate took longer to produce results but, unlike NSAIDs, pain relief lasted three months after treatment was stopped.[14]

There is evidence that chondroitin supplementation may actually slow the progression of osteoarthritis. When researchers looked at the effects of chondroitin in 119 people with osteoarthritis, they found that those using chondroitin experienced much less joint damage over three years compared with the placebo treatment.[15]

Chondroitin may work by providing joints with the building blocks they need to repair cartilage. Some experts believe that chondroitin increases the amount of hyaluronic acid (a lubricating fluid) in the joints. Chondroitin may also inhibit the activity of enzymes that break down cartilage. Chondroitin also possesses anti-inflammatory properties, which may provide pain relief.

The recommended dose is 400 milligrams taken three times daily. One study found that 1200 milligrams taken once daily was equally effective and well tolerated.[16] It may take two to four months of treatment to notice significant improvement in osteoarthritis symptoms. Although chondroitin sulfate and glucosamine sulfate are frequently sold together in combination products, at this time there is no evidence from human studies that the combination works better than either product alone. However, if you are taking a combination product, be sure to take the appropriate doses to achieve a therapeutic effect. Products such as Arthri-Logic™ by Quest® Vitamins supplies 500 milligrams of glucosamine and 400 milligrams of chondroitin. The recommended dosage is one tablet three times daily for a total of 1500 milligrams glucosamine and 1200 milligrams chondroitin.

Occasionally, chondroitin supplements may cause stomach upset and nausea. There is a potential for allergic reaction from chondroitin supplements made from animal sources. See Chapter 8 for information about chondroitin safety.

Glucosamine Sulfate
The body uses glucosamine sulfate to make a family of compounds called mucopolysaccharides, which are a normal part of cartilage. Findings from studies lasting one month to three years have

shown that glucosamine significantly improved pain and mobility in people with osteoarthritis of the knee.[17-23] The supplement appears to be as effective as ibuprofen and piroxicam (Feldene®), two nonsteroidal anti-inflammatory drugs used to manage osteoarthritis. Whereas conventional medications appear to take two weeks to improve symptoms, glucosamine takes four weeks to have an effect. In one study, after eight weeks of treatment, glucosamine was superior to ibuprofen. Research suggests that glucosamine supplements stop and possibly even reverse degenerative diseases of the joints.[24]

The recommended dose is 500 milligrams taken three times daily. One three-year study found that 1500 milligrams taken once daily was effective. Glucosamine supplements may cause nausea, heartburn, diarrhea and/or constipation. See Chapter 8 for information about glucosamine safety.

Glucosamine supplements are made from chitin, a substance found in shrimp, lobsters and crab, or are produced synthetically. There is potential for glucosamine supplements made from shellfish to cause allergic reactions in people with a shellfish allergy. If you have such an allergy, call the manufacturer to determine the source of glucosamine if it is not stated on the label.

SAMe (S-Adenosyl-Methionine)
SAMe is a compound found in virtually all body tissues and fluids. The body makes SAMe from certain amino acids in high-protein foods like fish and meat. In the body, SAMe is used to synthesize hormones, brain neurotransmitters, proteins and cell membranes.

SAMe has analgesic and anti-inflammatory properties, which are thought to be responsible for its beneficial effects in osteoarthritis. Several studies lasting from two weeks to two years have found SAMe to be significantly better than placebo and comparable to nonsteroidal anti-inflammatory drugs (NSAIDs) for decreasing symptoms of osteoarthritis.[25-31] Some evidence even suggests that SAMe might stimulate the growth and repair of cartilage.[32]

Take 200 milligrams three times daily on an empty stomach. Buy an enteric-coated product. SAMe is very well tolerated at the recommended doses, but daily doses greater than 1600 milligrams may cause nausea, gastrointestinal upset and headache. Refer to Chapter 8 for information on SAMe safety.

Nutrition Strategy Checklist for Osteoarthritis

- ☐ Weight control
- ☐ Vitamin C
- ☐ Vitamin D
- ☐ Capsaicin cream
- ☐ Chondroitin OR Glucosamine
- ☐ SAMe

Recommended Resources

www.rheumatology.org
American College of Rheumatology
1800 Century Place, Suite 250
Atlanta, GA, USA 30345
Tel: 404-633-3777
Fax: 404-633-1870

www.arthritis.org
Arthritis Foundation
1330 W Peachtree Street
Atlanta, GA, USA 30309
Tel: 404-872-7100 or 1-800-283-7800

www.arthritis.ca
The Arthritis Society
393 University Avenue, Suite 1700
Toronto, ON, Canada M5G 1E6
Tel: 416-979-7228
Fax: 416-979-8366
E-mail: info@arthritis.ca

www.nih.gov.niams/healthinfo
National Institute of Arthritis and Musculoskeletal and Skin Diseases Information Clearinghouse
National Institutes of Health
1 AMS Circle
Bethesda, MD, USA 20892-3675
Tel: 301-495-4484 or 1-877-22-NIAMS (1-877-226-4267)
Fax: 301-718-6366

Osteoporosis

It is estimated that 1.4 million Canadians have osteoporosis, a disease of fragile, brittle bones that are more likely to break than normal, healthy bones. Osteoporosis can strike at any age, but it is more likely to occur in later years, affecting one in four women and one in eight men over the age of 50.[1]

Osteoporosis is characterized by low bone mass and deterioration of existing bone tissue. Bones become weaker and more susceptible to fractures. The definition of osteoporosis emphasizes fracture risk, not only low bone density. While many bone fractures are not life threatening, the impact that fractures have on health is underappreciated. For instance, hip fractures lead to death in 20 percent of cases. Close to 50 percent of elderly women who fracture their hips lose their ability to live independently.

What Causes Osteoporosis?

Throughout childhood, bones grow in length and density. At some point in adolescence, bones stop growing in length but continue to increase in density, though at a slower rate. Then, some time in your 20s, bones achieve what's called their peak mass. Once this occurs, they stop building density. This happens when you are between 20 and 30 years old. Peak bone mass is determined largely by genetics, but nutrition and other lifestyle factors determine whether or not you will achieve your body's genetically programmed peak bone mass.

After you achieve your peak bone mass, natural bone loss begins. Before menopause, women lose bone at a rate of 1 percent per year, the same rate as men. Within the first five years after menopause, women lose bone two to six times faster than premenopausal women do. Then, ten years after menopause, bone loss returns to 1 percent per year. During this ten-year period, women have the potential to lose bone very quickly.

Despite its "dead" appearance, bone is very active tissue that contains two types of cells. *Osteoclasts* are always breaking down the bone in areas where it is not needed. For example, osteoclasts go to work when your diet lacks calcium. These bone cells release calcium into the blood from the bone for important body functions. *Osteoblasts* are responsible for building the support structure of bones, as well as adding minerals to strengthen bones. Your bones are constantly going through a bone remodeling cycle. Osteoclast cells break down bone and osteoblast cells rebuild it.

Symptoms

Osteoporosis is a silent disease because bone loss occurs without symptoms. You may not know you have the disease until you break a bone. The outward signs of osteoporosis are usually not apparent until the disease is quite advanced. Signs that you may have osteoporosis include

- a broken wrist or rib from a slight blow
- a broken hip
- back pain in the mid to lower spine
- loss of more than one inch of height
- a stooped or hunched-over appearance
- a hump forming in the upper back

Who's at Risk?

The strength of your bones is determined by 1) their bone mineral density, 2) their rate of self-healing and 3) the integrity of their support structures. Any factor that jeopardizes these three factors can increase the odds of getting osteoporosis. Risk factors include

- older age
- low bone density
- being female
- slender or petite body structure
- deficiency of estrogen (early or surgical menopause)
- cigarette smoking
- low calcium and vitamin D
- excessive alcohol and caffeine
- sedentary lifestyle
- certain medications (e.g., corticosteroids)
- prolonged immobilization
- family history of maternal hip fracture
- previous bone fracture of any type after the age of 50
- certain health conditions (e.g., kidney failure, hyperthyroid, malabsorption states)

Conventional Treatment

Estrogen Therapy

Many studies have shown that hormone replacement therapy (HRT) protects the bones of women. Both estrogen pills and estrogen patches have been found to decrease bone loss, reduce fractures and prevent the loss of height. Estrogen replacement prevents bone loss at any point a woman starts to take it. However, the longer a woman waits after menopause, the greater the chance she will lose some bone permanently. And once a woman stops taking estrogen, bone loss occurs: estrogen's protective effect lasts only as long as the estrogen is taken.

While studies do find that estrogen delays bone loss, recent clinical trials have not found this medication to be effective at preventing bone fractures. The Heart and Estrogen-Progestin Replacement Study (HERS) followed over 2700 postmenopausal women who did not have osteoporosis and found no significant difference in hip or spine fracture rates among women taking HRT and those not taking the drugs.[2] Experts believe that HRT may reduce bone fractures only in women who have defined osteoporosis when they start on the medication.

Bisphosphonates

This newer class of nonhormonal drugs offers both men and women with low bone density or osteoporosis an alternative to HRT. Biphosphonate drugs prevent bone breakdown by binding to the bone surface and inhibiting the activity of the osteoclasts, the cells that strip down old bone. Types of bisphosphonates include Didrocal® (etidronate and calcium carbonate) and Fosamax® (aldendronate).

Selective Estrogen Receptor Modulators (SERMs)

Often called "designer estrogen" drugs, these medications offer all the beneficial effects of estrogen (bone protection, cholesterol lowering) without any of its negative effects (increased breast cancer risk, endometrial bleeding). SERMs such as Evista® (raloxifene) offer the favorable effects of estrogen on bone and blood cholesterol levels and act as an antiestrogen in the breast and the uterus.

Preventing and Managing Osteoporosis

Dietary Strategies

Soy Foods

Soybeans contain naturally occurring compounds called isoflavones, a type of plant estrogen. Genistein and daidzein are the most active isoflavones in soy and have been the focus of much research. Isoflavones have a chemical structure similar to estrogen and so are able to bind to estrogen receptors in the body. It is the action of isoflavones on estrogen receptors in the bone that scientists believe may be responsible for soy's potential bone-preserving effect.

The interest in soybeans and osteoporosis began when researchers observed that populations that consume soy foods on a regular basis report much lower rates of hip fracture. Since then, soy foods and their naturally occurring phytoestrogens have been the focus of many studies. A three-month study conducted at Iowa State University found that 40 grams of phytoestrogen-rich soy protein providing 90 milligrams of isoflavones prevented bone loss in postmenopausal women.[3] Women in this study who were given whey protein powder (a protein made from milk) instead showed significant bone loss in the lower spine. Another study from the University of Cincinnati's College of Medicine found that 60 to 70 milligrams of soy isoflavones consumed as So Good® soy beverage and soy nuts significantly decreased bone turnover in postmenopausal women after 12 weeks.[4]

Based on the research so far, a minimum intake of 50 milligrams of isoflavones is needed to benefit bones. Ideally, consume soy foods twice daily. Soy foods vary in terms of the amount of isoflavones they contain. Even the same type of food made by different manufacturers can differ in isoflavone content.

Soy Food	Serving Size	Isoflavone Content (milligrams)
Roasted soy nuts	1/4 cup (60 ml)	40–50 mg
Green soybeans, uncooked	1/2 cup (125 ml)	70 mg
Tempeh, uncooked	3 oz (90 g)	38 mg
Soy flour	1/4 cup (60 ml)	37 mg
Tofu, firm	1/2 cup (125 ml)	27 mg
Texturized vegetable protein, dry	1/2 cup (125 ml)	30–120 mg
Soy milk	1 cup (250 ml)	24 mg
Soy protein powder, isolate	1 oz (30 g)	28 mg
Soy sauce		none
Soya oil		none
Yves Veggie Cuisine Good Dog	1 (52 g)	12–19 mg
Yves Veggie Cuisine Veggie Dog	1 (46 g)	12–19 mg
Yves Veggie Cuisine Deli Slices	3 slices (62 g)	12–19 mg

USDA: Iowa State University Database on the Isoflavone Content of Foods, 1999.

Protein Foods

High levels of dietary protein cause calcium to be excreted by the kidneys. An average increase in dietary protein of 7 grams (1 ounce of meat) causes 7 grams of calcium to be lost in the urine. The effect of eating large quantities of protein is rapid, and it appears that the body doesn't correct for this by absorbing more calcium from food. The protein effect may be very important for people who consume very little calcium or for those who, because of intestinal problems, absorb very little calcium.

While eating very large amounts of protein may not be good for your bones, eating too little isn't healthy either. Protein is an important structural component of bone, and research suggests that a lack of protein increases the risk of hip frac-ture. The Iowa Women's Health Study found that dietary protein protected postmenopausal women from hip fracture.[5] Women who ate the most protein had a 69 percent reduced risk of hip fracture compared with women who ate the least. Studies have also found that when protein supplements are given to patients with hip fracture, the rate of complications and death are reduced immediately after surgery and for six months afterward.[6]

To determine your protein requirements, see Chapter 2. There you will also find a list of foods and their protein content.

Caffeine

Drinking coffee, tea or colas increases the amount of calcium your kidneys excrete in the urine for up to three hours after consuming caffeine. For every 6-ounce cup of coffee you drink, approximately 48 milligrams of calcium is leached from your bones. The effects of caffeine are likely most detrimental for women who are not meeting their daily calcium requirements. One study found that 400 milligrams of caffeine caused calcium loss in women whose daily diet had less than 600 milligrams of calcium.[7] Another study, from Tufts University in Boston, found that women who consumed less than 800 milligrams of calcium and 450 milligrams of caffeine (about three small cups of coffee) had significantly lower bone densities than women who consumed the same amount of caffeine but more than 800 milligrams of calcium.[8]

Here's what you need to know:

- If you drink coffee, make sure you're meeting your calcium requirements of 1000 to 1200 milligrams a day.

- Add 3 tablespoons of milk (58 mg calcium) or calcium-fortified soy beverage to each cup of coffee you drink.

- Do not consume more than 450 milligrams of caffeine a day (see page 82, Chapter 5). If you have osteoporosis, aim for no more than 200 milligrams.

- Replace regular coffee with water, tea, herbal tea, vegetable juice, lattes (coffee with milk) and soy beverage. All have substantially less caffeine than coffee.

Sodium

Like caffeine, sodium also causes the kidneys to excrete calcium. This means that you need to replace the calcium you are losing. However, a study of postmenopausal women determined that a maximum intake of 2000 milligrams of sodium (the amount in 3/4 teaspoon of salt) and 1000 milligrams of calcium *minimized* bone loss.[9] Unfortunately, most of us get more than double that amount of sodium in our daily diets.

To reduce sodium intake, avoid the saltshaker at the table, minimize your use of salt in cooking and buy commercial food products that are low in added salt. Most of the salt we eat every day comes from processed and prepared foods. You'll find the sodium content of foods listed on page 80, Chapter 5.

Vitamins and Minerals

Calcium

The fact that calcium is the most abundant mineral in the body and that 99 percent of it is housed within the bones and teeth underlines the importance of dietary calcium to bone health. During the bone-building process, the osteoblast cells secrete bone mineral, consisting of calcium and phosphorus, which strengthens the bone. By providing structural integrity to bones, dietary calcium plays a critical role in preventing osteoporosis.

The remaining 1 percent of the body's calcium circulates in the bloodstream and is vital to the functioning of the heart, nervous system and muscles. The body keeps this circulating pool of calcium at a constant level. If your diet lacks cal-

cium and your blood calcium level drops, your body releases parathyroid hormone (PTH), which returns calcium to your blood by taking it from the bones. When you shortchange your diet of calcium, you shortchange your bones too.

Calcium Supplements

Research supports using calcium supplements to lower the risk of osteoporosis. Researchers at the University of Texas Southwestern Medical Center in Dallas found that a 400 milligram calcium citrate supplement taken twice daily increased bone density in healthy postmenopausal women.[10] In contrast, women in the placebo group experienced a 2.38 percent bone reduction in the lower spine.

Scientists at the University of Massachusetts studied 98 premenopausal women (average age 39 years) and found that those who received 500 milligrams of calcium carbonate had increased bone density by 0.3 percent per year.[11] The women in the placebo group lost bone at a rate of 0.4 percent per year in the hip and 0.7 percent in the neck. A number of studies have also shown that older women and men who take calcium and vitamin D supplements have a lower incidence of nonvertebral fractures.

The recommended dietary allowance (RDA) for calcium is 1000 to 1300 milligrams, depending on your age. Older adults at risk for osteoporosis need 1500 milligrams. The best food sources include milk, yogurt, cheese, fortified soy and rice beverages, fortified orange juice, tofu, salmon (with bones), kale, bok choy, broccoli and Swiss chard. If you take calcium supplements, buy calcium citrate with vitamin D and magnesium added. See page 43, Chapter 4, for more information on calcium requirements, calcium-rich foods and calcium supplements.

Vitamin D

Experts cite a silent epidemic of vitamin D deficiency, in addition to getting too little calcium, as a contributing factor to osteoporosis. Vitamin D makes calcium and phosphorus available in the blood that bathes the bones, so that it can be deposited as bones harden or mineralize. Vitamin D raises blood levels of calcium in three ways: it stimulates your intestine to absorb more dietary calcium, it tells your kidneys to retain calcium and it withdraws calcium from your bones if your diet is lacking this mineral. A vitamin D deficiency will speed up bone loss and increase the risk of fracture at a younger age.

Vitamin D is different from any other nutrient because the body can synthesize it from sunlight. When ultraviolet light hits the skin, a pre–vitamin D is formed. This compound eventually makes its way to the kidneys, where it's transformed into active vitamin D. The long winter months in Canada result in very little vitamin D being synthesized by the skin. Researchers from Tufts University in Boston have demonstrated that blood levels of vitamin D are at their lowest point between February and March and peak in June and July.[12] (Although this is an American study, the findings hold true for Canadians.) But even in the summer, your body might not be making enough vitamin D, since sun protection factor (SPF) in sunscreen blocks the production of the vitamin. To help you meet your vitamin D requirements, expose your hands, face and arms to sunlight for 10 to 15 minutes, two or three times a week, without sunscreen.

The daily adequate intake for vitamin D is 200 to 600 international units (IU). Postmenopausal women should consume 400 to 800 IU of vitamin D each day to minimize bone loss. The best food sources include fluid milk, fortified soy and rice beverages, oily fish, egg yolks, butter and margarine.

Vitamin D Supplements
Most multivitamin and mineral supplements provide 200 to 400 IU of vitamin D. If you take calcium supplements, buy a product with vitamin D added.

Fish liver oil can be used to supplement your diet with vitamin D; 1 teaspoon (5 ml) of cod liver oil provides 1100 IU. If you take fish oil capsules, follow the manufacturer's dosage recommendations. When taken in large doses over a period, fish oil supplements have the potential to cause vitamin D (and vitamin A) toxicity.

Vitamin D supplements are also available. Do not exceed 2000 IU of vitamin D per day.

Other Nutrients
While calcium and vitamin D are critical to healthy bones, other nutrients are also important players in bone building. Together with calcium and vitamin D, they comprise the nutrient team that orchestrates the continual process of bone building and bone breakdown.

Vitamin A
This vitamin supports bone growth and development. It is used by degradative enzymes in osteoclast cells that break down old bone in order to build new bone. That bone growth relies on vitamin A is witnessed by the fact that children who are deficient in vitamin A fail to grow properly.

Vitamin A is found preformed in animal foods such as fortified milk, cheese, butter, eggs and liver. Do not take single vitamin A supplements. Beta-carotene-rich fruits and vegetables also contribute to our daily vitamin A requirements. The beta-carotene in these plant foods is converted to vitamin A in the body. The best sources of beta-carotene include carrots, winter squash, sweet potatoes, spinach, broccoli, rapini, romaine lettuce, apricots, peaches, mango, papaya and cantaloupe.

Vitamin C
A number of studies involving postmenopausal women have linked higher intakes of vitamin C with higher bone density. One study revealed that women aged 55 to 64 years who had taken vitamin C supplements for at least ten years had significantly higher bone mass compared with

women who did not supplement their diet.[13] Vitamin C is important for the formation of collagen, a tissue that lends support to bones. This vitamin may also protect bones by acting as an antioxidant and modifying the negative effect of cigarette smoking on bones. Cigarette smoking inactivates circulating estrogen so that it cannot exert its protective effect on bone.

The RDA for vitamin C is 75 and 90 milligrams for women and men respectively (smokers need an additional 35 milligrams). Best food sources include citrus fruit, citrus juices, cantaloupe, kiwi, mango, strawberries, broccoli, Brussels sprouts, cauliflower, red pepper and tomato juice. To supplement, take 500 milligrams of Ester C once or twice daily. The daily upper limit is 2000 milligrams.

Vitamin K

This fat-soluble vitamin is used to make a bone protein called osteocalcin. A high level of osteocalcin in the blood indicates that osteoblast cells are busy making new bone. Without enough vitamin K, the bones produce an abnormal protein that cannot bind to the minerals that form the bones.

The famous Nurse's Health Study from Harvard University found that women with the highest intake of vitamin K had a significantly lower rate of hip fracture compared with women who consumed the least.[14] Eating lettuce was also linked with fewer hip fractures. Lettuce accounted for most of the vitamin K in their diet. Those women who ate one or more servings of the leafy green each day (versus one or fewer servings a week) had a 45 percent lower risk of hip fractures.

The best food sources of vitamin K are leafy green vegetables, cabbage, milk and liver.

Boron

While there's no daily recommended intake for boron, research suggests that higher intakes of this trace mineral may slow down loss of calcium,

magnesium and phosphorus from the urine. Scientists aren't exactly sure how boron keeps calcium in balance, but they think that boron is needed for activation of vitamin D.

A daily intake of 1.5 to 3 milligrams of boron is more than adequate to meet your requirements for bone growth and development. The main food sources are fruits and vegetables, but their boron content will depend on how much of the mineral is in the soil in which they grew. If you want to take a supplement, 3 to 9 milligrams per day is a very safe amount. Intakes greater than 500 milligrams a day can cause nausea, vomiting and diarrhea. However, boron supplements are not available in Canada (but are in the United States).

Magnesium

One-half of the body's magnesium stores are in the bone. The mineral helps make parathyroid hormone, an important regulator of bone building. Animal studies show that a lack of dietary magnesium causes increased bone breakdown and decreased bone synthesis.

It's difficult to say to what extent magnesium plays a role in osteoporosis, since very few studies have actually looked at the effect of dietary magnesium and bone loss. Most of the studies that support the use of magnesium supplements found that osteoporosis is more common in people who have other health problems that cause a magnesium deficiency, such as alcoholism and hyperthyroidism.

The recommended daily intake for women is 310 to 420 milligrams (see page 47, Chapter 4). The best food sources are wheat bran, whole-grain breads, cereals and pasta, legumes, nuts, seeds and leafy green vegetables.

If you use calcium supplements, buy one with magnesium added. Buy a calcium supplement with magnesium in a 2:1 ratio (two parts calcium for one part magnesium) to avoid gastrointestinal upset. The daily upper limit for magnesium from a supplement is 350 milligrams.

Phosphorus

This mineral is an important component of the bone mineral complex. Indeed, 85 percent of the body's phosphorus is stored in the bones. It appears that both too little and too much dietary phosphorus can result in bone loss. Scientists believe that a long-standing imbalance of phosphorus and calcium, caused by too much dietary phosphorus and too little dietary calcium, may contribute to bone breakdown.

On the other hand, if your diet lacks phosphorus and your blood levels of the mineral become low, your body will release the mineral from your bones in an effort to keep your blood level constant (in the same way that calcium blood levels remain stable at the expense of your bone). One of the symptoms of a phosphorus deficiency is bone pain. A low blood phosphorus level can result from poor eating habits, excessive use of phosphorus-binding antacids and intestinal malabsorption.

The daily recommended intake for adults is 700 milligrams of phosphorus. Most of the phosphorus in our diet comes from additives in cheese, bakery products, processed meats and soft drinks. Other food sources include wheat bran, milk, fish, eggs, poultry, beef and pork. Most people don't have a problem getting enough phosphorus. Just make sure you meet your daily calcium requirements so that these two minerals are kept in balance.

Manganese, Zinc and Copper

These trace minerals are important helpers (cofactors) for enzymes that are essential to making bone tissue. Postmenopausal women who received a daily supplement of calcium, manganese, copper and zinc did not experience any bone loss of the spine at the end of a two-year study.[15] The placebo group, on the other hand, lost 3.5 percent of their bone mass. Manganese is widely available in foods and deficiencies have

not been seen in humans. Meat and drinking water are your best bets for copper. When it comes to zinc, wheat bran, wheat germ, oysters, seafood, lean red meat and milk are good sources.

Other Natural Health Products

Ipriflavone

This supplement is made from daidzein, one of the main phytoestrogens found in soybeans. Numerous clinical trials suggest that ipriflavone is an effective alternative to estrogen therapy in the prevention and treatment of osteoporosis.[16-19] Studies have shown that when ipriflavone is taken alone or with calcium, it is more effective at maintaining bone density than calcium alone. Researchers have also evaluated the effects of combining ipriflavone with low doses of estrogen and found positive effects on bone health.[20]

Ipriflavone enhances the effects of calcium and vitamin D in preventing osteoporosis when they are taken together. Ipriflavone stimulates the action of cells that build bone and inhibits the activity of cells that break down bone.

Advanced calcium supplements that contain ipriflavone are available. Look for a supplement that contains a branded form of ipriflavone called Iprigen™ (Osteo-Logic™ by Quest® Vitamins is one such supplement). Studies show that Iprigen™ is more available to the body than generic ipriflavone.[21]

The recommended dose of ipriflavone is 200 milligrams taken three times daily with food. If you choose a product that contains a more bioavailable form of ipriflavone, such as Iprigen™, you might use a lower dose, with adequate monitoring by your doctor. Choose a product that has other nutrients important for bone health, including calcium, vitamin D, magnesium and vitamin C. Such a supplement can replace your standard calcium pill. For instance, each

Osteo-Logic™ pill provides 300 milligrams of calcium, 100 IU of vitamin D, 150 milligrams of magnesium and 25 milligrams of vitamin C in addition to 150 milligrams of Iprigen™.

Side effects of ipriflavone are uncommon but may include stomach upset, diarrhea and dizziness. One recent American study found that ipriflavone reduced the number of certain white blood cells in some women.[22] So far this is the only study to report this side effect; more than 60 clinical trials have not shown this effect.

Women with hormone-sensitive health conditions such as breast, uterine and ovarian cancer, endometriosis and uterine fibroids should seek the advice of a doctor, since it may enhance some effects of estrogen. As with many natural health products, women with liver or kidney disease should use the supplement with caution.

Other Lifestyle Factors

Weight-Bearing Exercise

Until the age of 30, regular exercise helps women get a head start on building peak bone mass. Children who spend the most amount of time being physically active have stronger bones compared with those who are sedentary. But the effect of exercise doesn't stop once you've achieved your peak mass. Bone cells are constantly active, tearing up old bone and laying down new bone. Participating in weight-bearing activities like brisk walking, stair climbing or weight training stimulates bones to increase in strength and density during the pre- and postmenopausal years. One study found that postmenopausal women who worked out three times a week for nine months actually increased their bone mass by 5.2 percent.[23]

If you have osteoporosis, a safe exercise program can help you slow bone loss, improve posture and balance and build muscle strength and tone. The benefits of exercise can reduce your risk for falling and fracturing a bone.

It's best to incorporate a mix of activities in your week. If you have never used weights before, consult a certified personal trainer. Personal trainers work in fitness clubs and many will come to your home. They'll design a safe and effective program for you.

Nutrition Strategy Checklist for Osteoporosis

☐ Soy foods

☐ Protein-rich foods

☐ Limit caffeine

☐ Limit sodium

☐ Calcium

☐ Vitamin D

☐ Vitamin A

☐ Vitamin C

☐ Vitamin K

☐ Boron

☐ Magnesium

☐ Phosphorus

☐ Ipriflavone

☐ Weight-bearing exercise

Recommended Resources

www.osteoporosis.ca
Osteoporosis Society of Canada
33 Laird Drive
Toronto, ON, Canada M4G 3S9
Tel: 1-800-463-6842

www.osteo.org
NIH Osteoporosis and Related Bone Diseases National Resource Center
1232 22nd Street NW
Washington, DC, USA 20037
Tel: 1-800-624-BONE (1-800-624-2663)

www.womenshealthmatters.ca
A Web site developed by Sunnybrook, the Women's College Health Sciences Centre and the Centre for Research in Women's Health.
E-mail: info@womenshealthmatters.ca

Parkinson's Disease

Identifiable by the characteristic tremors that it causes, Parkinson's disease is a degenerative disorder that affects the part of the brain that controls muscle movement. The disease damages nerve cells in the substania nigra, an area deep within the brain. These nerve cells produce dopamine, a neurotransmitter that carries messages along nerve pathways from one part of the nervous system to another. These messages enable muscles to make smooth, relaxed, well-controlled movements. In Parkinson's disease, the nerve cells in the substania nigra begin to degenerate rapidly, resulting in a shortage of dopamine. Without adequate supplies of dopamine, the brain loses the ability to communicate effectively with the nerves and muscles. This loss of communication interferes with the regulation of normal muscle actions, such as walking, sitting and standing.

Parkinson's disease usually begins with a slight tremor or shaking in a limb, often in the hand. The disease progresses quite slowly, but, eventually, the tremor becomes worse, affecting the arms, legs and other parts of the body. Balance deteriorates, automatic movements, such as blinking and smiling, are lost and daily activities, such as walking, talking and writing, become difficult and time-consuming.

What Causes Parkinson's Disease?

Scientists are working intensively to determine what causes Parkinson's disease. While we all lose some dopamine-producing cells as a normal part of aging, people with Parkinson's disease lose at least 60 percent of the cells in the substania nigra.

Researchers believe that the disease might be caused by a combination of genetic and environmental factors. Certain drugs, degenerative diseases and toxins are known to inhibit the action of dopamine in the brain, producing symptoms similar to Parkinson's disease.

Symptoms

- *Tremor* Tremors begin as a slight shaking in one finger or hand and may spread to other parts of the body, including the head, eyelids and feet. Tremors in the hand may cause your finger and thumb to rub back and forth in a motion known as pill rolling. Tremors are more noticeable when you are fatigued or under stress and often disappear when you sleep.

- *Difficulty moving* Walking is slow and shuffling, gait is unsteady and posture becomes stooped. Balance problems result in a tendency to fall. Muscles may freeze up, making it difficult to begin moving again. The digestive tract slows down, causing swallowing problems, indigestion and constipation.

- *Rigid muscles* Muscles become stiff and unresponsive, which limits movement and causes fatigue and aching. Handwriting becomes small and cramped and daily tasks become difficult.

- *Loss of automatic facial movements* The face becomes less expressive because facial muscles don't move. A fixed, staring expression with no blinking develops. Arms don't swing while walking and there are no gestures when talking.

- *Impaired speech* The voice becomes monotonous and soft, and speech becomes slower. Dementia can develop late in the disease.

Other symptoms include depression, lack of energy, difficulty sleeping and decreased sexual desire.

Who's at Risk?

Over one million people in North America live with the disease, and at least 50,000 more people are diagnosed with it every year.[1] Risk factors for Parkinson's disease include

- *Age* Symptoms usually appear later in life. The average age of diagnosis is 60, and rates continue to rise as people enter their 70s and 80s.

- *Gender* Men are slightly more at risk than women. A loss of estrogen levels after menopause may elevate the risk for women.

- *Heredity* Individuals with a close family relative with Parkinson's disease are three times more likely to develop the disease.[2]

- *Environmental factors* People exposed to herbicides and pesticides have a threefold higher risk of developing Parkinson's disease.[3]

- *Medications* Drugs used for psychiatric disorders, epilepsy or nausea may cause symptoms of Parkinson's disease.

- *Toxins* Manganese dust or the chemical MPTP used in heroin production can trigger symptoms, though these cases are very rare.

Conventional Treatment

At this time there is no cure for Parkinson's disease. Fortunately, people often need little or no treatment for quite a while after their diagnosis. When symptoms grow more severe, lifestyle changes and medications can provide some relief, including

- *physical therapy* to improve mobility, range of motion and muscle tone

- *regular weight-bearing exercise* to improve gait, balance and strengthen muscles

- *eating a healthy diet* to provide antioxidants to protect against free radical damage (see below)

- *minimizing stress* to help plan and manage daily tasks at times of peak energy and ability

- *medications* to manage symptoms in later stages of the disease:

  - *Levodopa* is a naturally occurring chemical that is converted into dopamine by nerve cells in the brain. The drug becomes less effective as the disease progresses.

  - *Dopamine agonists* imitate the effects of dopamine on the brain. It is usually used in combination with levodopa.

  - *Selegiline* prevents the breakdown of natural dopamine and dopamine formed from levodopa.

  - *Anticholinergics* help control tremors in the early stages of the disease.

  - *Amantadine* is an antiviral drug prescribed in the later stages of the disease for treatment of involuntary movements.

- *surgery* to reduce tremors, but it can cause complications and the beneficial effects of the surgery may not last

- *deep brain stimulation,* in which a deep brain stimulator is implanted in the chest and sends electrical impulses to the brain through a wire. The impulses interrupt signals from the thalamus in the brain that may cause symptoms.

- *fetal cell transplantation,* in which cells from fetuses or embryos are transplanted into the brains of people with Parkinson's disease. This is still an experimental therapy, because of the medical, moral and ethical considerations.

Managing Parkinson's Disease

Dietary Strategies

It is important to eat a healthy diet that is low in fat and contains plenty of whole grains, vegetables and fruits. These foods provide important vitamins, minerals and antioxidants that help protect from free radical damage to the brain. Weight loss can also be a problem for people with difficulty swallowing, loss of appetite or loss of their sense of taste. You'll find dietary guidelines in Chapter 5.

In the later stages of the disease, you may experience swallowing problems. To make eating and swallowing easier, take small bites of food and chew each mouthful thoroughly. Swallow each mouthful before putting more food into your mouth. Eat slowly. If your food tends to get cold before you are finished eating, use a warming tray under your plate. Foods that are chopped or puréed in the blender are easier to swallow. Hot cereals, soft bread, scrambled and poached eggs, yogurt, milk, low-fat puddings, applesauce, bananas, baked potatoes without the skin, cooked winter squash, ground meat and poultry are relatively easy to chew and swallow. Avoid nuts and hard candies.

Dietary Fat

Numerous studies report a much higher risk of Parkinson's disease among people who have high intakes of animal fat, with some studies showing as much as a ninefold greater risk.[4-7] Animal fat may increase free radical formation in the brain and, as result, cause oxidative damage to nerve cells in the substania nigra.

To reduce your intake of animal fat, choose the leanest cuts of meat (flank steak, inside round, pork tenderloin), poultry breast without the skin, skim or 1 percent milk and yogurt and skim-milk cheese. Use butter sparingly. More often, substitute animal protein with vegetarian protein foods such as legumes and soy foods. Eat fish at least three times a week.

Dietary Protein

Amino acids from high-protein foods such as meat, poultry, fish, eggs and dairy products can affect brain levels of levadopa by competing for entry into the brain. You may need to cut down on high-protein foods, or plan to eat those foods only at times that won't affect your medication. Some studies have found that patients who virtually eliminate protein during the daytime (no more than 10 grams) and have unrestricted intake after 5 p.m. show a more constant response to levadopa and experience symptom improvement.[8-10] Your doctor will advise you if this dietary approach will enhance your treatment.

Redistributing your protein intake may reduce your daily intake of calcium, iron and B vitamins. Consult with a registered dietitian (**www.dietitians.ca**) to help you develop a meal plan that limits protein during the daytime but provides all essential nutrients.

Dietary Fiber

Because the digestive tract works more slowly in Parkinson's disease, constipation is a common complaint. Constipation may also be a side effect of certain medications. Foods that have a greater proportion of insoluble fibers, such as wheat bran, whole grains, nuts, seeds and certain fruits and vegetables, are used to treat and prevent constipation. One study found that a diet high in insoluble fiber improved constipation and the absorption of levadopa in Parkinson's patients with marked constipation.[11] Psyllium, a type of soluble fiber, also adds bulk to stools and can be used to treat constipation.

Aim to consume 25 to 35 grams of fiber per day. Refer to page 243, Constipation, for a list of high-fiber foods used to treat constipation. Increase your fluid intake to 8 to 12 cups (2 to 3 liters) per day; otherwise constipation may worsen.

Coffee

Drinking coffee and other caffeine-containing beverages may help protect from Parkinson's disease. Researchers from the Mayo Clinic noted that compared with coffee abstainers, coffee drinking was associated with a 65 percent lower risk of Parkinson's disease and a later age of onset.[12] A larger trial that followed 8000 Japanese-American men for 30 years found a similar effect of coffee and caffeine.[13] The more coffee consumed, the lower the risk of Parkinson's disease. Precisely how caffeine might protect the nervous system remains unknown.

These findings do not imply that coffee can delay the progression of Parkinson's disease once you have it—this has not been studied. Rather, coffee may prevent the disease from developing in the first place. If your symptoms include difficulty sleeping, limit your intake of caffeine to no more than one cup of coffee per day. Refer to page 82, Chapter 5, for a list of caffeine-containing beverages and foods.

Vitamins and Minerals

Vitamin E

Free radical damage may cause nerve cell death in the substania nigra, possibly causing Parkinson's disease or worsening it. There is evidence of increased free radical damage in the brain tissue of people with Parkinson's disease.[14] Researchers have also noted a higher risk of the disease among people with lower dietary intakes and blood levels of vitamin E.[15,16]

Scientists have tested the effects of high-dose vitamin E supplementation on the progression of the disease with disappointing results. An American study found that vitamin E added no benefit to the treatment of Parkinson's disease.[17]

The evidence suggests that vitamin E must be present in the brain and nervous system before the disease takes hold.

If you have a close relative with Parkinson's disease, consider increasing your vitamin E intake. The recommended dietary allowance is 22 international units (IU). The best food sources include wheat germ, nuts, seeds, vegetable oils, whole grains and kale. To supplement, take 200 to 800 IU of natural source vitamin E. Buy a "mixed" vitamin E supplement if possible. The daily upper limit is 1500 IU.

Herbal Remedies

Psyllium Seed Husks

Psyllium is a bulk-forming laxative and is high in both insoluble and soluble fibers. Once consumed, psyllium forms a gelatinous mass and keeps the stool hydrated and soft. The increased bulk stimulates a reflex contraction of the walls of the bowel. Take 5 to 10 grams of the husks with 2 cups (500 ml) water, one to three times per day.

Other Natural Health Products

Acetyl-L-Carnitine

Carnitine is an amino acid found in all body cells, where it is used to metabolize fatty acids into energy. Carnitine also clears toxic accumulations of fatty acids from cells and serves as a building block for acetylcholine, a memory neurotransmitter. Based on the positive effects seen in studies of Alzheimer's patients, acetyl-L-carnitine has been suggested for Parkinson's disease. The research is scant, but one short-term study conducted among 20 patients with Parkinson's found that the supplement improved motor function symptoms and sleep patterns.[18]

The typical dosage is 1000 milligrams (1 gram) taken two or three times daily. Be sure to buy acetyl-L-carnitine and not one of its other chemical forms (L-carnitine, propionyl-carnitine). L-carnitine is available in the United States but is not legally available in Canada. However, some health food stores do stock it.

Do not take "D-carnitine" or "DL-carnitine," which can cause heart and muscle dysfunction.

Nutrition Strategy Checklist for Parkinson's Disease

- ☐ Low animal fat
- ☐ Protein redistribution
- ☐ Dietary fiber
- ☐ Coffee
- ☐ Vitamin E
- ☐ Acetyl-l-carnitine

Recommended Resources

www.apdaparkinson.com
American Parkinson's Disease Association, Inc.
1250 Hylan Boulevard, Suite 4B
Staten Island, NY, USA 10305-1946
Tel: 718-981-8001 or 1-800-223-2732
Fax: 718-981-4399

www.michaeljfox.org
The Michael J. Fox Foundation for Parkinson's Research
Grand Central Station
P.O. Box 4777
New York, NY, USA 10163
Tel: 1-800-708-7644

www.ninds.nih.gov
National Institute of Neurological Disorders and Stroke, NIH, HHS
P.O. Box 5801
Bethesda, MD, USA 20824
Tel: 301-496-5751
Fax: 301-402-2186

www.parkinson.ca
The Parkinson Foundation of Canada
4211 Yonge Street, Suite 316
Toronto, ON, Canada M2P 2A9
Tel: 416-227-9700 or 1-800-565-3000
Fax: 416-227-9600

Perimenopause

The signs and symptoms associated with menopause occur over a period of time, called perimenopause, which literally means "around menopause." For many women, the first sign of perimenopause is an erratic menstrual cycle—either skipped, lighter or shorter periods. The hallmark of this countdown to menopause is a fluctuating level of the female sex hormones, estrogen and progesterone. Estrogen highs can bring on PMS-like symptoms, including mood swings, fluid retention and headaches, whereas estrogen lows promise hot flashes, vaginal dryness and forgetfulness.

A woman is considered to have reached menopause when a year has passed since her last period. Although it can vary, the average age a Canadian woman hits menopause is 51. It's at this time that women enter post menopause, the phase of life in which the risks for heart disease, osteoporosis and breast cancer increase.

Your Menstrual Cycle

In order to understand what happens to your body during menopause, it helps to know how your hormones normally act during the childbearing years. During the early part of your monthly cycle, the ovaries produce estrogen. The brain responds to this increasing estrogen level by telling the pituitary gland to release follicle stimulating hormone (FSH) and luteinizing hormone (LH). These two hormones, in turn, act on your ovaries. FSH causes egg follicles to develop and release estrogen. When the circulating estrogen rises to a critical level, the pituitary gland releases a surge of LH. This influx of LH causes ovulation by telling the follicle to release a mature egg.

The empty egg follicle turns into something called the corpus luteum, a gland that produces progesterone after ovulation. During the last 14 days of the menstrual cycle, progesterone prepares your body for pregnancy by thickening the lining of your uterus. If conception does not occur, the corpus luteum becomes smaller, estrogen and progesterone levels fall and the uterine lining sheds, resulting in your period. Lower levels of estrogen and progesterone signal your pituitary to release FSH and LH and the cycle continues.

What Causes Perimenopause?

As you get older, your supply of eggs and follicles dwindles. Fewer follicles mean that your ovaries are producing less estrogen. Lower levels of estrogen and progesterone tell the pituitary gland that it's time to release FSH and then LH. But now your ovaries are unable to respond to FSH and LH. They can't produce much estrogen and release an egg, and, as a result, the pituitary gland keeps on releasing more and more FSH. This constant production of FSH can trigger hot flashes. With no egg being released from your ovary, there is no corpus luteum and, consequently, no progesterone secretion. Without progesterone, the body won't shed its uterine lining and you'll skip a period. With lower levels of hormones, your periods will become shorter and eventually they will cease.

Symptoms

Vaginal Changes

The tissues of the vagina and urethra (opening to the bladder) become thinner, less elastic and drier with declining estrogen levels. This can result in decreased lubrication, burning, itching, urinary tract infections and uncomfortable sexual intercourse.

Hot Flashes and Night Sweats

Hot flashes occur in up to 85 percent of North American women.[1,2] It's estimated that 10 to 15 percent of women have them severely enough to interfere with their daily life. On average, hot flashes persist for three to five years, but in 50 percent of women, they last up to five years.

A warning signal or aura often precedes a hot flash. A hot flash may begin as a pressure in the head, a headache or a wave of nausea. A sensation of heat then starts in the head and neck and spreads to the torso, arms and entire body. Sweating follows and is most intense in the upper body. Clothing may become soaked, particularly if hot flashes occur during sleep. (Night sweats are another term for hot flashes that occur during sleep.) Chills or shakes may follow as a result of a drop in body temperature. The entire event can last a few seconds to several minutes, and it may take an hour for chills to subside.

Insomnia

Night sweats often cause disrupted sleep. While many women have no difficulty falling back to sleep, some simply cannot. Fatigue caused by lack of sleep can lead to irritability, depression and forgetfulness. Many experts believe that there is something else going on to interrupt sleep, something that's not related to hot flashes during sleep.

Mood Swings

Most women describe the mood swings of perimenopause like those of premenstrual syndrome (PMS). Feelings of depression, anxiety and irritability can be disruptive to personal and work life.

Memory Problems

During perimenopause there are a few things happening to your body that may cause forgetfulness. For one, there's an aging process going on. The older we get, the more short-term memory we lose. Menopausal symptoms such as insomnia and fatigue can also cause memory problems. Evidence suggests that estrogen affects the brain chemistry and structure that's involved in memory, and that the loss of estrogen associated with menopause may be largely responsible for memory decline.

Heavy Bleeding

Most women will experience some change to their monthly cycle. The first sign of perimenopause is irregular menstruation. Your periods may stop suddenly or may become lighter and closer together, and then stop. Some women, on the other hand, experience heavy bleeding during their periods. Heavy bleeding is usually caused by an imbalance of estrogen and progesterone. When ovulation does not occur, progesterone is not produced. This means that estrogen is allowed to continue to build up the uterine lining. The lining becomes very thick and releases a lot of blood when it sheds in response to a drop in estrogen levels. As estrogen levels decline with approaching menopause, heavy bleeding will become less of an issue.

In some cases, heavy bleeding can be the sign of another health disorder: polyps, a fibroid or, less commonly, cancer. Alert your gynecologist if your periods last more than seven days, if you bleed between your periods, or if your menstrual flow becomes much heavier than usual.

Who's at Risk?

Perimenopausal symptoms can affect women ten years before actual menopause. Today in Canada, almost 3.5 million women are between the ages of 40 and 54, the phase of life when levels of certain hormones are changing and dwindling. While perimenopause can start in the late 30s, most women begin noticing symptoms in their 40s.

Not all women experience uncomfortable symptoms associated with perimenopause. Although research is lacking in this area, there are a few factors that may increase your risk for suffering one or more of the symptoms of perimenopause. Ask yourself the following:

- Are you in your mid to late 40s?
- Did your mother experience any perimenopausal symptoms?
- Do you suffer from premenstrual symptoms, especially mood swings?
- Do you eat a diet that's high in animal fat and lacking fruits, vegetables and fiber?
- Do you drink too much alcohol and coffee?
- Is your life full of stress and tension?
- Do you lack adequate sleep on a regular basis?
- Do you lack regular exercise?

Conventional Treatment

Perimenopause itself requires no medical treatment. Instead, treatments focus on relieving symptoms and reducing the risk of osteoporosis and heart disease that may occur during the postmenopausal years.

Hormone Replacement Therapy (HRT)

A combination of estrogen and progestin may be used to relieve hot flashes, mood swings and vaginal dryness. Women who have had a hysterectomy use estrogen alone. Hormone Replacement Therapy (HRT) prevents bone loss and may prevent bone fracture in women with osteoporosis. HRT may also reduce the risk of heart disease by lowering bad LDL cholesterol and raising good HDL cholesterol.

The protective effects of HRT last only as long as you take the medication. Surveys show that adherence to HRT is low. Side effects such as bloating, fluid retention, weight gain, irregular bleeding and nausea are frequently cited reasons for stopping the medication. Taking hormone replacement by pill, cream or patch can influence the potential for side effects. Changing the dosage can also make a difference. Depending on your body size, lower doses may be able to eliminate side effects and offer as much protection as the higher dose. If you are taking HRT and finding it difficult to tolerate the side effects, or the medication is not relieving your symptoms, ask your doctor about your options.

HRT is not without risks. When taken for more than five or ten years, HRT may increase the risk of breast cancer. And HRT may actually increase the risk of heart disease in women who have the disease. The long-term benefits of HRT on breast and heart health are under investigation.

Biphosphonates

These nonhormonal drugs are used to prevent osteoporosis and reduce the risk of bone fractures. Types of biphosphonates include Didrocal® (etidronate and calcium carbonate) and Fosomax® (aldendronate). Fosomax® may cause gastrointestinal upset and irritation of the esophagus.

Selective Estrogen Receptor Modulators (SERMs)

Often called "designer estrogen" drugs, these medications offer some of the beneficial effects of estrogen (bone protection, cholesterol lowering) without any of its negative effects (increased breast cancer risk, endometrial bleeding).

Evista® (raloxifene) is one SERM. These medications may increase the risk of blood clots and gallstones.

Managing Perimenopause

Today, more and more Canadian women are seeking alternative approaches to HRT. While the list below is not all-encompassing, it highlights a few important strategies that can help ease perimenopausal symptoms. If you're looking for a more comprehensive guide to managing perimenopausal symptoms, pick up a copy of my book *Managing Menopause with Diet, Vitamins and Herbs* (Prentice Hall Canada, 2000).

Dietary Strategies

Trigger Foods

Eliminate foods in the diet that can worsen hot flashes, insomnia or mood swings. Caffeine-containing foods and beverages like coffee, tea, dark chocolate, colas, certain orange sodas and root beers trigger hot flashes and can affect the quality of your sleep. Start by avoiding caffeine in the afternoon. Replace these beverages with caffeine-free or decaffeinated beverages like herbal tea, mineral water, fruit and vegetable juice or decaf coffee. Medications such as Midol®, Excedrin® and Anacin® also provide a fair amount of caffeine. The caffeine content of various beverages, foods and medications can be found on page 82, Chapter 5.

Reduce alcohol intake to no more than one drink a day, preferably none if you are experiencing hot flashes or you are under stress. Drinking alcoholic beverages can bring on a hot flash, interrupt sleep and affect mood. To lessen the effect of alcohol, drink alcohol only with a meal. When alcohol is consumed on an empty stomach, 20 percent is absorbed directly across the walls of your stomach, reaching your brain within a minute. When the stomach is full of food, alcohol is less able to reach the stomach wall and pass through, so its effect on the brain is delayed. When you are out socializing, have no more than one drink per hour. Since the liver can't metabolize alcohol any faster than this, drinking slowly will ensure that your blood alcohol concentration doesn't rise. To slow your pace, alternate one alcoholic drink with a nonalcoholic drink. One drink is equivalent to 5 ounces of wine, 12 ounces of beer, 10 ounces of wine cooler or 1.5 ounces of liquor.

If you are experiencing hot flashes, avoid spicy foods. Many women complain that certain spices can trigger a hot flash.

Soy Foods and Isoflavones

Diets rich in soy may explain why women living in China and Japan have a 20 percent incidence of hot flashes compared with women in Western countries who have an 85 percent incidence.[3] Well-controlled studies have found that soy foods can modestly ease hot flashes.[4-6] A 12-week Italian study looked at the effects of soy protein and hot flashes in 104 women aged 48 to 61 years. The study found that, compared with the placebo group, the women who consumed 60 grams of soy protein powder reported a 26 percent reduction in the average number of hot flashes by week three and a 33 percent reduction by week four.

Soybeans contain naturally occurring compounds called isoflavones, a type of phyto (plant) estrogen. Genistein and daidzein are the most active soy isoflavones and have been the focus of much research. Isoflavones have a similar structure to the hormone estrogen and, as a result, they have a weak estrogenic effect in the body. Even though isoflavones in soy are about 50 times less potent than estrogen, they are able to offer women a source of estrogen. When a woman's estrogen levels are low during perimenopause, a regular intake of foods like roasted soy nuts, soy beverages and tofu can help reduce hot flashes.

Experts believe that a daily intake of 40 to 80 milligrams of phytoestrogens is required to help alleviate hot flashes and reduce other health risks.[7]

Soy Food	Serving Size	Isoflavone Content (milligrams)
Roasted soy nuts	1/4 cup (60 ml)	40–50 mg
Green soybeans, uncooked	1/2 cup (125 ml)	70 mg
Tempeh, uncooked	3 oz (90 g)	38 mg
Soy flour	1/4 cup (60 ml)	37 mg
Tofu, firm	1/2 cup (125 ml)	27 mg
Texturized vegetable protein, dry	1/2 cup (125 ml)	30–120 mg
Soy milk	1 cup (250 ml)	24 mg
Soy protein powder, isolate	1 oz (28 g)	28 mg
Soy sauce		none
Soya oil		none
Yves Veggie Cuisine Good Dog	1 (52 g)	12–19 mg
Yves Veggie Cuisine Veggie Dog	1 (46 g)	12–19 mg
Yves Veggie Cuisine Deli Slices	3 slices (62 g)	12–19 mg

USDA: Iowa State University Database on the Isoflavone Content of Foods, 1999.

See page 72, Chapter 5, for ways to incorporate soy into your diet.

Carbohydrates

If you are experiencing sleep problems, try eating a small serving of a carbohydrate-rich food before bed. Carbohydrate-containing foods, such as milk, cereal or a slice of toast, provide the brain with an amino acid called tryptophan. The brain uses tryptophan as a building block to manufacture serotonin, a brain chemical that has been shown to facilitate sleep, improve mood, diminish pain and even reduce appetite.

This recommendation is not intended to make you gain weight. Eat something small or drink a glass of low-fat milk or soy beverage. If your insomnia has not improved after one week, look at other factors that may be disrupting sleep.

If you're feeling depressed or irritable, eat high-carbohydrate meals that contain very little protein. Protein foods such as chicken, meat or fish provide the body with many different amino acids that compete with tryptophan for entry into the brain. Try pasta with tomato sauce, a toasted whole-grain bagel with jam or a bowl of cereal with low-fat milk.

If you're suffering from fuzzy thinking, include carbohydrates in your breakfast. Studies in children and adults have shown that compared with breakfast skippers, individuals who eat the morning meal score higher on tests of mental performance that same morning.[8-10] The speed of information retrieval (a component of memory) seems to be affected the most by breakfast skipping. Breakfast foods such as whole-grain cereal, fruit, yogurt and whole-grain toast supply brain cells with glucose, their primary energy source. A low blood-glucose level that occurs after a night of fasting needs to be replenished in the morning.

Vitamins and Minerals

Vitamin B12

Many studies have found that vitamin B12 promotes sleep, especially in people with sleep disorders.[11-14] Researchers in Japan have used 1.5 to 3 milligrams of the vitamin each day to restore normal sleep patterns in patients. B12 is thought to restore sleep by working with melatonin, a hormone that's involved in maintaining the body's internal clock. A deficiency of vitamin B12 may cause disturbances in melatonin release.

The recommended dietary intake for vitamin B12 for healthy women is 2.4 micrograms. Vitamin B12 is found in all animal foods: meat, poultry, fish, eggs and dairy products. If you're eating these foods every day, chances are you are meeting your B12 needs. Foods fortified with the vitamin include soy beverages, rice beverages and breakfast cereals (but check labels to be sure).

Strict vegetarians, women who take acid-blocking medication and women over the age of 50 must get B12 from foods fortified with the vitamin or by taking a supplement. As we age, we produce less stomach acid, which results in an inability to properly absorb B12 in foods. Vitamin B12 supplements come in 500 or 1000 microgram strengths. B complex supplements provide 25 to 100 micrograms of B12 along with the family of B vitamins.

Choline

Although not an official vitamin, choline is a member of the B vitamin family. It's found in egg yolks, organ meats and legumes, and it's used as a building block for a memory neurotransmitter called acetylcholine. Supplements of choline have been shown to enhance memory and reaction time in animals, particularly aging animals. Researchers believe that choline supplements will improve brain tasks only if you're deficient in the nutrient. Stress and aging can deplete choline levels.

Although it's not known if supplemental choline can improve memory in people who have normal levels of choline, it is important to meet your daily requirements. Healthy women need 425 milligrams of choline each day. The best food sources are egg yolks, liver and other organ meats, Brewer's yeast, wheat germ, soybeans, peanuts and green peas.

Supplemental choline is available as lecithin supplements. The maximum safe limit is 3500 milligrams (3.5 grams) of choline a day. High doses of choline can cause low blood pressure and a fishy body odor in some people.

Iron

If you're experiencing heavy menstrual flow, it's extremely important to eat an iron-rich diet. Iron is used by red blood cells to form hemoglobin, the molecule that transports oxygen from your lungs to your cells. If your diet falls short of iron, or if your body loses iron faster than your diet can replace it, red blood cell levels drop and less oxygen is delivered to your tissues. Symptoms of iron deficiency include weakness, lethargy and fatigue on exertion. Iron deficiency is a progressive condition. Even if your iron stores aren't low enough to diagnose anemia, symptoms of iron deficiency can still be felt.

Women who are menstruating require 18 milligrams of iron per day. Postmenopausal women need 8 milligrams. The best iron sources are lean beef, tofu, legumes, enriched breakfast cereals, whole-grain breads, raisins, dried apricots, prune juice, spinach and peas. Iron in food comes in two forms: heme iron in animal foods and non-heme iron in plant foods. Heme iron is the most efficiently absorbed and is found in red meat, chicken, eggs and fish. Nonheme iron is less efficiently absorbed. Refer to page 56, Chapter 4, for tips on how to enhance iron absorption.

A multivitamin and mineral supplement is recommended for women with higher iron requirements. Most formulas provide 10 milligrams, but you can find some that provide up to 18 milligrams. If you're experiencing persistent heavy bleeding, the recommended daily intake might not be enough to meet your needs. Sometimes 100 milligram tablets of supplemental iron are recommended to rebuild your iron stores. Single iron supplements are toxic in large doses and should be taken only under supervision by your doctor. Take single iron supplements for one to three months and then have your blood retested by your doctor. Once iron stores are replenished, iron supplements should be discontinued. To prevent constipation associated with high doses of iron, increase your fiber and fluid intake.

Herbal Remedies
Black Cohosh *(Cimicifuga racemosa)* for Hot Flashes
Based on clinical experience and findings from controlled scientific studies, black cohosh is the most promising herbal remedy for treating hot flashes. A number of randomized controlled trials have found black cohosh to be as effective as estrogen therapy at relieving flashes.[15-19] Black cohosh does not cause the uncomfortable side effects associated with hormone therapy. And unlike estrogen, laboratory research has found that black cohosh inhibits the growth of breast cancer cells.[20]

Exactly how the herb works is under scientific debate. While some studies suggest it may bind to estrogen receptors, others do not.[21,22] Black cohosh may exert its effect by interacting with certain brain receptors. The herb contains naturally occurring compounds called triterpene glycosides that are thought to be responsible for its effect.

The recommended dose is 40 milligrams twice daily. Buy a product standardized to contain 2.5 percent triterpene glycosides. The specific black cohosh evaluated in much of the scientific research is sold under the name Remifemin® Menopause. This product is sold as a 20 milligram tablet, since a recent study showing that a lower dose of the herb is equally effective.

Once you start black cohosh, it may take up to four weeks to notice an effect. Mild stomach upset and headache may occur.

Herbal Combination Formulas
These products combine black cohosh with a number of herbs known to ease a variety of perimenopausal symptoms. These may be used instead of taking black cohosh alone. Estro-Logic™ (Quest® Vitamins) contains standardized black cohosh, soy isoflavones and a number of

other herbs supportive to menopause. It was developed by American gynecologist Dr. Kathleen Fry and medical herbalist Claudia Wingo. The product is currently being studied in a trial of 100 menopausal women. Preliminary findings show the product to be effective at easing a number of common menopausal complaints. Other products include Menopause Formula (Natural Factors®), Meno+ (ehn®) and Life® Menopause Formula (Shoppers Drug Mart).

Valerian (*Valeriana officinalis*) for Insomnia

A number of European studies have shown that valerian makes getting to sleep easier and that it increases deep sleep.[23-25] Unlike popular prescribed sleeping pills, valerian does not lead to dependence or addiction. Nor does it cause a morning drug hangover. Scientists have learned that valerian promotes sleep by binding weakly to two brain receptors, GABA receptors and benzodiazepine receptors.

The recommended dose is 400 to 900 milligrams, taken 30 minutes to one hour before bedtime. Buy a product that is standardized to contain at least 0.5 percent essential oils or 0.8 percent valerenic acid. If you wake up feeling groggy, reduce the dose. The herb is most effective when used over a period.

Do not take valerian with alcohol or sedative medications. The herb is not recommended for use during pregnancy and breastfeeding.

Kava Kava (*Piper methysticum*) for Anxiety

Anxiety is a mood change often reported by many perimenopausal women. It's described as a feeling of apprehension, uncertainty and fear and is often accompanied by an increased heart rate, sweating and even tremors. Kava kava is used to calm the nerves. In higher doses, it's used as a sleeping aid.

The plant contains kavalactones, components that exert their effect by working on the limbic system of the brain, the center of our emotions. Research has deemed kava to be effective in the treatment of anxiety. One study found that menopausal women with anxiety disorders obtained significant relief with kava, without the negative side effects of conventional drugs like Valium.[26]

Until recently kava was thought to have a wide margin of safety. The only side effects reported were mild stomach upset, headache, or dizziness. If you are already taking kava, *read the following section very carefully.* There is growing concern over reports from Europe that describe liver damage in some people taking kava. Individuals at particular risk for liver damage associated with use of kava include those who have compromised liver function due to liver disease, age factors, or prior or current drug/alcohol abuse.

In August 2002, Health Canada issued a stop-sale for kava products and recalled the supplement from the market. If you have a bottle at home, I advise you to throw it out.

Nutrition Strategy Checklist for Perimenopause

☐ Avoid alcohol and caffeine
☐ Carbohydrates
☐ Soy foods
☐ Vitamin B12
☐ Choline
☐ Iron
☐ Black cohosh
☐ Valerian

Recommended Resources

www.healthywomen.org
National Women's Health Resource Center
120 Albany Street, Suite 820
New Brunswick, NJ, USA 08901
Tel: 1-877-986-9472
Fax: 732-249-4671
E-mail: vngethe@healthywomen.org

www.menopause.org
The North American Menopause Society
P.O. Box 94527
Cleveland, OH, USA 44101
Tel: 440-442-7550
Fax: 440-442-2660
E-mail: info@menopause.org

Phlebitis

Thrombophlebitis, or phlebitis as it is more commonly known, is an inflammation that develops in a vein, usually accompanied by a blood clot called a thrombus. Phlebitis typically occurs in the veins of the legs, although, rarely, it has also been known to affect the veins in the arms. When the affected vein is close to the surface of the skin, the condition is called *superficial thrombophlebitis*. If the affected vein lies deeper in the body, often within a muscle, the condition is known as *deep vein thrombosis*.

Blot clots that occur in superficial thrombophlebitis do not pose a serious health risk. When phlebitis affects a superficial vein, the inflammatory reaction is sudden and acute, which tends to bind the blood clot firmly to the wall of the vein. Since veins that lie close to the surface of the skin have no surrounding muscles that might squeeze the blood clot and dislodge it, there is little likelihood of a pulmonary embolism (see below). Superficial thrombophlebitis usually resolves by itself in one or two weeks. The blood clot will be gradually absorbed by the body, causing no harm.

When a blood clot develops in a deep vein in the leg, however, the condition can be very dangerous as there may not be enough inflammation to make the blood clot adhere to the vein wall. The squeezing action of the calf muscles can dislodge all or part of the blood clot, allowing it to circulate through the bloodstream until it reaches the lungs, where it can block one or more arteries and cause a life-threatening condition called pulmonary embolism.

What Causes Phlebitis?

Phlebitis usually develops because of an irritation or injury to the vein such as an injection into a vein or a varicose vein that becomes irritated.

Blood clots that form in deeper veins are often the result of poor blood flow or aggregation of cells called platelets that increase the stickiness of the blood. Sluggish blood flow can be caused by

- extended periods of inactivity, such as sitting during a long car or airplane trip
- long periods of standing in one spot, often job-related
- prolonged bed rest, such as during a lengthy illness or surgical recovery
- restrictive clothing that interferes with circulation

Increased stickiness in the blood can be caused by

- severe infection
- liver disease
- some types of cancer
- recent surgery or childbirth
- estrogen or oral contraceptives

Symptoms

Deep vein thrombosis can be difficult to diagnose because there may be no signs of a problem until the blood clot reaches the lungs. Any symptoms of swelling, pain or warmth in the leg or foot should be considered as possible warning signs of a thrombosis and should receive medical attention immediately. Do not attempt to self-treat phlebitis as it is a potentially fatal disease. Symptoms of deep vein thrombosis include

- redness, swelling and a feeling of heat in the area of the affected vein

- a vein close to the surface of the skin appearing more noticeable than usual

- a vein that feels hard, like a piece of rope

- pain or discomfort in the area of the affected vein

- discoloration or ulcers on the skin

- swelling in the leg, calf, ankle or foot

Who's at Risk?

The risk of developing phlebitis increases after surgery, childbirth, long periods of illness involving bed rest and long periods of inactivity such as sitting or standing still. People with varicose veins are also more susceptible to phlebitis.

Medical treatments such as having injections or intravenous catheters inserted into a vein may cause irritations that will provoke phlebitis. Medications such as estrogen or oral contraceptives can also increase the likelihood of blood clots.

Conventional Treatment

Pain relievers and warm compresses are often used to ease discomfort. Compression bandages or stockings may be recommended to increase blood flow in the veins. More aggressive therapy may be needed for deep vein thrombosis, including

- anticoagulants (blood thinners) given intravenously or in oral tablets

- restricting activity to prevent the clot from dislodging

- elevating the affected limb

- surgery

- hospitalization

To help prevent blood clots and phlebitis from developing, you should

- maintain a healthy weight; lose weight, if necessary

- exercise regularly

- limit salt intake

- stop smoking

- when sitting or standing for long periods, take frequent breaks to walk around and get your blood circulating

Preventing and Managing Phlebitis

Dietary Strategies

Weight Control

Swedish researchers demonstrated that following a healthy diet, getting regular exercise and achieving a healthy weight can improve properties of the blood and reduce the chances that thromboembolism, a blood clot traveling to the lung, will reoccur.[1] To determine whether or not you are at an acceptable weight, turn to page 439, Obesity and Weight Loss, to calculate your body mass index (BMI). Having a BMI over 25 indicates overweight and a BMI greater than 27 is defined as obese. Weight loss is best achieved by a combination of reducing calorie intake and increasing physical exercise. Refer to page 442, Obesity and Weight Loss, for strategies to help you lose weight.

Fluids and Alcohol

People with phlebitis who travel long distances in an airplane are at increased risk for pulmonary embolism. Scientists speculate that insufficient fluid intake and drinking alcohol can increase the risk of a blood clot dislodging and causing harm.[2] Other risk factors associated with prolonged air travel include low humidity, low oxygen levels, immobilization and the coach or economy-class seat that does not allow elevation of the legs.

If you have phlebitis and you travel by air, be sure to drink plenty of water during the flight. Drinking water will keep your circulation efficient and get you out of your seat to use the washroom, allowing you to walk and move your legs.

Research suggests that higher intakes of alcohol are linked with a greater risk of phlebitis.[3] Women should have no more than one drink a day, and men no more than two drinks per day, to a limit of nine per week. However, it is best to avoid alcoholic beverages altogether, since they cause fluid to be lost from the body.

Dietary Fiber

Some researchers believe that vein problems in the legs are caused by constipation resulting from a low-fiber diet.[4] Straining to evacuate small, firm stools puts pressure on the abdominal muscles, which can be transmitted to the veins in the leg. To avoid constipation, aim to include 25 to 35 grams of fiber in your daily diet.

Foods contain varying amounts of insoluble fibers and soluble fibers. Foods that have a greater proportion of insoluble fibers, such as wheat bran, whole grains, nuts, seeds and certain fruits and vegetables, are used to treat and prevent constipation. Once consumed, insoluble fibers make their way to the intestinal tract, where they absorb water, help form larger, softer stools and speed evacuation. Psyllium, a type of soluble fiber, also adds bulk to stools and can be used to treat constipation. Refer to page 245, Constipation, for strategies to increase fiber intake.

Herbal Remedies

Horse Chestnut
(*Aesculus hippocastanum*)

Many studies have found this herbal remedy to be effective in the treatment of varicose veins and poor circulation in the veins (see Chapter 7). While no studies have been conducted in people with phlebitis, this herb is often recommended for the condition.

An active compound called aesin in the horse chestnut seeds enhances circulation through the veins. The herb appears to constrict and promote normal tone in the veins so that blood returns to the heart. The compound also has anti-inflammatory properties and may reduce swelling in the legs.

Buy a product standardized to 16 to 21 percent aescin. Take one capsule up to three times per day. The extract used in the clinical studies is sold as Venastat® (Pharmaton®) in Canada and the United States. The safety of horse chestnut during pregnancy and breastfeeding has not been established; avoid using the herb at these times. Do not take horse chestnut if you have liver or kidney disease.

Other Natural Health Products
Bromelain

This natural product is a collection of enzymes extracted from the juice and stems of pineapple. Once bromelain is absorbed into the bloodstream, it causes the release of kinin, a substance that has anti-inflammatory and blood-thinning properties. Based on its action in the body, bromelain is often recommended for vein problems, including phlebitis.[5,6]

The typical dose of bromelain is 80 to 320 milligrams taken two to three times per day. However, dosage will vary with the form used, so follow the manufacturer's directions. Bromelain may cause diarrhea in some individuals and an allergic reaction in those people allergic to pineapple and wheat.

Bromelain may increase the risk of bleeding if you take blood-thinning medications and herbs such as aspirin, warfarin (Coumadin®), heparin, garlic, ginger, ginkgo biloba, horse chestnut and red clover. Consult your doctor before using bromelain. Taking zinc supplements concurrently with bromelain can inhibit the enzyme's action.

Aortic Glycosaminoglycans (GAGs)

These compounds are made by the body and are found in the joints and the lining of the arteries. Related to the anticoagulant drug heparin, aortic GAGs appear to reduce the risk of blood clotting. Italian researchers have shown GAGs supplements to improve the symptoms of many vein conditions, including phlebitis.[7-10] While GAGs may ease the pain and discomfort of phlebitis, one study found that the supplement was not effective at preventing a recurrence of deep vein thrombosis or pulmonary embolism.[11]

The recommended dose is 100 milligrams per day. Using aortic GAGs with aspirin or prescription blood-thinning medications may increase the risk of bleeding; consult your physician before taking GAGs. This supplement may cause gastrointestinal upset and headache in some individuals.

Aortic GAGs supplements are manufactured from the large artery (aorta) of cows. Since GAGs are derived from animals, there is some concern about contamination with diseased animal parts. However, so far there have been no reports of disease transmission to humans from GAGs supplements. If you are concerned, contact the manufacturer to ask what steps are being taken to ensure that its product is not contaminated.

Nutrition Strategy Checklist for Phlebitis

☐ Weight control
☐ Fluids
☐ Avoid alcohol
☐ Dietary fiber

☐ Horse chestnut
☐ Bromelain OR Aortic GAGs

Recommended Resources

www.crha-health.ab.ca
Calgary Regional Health Authority Communications
1035-7th Avenue SW
Calgary, AB, Canada T2P 3E9
Tel: 403-265-INFO (403-265-4636) or 1-800-860-2742 (Alberta only)
E-mail: publicweb@crha-health.ab.ca

www.mayoclinic.com
Mayo Foundation for Medical Education and Research

Polycystic Ovary Syndrome (PCOS)

Sometimes referred to as Stein-Leventhal syndrome, polycystic ovary syndrome (PCOS) is the most common cause of menstrual problems in women. The disorder affects 4 to 7 percent of all premenopausal women, and many don't even know they have it. For reasons not fully understood, women with PCOS produce unusually high levels of estrogen, luteinizing hormone and male hormones called androgens. This disrupts the normal menstrual cycle and encourages the formation of cysts in the ovaries, making PCOS one of the leading causes of infertility.

What Causes Polycystic Ovary Syndrome?

Hormones are produced and regulated by an interrelated series of glands called the endocrine system. Two tiny glands located in the brain, the hypothalamus and the pituitary gland, are responsible for monitoring and balancing the normal activity of the endocrine system. The pituitary gland helps control the cycles of the female reproductive system. This gland secretes luteinizing hormone (LH), which stimulates the ovaries to release mature eggs and to produce the female sex hormones estrogen and progesterone. LH is also necessary for the production of androgens, male sex hormones that are present in small quantities in every woman.

PCOS is thought to develop when the pituitary gland malfunctions and secretes an overabundance of LH. This abnormally high level of LH triggers an increase in the production of androgens, which results in a corresponding increase in estrogen levels. PCOS causes the production of these three hormones to remain at high levels, disrupting the natural hormonal balance of the menstrual cycle.

PCOS usually develops during puberty at the time when menstruation would normally begin. The elevated level of LH in the bloodstream interferes with the normal functioning of the ovaries. The excess hormones prevent eggs from maturing properly, which often results in the failure to ovulate, called anovulation. Failure to release an egg will prevent or delay the onset of menstruation in young girls and may cause mature women to experience irregular periods or skipped periods. PCOS can also cause heavy vaginal bleeding that can lead to iron-deficiency anemia.

The hormonal imbalance seen in women with PCOS also causes cysts (fluid-filled sacs) to accumulate in the ovaries. These cysts are eggs that have matured, but because of abnormal hormone levels, were never released. Polycystic (meaning "many cysts") ovaries are covered with a tough, thick outer layer and may grow to become as much as two to five times larger than normal. These cysts interfere with the activity of the ovaries and contribute to the infertility problems associated with PCOS.

Symptoms and Associated Medical Conditions

PCOS progresses fairly slowly, but, unfortunately, the symptoms tend to worsen over time. Although the syndrome affects each woman a little differently, the primary symptoms include

- infertility
- abnormal, irregular or absent periods
- mood swings
- weight problems or obesity
- high blood pressure
- increased hair growth (hirsutism)
- male-pattern baldness
- aggravated acne
- heavy, persistent vaginal bleeding
- iron-deficiency anemia

In addition to infertility, women with PCOS face other reproductive concerns. Approximately one-third of all pregnancies in women with PCOS end in miscarriage. There's also an increased risk of pregnancy disorders such as preeclampsia, gestational diabetes, premature labor and stillbirth.

PCOS also disrupts normal physical development by stimulating the production of higher levels of androgens, the male hormones. This causes some women to acquire secondary male characteristics such as frontal balding, deepening of the voice and increased muscle mass. One of the most common symptoms in women with PCOS is hirsutism, a condition that causes body and facial hair to follow a male growth pattern. Women with hirsutism grow excessive amounts of coarse hair on their face, legs, chest and groin.

Obesity affects nearly 50 percent of all women with PCOS and contributes to the already high levels of estrogen associated with this disorder.[1] Androgens are converted to estrogen in body fat, and the greater the amount of body fat a woman has, the higher the level of estrogen. Excess estrogen in the bloodstream can trigger severe acne and has been associated with increased risk of endometrial, ovarian and breast cancer.

Women with PCOS have a higher risk of developing insulin resistance, a condition that is further aggravated by obesity. Insulin is a hormone secreted by the pancreas. By attaching to special receptors on body cells, insulin enables cells to take in and store glucose and protein. Insulin resistance is caused by defective insulin receptors so that insulin cannot attach properly to these sites. As a result, insulin is not able to do its job properly and sugar (glucose) is unable to enter the cells where it is needed for energy. Insulin resistance causes a high level of insulin to remain in the bloodstream, causing hyperinsulinemia. These high insulin levels can lead to diabetes and heart disease. High blood insulin can also cause weight gain.

Most women with PCOS have some degree of insulin resistance and many go on to develop glucose intolerance or diabetes. It's estimated that by the age of 40, as many as 40 percent of women with PCOS will have type 2 diabetes or impaired glucose tolerance.[2] Treatment directed at reducing insulin resistance can restore ovulation, decrease the levels of male hormones, lower triglycerides and elevated blood pressure and promote weight loss.

Who's at Risk?

Women can develop PCOS as early as their pre-teens, or the condition may appear at any time throughout their childbearing years. Most women, however, begin to experience symptoms at menarche, the onset of menstruation. PCOS becomes less common as women get older and rarely develops after menopause. But the health consequences of the disorder, such as diabetes resulting from insulin resistance, persist into the menopausal years.

Although there is not enough evidence to prove a genetic link to the disease, many women with PCOS have a mother or a sister with similar symptoms.

Conventional Treatment

Since PCOS has no cure, treatment is usually directed at managing the primary symptoms, especially hirsutism, menstrual irregularities and infertility. The choice of treatment will depend on the type and severity of symptoms, a woman's age and her plans regarding pregnancy.

For women not planning to become pregnant, oral contraceptives can control menstrual irregularities. Birth control pills inhibit the production and activity of androgens and therefore help reduce acne, lower the risk of ovarian and endometrial cancer and slow hair growth for women with hirsutism. Oral contraceptives are not recommended for menopausal women or for women with risk factors for certain heart or blood diseases.

Antiandrogen drugs (e.g., spironolactone, Diane 35®) are also effective in reducing growth of unwanted hair. To further minimize the effects of hirsutism, many women remove excessive hair by shaving, waxing, using depilatories or electrolysis.

For women planning to have children, the treatment of choice is usually the fertility drug clomiphene citrate (Clomid®). Clomiphene is effective in stimulating the ovaries to release eggs. Studies indicate that 80 percent of women with PCOS ovulate in response to clomiphene but only 50 percent of these women become pregnant.[3] If clomiphene does not work well for you, your physician may try to induce ovulation with a variety of hormone supplements, including follicle-stimulating hormone (FSH) and gonadotropin-releasing hormone (GnRH) drugs such as leuprolide (Lupron®) and nafarelin (Synarel®).

To lower health risks such as diabetes and heart disease, your doctor may prescribe an insulin-sensitizing drug to decrease insulin resistance (e.g., Metformin®, Avandia®). These medications also reduce androgen production and restore normal menstrual cycles.

Managing Polycystic Ovary Syndrome

Dietary Strategies

Weight Control

Obesity is present in as many as 50 percent of women with PCOS. Being overweight worsens the symptoms of PCOS by increasing insulin resistance and further elevating levels of male hormones. As a result, weight loss is one of the most important treatment strategies for PCOS. Research has demonstrated that losing weight if you are obese enhances the body's sensitivity to insulin and normalizes hormone levels.[4-7] Studies have shown that losing more than 5 percent of body weight can restore fertility in obese women with PCOS.[8,9]

To determine if you are at a healthy weight, refer to page 439, Obesity and Weight Loss, to calculate your body mass index (BMI). Having a BMI over 25 indicates overweight and a BMI greater than 27 is defined as obese. If you determine that your BMI is greater than 25, use the strategies outlined on page 442, Obesity and Weight Loss, to promote safe, gradual weight loss.

Low Glycemic Carbohydrates

Unfortunately, insulin resistance makes weight loss more difficult to achieve. To help improve insulin resistance and lower blood insulin levels, it is important to eat smaller portions of carbohydrate-rich foods *and* to choose the right types of carbohydrate foods. When you eat a carbohydrate-rich food, whether it's pasta, yogurt, an apple or fruit juice, the carbohydrate is broken down into glucose and absorbed into your bloodstream. Blood sugar (glucose) rises, signaling the pancreas to release insulin into the bloodstream. Insulin then clears sugar from your

blood, taking it into your cells, where it's used for energy. If you have insulin resistance, insulin cannot perform this task properly. Some sugar remains in the blood, causing more insulin to be released, resulting in a chronically high insulin level.

Carbohydrate foods are digested and absorbed at different rates. Some foods are digested slowly and result in a steady, slow rise in blood sugar. This means that less insulin will be secreted into the blood. Slow carbohydrates have what is called a low glycemic index. Foods with a high glycemic index are digested and absorbed more quickly and cause much higher insulin levels.

To prevent an excessive surge of insulin after eating, meals and snacks should emphasize foods with a low glycemic index. Foods such as whole-grain pumpernickel bread, oatmeal, 100 percent bran cereal, legumes, yogurt and soy milk all have a low glycemic index value. See page 7, Chapter 1, for a list of foods ranked by their glycemic index value.

Vitamins and Minerals

Calcium and Vitamin D

Gonadotropin-releasing hormone (GnRH) drugs such as leuprolide (Lupron®) and nafarelin (Synarel®) that are used to improve PCOS symptoms work by causing a deficiency of estrogen, a hormone that prevents bones from losing calcium. As a result, GnRH drugs cause accelerated bone loss, which may be partially irreversible.

A six-month Italian study of 44 women with PCOS showed that those women receiving such a medication experienced a significant decrease in bone density.[10] Women given the drug in combination with the antiandrogen drug spironolactone did not show any change in bone density. It seems that spironolactone offers a bone-sparing effect in this situation. Your doctor may prescribe another medication along with a GnRH drug to offset the bone loss. The jury is still out on whether some of these drug combinations (called addback regimens) actually prevent bone loss.

If you are taking a GnRH drug, it is very important to meet your daily recommended intakes for calcium and vitamin D, two nutrients critical for bone health. This is important to help minimize bone loss.

- *Calcium* The recommended dietary allowance (RDA) is 1000 to 1300 milligrams, depending on your age. The best food sources are milk, yogurt, cheese, fortified soy and rice beverages, fortified orange juice, tofu, salmon (with bones), kale, bok choy, broccoli and Swiss chard. If you take calcium supplements, buy calcium citrate with vitamin D and magnesium added. See page 45, Chapter 4, for more information about calcium supplements.

- *Vitamin D* The daily adequate intake is 200 to 600 international units (IU) depending on your age. The best food sources are fluid milk, fortified soy and rice beverages, oily fish, egg yolks, butter and margarine. Most multivitamin and mineral supplements provide 200 to 400 IU of vitamin D.

Chromium

The body uses this mineral to make glucose tolerance factor (GTF), a compound thought to maintain normal blood-sugar levels by increasing insulin receptor sensitivity. A deficiency of chromium causes impaired glucose tolerance, increased cholesterol and triglyceride levels and decreased good HDL cholesterol levels. Studies suggest that when taken as a supplement, chromium can help reduce high blood cholesterol and triglycerides and stabilize blood-sugar levels.[11]

The recommended dietary intake for women is 25 micrograms of chromium. Good food sources include apples with the skin, green peas, chicken breast, refried beans, mushrooms, oysters, wheat germ and Brewer's yeast. Processed foods and refined foods like white bread, rice, pasta, sugar and sweets contain very little chromium.

If you're concerned you're not getting enough chromium in your diet, check your multivitamin and mineral to see how much it contains. Most brands supply 25 to 50 micrograms. If you choose to take a separate chromium supplement, *do not exceed 200 micrograms* per day. High doses of chromium can cause cognitive impairment, anemia and kidney damage. Supplements made from chromium picinolate are thought to be absorbed more efficiently than those made from chromium chloride or chromium nicotinate.

Other Natural Health Products

Ipriflavone

Ipriflavone is a supplement manufactured from daidzein, a natural plant estrogen found in soybeans. Ipriflavone enhances the action of cells that build bone and inhibits the activity of cells that break down bone. Research suggests that ipriflavone, taken alone or with calcium, is more effective at maintaining bone density than calcium alone. Ipriflavone appears to enhance the effects of calcium and vitamin D in preventing osteoporosis.

If you are taking a medication that causes bone loss, consider taking a calcium supplement with ipriflavone added. In a double-blind study, ipriflavone taken in combination with calcium prevented loss of bone density in women taking leuprolide (Lupron®).[12]

Choose a calcium supplement that contains a branded form of ipriflavone called Iprigen™ (e.g., Osteo-Logic™ by Quest® Vitamins). Laboratory research has revealed that Iprigen™ is more available to the body than generic ipriflavone.[13]

The recommended dose is 200 milligrams taken three times daily with food. If you take a more bioavailable form of ipriflavone, such as Iprigen™, a lower dose may be used. Choose a product that has other nutrients important for bone health, including calcium, vitamin D, magnesium and vitamin C. Such a supplement can replace your standard calcium pill. For instance, each Osteo-Logic™ pill provides 300 milligrams of calcium, 100 IU of vitamin D, 150 milligrams of magnesium and 25 milligrams of vitamin C in addition to 150 milligrams of Iprigen™.

Women with hormone-sensitive health conditions such as breast, uterine or ovarian cancer, endometriosis or uterine fibroids should seek the advice of a physician as ipriflavone may potentiate some effects of estrogen. As with many natural health products, women with liver and kidney disease should use the supplement with caution; inform your doctor if you start taking ipriflavone.

Inositol

Although not an official vitamin, this natural compound is closely related to the B vitamin family. Inositol is found in foods mainly as phytic acid, a fibrous compound. Good sources include citrus fruits, whole grains, legumes, nuts and seeds. When you eat these foods, intestinal bacteria liberate inositol from phytic acid.

Once in the body, inositol is an essential component of cell membranes. It promotes the export of fat from cells in the liver and intestine. Supplements of inositol are thought to improve insulin sensitivity and have been used to treat symptoms of PCOS. In one study of 44 obese women, 1200 milligrams of inositol taken once daily for six to eight weeks decreased blood triglycerides and testosterone levels, reduced blood pressure and caused ovulation.[14] Previous studies suggest that people with insulin resistance and type 2 diabetes might be deficient in inositol.

The recommended dose for PCOS is 1200 milligrams per day. When choosing a supplement, look for D-chiro-inositol. No adverse effects of inositol have been reported. Inositol supplements may be difficult to find, since few companies manufacture them (see Chapter 8).

Nutrition Strategy Checklist for PCOS

☐ Weight control   ☐ Chromium
☐ Low GI carbohydrates ☐ Ipriflavone
☐ Calcium   ☐ Inositol
☐ Vitamin D

Recommended Resources

www.askdrkoop.com
Founded by former US Surgeon General Dr. Everett Koop.

www.hormone.org
The Hormone Foundation
4350 E West Highway, Suite 500
Bethesda, MD, USA 20814-4426
Tel: 1-800-HORMONE (1-800-467-6663)
Fax: 301-941-0259

www.pcosupport.org
Polycystic Ovarian Syndrome Association
P.O. Box 80517
Portland, OR, USA 97280
Tel: 1-877-775-PCOS (1-877-775-7267)

Premenstrual Syndrome (PMS)

Premenstrual syndrome (PMS) is a collection of emotional, psychological and physical symptoms that develop during the 7 to 14 days before the start of your menstrual period and resolve once your period begins on day one of your menstrual cycle.

For some women, the physical and emotional changes caused by PMS are so severe that they interfere with the ability to function at work or interact with family and friends. When PMS symptoms seriously undermine quality of life, the condition is called premenstrual dysphoric disorder—a complex medical disorder that affects only a small percentage of women. It's thought to be an excessive reaction to the normal hormonal changes associated with the menstrual cycle.

Your Monthly Cycle

The symptoms of PMS appear during the last two weeks of the menstrual cycle. These two weeks are referred to as the luteal phase of your cycle. There are three distinct phases in each menstrual cycle: the follicular phase, ovulation and the luteal phase. Two areas of the brain, the hypothalamus and the pituitary gland, control all the hormonal changes that regulate each of these distinct stages.

The menstrual cycle begins when the hypothalamus produces gonadotropin-releasing hormones (GnRH). These hormones pass into the pituitary gland and trigger the release of luteinizing hormone (LH) and follicle-stimulating hormone (FSH). Working in combination, these two hormones promote the growth of follicles, tiny sac-like structures located in the ovaries. Each follicle surrounds an ovum, or egg. Between 10 to 20 follicles will enlarge, but normally only one egg is released during each menstrual cycle. Throughout this time of growth, the follicles produce most of the female sex hormone estrogen, which circulates in your body. This is the follicular phase of your cycle, and it lasts from the first day of your period until you ovulate.

Ovulation occurs in the middle of the menstrual cycle, near day 14. It's at this time that hormone surges trigger one follicle to burst and release its egg. Over the next 36 hours, the egg will travel through your fallopian tubes to reach the uterus.

After ovulation, your body enters the luteal phase. The outer wall of the burst follicle remains in the ovary and transforms into a mass of tissue called the corpus luteum. This tissue begins to secrete another female sex hormone, progesterone, which prepares the uterus for pregnancy. If the egg is not fertilized and pregnancy doesn't occur, the levels of estrogen and progesterone immediately begin to drop. The lining of the uterus and the unfertilized egg are no longer needed and are eliminated from the body through menstruation. This completes the menstrual cycle and the entire process starts all over again.

What Causes PMS?

Researchers don't know exactly what triggers PMS. One of the most popular theories suggests that PMS is caused by an imbalance in the levels of estrogen and progesterone. Symptoms may develop because you have too much estrogen and not enough progesterone in your system during the last two weeks of the menstrual cycle. Estrogen affects the kidneys and causes sodium and water retention. Alterations in estrogen and progesterone can also affect the levels of natural brain chemicals called neurotransmitters. It's thought that deficiencies in serotonin and dopamine, two neurotransmitters that affect mood and emotion, may be responsible for the mood swings typical of PMS.

Excessive levels of a hormone called prolactin may be responsible for breast tenderness and swelling. Prolactin is responsible for stimulating the breast changes and milk production necessary for breastfeeding.

Nutrient deficiencies may also account for certain symptoms of PMS. For instance, breast tenderness may also be caused by a lack of essential fats in the diet, which play an important role in regulating pain and inflammation. A deficiency of calcium may cause agitation, irritability and depression. Low calcium levels may also stimulate an overproduction of parathyroid hormones, which are believed to influence mood and mental function by interacting with the brain chemical serotonin. Dietary deficiencies of vitamin B6, magnesium and zinc or excessive consumption of caffeine, salt, alcohol and red meat may also trigger PMS.

Symptoms

There are more than 150 documented symptoms with the most common being depression. PMS symptoms tend to fall into two main categories:

1. *Physical symptoms* include breast tenderness and swelling, bloating, fluid retention, weight gain, headaches, food cravings (especially for sweet or salty foods), acne, muscle pain, backaches, fatigue, dizziness, sleep disturbances, constipation or diarrhea. Many women gain an average of 2 to 4 pounds during the premenstrual week because of fluid retention. Heavier women may gain as much as 8 pounds.

2. *Emotional or psychological symptoms* include mood swings, depression, irritability, aggressiveness or hostility, anxiety, crying spells, changes in sex drive, difficulty concentrating and feelings of low self-esteem.

PMS symptoms vary from woman to woman, and they can also be different from one menstrual cycle to the next. PMS symptoms tend to get worse as your menstrual cycle progresses and are then relieved when your period begins.

Who's at Risk?

As many as 75 percent of all women experience one or more of the symptoms associated with PMS.[1] But research indicates that only 30 to 40 percent of women between the ages of 25 and 50 years report the recurring symptoms indicative of PMS. And only 5 to 10 percent of women develop symptoms severe enough to disrupt lifestyle and daily functioning.[2]

PMS can begin any time after puberty. Research suggests that you're more susceptible to PMS if you're under a lot of stress, you're younger than 34 years or you drink alcohol.[3] Although heredity may also play a role, PMS symptoms are not consistent in families and vary considerably among female relatives.

Conventional Treatment

Most treatment approaches are directed at relieving symptoms and improving the quality of life. Before you embark on a medication to treat a symptom, try implementing the nutritional approaches suggested below for three consecutive menstrual cycles. If dietary and/or other lifestyle changes don't improve your PMS within three months, you may want to talk to your doctor about medications to reduce your symptoms. Keep in mind that the drugs below can help alleviate symptoms, but some of them have side effects that may cause problems of their own.

- *Diuretics* The drugs eliminate excess fluid from your body through increased urine production; they are often used to treat premenstrual swelling of hands, feet and face.

- *Analgesics (pain killers)* The most effective of these are nonsteroidal anti-inflammatory medications (NSAIDs) such as Anaprox® for headaches, menstrual cramps and pelvic pain.

- *Antidepressants* Used to treat depression and mood disorders associated with PMS, these drugs work by increasing the level of natural brain chemicals that are affected by the female sex hormones. Selective serotonin reuptake inhibitors (SSRIs) such as Prozac® and Zoloft® are the most effective in reducing the psychological symptoms of PMS.

- *Oral contraceptives* These are often prescribed to even out hormonal fluctuations. Some women find that their symptoms are worsened by birth control pills.

- *Ovarian suppressors* Drugs such as Danocrine® (a synthetic hormone related to the male sex hormone testosterone) may be used to stop the menstrual cycle. Side effects of ovarian suppressors include the development of menopausal symptoms, such as vaginal dryness and hot flashes.

Managing PMS

Dietary Strategies

Meal Timing

Plan to eat three meals *and* one or two midday snacks. Levels of neurotransmitters in the brain are susceptible to fluctuations in the levels of nutrients in your bloodstream. So any drastic change in normal eating patterns, such as crash dieting, bingeing, or meal or snack skipping, can alter neurotransmitter levels and mood. The hormonal fluctuations of PMS also make you more susceptible to having a low blood-sugar level, which can cause low energy, increased appetite and hunger, irritability and headache.

Carbohydrates

Studies have found that high-carbohydrate meals produce a calming, relaxing effect by influencing the level of serotonin in the brain. Researchers have linked high serotonin levels with happier moods and low levels with mild depression and irritability in women with PMS. One study found that meals high in carbohydrates improved mood in young women within 30 minutes of consumption.[4] Another study found that when women with PMS took a high-carbohydrate drink, their mood improved within 90 minutes.[5]

Carbohydrate-rich foods like whole-grain bread, cereal, rice and pasta contain an amino acid called tryptophan; eating these foods allows tryptophan to get into the brain. The brain uses tryptophan to make the neurotransmitter serotonin.

If your mood is affected by PMS, eat high-carbohydrate meals that contain very little protein. High-protein foods like chicken, meat or fish supply the body with other amino acids that compete with tryptophan for entry into the brain. Try pasta with tomato sauce, a toasted whole-grain bagel with jam or a bowl of cereal with low-fat milk.

If your mood needs a boost between meals, drink a high-carbohydrate beverage. The next time you're in the United States, drop by a pharmacy and pick up a liquid dietary supplement called PMS Escape™. It's a flavored, powdered drink mix made from a blend of carbohydrates, vitamins and minerals that's thought to act by boosting the normal level of serotonin in the brain. You might also consider trying sports carbohydrate replacement drinks. These are sold at health food stores and sporting good stores as powder mixes or ready-to-drink and come in a variety of flavors.

Low Glycemic Carbohydrates

Nutritionists now classify carbohydrate foods according to their glycemic index (GI), or, their ability to cause a rise in blood sugar. Foods with a low GI value raise blood-sugar levels more slowly than do foods with a high GI value. When you eat a food that raises your blood sugar quickly, you will get a burst of energy. But this spike in sugar also causes your pancreas to release a large amount of insulin into the bloodstream. Since insulin's job is to lower your blood sugar, your quick energy boost will be followed by a crash. That can lead to increased hunger and carbohydrate cravings.

Foods with a low GI value take longer to digest and lead to a gradual, slow rise in blood glucose. You don't get that insulin surge, so the energy from that food lasts longer. The glycemic index of a food depends on cooking time, fiber content, fat content and ripeness. Refer to page 7 Chapter 1, for a list of low glycemic foods.

Dietary Fat

A few studies have found that when women with PMS are put on a low-fat diet, they suffer fewer and less intense PMS symptoms.[6-8] Diets consisting of 15 to 20 percent calories from fat are associated with less water retention, less weight gain and fewer menstrual cramps. A low-fat diet may affect PMS symptoms by influencing the levels of hormones in the body, especially estrogen.

To reduce your intake of dietary fat, choose lower-fat animal foods such as lean meat and poultry breast, and milk and yogurt with 1 percent or less milk fat. Use added fats and oils sparingly. Choose packaged foods with no more than 3 grams of fat per serving. See Chapter 3 for sources of saturated fat and cholesterol.

Sodium

High levels of estrogen associated with PMS can cause the kidneys to retain water and sodium. Eliminating table salt and foods high in sodium the week before your period will help prevent swollen hands and feet.

To help cut back on sodium, avoid the salt-shaker at the table, minimize the use of salt when you cook and buy commercial food products that are low in added salt. Eating fewer processed foods is one of the key strategies to desalt your diet. Most of the salt we consume every day comes from processed and prepared foods—only one-fourth comes from the saltshaker. Aim for no more than 2400 milligrams of sodium each day (that's 1 teaspoon worth of salt). Season your foods with herbs, spices, flavored vinegars and fruit juices. You'll find the sodium content of selected foods on page 80, Chapter 5.

Alcohol and Caffeine

You read earlier that women who drink alcohol are at greater risk for PMS. Alcoholic beverages can trigger or worsen many PMS symptoms, including fatigue, irritability, depression, bowel function, appetite and fluid retention. Alcohol has a dehydrating effect on the body, which can leave you feeling sluggish. Alcohol can also cause fatigue by interfering with the body's ability to fall into REM (rapid eye movement) sleep. This is the restorative phase of sleep that leaves you feeling refreshed and energetic. If you suffer with PMS, avoid alcohol completely during the 7 to 14 days before your menstrual period. During the rest of the month, you should consume no more than seven drinks per week (one a day).

Caffeine can also aggravate irritability, anxiety, headaches, diarrhea, fatigue and breast tenderness. Drinking too much coffee during the day can overstimulate the body, causing irritability, nervousness, anxiety, insomnia and fatigue. As little as two small cups of coffee in the morning can affect your sleep that same night by blocking the brain's production of a natural sleep-inducing chemical called adenosine.

If your PMS symptoms include irritability, anxiousness or general fatigue, consume no more than 200 milligrams of caffeine daily, and preferably none. Switch to low-caffeine beverages like tea or hot chocolate or caffeine-free alternatives such as decaf coffee, herbal tea, cereal coffee, juice, milk or water. The caffeine content of beverages and foods is outlined on page 82, Chapter 5.

Vitamins and Minerals

Vitamin B6

In 1999, British researchers analyzed the results from nine clinical trials involving 940 women with PMS.[9] They concluded that B6 was significantly better than the placebo treatment in relieving PMS-related depression. However, since many of these studies were considered to have flaws, it is not possible to say with certainty that the vitamin is an effective treatment for PMS.

The studies do suggest, however, that doses of B6 up to 100 milligrams per day are likely to benefit women who experience premenstrual depression. A recent study published in 1999 from the University of Reading in Great Britain found that 50 milligrams of B6 combined with 200 milligrams of magnesium had a significant but modest effect on reducing anxiety-related PMS symptoms, including nervous tension, mood swings, irritability and anxiety.[10]

B6 is needed in the body for the production of two brain chemicals, serotonin and dopamine, which have a potent effect on mood. Dopamine also regulates the secretion of prolactin, a hormone that may be linked to PMS.

To use B6 for PMS-related depression, take 50 to 100 milligrams of vitamin B6 three days before the expected onset of your symptoms. Stop taking it one or two days after your period begins (i.e., day 2 or 3 of your menstrual cycle). Not only have studies *not* demonstrated a better effect by taking more B6, but supplementing with too much B6 for a period of time has toxic effects, including irreversible nerve damage.

Vitamin E

Three randomized clinical trials revealed that vitamin E supplements improved PMS-related mood swings, anxiety, headache, food cravings and insomnia.[11-13] In one study, women with PMS were given either 150 international units (IU), 300 IU or 600 IU of vitamin E. All doses were more effective at relieving symptoms than the placebo pill.

How vitamin E works to help your PMS is not understood. The richest sources of vitamin E are vegetable oils, nuts, seeds and wheat germ. Leafy green vegetables (especially kale) are also good sources. But if you consider that 1 tablespoon (15 ml) of olive oil provides only 2.6 IU of the vita-

min, you can see why you must rely on a supplement to get 400 to 600 IU. Even 2 tablespoons (30 ml) of toasted wheat germ gives you a mere 4 IU.

To supplement, take 200 to 800 IU of natural source vitamin E. Buy a "mixed" vitamin E supplement if possible. The daily upper limit is 1500 IU.

Calcium

A well-designed study of 466 women found that those who took 1200 milligrams of supplemental calcium daily for three months had a significant reduction in PMS symptoms, especially mood swings, low back pain, food cravings and fluid retention.[14] The majority of women experienced a 50 percent reduction in overall symptoms (compared with a 36 percent improvement among women who took the placebo pill). The strongest improvement was observed during the third menstrual cycle, which implies that the effect of calcium supplements increases with continued use.

Many of the symptoms of a calcium deficiency are similar to those of PMS. Researchers have found that blood levels of calcium are low in women with PMS. Low calcium levels cause an overproduction of parathyroid hormone, which interacts with serotonin in the brain to affect mood. Calcium supplements may ease PMS symptoms by replenishing a deficiency of the mineral.

The recommended dietary allowance (RDA) for calcium is 1000 to 1300 milligrams. The best food sources are milk, yogurt, cheese, fortified soy and rice beverages, fortified orange juice, tofu, salmon (with bones), kale, bok choy, broccoli and Swiss chard. To supplement, take 300 milligrams of calcium citrate one to three times daily, depending on your dietary calcium intake. See Chapter 4 for more information about calcium supplements.

Magnesium

Research has found that increasing your intake of this mineral can improve symptoms of depression, anxiety, fluid retention and breast tenderness.[15,16] Magnesium is found in all body cells and fluids, where it is needed to maintain fluid balance by pumping sodium and potassium in and out of cells. It's also used by over 300 enzymes, including those that produce energy. Studies have found that women with PMS tend to have lower blood levels of magnesium.[17,18]

The best sources of magnesium are whole foods, including unrefined grains, nuts, seeds, legumes, dried fruit and green vegetables. Studies have determined a daily dose of 200 to 360 milligrams of supplemental magnesium to be effective in easing PMS symptoms. If you take calcium supplements, buy one with magnesium added. A 2:1 calcium citrate supplement will generally give you 300 milligrams of calcium and 150 milligrams of magnesium. Depending on your diet, you might need to take one of these supplements two or three times a day.

If you don't need supplemental calcium, buy a supplement made from magnesium citrate, aspartate, succinate, fumarte or gluconate. The body absorbs these forms of the mineral more efficiently. The daily upper safe limit for magnesium is 350 milligrams per day from a supplement—more than this can cause diarrhea, nausea and stomach cramps.

Herbal Remedies

Chasteberry (*Vitex angus-castus*)
European physicians have been prescribing this herbal remedy for more than 40 years to regulate the menstrual cycle and ease PMS symptoms. One German study, which followed more than 1600 women with PMS for three months, found that 93 percent of women taking chasteberry reported symptom improvement or complete relief of mood swings, anxiety, food cravings and/or fluid retention.[19] While there are a limited number of well-controlled clinical studies assessing the effectiveness of chasteberry, the experience of physicians has long established the practical use of the herb in women with PMS.

The recommended dose is 175 to 225 milligrams once daily. Buy a product standardized to contain 0.5 percent agnuside and 0.6 percent aucubin. It takes at least four weeks for the herb to start working and several months for it to reach its full effect. Mild side effects may include nausea, headache and skin rash.

Since chasteberry inhibits prolactin secretion (prolactin is necessary for milk production), the herb should not be used during breastfeeding. The herb may interact with medications that influence the brain chemical dopamine, such as the antidepressants Wellbutrin® and Effexor®. Inform your doctor if you take such a medication and chasteberry. Use caution if you are taking birth control pills or hormone replacement therapy, since it is possible that the herb could interfere with the effectiveness of these medications.

Evening Primrose Oil (*Oenothera biennis*)
Supplements of evening primrose oil are a rich source of gamma linolenic acid (GLA). GLA is a fatty acid the body uses to make special compounds called prostaglandins that decrease inflammation and pain. Researchers studying women with PMS have focused on a beneficial prostaglandin called PGE_1.

GLA is formed in the body from linoleic acid, an essential fatty acid found in vegetable oils, nuts and seeds. Some experts believe that women with PMS have a reduced ability to make PGE_1 from linoleic acid in the diet and that this can cause symptoms such as breast pain and tenderness, irritability, depression and headache. Many dietary factors, such as animal fat, alcohol and hydrogenated vegetable oils, can also interfere with the conversion of linoleic acid to GLA. The enzyme responsible for this conversion requires zinc, magnesium and vitamins B6 and C to function properly. So a high-fat diet that's missing important vitamins and minerals can hamper GLA production and contribute to low levels of PGE_1.

A number of studies have investigated the effectiveness of evening primrose oil in alleviating PMS symptoms. A handful of studies in the 1980s found that daily supplements of evening primrose oil outperformed the placebo treatment in improving PMS symptoms of breast tenderness, irritability and depression. However, studies performed over the past ten years have not found evening primrose oil to be an effective treatment for PMS as a whole, possibly because the doses used were too low or the supplement was not taken long enough.

Evening primrose oil does appear to offer promise for treating breast pain and tenderness. Research has shown the supplement to be as effective as certain drugs used to treat cyclic breast pain. Investigators from the University of Wales in Great Britain concluded that evening primrose oil was the best first-line therapy for cyclic breast pain, providing relief with essentially no side effects.[20]

To treat PMS breast pain and tenderness, the effective dose is 1.5 to 2 grams taken twice daily. Buy a supplement standardized to contain 9 percent GLA. It can take three menstrual cycles to feel the effects of evening primrose oil and up to eight months for full effectiveness.

Ginkgo Biloba

The finding that ginkgo helped women with PMS occurred by accident. Women who were taking ginkgo for brain health noticed that fluid retention associated with their menstrual cycle lessened while on the herb. Then, in 1993, researchers from France conducted a formal study of 143 women with PMS.[21] They found ginkgo to be significantly more effective than the placebo in treating PMS-related breast tenderness, abdominal bloating and swollen hands, legs and feet. The women in the study took ginkgo on day 16 of

their cycle and continued until day 5 of their next cycle, at which time they stopped. They resumed taking the herbal remedy again on day 16.

The recommended dose of ginkgo is 40 to 80 milligrams three times daily. Start on day 16 (ovulation) and continue until the end of your next period (day 5 to 7). Buy a product standardized to contain 24 percent ginkgo flavone glycosides.

A small number of women have reported that the herb caused mild stomach upset. Ginkgo should not be taken with blood-thinning drugs such as warfarin (Coumadin®), heparin or Trental® unless your doctor is monitoring you. It is also possible that ginkgo can enhance the effect of other natural health products that also thin the blood, such as vitamin E or garlic. Inform your physician and pharmacist if you are taking more than one of these products.

St. John's Wort (*Hypericum perforatum*)

This yellow-flowered plant has long been heralded for its ability to balance emotions. It is widely used in Europe to treat both mild depression and seasonal affective disorder. An analysis of 26 controlled studies conducted in 1700 patients concluded that the herb was as effective as certain antidepressant drugs in treating mild to moderate depression.[22] More recently, a small pilot study found that St. John's wort taken daily for two months yielded significant improvements in PMS-related depression.[23]

Experts believe the herb eases depression by keeping brain serotonin levels high for a longer period of time, the same way that the antidepressant drugs Paxil®, Zoloft® and Prozac® do. The effective dosage is 300 milligrams taken three times daily. Buy a product standardized to 0.3 percent hypericin and 3 to 5 percent hyperforin. The European formula used in the clinical research is sold as Movana® (Pharmaton® Natural Health Products) in North America. This extract has been used in clinical studies.

St. John's wort has been reported to cause sensitivity to sunlight in very light-skinned individuals. The herb also has the potential to interact with a number of medications. Do not take the herb if you are taking indinavir, cyclosporine, theophylline, warfarin, birth control pills or digoxin. St. John's wort is not recommended for use during pregnancy and breastfeeding. If you are currently taking a prescription antidepressant drug, do not take it concurrently with St. John's wort. Be sure to consult your physician before stopping any medication.

Kava Kava (*Piper methysticum*)

This herb may relieve PMS-related anxiety, apprehension or nervousness. Three double-blind, randomized, placebo-controlled trials proved the effectiveness of kava against the Hamilton Rating Scale for Anxiety, a tool used by psychiatrists to measure levels of anxiety.[24] Another study found that menopausal women with anxiety disorders obtained significant relief with kava, without the negative side effects of conventional drugs like Valium.[25] Experts believe that kava's active ingredients, kavalactones, exert their effect by working on the limbic system of the brain, the center of emotions.

The daily dose of kava used in the studies ranges from 60 to 120 milligrams of kavalactones. Buy a product standardized to 30 percent kavalactones. This means that every 100 milligram capsule provides 30 milligrams of kavalactones. To achieve a dose of 60 to 120 milligrams of kavalactones, you will need to take two to four capsules per day. You should notice relief in one week, but it can take up to a month for the herb to reach its full effect.

The herb should not be used with alcohol, tranquilizers, antidepressants or sedatives. Its safety has not been evaluated in pregnant or nursing women or people with liver or kidney disease.

Nutrition Strategy Checklist for PMS

- ☐ Three meals plus two snacks
- ☐ Low GI carbohydrates
- ☐ Low fat
- ☐ Low sodium
- ☐ Avoid caffeine and alcohol
- ☐ Vitamin B6 OR St John's wort (if depression is only symptom)
- ☐ Vitamin E
- ☐ Calcium
- ☐ Magnesium
- ☐ Chasteberry (overall symptom relief)
- ☐ Evening primrose oil
- ☐ Kava kava (for anxiety)

Recommended Resources

www.askdrkoop.com
Founded by former US Surgeon General Dr. Everett Koop.

www.mayoclinic.com
Mayo Foundation for Medical Education and Research

www.pms.org.uk
National Association for Premenstrual Syndrome
7 Swift's Court, High Street
Seal, Kent, UK TN15 0EG
Tel: 01-732-760011 or 01-732-760012 (helpline)

Prostate Cancer

Prostate cancer is now the most commonly diagnosed form of cancer in Canadian men.[1] Since 1994, the incidence of prostate cancer has begun to decline, after several decades of rapid increase. By the age of 50, as many as one in four men will have some cancerous cells in their prostate gland. That number increases to one in two by the time men reach the age of 70, and it is estimated that almost every male over the age of 90 has the disease.[2]

What Causes Prostate Cancer?

The prostate is a male sex gland located below the bladder and in front of the rectum. It surrounds the urethra, which is the tube that carries both urine and semen out of the body. The prostate gland contributes to reproductive function by producing a milky fluid that helps to keep the sperm nourished, mobile and healthy. This fluid forms part of the semen, the sperm-carrying fluid released during ejaculation.

Cancer develops when abnormal or mutated cells go out of control, damaging the body's vital organs or tissues. As mutated cells accumulate, they form a mass or clump that is known as a tumor. In the case of prostate cancer, the tumor often remains inside the prostate gland, causing few symptoms until the cancer has reached an advanced stage. Sometimes, however, the cancer cells invade and destroy normal tissue, spreading to other organs and bones, where they can cause life-threatening problems. Very often, prostate cancer spreads to the lymph nodes, to the bones of the pelvis, ribs and spine or to the kidneys, where it causes kidney failure.

Scientists have not yet determined what causes abnormal cell growth in prostate tissues. Theories focus on genetics, hormones, environment and diet as key factors that influence prostate cancer risk.

Screening for Prostate Cancer

Considerable progress has been made in both the diagnosis and treatment of prostate cancer. If diagnosed at an early stage, prostate cancer can be cured. Unfortunately, more than 40 percent of all cases are not diagnosed until the cancer is advanced and has spread beyond the prostate gland.[3] To help improve the chances of early detection, doctors routinely screen for prostate cancer in men over the age of 40. A digital rectal exam is the most common and simplest diagnostic test for prostate cancer. Your doctor will manually check your prostate, using a gloved finger to feel for unusual bumps or hard spots on the gland wall. While the majority of tumors can be felt this way, approximately one-third of all prostate tumors develop deeper within the gland and cannot be detected during a digital rectal exam.

The prostate-specific antigen (PSA) blood test is rapidly becoming one of the most reliable indicators of prostate cancer. Normally, the prostate generates PSA as part of the fluid production process necessary for healthy semen. A small amount of this substance also circulates in the bloodstream. In approximately one-third of all cases, elevated blood PSA levels indicate prostate cancer. High levels may also be the result of less serious conditions such as prostate enlargement, prostate infections and the use of certain drugs or herbal medications.

Symptoms

Often there are no symptoms in the early stages of the disease. The symptoms that do occur are very similar to those of benign prostatic hyperplasia (BPH), commonly known as prostate enlargement (see page 494). These symptoms include

- chronic, dull pain in the lower pelvis, lower back or upper thighs
- pain during urination
- sudden need to urinate
- frequent urination during the night
- difficulty starting to urinate, dribbling, weak urine flow
- blood or pus in the urine

- painful ejaculation
- loss of appetite and weight

Who's at Risk?

- *Older men* Most cases are diagnosed in men over the age of 65.
- *Certain racial or ethnic groups* Black men have a 60 percent higher incidence of prostate cancer than white men, and Asian men have the lowest incidence.
- *Men with a family history of the disease* Having a father or brother with the disease doubles the risk and is associated with developing the prostate cancer at an earlier age.
- Men who eat *a high-fat diet.*

Conventional Treatment

Prostate cancer is very slow growing and is not usually an aggressive type of cancer. Only 3 percent of the men diagnosed with prostate cancer actually die of the disease. Treatment for prostate cancer will vary, depending on how far the cancer has spread, how fast the cancer is growing, your age and your general health.

Older men with early-stage, slow-growing cancer may not need treatment because their risk of dying from the disease is not high. Watchful waiting for symptoms and a regular program of PSA tests and rectal exams may be sufficient to monitor the disease. For younger men, the most effective treatment involves surgery to remove the prostate gland. This procedure is known as radical prostatectomy. However, research indicates that cancer recurs in 30 percent of all men who have surgery.

Radiation therapy to kill cancerous cells may be used for older men in poor health who may have difficulty withstanding surgery. Cryotherapy, a procedure in which liquid nitrogen is used to freeze and destroy cancerous cells, may also be used. Impotence results from cryotherapy in 90 percent of cases. Hormone therapy may be used to prevent male sex hormones from speeding up the growth of cancer cells.

Prostate cancer and the treatments used to control the disease can cause a number of complications, including incontinence, impotence, reduced libido, breast enlargement and depression.

Preventing and Managing Prostate Cancer

Most of the nutritional recommendations focus on reducing the risk of prostate cancer. A few strategies, however, may also prevent the progression of cancer. The herbal remedy PC-SPES, which is discussed below, is being studied as an alternative form of prostate cancer treatment. For an excellent summary on the effectiveness of various alternative therapies used to treat cancer, visit **www.cancer.nci.nih.gov/treatment/cam.html**.

Dietary Strategies
A Healthy Diet
Dietary Fat
Studies comparing the diets of men with prostate cancer to those of men free of the disease have found a number of foods linked to development and progression of the cancer. Most notable is the link between saturated animal fat and prostate cancer. Many studies have found that men who have higher intakes of total fat and of animal fat increase their risk for the disease and also have more advanced forms of prostate cancer.[4-9] When mice are injected with human prostate cancer cells and fed a high-fat diet, the cancer grows faster. Dietary fat is believed to increase the level of circulating hormones that may cause prostate cancer.

Follow a low-fat diet by choosing lean cuts of meat (flank steak, inside round, pork tenderloin), poultry breast without the skin, skim or 1 percent milk and yogurt and skim-milk cheese. Use butter sparingly. If you eat meat, consume no more than 3 ounces (90 grams) per day.

Vegetable Protein

More often, substitute animal protein with vegetarian protein foods such as legumes and soy foods. Eating more legumes, such as kidney beans, chickpeas and lentils, has been associated with a lower risk of prostate cancer.[10,11] As well, beans contain phyto (plant) estrogens called isoflavones that may slow the growth of prostate tumors.

Fish

Eating more fish will also help you reduce animal fat in your diet. Fish contains omega-3 fatty acids, compounds that have been shown in the laboratory to inhibit cancer growth. Some evidence suggests that men with higher levels of these fatty acids in their blood have a lower risk of prostate cancer.[12] Aim to eat fish at least three times per week.

Whole Grains

Consuming plenty of whole-grain breads, cereals, brown rice, whole-wheat pasta and other whole grains has also been linked with protection from prostate cancer.[13] These foods offer fiber, phytoestrogens, vitamin E, selenium, flavonoids and antioxidants—all of which may play a role in prostate cancer prevention.

Vegetables and Fruits

When it comes to fruits and vegetables, cruciferous vegetables appear to offer the most protection from prostate cancer. One large study found that men with the highest intake of these vegetables had a 39 percent lower risk of the cancer.[14] Broccoli, bok choy, cabbage, cauliflower, kale and turnip contain isothiocyanates, natural chemicals that have been shown to help the liver detoxify cancer-causing substances. Orange and yellow vegetables and tomatoes are also protective (see more on lycopene-rich foods below).

Alcohol, Green Tea

Some research suggests that drinking alcohol, regardless of the type, increases prostate cancer risk.[15] If you drink, consume no more than nine drinks per week.

Green tea may be beneficial. Studies have found that populations that drink green tea regularly have lower rates of prostate cancer. Laboratory studies have determined that natural chemicals in green tea, called flavonoids, have anticancer properties.

Lycopene

Lycopene is an antioxidant compound found in red-colored vegetables and fruits; it is especially abundant in tomatoes. One large study from Harvard University found that men who consumed ten or more servings of tomato-based foods per week had a 35 percent lower risk of prostate cancer compared with those who ate less than 1.5 servings per week.[16] Eating tomatoes, tomato sauce, tomato juice and pizza offered protection. Other studies have also related tomato-based foods to a lower risk of prostate cancer.[17-19]

Researchers have also learned that prostate cancer risk is significantly higher in men who have low blood and tissue levels of lycopene.[20-22] Lycopene taken in high supplemental doses is currently being studied for its potential as a treatment for prostate cancer.

A daily intake of 5 to 7 milligrams of lycopene appears to offer protection. While the foods below are all good sources of lycopene, heat-processed tomato products provide a source of lycopene that is much more available to the body. Lycopene is a fat-soluble compound, which means it is better absorbed when eaten with a little fat.

Food	Lycopene (milligrams)
Tomato, raw, 1 small	0.8–3.8 mg
Tomatoes, cooked, 1 cup (250 ml)	9.25 mg
Tomato sauce, 1/2 cup (125 ml)	3.1 mg
Tomato paste, 2 tbsp (30 ml)	8.0 mg
Tomato juice, 1 cup (250 ml)	23.0 mg
Ketchup, 2 tbsp (30 ml)	3.1–4.2 mg
Apricots, dried, 10 halves	0.3 mg
Grapefruit, pink, 1/2	4.2 mg
Papaya, 1 whole	6.2–16.5 mg
Watermelon, 1 slice (25 cm × 2 cm)	8.5–26.4 mg

Soy Foods

Asian men and vegetarian men have much lower rates of prostate cancer, an observation that has been linked to a higher intake of soy foods. A study of California Seventh-Day Adventist men found that drinking soy milk more than once a day was associated with a 70 percent lower risk of prostate cancer.[23]

Soybeans contain isoflavones, phytoestrogens that have been shown to inhibit the growth of prostate tumors in animal studies and laboratory studies using human prostate cancer cells. One study is underway at the University of New York to determine if eating soy on a regular basis will reduce the risk of prostate cancer recurrence in men. American researchers are also in the midst of investigating the effect of soy food consumption on markers of prostate cancer in men.

So far, however, the evidence looks promising that soy foods may protect the prostate. To increase your intake, begin by replacing three animal-based meals each week with soy. Tofu, soy meats, soy nuts, soy milk, canned soybeans and tempeh are all good choices. Read page 72, Chapter 5, to learn how to incorporate these foods into your diet.

Vitamins and Minerals

Vitamin D

Our requirements for this vitamin are met through food intake and exposure to sunlight. The sun's ultraviolet rays trigger the skin to produce vitamin D. The fact that populations that get little exposure to sunlight have higher rates of prostate cancer has led researchers to speculate that vitamin D is somehow involved. The recent finding that the prostate can also metabolize vitamin D has opened up investigations into vitamin D and cancer prevention. Laboratory studies have found that vitamin D inhibits the growth of human prostate cancer cells.

As we age, our skin becomes less efficient at producing vitamin D, and this may contribute to prostate cancer risk. The adequate daily intake for vitamin D is 200 to 600 international units (IU), depending on your age (see page 39, Chapter 4). Food sources of vitamin D are limited to fluid milk, fortified soy and rice beverages, oily fish, egg yolks, butter and margarine. Your multivitamin and mineral should provide 400 IU of vitamin D. High supplemental intakes of vitamin D have the potential for harm and should be used under the guidance of your doctor. The upper daily limit is 2000 IU.

Vitamin E

Higher intakes of vitamin E are linked with a lower risk of prostate cancer. Researchers have also observed that men, especially those who smoke, with lower blood levels of this nutrient are at increased risk.[24,25] A number of studies suggest that vitamin E supplements help prevent prostate cancer. One large trial from Finland found that male smokers who took 50 milligrams of vitamin E had a 32 percent lower risk of the cancer compared with nonsupplement users.[26] Harvard researchers also learned that 100 IU of vitamin E protected current smokers and recent quitters from fatal prostate cancer.[27]

Vitamin E is a potent antioxidant and may protect prostate cells from free radical damage, which can lead to cancer. The vitamin may also prevent prostate cancer by altering the levels of sex hormones in the blood. An American study conducted among 100 older men found that taking 100 IU of vitamin E per day resulted in significantly lower levels of androstenedione and testosterone, two hormones implicated in prostate cancer development.[28]

The recommended dietary intake for vitamin E is 22 IU. Foods rich in vitamin E include wheat germ, nuts, seeds, vegetable oils, whole grains and kale. To supplement, take 100 to 800 IU of natural source vitamin E. Buy a "mixed" vitamin E supplement that contains gamma-tocopherol, a form of vitamin E that may offer added protection from prostate cancer.[29] The daily upper limit is 1500 IU.

Selenium

The protective effects of this mineral were discovered by accident when researchers from Arizona investigated the effect of selenium supplement on skin cancer recurrence.[30] Men with a history of skin cancer were given 200 micrograms of selenium or a placebo and followed for four and a half years. While the risk of skin cancer was unaffected, there was a significant reduction in prostate cancer among men taking selenium supplements. In areas like the northeastern United States and Canada, where the selenium level in the soil is low, rates of prostate cancer are higher.

Selenium acts as an antioxidant in the body, protecting cells from the damaging effects of free radicals. The recommended dietary intake for selenium is 55 micrograms, an amount easy to get from the diet by consuming foods like seafood, chicken, organ meats, whole grains, nuts, onions, garlic and mushrooms.

To prevent prostate cancer, a dose of 200 micrograms is recommended. Buy a supplement made from selenium-rich yeast. Do not exceed 400 micrograms per day.

Herbal Remedies

Garlic (*Allium sativum*)

Eating more garlic and taking garlic supplements may offer protection from prostate cancer. Researchers from the United Kingdom studied 328 men with prostate cancer and found that those who ate garlic at least twice weekly had a 44 percent lower risk of prostate cancer compared with those who never consumed it.[31] Compared with men who never used garlic supplements, those who used supplements at least twice weekly had a 60 percent lower risk of the cancer.

Garlic contains natural sulfur compounds that have been shown in the laboratory to enhance the immune system and inhibit the growth of prostate cancer cells. One study found that compounds in aged garlic extract suppress the growth of hormone-responsive prostate cancer cells.[32,33]

To boost your intake of garlic, reach for it when you are cooking. To supplement, buy a product made with aged garlic extract. Take two to six capsules a day in divided doses. Aged garlic extract is odorless and less irritating to the gastrointestinal tract than other forms of garlic supplements. Garlic (both fresh and supplements) may enhance the effects of blood-thinning medications like warfarin (Coumadin®). If you are taking this drug and garlic at the same time, be sure to inform your doctor.

PC-SPES

This Chinese herbal supplement is being increasingly used by prostate cancer patients in whom conventional treatments have failed or by those who opt for alternative therapy. PC-SPES is a formula containing eight different herbs: chrysanthemum, dyers woad, licorice, reishi, panax pseudo-ginseng, rabdosia, saw palmetto and baikal skullcap.

Studies have found the formula to be useful in the treatment of advanced metastatic prostate cancer, hormone-dependent prostate cancer and in cases where conventional therapy has failed.[34-36] The herbal supplement has been shown to reduce PSA levels, ease pain and improve quality of life. As well, laboratory studies have demonstrated the herb's anticancer effects on human prostate cells.[37-39]

PC-SPES will cause side effects and should be used only under your doctor's supervision. If you are interested in learning more about this alternative treatment, consult your specialist.

Nutrition Strategy Checklist for Preventing Prostate Cancer

- ☐ Low animal fat
- ☐ Fish
- ☐ Whole grains
- ☐ Vegetables and fruit
- ☐ Limit alcohol
- ☐ Green tea
- ☐ Lycopene-rich foods
- ☐ Soy foods
- ☐ Vitamin D
- ☐ Vitamin E
- ☐ Selenium
- ☐ Garlic

Recommended Resources

www.cancer.ca
Canadian Cancer Society
10 Alcorn Avenue, Suite 200
Toronto, ON, Canada M4V 3B1
Tel: 416-961-7223
Fax: 416-961-4189

cancernet.nci.nih.gov
A service provided by the National Cancer Institute
Public Inquiries Office
Building 31, Room 10A31, 31 Center Drive, MSC 2580
Bethesda, MD, USA 20892-2580
Tel: 301-435-3848 or 1-800-4-CANCER (1-800-422-6237) (help-line)

www.mayoclinic.com
Mayo Foundation for Medical Education and Research

Prostate Enlargement (Benign Prostatic Hyperplasia)

The causes of prostate enlargement, or benign prostatic hyperplasia (BPH), are not fully understood. The prostate is responsible for making the fluid that nourishes the sperm and helps them move through the reproductive system. The fluid forms part of the semen, which is the milky sperm-carrying substance released during ejaculation. The prostate gland develops steadily throughout childhood and adolescence, growing to the size of a walnut by the time a child reaches adulthood.

As a man approaches his 40s, the prostate often enters a new growth phase, which might be a response to the natural drop in production of the male hormone testosterone. This reduction in testosterone production allows higher levels of estrogen to circulate in the bloodstream. Researchers speculate that this increase in estrogen may somehow trigger prostate cells to begin growing again. An accumulation of dihydrotestosterone (DHT), a substance derived from testosterone, has also been shown to stimulate new cell growth. The growing tissues of the prostate gland can swell up to three times their normal size, interfering with urine flow.

Because the prostate gland surrounds the urethra, the tube that carries both urine and semen out of the body, changes in the prostate gland almost inevitably affect the urinary tract. As prostate tissues grow, they begin to press on the urethra. This blocks the flow of urine, forcing the bladder muscles to work harder to push the urine out through the tube. The bladder wall thickens and becomes more irritable. Once this happens, the bladder starts to contract more often, leading to frequent urination, especially at night. Eventually, the bladder muscles weaken, preventing the bladder from emptying completely. Urine that remains in the bladder usually becomes stagnant, increasing the risk of bladder infections, incontinence and kidney problems. Sometimes, the prostate can grow so large that it blocks the flow of urine completely, a situation that requires immediate medical attention.

Symptoms

The symptoms of BPH are very similar to those of prostate cancer, and your doctor will suggest diagnostic tests, including a digital rectal exam and a prostate-specific antigen (PSA) blood test, to rule out cancer as a cause of your urinary problems. Fortunately, having BPH does not seem to increase the risk of developing prostate cancer. Early diagnosis and treatment does decrease the likelihood of developing the other complications associated with this condition.

Symptoms of prostate enlargement rarely develop before age 40. The size of the swelling or obstruction does not determine how severe the symptoms will be. Men with only a small amount of enlargement may have greater problems than men with significant swelling. Symptoms can include

- difficulty starting to urinate
- more frequent urination, especially at night
- urgent need to urinate
- weak urine stream
- dribbling and leaking at the end of urination
- urinary incontinence
- blocked urination

Who's at Risk?

More than half of all men in their 60s and 90 percent of all men in their 80s have some signs of the urinary complications associated with prostate enlargement.[1] This condition develops in older men, usually after age 40. It is more common in North American and European men and less common among Asian men. Married men seem to suffer from prostate enlargement more often than single men. Men with a family history of prostate enlargement appear to have a higher risk of developing the condition themselves.

Conventional Treatment

If symptoms are not bothersome, watchful waiting may be the recommended approach. Lifestyle changes can help control symptoms, including

- limiting the amount of liquid you drink after 7 p.m. to reduce the need to urinate at night
- emptying your bladder completely when you urinate
- reducing alcohol intake, since alcohol increases urine production
- avoiding over-the-counter cold medicines and antihistamines, which can cause muscles to tighten, reducing urine flow
- exercising regularly
- staying warm, since cold temperatures can lead to urine retention

Various medications may be used to shrink or stop the growth of the prostate. Alpha-blockers relax muscles in the pelvis, making it easier to urinate. Finasteride inhibits the production of DHT, which helps shrink the prostate.

Heat therapy, in which heat energy is sent to the prostate tissue through the urethra, may also be recommended. Heat therapy is more effective than drugs in treating moderate to severe symptoms.

Surgery is the most effective treatment for relieving symptoms; however, it's not used often because other treatments are now available. Surgery is the treatment most likely to produce side effects, including loss of bladder control and impotence, which are usually temporary.

Managing Prostate Enlargement

Dietary Strategies

A Healthy Diet

Dietary factors that increase the risk of prostate cancer also increase the risk of prostate enlargement. Studies have revealed that men with the condition have higher intakes of fat, especially animal fat, and lower intakes of vegetables, fruit and omega-3 fats found in fish.[2-4] For optimal prostate health, follow the dietary guidelines outlined on page 490, Prostate Cancer. Pay particular attention to reducing animal fat and increasing your intake of fruits and vegetables.

Soy foods also play a role in preventing prostate enlargement. Populations that consume soy on a regular basis have much lower rates of prostate disease, including prostate enlargement. Foods made from soybeans contain natural plant estrogens called isoflavones. One of the main isoflavones in soybeans, genistein, has been shown to decrease the growth of prostate tissue. Soy isoflavones may protect the prostate by inhibiting the action of growth-promoting hormones. Include soy foods in your diet at least three times per week, preferably daily. Refer to Chapter 5 for ways to incorporate a variety of soy foods into your diet.

Flaxseed is a source of plant estrogens called lignans. Although studies have not examined the influence of flaxseed on prostate enlargement, it is thought to work in the same manner as soy isoflavones. Include 1 to 2 tablespoons (15 to 30 ml) of ground flaxseed in your daily diet. Ground flaxseed can be added to hot cereal, smoothies, yogurt, applesauce and pancake and quick bread batters.

Vitamins and Minerals

Zinc

The prostate gland contains more zinc than any other tissue in the body. And it appears to be very important for prostate health, although its exact role in prostate enlargement is still unclear. Researchers do know that the mineral helps many enzymes perform their tasks. Zinc also seems to inhibit male sex hormone metabolism in the prostate.

The recommended dietary intake of zinc for men is 11 milligrams per day. To prevent a deficiency, include zinc-rich foods in your daily diet. Foods such as oysters, seafood, lean red meat, poultry, yogurt, wheat bran, wheat germ, whole grains and enriched breakfast cereals are all good sources. A detailed list of foods and their zinc content can be found on page 62, Chapter 4.

Most adult multivitamin and mineral formulas provide 10 to 20 milligrams of zinc. Single zinc supplements are rarely appropriate. Too much zinc has toxic effects, including copper deficiency, heart problems and anemia.

Herbal Remedies

Saw Palmetto (*Serenoa repens*)

Of all the herbal extracts found to improve symptoms of prostate enlargement, saw palmetto has been the most heavily studied. A review of 18 randomized controlled trials involving 2939 men concluded that the herb was significantly better than a placebo and as effective as the drug finasteride at improving urologic symptoms.[5]

Saw palmetto has been shown to improve overall urinary symptom scores. Men taking the herb experience increased urine flow and reduced frequency of nighttime urination. Compared with standard drug treatment, saw palmetto is associated with fewer side effects.

Saw palmetto appears to block the conversion of testosterone to DHT and prevents DHT from binding to prostate cells. The herb may also have anti-inflammatory and antiestrogenic properties.

The recommended dose is 160 milligrams taken twice daily. Buy a product standardized to contain 85 to 95 percent fatty acids and sterols. Improvement may take up to two months of treatment. On rare occasions, saw palmetto may cause stomach upset and headache.

Pygeum (*Pygeum africanum*)

This herb may be used instead of saw palmetto to treat prostate enlargement. Pygeum comes from the bark of an African tree and has a long history of use for urinary problems. A review of 18 trials conducted among 1562 men found that the herb achieved modestly large improvements in symptoms such as urinary flow and nighttime urination.[6]

Unlike saw palmetto, pygeum is not thought to affect DHT levels. Rather, it is thought to have anti-inflammatory effects in the prostate and to inhibit the action of growth factors.

The recommended dose is 50 milligrams taken twice daily or 100 milligrams taken once daily. Buy a product standardized to contain 14 percent triterpenes and 0.5 percent n-docosanol. Pygeum is very safe. It may cause mild stomach upset in some individuals.

Researchers have also found that pygeum is more effective at relieving symptoms when it is combined with stinging nettle root (see below).[7] The recommended dose of such a combination product is 25 milligrams of pygeum and 300 milligrams of stinging nettle, taken twice daily. One study found that half of this dosage was equally effective.[8] Prostatonin® (Pharmaton® Natural Health Products) provides the combination extract used in the clinical research and is available in Canada and the United States.

Stinging Nettle (*Urtica dioica*)

This herb is often recommended as a stand-alone treatment for prostate enlargement, despite the limited number of studies evaluating its use. At this time, there is no good evidence that stinging nettle is effective except in combination with pygeum.[9] Stinging nettle is thought to affect prostate cell membranes in such a way that cell growth is suppressed. It has also been shown to prevent sex hormones from binding to prostate cell receptors.[10]

Rye Grass Pollen (*Secale cereale*)

Cernilton is a product made from rye grass pollen that has been used in Europe to treat prostate enlargement. A review of two well-controlled trials enrolling 444 men found that rye grass pollen improves overall urinary symptoms, including nighttime urination.[11] In one study, researchers noted that men taking the supplement had significantly reduced prostate size. How rye grass pollen works is unclear. It is thought that it may have anti-inflammatory effects and relieve fluid build-up in the prostate.

The recommended dose is 80 to 120 milligrams per day. No side effects have been noted other than occasional stomach upset. This product has been processed to remove allergy-causing proteins, so individuals with an allergy to grass pollen should not react.

Other Natural Health Products

Beta-Sitosterol

Fruits, vegetables, grains, nuts and seeds contain naturally occurring compounds called sterols. Beta-sitosterol is one plant sterol that has been used to treat symptoms of prostate enlargement. A review of four trials conducted among 519 men found beta-sitosterol effective at improving urinary symptoms and flow measures.[12] The supplement has not been shown to affect prostate size. Beta-sitosterol binds to prostate cell receptors and appears to exert anti-inflammatory effects in the prostate.

The recommended dose is 20 to 130 milligrams taken two to three times per day. Beta-sitosterol may take up to four weeks to have an effect. Most clinical studies have used 60 milligrams per day. After improvement, the dose can be reduced to 10 to 65 milligrams two or three times daily. No significant adverse effects have been reported.

Products sold in Canada and the United States contain a combination of plant sterols. Moducare™ (by Dynapro) contains 20.2 milligrams of plant sterols from soy and pine and is readily available in supplement stores.

Nutrition Strategy Checklist for Prostate Enlargement

- ☐ Low animal fat
- ☐ Fruit and vegetables
- ☐ Soy foods
- ☐ Zinc
- ☐ Saw palmetto OR Pygeum/Stinging nettle
- ☐ Rye grass pollen
- ☐ Beta-sitosterol

Recommended Resources

www.mayoclinic.com
Mayo Foundation for Medical Education and Research

www.niddk.nih.gov/
National Kidney and Urologic Diseases Information Clearinghouse
The National Institute of Diabetes and Digestive and Kidney Diseases
Office of Communications and Public Liaison
NIDDK, NIH, 31 Center Drive, MSC 2560
Bethesda, MD, USA 20892-2560
Tel: 1-800-622-9010

Psoriasis

Psoriasis is a chronic skin disease that is easily identified by the presence of rough, red patches and thick, silvery scaling on the skin. Psoriasis typically starts to develop during the teenage years and flare-ups may be lifelong. Although some people are only mildly affected by psoriasis, it is a persistent disease that can be the source of considerable discomfort, disability and emotional distress.

What Causes Psoriasis?

Psoriasis is probably caused by a disorder of the immune system that disrupts the activity of the skin cells. The upper layer of the skin, the epidermis, acts as a strong, protective barrier for the body. For most people, the life cycle of the skin is about 28 days long. During this 28-day cycle, new skin cells move from the lowest layer of the epidermis to the top layer, where they die and flake off. For people suffering from psoriasis, the life cycle of the skin progresses much more rapidly. Skin cells multiply nearly ten times faster than necessary and the life cycle is reduced to only four or five days. The rapidly dividing cells accumulate on the outer layer of the epidermis, resulting in the rough scaling and inflammation.

Psoriasis usually occurs on areas of the body that are exposed to irritation, friction or injury. The knees and elbows are common pressure points, but scaling can also develop on the scalp, lower back, hands, feet and nails and may even be found inside the mouth or on the genitals. The red, scaly patches, called plaques, may become cracked and sore, especially on the skin over the joints. Gradually, the skin will heal and return to normal, but the scaling tends to reappear again and again in the same areas. Some people also experience itching skin or burning sensations when psoriasis develops in the body creases. In more serious cases, pus-filled blisters may develop or inflammation may attack the joints, causing psoriatic arthritis.

Psoriasis is not contagious. The disease tends to flare up for weeks or months at a time and then subside. During these periods of remission, there are usually no symptoms. While scientists do not fully understand the causes of this disease, certain factors are known to trigger psoriasis attacks. These trigger factors include changes in climate, stress, infections, skin injuries, severe sunburn, exposure to household chemicals and reactions to medications.

Symptoms

Symptoms of psoriasis include

- dry, red patches of skin covered with thick, silvery scales

- pitted and discolored finger and toenails; nails may also lift and crack

- itching or burning sensations and minor bleeding, especially on the skin in the body creases

- stiff, swollen joints

- pus-filled blisters

Who's at Risk?

Psoriasis affects at least one in every 100 Canadians.[1] In one-third of all cases, the skin condition is inherited. Psoriasis usually develops gradually between the ages of 15 and 35 but can occur at any age. Approximately one in 20 people with psoriasis go on to develop psoriatic arthritis.[2] Psoriatic arthritis causes joint inflammation —pain and swelling of joints in the knees, ankles, fingers and toes—as well as skin rashes.

Conventional Treatment

Treatment usually depends on the severity of the disease, the extent of the areas affected, the type of psoriasis and the disease's response to initial treatment. Over time, affected skin may become resistant to treatments. Some doctors rotate or switch treatments periodically to avoid adverse effects and a resistance. Common treatments include one or a combination of the following:

- *Topical creams or ointments* These are used to improve the patchy areas and remove scales. Creams may be derived from vitamins D or A, coal tar, salicylic acid or anthralin or may contain corticosteroids.

- *Bath oils* and *moisturizers* These are used to soothe the skin and reduce itching.

- *Phototherapy* A procedure done to reduce the overproduction of skin cells and improve psoriasis.

- *Oral medications* Drugs used in more severe cases include retinoids (derived from vitamin A) or methotrexate to block the rapid growth of cells and cyclosporine to suppress the immune system.

To improve the symptoms of psoriasis, it is also important to eat a nutritionally balanced diet (see below), get adequate rest and exercise regularly. Avoid scratching or rubbing dry patches of skin. Bathe often to soak off scales—mineral or sea salt baths may be beneficial. After bathing, pat skin dry rather than rubbing it with a towel. Use a moisturizer after bathing, but avoid creams with alcohol. It is also helpful to expose your skin to sunlight every day, but avoid sunburn.

Managing Psoriasis

Dietary Strategies

Fish

Oily fish is a rich source of two omega-3 fatty acids: EPA (eicosapentaenoic acid) and DHA (docosahexanaenoic acid). EPA and DHA are used in the body to produce noninflammatory immune compounds and therefore may be useful in psoriasis. Research suggests that people with psoriatic arthritis have lower levels of these fatty acids in their bloodstream.[3] While the use of fish oil taken either intravenously or as supplements to treat psoriasis has been the most widely studied (see below), some studies suggest that eating fish can be just as beneficial.

One study found that eating fish four to seven times per week resulted in a significant increase in blood levels of EPA and DHA.[4] Another report found that patients taking medication for their psoriasis who ate a daily 170-gram portion of oily fish for four weeks experienced a modest improvement in symptoms.[5] Eating the same amount of white fish (non-oily) had no effect on psoriasis.

Eating fish on a daily basis may not be feasible or desirable for many people. Aim to eat oily fish at least four times per week. Good choices include salmon, trout, herring, mackerel, sardines and kipper.

Gluten

Researchers have observed that some people with psoriasis do well on a gluten-free diet. Blood tests have revealed that some people have antibodies to gluten, the protein found in wheat and other cereals.[6,7] A study from Sweden found that when psoriasis patients with gluten antibodies were placed on a gluten-free diet for three months, there was a significant improvement in itching, redness, scaling and the size of plaques.[8] When their ordinary diet was resumed, their psoriasis worsened.

Gluten is found in wheat, oats, rye, barley and triticale. If your doctor determines that you have gluten antibodies, you should eliminate gluten-containing foods, such as bread, cereal, pasta, crackers, cookies and cakes, from your diet. See page 209, Celiac Disease, for detailed information on a gluten-free diet.

Vitamins and Minerals

Beta-Carotene

This nutrient is sometimes cited as a remedy for psoriasis; however, there is very little evidence to support such claims. It appears they are largely based on an Italian study of 316 newly diagnosed psoriasis patients.[9] The researchers found that compared with healthy controls, the psoriasis sufferers consumed significantly less beta-carotene—their diet was low in carrots, tomatoes and fresh fruit.

Based on these findings, a poor intake of beta-carotene may increase your risk for developing psoriasis, but it is not known whether the nutrient can improve the condition. Beta-carotene is converted to vitamin A in the body; vitamin A is needed to maintain healthy skin and support the immune system.

There is no recommended dietary intake for beta-carotene. To increase your intake, reach for orange and dark green produce. The best sources include carrots, sweet potato, winter squash, broccoli, collard greens, kale, spinach, apricots, cantaloupe, peaches, nectarines, mango and papaya.

Zinc

A handful of studies have found lower levels of zinc in the blood and skin of people with psoriasis.[10,11] This has led researchers to speculate about the benefits of zinc supplements in managing the condition. Unfortunately, two trials found that zinc supplements were ineffective at improving clinical symptoms.[12,13] One study did find, however, that zinc influenced the activity of white blood cells, suggesting that the mineral might help decrease inflammation.

Zinc is essential for a healthy immune system and it also helps the body transport vitamin A. The best food sources include oysters, seafood, red meat, poultry, yogurt, wheat bran, wheat germ, whole grains and enriched breakfast cereals. See page 62, Chapter 4, for a list of the zinc content of selected foods.

Most adult multivitamin and mineral formulas provide 10 to 20 milligrams (children's formulas may or may not contain zinc). Single zinc supplements are rarely appropriate. Too much zinc has toxic effects, including copper deficiency, heart problems and anemia.

Herbal Creams
Aloe Vera
Aloe vera seems to reduce inflammation and possess antibacterial and antifungal properties. According to one study conducted among 60 patients with mild to moderate psoriasis, aloe vera cream is very effective at reducing symptoms.[14] Patients used the cream three times daily for a maximum of four weeks. At the end of the study, the cream had cured 83 percent of the patients, whereas the placebo cream had cured only 6.6 percent.

Use a cream that contains 0.5 percent aloe. Apply liberally as needed three times per day.

Oregon Grape (*Mahonia aquifolium*)
One study found that a cream made from Oregon grape extract reduced psoriasis symptoms.[15] Active components of Oregon grape appear to relieve symptoms of psoriasis by slowing the rate of abnormal cell growth and reducing inflammation.

Other Natural Health Products
Fish Oil Supplements
Most of the studies that show the benefits of fish oil have given patients with severe psoriasis fish oil intravenously. However, a few studies suggest that fish oil capsules rich in EPA help reduce pso-

riasis symptoms.[16,17] Researchers have also found that when fish oil is taken in combination with medication or phototherapy, greater improvements are seen.[18,19] There is also a possibility that taking fish oil capsules together with cyclosporine may reduce kidney problems associated with that drug's use.[20]

The typical dosage is 2 to 9 grams of fish oil per day, often taken in divided doses. Look for a product rich in EPA. Fish oil supplements can cause belching and a fishy taste. Because fish oil has a thinning effect on the blood, use caution if you are taking blood-thinning medication such as aspirin, warfarin (Coumadin®) or heparin.

Nutrition Strategy Checklist for Psoriasis

☐ Fish
☐ Gluten
☐ Beta-carotene
☐ Zinc
☐ Aloe vera cream OR Oregon grape cream
☐ Fish oil supplements

Recommended Resources

www.nih.gov/niams/
National Institute of Arthritis and Musculoskeletal and Skin Diseases Information Clearinghouse
1 AMS Circle
Bethesda, MD, USA 20892-3675
Tel: 301-495-4484
Fax: 301-718-6366

www.psoriasis.org
National Psoriasis Foundation
6600 SW 92nd Avenue, Suite 300
Portland, OR, USA 97223
Tel: 503-244-7404 or 1-800-723-9166
Fax: 503-245-0626

www.psoriasissociety.org/index.html
Psoriasis Society of Canada
P.O. Box 25015
Halifax, NS, Canada B3M 4H4
Tel: 902-443-8680 or 1-800-656-4494
Fax: 902-457-1664
E-mail: info@psoriasissociety.org

Rheumatoid Arthritis

One in every 100 Canadians suffers from arthritis.[1] Arthritis attacks the joints and connective tissue of the body and can lead to immobility and serious disability. There are several types of chronic arthritis, but one of the most severe forms is rheumatoid arthritis, a debilitating and often crippling disease that causes painful inflammation of the joints. At present, there is no cure for rheumatoid arthritis.

What Causes Rheumatoid Arthritis?

Rheumatoid arthritis is an autoimmune disease. An autoimmune disease develops when something in the body triggers the immune system to attack its own tissues. The result is a painful and chronic inflammation that can damage normal tissues.

Rheumatoid arthritis usually begins with an attack on the synovial membrane of the joint. The synovial membrane is a thin layer of tissue that surrounds each joint. It secretes synovial fluid, which helps the joint to move smoothly and carries nutrients to the bones and cartilage. Rheumatoid arthritis inflames the synovial membrane, causing it to grow and thicken. As the disease progresses, the thickening tissue squeezes the bones, cartilage and ligaments, resulting in loss of movement, severe pain and deformity of the joint. The synovial membrane and white blood cells release enzymes and growth factors, which contribute to the destruction of joint function.

Symptoms

Rheumatoid arthritis is considered to be a systemic disease because it affects the body as a whole. Because it triggers an autoimmune response in the body, the impact of the disease is not limited to the joints. Often, arthritic pain will be accompanied by flu-like symptoms, such as fatigue, general aches and pains and weakness. Weight loss and anemia may also occur. The main symptoms of arthritis are

- painful, stiff, swollen and tender joints, especially in the hands and feet
- joint pain that is often worse in the morning
- joint pain that occurs all night long
- morning stiffness that lasts longer than 30 minutes
- pain in three or more joints at the same time
- pain in the same joint on both sides of the body

Rheumatoid arthritis may flare up suddenly, affecting many joints at once. More often, it starts slowly. Once the symptoms begin, it may be only a matter of months before there is serious joint destruction. Often, affected joints will freeze in one position, which prevents them from opening or extending properly. Cysts may develop behind the knees, causing pain and swelling in the lower legs. You may also develop rheumatoid nodules, small lumps of tissue that form under the skin near the joints.

Rheumatoid arthritis may occasionally go into spontaneous remission, although this is fairly rare. Nearly half of all people diagnosed with this disease develop some pattern of remission and relapse, and experience symptoms that vary from mild to moderate. However, if the symptoms of rheumatoid arthritis are persistent and the disease remains active for a longer period, there is a much greater risk for permanent joint damage and eventual disability.

Who's at Risk?

Arthritis affects twice as many women as men. Although rheumatoid arthritis can strike at any age, it usually affects people between the ages of 25 and 50. Scientists suspect that some people have a genetic predisposition to rheumatoid arthritis. If your parents or siblings suffer from rheumatoid arthritis, there is a greater chance that you will develop the disease.

Conventional Treatment

Treatment for rheumatoid arthritis may be as simple as rest and healthy eating or as complex as drugs and surgery. Usually physicians will start with the most conservative treatment, moving on to more aggressive therapies only when necessary.

There are four main types of drugs used to treat arthritis:

1. *Nonsteroidal anti-inflammatory drugs (NSAIDs)* to reduce joint pain and swelling. Nonprescription NSAIDs include aspirin, Anacin® and Advil®. Prescription NSAIDs include Naprosyn®, Relafen®, Indocid® and Voltaren®. These drugs may cause stomach upset, heartburn, ulcers and possibly high blood pressure.

2. *Disease-modifying antirheumatic drugs (DMARDs)* stop arthritis from getting worse by suppressing the immune system, but they do not reverse joint damage. They include gold salts, methotrexate, hydroxychloroquine, sulfasalazine, chloroquinone and azathioprine. Rashes, suppressed blood cell production and liver, kidney and eye problems are a few possible side effects.

3. *Corticosteroids* (e.g., prednisone) suppress the activity of the immune system and significantly reduce inflammation anywhere in your body. They may be injected directly into your affected joints for fast, short-term relief of pain or may be used intermittently, in combination with other types of treatment. Corticosteroids are recommended only for short-term use. Long-term use of corticosteroids can cause osteoporosis, weight gain, high blood pressure, cataracts and susceptibility to infection.

4. *Biological response modifiers* block specific hormones involved in inflammation. Two of these drugs, etanercept (Enbrel®) and infliximab (Remicade®), are available in the United States. They are awaiting approval in Canada. These drugs target tumor necrosis factor (TNF), a substance responsible for joint inflammation and pain. By interfering with TNF function, etanercept and infliximab reduce inflammation and slow joint destruction.

While drugs may help reduce the symptoms of rheumatoid arthritis, your treatment plan should also include regular rest periods, gentle exercise to keep joints from freezing in one position and a healthy diet. Applying heat to affected joints can also ease discomfort.

When the disease is advanced and drugs are not effective, you may want to consider surgery. Surgery to replace knee or hip joints may restore function and mobility. In some cases, joint removal or fusion may also help improve walking and reduce your daily discomfort.

Managing Rheumatoid Arthritis

Dietary Strategies

Food Triggers

There is evidence that a small percentage of people with arthritis have food allergies that exacerbate joint symptoms.[2-6] Researchers have found that when allergy-causing foods are removed from the diet, arthritis patients have significantly less pain and stiffness and fewer painful joints.

Foods identified to cause problems include milk, wheat, corn, pork and oranges.

There is a widespread belief that nightshade vegetables such as eggplant, bell peppers, tomatoes and potatoes may aggravate arthritis. No studies have proven this, however.

If you think a certain food is triggering your joint pain, remove it from your diet for two weeks. Keep a diary to document any change in symptoms, along with what you ate and when. After two weeks, reintroduce the food and see if your symptoms worsen.

Vegetarian Diet

Researchers have found that fasting for seven to ten days, followed by a strict vegetarian diet for at least three months, can bring about significant long-term improvements in arthritis symptoms.[7-11] This dietary regimen may reduce inflammation in a number of ways. Vegetarian diets are plentiful in vegetables, fruits, legumes and whole grains, foods that supply the body with protective antioxidants (see below). These diets are very low in or free of animal fat, fat that promotes the production of inflammatory immune compounds. It is also thought that vegetarian diets encourage the growth of friendly bacteria in the intestinal tract. Such microbes provide a protective barrier from disease-causing organisms and may also enhance the immune system.

Most of the studies exploring the link between diet and arthritis have used a gluten-free, vegan diet to achieve results. Vegan diets exclude all animal foods, including milk, fish and eggs. This may be too extreme for many people. Such a diet also increases the risk of nutrient deficiencies, especially calcium and vitamin D. If you are interested in trying the fasting/vegan diet approach, consult with a registered dietitian for professional guidance (**www.dietitians.ca**).

You may decide to ease into a vegetarian diet by following a lacto-vegetarian eating plan. This diet includes dairy products but excludes meat, poultry and eggs.

Fish

You may also decide to add fish to your vegetarian diet. Fish contains omega-3 fats, which have consistently been shown to reduce arthritis joint pain and stiffness. Omega-3 fats inhibit the body's production of inflammatory immune compounds called leukotrienes. While the use of fish oil *supplements* (see below) to treat arthritis has been studied the most, some studies suggest that eating fish can be just as beneficial.

An American study found that women who ate at least two servings of baked or broiled fish per week were almost half as likely to have rheumatoid arthritis compared with women who ate fish less than once per week.[12] The best choices are oily fish: salmon, mackerel, herring, sardines, anchovies and (fresh) albacore tuna.

Sodium

Corticosteroid medications, which your doctor may prescribe to you in order to reduce inflammation, will cause you to retain sodium. To help prevent fluid weight gain and swelling, reduce the amount of sodium in your diet to no more than 2400 milligrams per day (about 1 teaspoon worth of salt). Avoid the saltshaker at the table, minimize the use of salt in cooking and buy commercial food products that are low in added salt. Season your foods with herbs, spices, flavored vinegars and fruit juices. Most of the salt we consume every day comes from processed and prepared foods—only one-quarter comes from the saltshaker. The sodium content of selected foods can be found on page 80, Chapter 5.

Vitamins and Minerals

Many of the drugs that are part of the conventional treatment of rheumatoid arthritis may deplete your body's store of certain vitamins and minerals. It is therefore important to ensure you are getting adequate amounts of these nutrients in your daily diet or through supplements.

Antioxidants

Free radicals generated by inflammatory immune compounds are thought to cause tissue damage in people with rheumatoid arthritis. When scientists examine the blood and joint fluid of arthritis suffers, they find increased free radical activity and lower levels of antioxidants such as vitamins C and E, beta-carotene and selenium.[13-22] A poor intake of these nutrients can contribute to further joint damage. A diet rich in fruits, vegetables and whole grains supplies a wide range of antioxidants that may help fight free radicals.

There is some evidence that vitamin E supplements have anti-inflammatory and pain-relieving properties in addition to their antioxidant properties. A study of arthritis patients who were given approximately 800 international units (IU) of vitamin E twice daily reported a small improvement in joint pain.[23]

- *Vitamin C* The recommended dietary allowance (RDA) is 75 and 90 milligrams for women and men respectively (smokers need an additional 35 milligrams). Best food sources include citrus fruit, citrus juices, cantaloupe, kiwi, mango, strawberries, broccoli, Brussels sprouts, cauliflower, red pepper and tomato juice. To supplement, take 500 milligrams of Ester C once or twice daily. The daily upper limit is 2000 milligrams.

- *Vitamin E* The RDA is 22 IU. Best food sources include wheat germ, nuts, seeds, vegetable oils, whole grains and kale. To supplement, take 200 to 800 IU of natural source vitamin E. Buy a "mixed" vitamin E supplement if possible. The daily upper limit is 1500 IU.

- *Selenium* The RDA is 55 micrograms. Best food sources are seafood, chicken, organ meats, whole grains, nuts, onions, garlic and mushrooms. To supplement, take 200 micrograms of selenium-rich yeast per day. The daily upper limit is 400 micrograms.

- *Beta-Carotene* No RDA has been established. Best food sources are orange and dark green produce, including carrots, sweet potato, winter squash, broccoli, collard greens, kale, spinach, apricots, cantaloupe, peaches, nectarines, mango and papaya. Avoid taking separate beta-carotene supplements if you smoke. If you're a nonsmoker, choose a multivitamin and mineral with beta-carotene added.

Folic Acid

Methotrexate, a potent DMARD (disease-modifying antirheumatic drug) used to treat arthritis, interferes with the body's metabolism of folic acid. This can lead to anemia and methotrexate toxicity, which can damage the liver. Taking a folic acid supplement can also help ease gastrointestinal upset associated with methotrexate use. Your doctor will prescribe a folic acid supplement if you take this drug, but you can also find this B vitamin in spinach, lentils, orange juice, whole grains, fortified breakfast cereals, asparagus, artichoke, avocado and seeds. You'll find a list of folate-rich foods on page 32, Chapter 4.

Calcium and Vitamin D

Corticosteroid drugs such as prednisone can thin the bones, and long-term use can lead to osteoporosis. If you are taking such a medication, it is critical that you consume 1000 to 1500 milligrams of calcium and 200 to 600 IU of vitamin D per day to preserve bone health. Some experts recommend that the elderly get as much as 1000 IU of vitamin D per day, especially during Canada's dark winter months, when little vitamin D is formed in the skin.

Many people don't meet the daily recommended or adequate intakes of calcium and vitamin D from their diet; you will most likely need to take supplements to achieve these intakes. A two-year study conducted among 96 patients with rheumatoid arthritis who were receiving low-dose corticosteroid therapy found that daily supplements providing 1000 milligrams of calcium and 500 IU of vitamin D prevented bone loss.[24] Patients in the study who did not supplement their diet lost bone from the spine at a rate of 2 percent per year. The supplement users gained 0.73 percent bone per year.

To learn more about your daily requirements and supplements, see Chapter 4.

Potassium

In addition to causing bone thinning, corticosteroid medications also cause the body to lose potassium, a mineral that helps maintain fluid balance. If taking such drugs, be sure to increase your intake of potassium by consuming bananas, oranges, orange juice, prune juice, potatoes, avocado, cantaloupe, peaches, tomatoes, low-sodium tomato juice, lima beans, nonfat yogurt and clams.

Herbal Remedies

Boswellia (*Boswellia serrata*)

This herbal product is derived from the resin of the Indian Boswellia tree. A few unpublished studies have demonstrated the effectiveness of boswellia in reducing joint pain and swelling when taken for three months. However, one study found that the herb offered no improvement.[25] Boswellia is thought to work by reducing inflammation.[26]

The recommended dose is 400 milligrams three times daily. Buy a product standardized to contain 37.5 percent boswellic acids. It may take up to eight weeks to notice improvement in arthritis symptoms. Boswellia has not been evaluated for safety in children or in pregnant or breastfeeding women.

Capsaicin Cream

Capsaicin, responsible for the heat of chili peppers, has a long history of use as a topical agent for pain disorders of the skin and joints. When applied to the skin surrounding the joint, capsaicin depletes substance P, a compound that transmits feelings of pain from the nerves to the spinal cord. As a result, pain relief is achieved.

Capsaicin creams are available with or without a prescription. Zostrix®, Capzasin-P® and Capsin® are all available over the counter. Buy a cream with 0.025 to 0.075 percent capsaicin (the greater strength may be more effective). Capsaicin cream will produce a burning sensation, which will diminish after several applications. Use a small amount to begin with. When you no longer feel burning upon application, increase the amount of cream you use. Be careful not to touch your eyes or other sensitive tissues after applying capsaicin cream. Wash your hands after using the product.

Devil's Claw (*Harpagophytum procumbens*)

A handful of studies have shown devil's claw to be helpful in rheumatoid arthritis. Several clinical studies have observed an improvement in mobility and reduction in pain in patients taking the herb.[27] Devil's claw may work by decreasing inflammation.

The recommended dose is 750 milligrams taken three times daily. Buy an extract standardized to contain 3 percent iridoid glycosides. People with ulcers should not use the herb. Its safety has not been established in people with liver or kidney disease.

Other Natural Health Products

Fish Oil Supplements

There is solid evidence to support adding fish oil supplements to your daily nutrition regime.

Many studies have found that omega-3 fats in fish oil capsules reduce the number of tender joints and the amount of morning stiffness, improve walking distance and reduce pain.[28-31] Researchers have even found that arthritis patients are able to reduce the dose or discontinue anti-inflammatory medication while taking fish oil without experiencing a flare-up of the disease.[32]

Buy a fish oil supplement that contains EPA and DHA, two omega-3 fatty acids responsible for fish oil's anti-inflammatory effect. Most studies have used a dose of fish oil that provides 3.8 grams EPA and 2 grams DHA per day. Fish oil supplements will vary in the amounts and ratios of EPA and DHA they contain. Many provide 18 percent EPA and 12 percent DHA. Take fish oil in divided doses. It may take three to four months to notice an improvement in symptoms.

Avoid fish *liver* oil capsules. These are concentrated in vitamins A and D and could cause toxicity symptoms if taken in high doses for a period of time. Fish oil supplements can cause belching and a fishy taste. High doses can cause nausea and diarrhea. Because fish oil has a thinning effect on the blood, use caution if you are taking blood-thinning medication such as aspirin, warfarin (Coumadin®) or heparin.

Nutrition Strategy Checklist for Rheumatoid Arthritis

- ☐ Food triggers
- ☐ Vegetarian diet
- ☐ Fish
- ☐ Fish oil supplements
- ☐ Low sodium
- ☐ Antioxidants
- ☐ Folic acid
- ☐ Calcium and vitamin D
- ☐ Potassium
- ☐ Boswellia OR Devil's claw*
- ☐ Capsaicin cream

*Stronger evidence—start here

Recommended Resources

www.rheumatology.org
American College of Rheumatology
1800 Century Place, Suite 250
Atlanta, GA, USA 30345
Tel: 404-633-3777
Fax: 404-633-1870

www.arthritis.org
Arthritis Foundation
1330 West Peachtree Street
Atlanta, GA, USA 30309
Tel: 404-872-7100 or 1-800-283-7800

www.arthritis.ca
The Arthritis Society
393 University Avenue, Suite 1700
Toronto, ON, Canada M5G 1E6
Tel: 416-979-7228
Fax: 416-979-8366
E-mail: info@arthritis.ca

www.nih.gov.niams/healthinfo/
National Institute of Arthritis and
Musculoskeletal and Skin Diseases
Information Clearinghouse
National Institutes of Health
1 AMS Circle
Bethesda, MD, USA 20892-3675
Tel: 301-495-4484 or 1-877-22-NIAMS (1-877-226-4267)
Fax: 301-718-6366

Shingles (Herpes Zoster)

Nearly 95 percent of North American children will contract chickenpox, otherwise known as the varicella virus, before they reach the age of 18.[1] Although the symptoms of chickenpox disappear within a week or two, the virus may linger in nerve cells long afterward. Often, the virus will remain there for a lifetime without causing any problems. But sometimes the virus will reactivate, causing a painful rash of blisters called shingles, or herpes zoster.

Shingles typically begins with a general feeling of illness, a slight fever and a tingling sensation along one side of your body. Within days, a rash of small, fluid-filled blisters will appear in the same general area. Unlike chickenpox, which produces itchy spots all over your body, the blisters caused by shingles will develop in a limited area only, along the path of the affected nerve root. Typically, this band of blisters will occur on the chest, abdomen, face or back, but it can also affect the neck, limbs or scalp. An outbreak of shingles can be excruciatingly painful, extremely itchy and tender. The blisters usually dry up and heal within a week or two but, while they are active, they carry the varicella virus and can infect anyone who has not been exposed to chickenpox before.

What Causes Shingles?

The cause of shingles is not clearly understood, but factors such as age, illness, medications and stress can trigger the virus to reactivate. Most people recover from the virus in approximately one month and never experience another outbreak. However, people with weakened immune systems, such as those with cancer or AIDS, may suffer repeated episodes.

Normally, shingles is not a serious condition. However, a shingles rash that develops anywhere near the eye could lead to an infection of the cornea and should be treated immediately. In rare cases, the virus may lead to ear damage or encephalitis (inflammation of the brain) or may attack nerves that control muscle movement, resulting in weakness and temporary paralysis.

One of the most common complications of shingles is a condition called postherpetic neuralgia (PHN). Nearly half of all people with shingles over the age of 60 and 75 percent of those over age 75 will go on to develop PHN.[2] Postherpetic neuralgia is an unrelenting, sometimes incapacitating, pain. It affects the areas of the skin that are supplied by the nerves infected with varicella zoster virus.

PHN develops when the shingles virus damages nerve fibers. The damaged fibers carry confused and exaggerated pain messages along the neural pathways connecting the skin to the brain. In some cases, even the touch of clothing, a light breeze or a simple change of temperature can trigger excruciating pain. PHN will normally subside within a few months but it can persist for over a year or more.

Symptoms

Common symptoms of shingles include

- chills, fever, general feeling of being unwell
- tingling or pain along one side of the body before any rash is visible
- red rash with blisters that last two to three weeks before drying out and scabbing over
- itching, tingling and pain in the area of the rash

Who's at Risk?

Anyone who has had chickenpox can develop shingles. In fact, one in five adults who have had chickenpox will experience shingles. Adults over the age of 50 are at greater risk of the condition, as are people with weakened immune systems.

The fluid in shingles blisters can infect people with the chickenpox virus. The risk of contracting chickenpox is higher for people who have never been exposed to chickenpox before, and for infants, people with weakened immune systems and pregnant women.

Conventional Treatment

Early medical treatment is crucial to minimize the intensity of the outbreak and lower the risk of nerve damage. Treatments may include

- Antiviral drugs (acyclovir, famciclovir and valacyclovir); these are most effective if taken within 72 hours of the development of the rash

- Aspirin or codeine to provide some pain relief

- Soaking in a tub of oatmeal or cornstarch or applying cool wet towels to the blisters to ease the pain and itching

- A chickenpox vaccine to help prevent shingles by reactivating the immune system response to varicella zoster virus in adults

PHN can be very difficult to treat. The following treatments may be used:

- Narcotics such as codeine to offer some pain relief (painkillers such as aspirin and ibuprofen are often ineffective)

- Creams containing lidocaine or capsaicin (an extract of hot peppers) to help relieve pain *after* the blisters have healed

- Antidepressant medications or epilepsy drugs to help calm the brain and blunt the perception of pain

- An injection of local anesthetic directly into the nerve causing the pain to provide relief (relief is very temporary)

- TENS (transcutaneous electrical nerve stimulator) unit to disrupt pain signals by sending a mild electrical current to the affected nerve

Vitamins and Minerals

Vitamins B1 and B12

These two B vitamins have been suggested often as possible treatments for shingles. However, there is very little evidence that high doses speed recovery from the herpes zoster virus. Nevertheless, because both B vitamins are essential to healthy nerve function, be sure to include foods rich in the two vitamins in your daily diet.

Vitamin B1 (thiamin) is found in pork, liver, whole grains, enriched breakfast cereals, legumes and nuts. Vitamin B12 is found in animal foods and foods that have been fortified with the nutrient. Good sources include meat, poultry, fish, eggs and dairy products, as well as fortified soy and rice beverages.

If you are over the age of 50, take a supplement that supplies vitamin B12. One-third of older adults produce inadequate amounts of stomach acid and have lost the ability to properly absorb B12 from food. To boost your intake of both B vitamins, take a high-potency multivitamin and mineral pill or a B complex supplement. Both formulas will supply anywhere from 25 to 100 milligrams of B1 and 25 to 100 micrograms of B12. Vitamin B1 and B12 supplements are very safe.

Vitamin C

This nutrient bolsters immunity by enhancing an antiviral agent in the body called interferon. Vitamin C is also needed for proper healing of skin blisters. The recommended dietary allowance (RDA) is 75 and 90 milligrams for women and men respectively (smokers need an additional 35 milligrams). The best food sources include citrus fruit, citrus juices, cantaloupe, kiwi, mango, strawberries, broccoli, Brussels sprouts, cauliflower, red pepper and tomato juice. To supplement, take 500 milligrams of Ester C once or twice daily. The daily upper limit is 2000 milligrams.

Vitamin E

Supplementation with vitamin E is sometimes recommended to reduce the pain associated with postherpetic neuralgia (PHN); however, there is not enough evidence to support its use. But vitamin E supplements *have* been shown to enhance the immune system of older adults by enhancing the action of certain white blood cells, called natural killer cells.[3,4] Consuming adequate amounts of the vitamin may help the body fight the herpes zoster virus.

The RDA is 22 international units (IU). The best food sources include wheat germ, nuts, seeds, vegetable oils, whole grains and kale. To supplement, take 200 to 800 IU of natural source vitamin E. Buy a "mixed" vitamin E supplement if possible. The daily upper limit is 1500 IU.

Zinc

This mineral is used to make antibodies, immune compounds that fight virus and bacteria. Ensuring a daily intake of zinc-rich foods will help you support your body's immune system. Good food sources include oysters, seafood, red meat, poultry, yogurt, wheat bran, wheat germ, whole grains and enriched breakfast cereals. See page 62, Chapter 4, for a list of zinc-rich foods. Most adult multivitamin and mineral formulas provide 10 to 20 milligrams. Single zinc supplements should be used only if your doctor has determined that you are deficient in this mineral. Too much zinc has toxic effects, including copper deficiency, heart problems and anemia.

Herbal Remedies

Capsaicin Cream

Capsaicin, the compound responsible for the heat of chili peppers, is used as a topical agent to relieve the pain of neuralgia that can follow an outbreak of shingles. A number of studies have found that capsaicin cream significantly reduces pain in people with PHN.[5-8] In one study, almost 50 percent of participants experienced a substantial reduction in pain severity and duration when using capsaicin cream. When applied to the skin, capsaicin depletes substance P, a compound that transmits feelings of pain from the nerves to the spinal cord. As a result, pain relief is achieved.

Capsaicin creams are available with or without a prescription. Zostrix®, Capzasin-P® and Capsin® are all available over the counter. Buy a cream with 0.025 to 0.075 percent capsaicin (the greater strength may be more effective). Capsaicin cream will produce a burning sensation, which will diminish after several applications. Use a small amount to begin with. When you no longer feel burning upon application, increase the amount of cream used. Be careful not to touch your eyes or other sensitive tissues after applying capsaicin cream. Wash your hands after using the product.

Other Natural Health Products
Digestive Enzymes

These enzymes are produced by the pancreas and released into the intestine after eating. Once in the gut, digestive enzymes break down protein, carbohydrate and fat into smaller units that can be absorbed into the bloodstream. When taken as a supplement, digestive enzymes are thought to have anti-inflammatory and immune-enhancing effects in the body.

Two studies compared digestive enzymes with the standard drug acyclovir in people with shingles. In each study, the enzyme group and the drug group had similar pain relief, but those taking the enzymes reported fewer side effects.[9,10]

When buying digestive enzymes, be aware that the strength is expressed in activity units rather than milligrams and refers to the enzyme's potency. The dosage will vary depending on the type of enzymes found in the product, so follow the manufacturer's directions.

Buy an enteric-coated broad-based enzyme supplement that contains protease (digests proteins), amylase (digests starch) and lipase (digests fat).

Nutrition Strategy Checklist for Shingles

☐ Vitamin B1   ☐ Zinc
☐ Vitamin B12   ☐ Capsaicin cream
☐ Vitamin C   ☐ Digestive enzymes
☐ Vitamin E

Recommended Resources

www.theacpa.org
The American Chronic Pain Association
P.O. Box 850
Rocklin, CA, USA 95677
Tel: 916-632-0922
Fax: 916-632-3208
E-mail: ACPA@pacbell.net

www.ninds.nih.gov
National Institute of Neurological Disorders and Stroke
National Institute of Health
NIH Neurological Institute
P.O. Box 5801
Bethesda, MD, USA 20824
Tel: 1-800-352-9424

www.vzvfoundation.org
VZV Research Foundation (for Research on Varicella Zoster)
40 E 72nd Street
New York, NY, USA 10021
Tel: 1-800-472-8478
Fax: 212-861-7033

Sinusitis (Sinus Infection)

Sinusitis is a persistent infection of the sinuses that is easily mistaken for the common cold. Sometimes, sinusitis clears up in a week or two.

But often, sinus infections can linger for months or even years, possibly causing other infections that can have much more serious consequences.

What Causes Sinusitis?

The sinuses are hollow air spaces or cavities located within the bones of the skull. You have four pairs of sinus cavities, called the paranasal sinuses, and they are all located in the vicinity of the nose. The sinuses are designed to lighten the weight of your skull and to add resonance to the sound of your voice. Each sinus opens into the nose for an efficient exchange of air. They are lined with the same type of mucus membrane that is found inside the nasal passages. The sinuses secrete a steady supply of mucus that helps to protect the lungs by trapping dirt and debris inhaled in the air we breathe. This mucus, along with other secretions, normally drains out of the sinuses through the openings into the nose and throat.

Anything that causes inflammation in the nose can also affect the sinuses. Infections or allergic reactions can cause the mucus membranes to swell, interfering with drainage flow from the sinuses to the nose. This forces mucus to back up into the sinuses, creating an ideal environment for bacteria to multiply. As infection and pus build up because of the clogged drainage passages, air also becomes trapped in the sinuses. The combination of swelling, pus and trapped air puts painful pressure on the sinus wall. The swollen mucous membranes can also prevent air from entering the sinuses, creating an unnatural vacuum in the nasal passages. The end result is the characteristic sinus headache.

Acute sinusitis is relatively short-lived, lasting for three weeks or less. Although acute sinusitis often mimics the symptoms of a cold, the causes and treatment are quite different. Anything that blocks drainage from the sinuses can ultimately lead to sinusitis. Factors that often lead to acute sinusitis include

- *Colds* Acute sinusitis often follows a common cold. The cold virus sets the stage for sinusitis by inflaming the mucous membranes. The drainage openings swell shut because of the inflammation, and bacterial sinusitis quickly takes hold.

- *Allergens* Breathing in airborne substances can cause allergic reactions that can lead to swollen nasal passages and sinusitis.

- *Smoking* Tobacco smoke can slow down the drainage action in the sinuses, causing mucus to back up in the sinuses.

Chronic sinusitis is much more persistent. It can linger for weeks or months at a time, despite treatment with antibiotics. It results from many of the same conditions that lead to acute sinusitis. Airborne allergens, such as dust mold and pollen, are prime causes of chronic sinusitis because they provoke persistent inflammation in the nasal passages. Other factors that trigger chronic sinus infections include

- *Fungal infections* Microscopic fungi are normally present in your nasal passages. However, people with malfunctioning immune systems may develop allergic reactions to them, leading to allergic fungal sinusitis.

- *Nasal obstructions* Nasal polyps, tiny tissue growths that sometimes block the nasal passages, can interfere with normal mucus drainage. A deviated septum, which is a condition that develops when the wall between the nostrils is crooked, can also block the openings to the sinuses.

- *Dental problems* Bacteria associated with dental infections or tooth problems may trigger sinusitis.

Although most cases of sinusitis do respond to antibiotics, sometimes the infection can spread to other sinus cavities or to the bones surrounding the sinuses. If the infection spreads to the membranes that protect your brain, it can lead to meningitis, a very dangerous condition that can cause brain damage or death. Occasionally, blood clots may develop in the veins around the sinuses, cutting off the blood supply to your brain. This causes symptoms similar to those of a stroke.

Symptoms

Symptoms may vary, depending on which sinus cavity is affected, and include

- tenderness or swelling over the affected sinus
- fever and chills
- fatigue
- cough that is more severe at night
- nasal congestion
- yellow or green discharge from the nose
- headache, especially in the morning
- pain in your forehead
- swelling or pain around the eyes
- aching in the jaw or teeth, cheeks feel tender to the touch
- earache, neck pain or deep aching at the top of your head

Who's at Risk?

- People who suffer from colds
- Cigarette smokers
- People with airborne allergies
- People with asthma
- People with immune deficiencies or abnormalities in mucus production

Conventional Treatment

Pain relievers may help reduce discomfort. Over-the-counter decongestants may help sinuses drain, but these should be used only for a few days, since longer use may lead to even more swelling and congestion. Applying warm facial packs may loosen congestion. Cautiously inhaling steam from a basin of boiling water may reduce swelling.

Antibiotics are prescribed to treat a bacterial infection. These may be required for a longer period to treat chronic sinusitis. Nasal sprays containing corticosteroids are often prescribed for severe inflammations. Antifungal medications may be used to treat allergic fungal sinusitis. Surgery may be necessary to remove nasal polyps, correct a deviated septum or manage other nasal obstructions.

Managing Sinusitis

Dietary Strategies

Alcohol   Avoid drinking alcoholic beverages while you have sinusitis. Alcohol worsens blockage by causing the nasal and sinus membranes to swell.

Other Fluids   Drink at least 8 to 12 cups (2 to 3 liters) of fluid such as water per day. Fluid helps to dilute secretions and promotes drainage of the sinuses.

Probiotics   Fermented milk products, such as yogurt, kefir and acidophilus milk, contain healthy bacteria called lactic acid bacteria that may help prevent bacterial sinus infection. Once ingested, these microbes take up residence in the gastrointestinal tract, where they exert their health benefits. A number of studies have shown that regular consumption of probiotic foods as well as a probiotic supplement enhances the activity of the immune system.

Include one fermented milk product in your daily diet. To supplement, buy a product that contains 1 to 10 billion live cells per dose (capsule). Take one capsule three times daily with food. Children's products are also available. These usually contain one-quarter to one-half the adult dose (250 to 500 billion live cells).

Vitamins and Minerals

Antioxidants

Damage caused by harmful free radical molecules has been implicated in many chronic inflammatory conditions of the upper respiratory tract.[1] There is some evidence to suggest that people with chronic sinusitis have reduced levels of antioxidants in the membranes of their sinuses. A reduced antioxidant defense may lead to further inflammation.

Dietary antioxidants include vitamins C and E and selenium. Vitamins C and E are also important for a healthy immune system, and higher doses have been shown to enhance the infection-fighting ability of the body.

- *Vitamin C*   The recommended dietary allowance (RDA) is 75 and 90 milligrams for women and men respectively (smokers need an additional 35 milligrams). The best food sources include citrus fruit, citrus juices, cantaloupe, kiwi, mango, strawberries, broccoli, Brussels sprouts, cauliflower, red pepper and tomato juice. To supplement, take 500 milligrams of Ester C once or twice daily. To treat a cold, take 1000 milligrams of time-released vitamin C twice daily. The daily upper limit is 2000 milligrams.

- *Vitamin E*   The RDA is 22 international units (IU). The best food sources include wheat germ, nuts, seeds, vegetable oils, whole grains and kale. To supplement, take 200 to 800 IU of natural source vitamin E. Buy a "mixed" vitamin E supplement if possible. The daily upper limit is 1500 IU.

- *Selenium* The RDA is 55 micrograms. The best food sources are seafood, chicken, organ meats, whole grains, nuts, onions, garlic and mushrooms. To supplement, take 200 micrograms of selenium-rich yeast per day. The daily upper limit is 400 micrograms.

Zinc

It is important to ensure that your daily diet contains zinc-rich foods, since the mineral is vital to a healthy immune system. Zinc-rich foods include oysters, seafood, red meat, poultry, yogurt, wheat bran, wheat germ, whole grains and enriched breakfast cereals. You'll find a detailed food list on page 62, Chapter 4.

Most adult multivitamin and mineral formulas provide 10 to 20 milligrams. Children's formulas may or may not contain zinc. Single zinc supplements are rarely appropriate. Too much zinc has toxic effects, including copper deficiency, heart problems and anemia.

Herbal Remedies

Echinacea

Many studies in the laboratory have shown the ability of echinacea to enhance the body's production of white blood cells that fight infection. This herb can be used to treat a cold before sinusitis sets in. Clinical trials in adults taking echinacea to treat a cold suggest that it may help lessen the duration of symptoms.[2] Echinacea may also be helpful in treating acute bacterial sinusitis.

To ensure quality, buy a product standardized to contain 4 percent echinacosides (*Echinacea angustifolia*) and 0.7 percent flavonoids (*Echinacea purpurea*), two of the herb's active ingredients. Take a total of 900 milligrams three to four times daily. For fluid extracts (1:1) take 0.25 to 1.0 milliliter three times daily. For tinctures (1:5), take 1 to 2 milliliters three times daily. For teas, take 125 to 250 milliliters three to four

times daily. Take until symptoms are relieved, then continue taking two to three times daily for one week. Guidelines for doses in children can be found in Chapter 7. Don't use echinacea if you are allergic to plants in the Asteracease/Compositae family (ragweed, daisy, marigold and chrysanthemum).

Garlic (*Allium sativum*)

The sulfur compounds in garlic have been shown to stimulate the body's immune system, making garlic a potential agent in the prevention of bacterial sinus infections.[3-5] A number of studies have focused on the specific sulfur compounds in aged garlic extract, a special supplement that is aged for up to 20 months. Whether garlic actually helps treat a cold remains to be proven. However, the herb does have a long history of use in the treatment of infection.

Use one-half to one clove each day in cooking. To supplement, buy a product made with aged garlic extract. Take two to six capsules a day in divided doses. Aged garlic extract is odorless and less irritating to the gastrointestinal tract than other forms of garlic supplements (garlic oil capsules, garlic powder tablets).

Panax Ginseng

This herbal remedy may help prevent sinus infection through its ability to stimulate the immune system. A well-controlled trial from Italy found that 100 milligrams of Panax ginseng (G115 extract) taken daily resulted in a significant decline in the frequency of colds and flus.[6]

To supplement, choose a product with a statement of standardization or "G115" printed on the label, such as Ginsana® (Pharmaton® Natural Health Products). Take 100 milligrams once daily. Take ginseng for three weeks to three months and follow with a one- to two-week rest period before you resume taking the herb. In some people, it may cause mild stomach upset, irritability and insomnia. To prevent overstimulation, avoid taking the herb with caffeine. Ginseng should not be used during pregnancy or breastfeeding or by individuals with poorly controlled high blood pressure.

Other Natural Health Products

Bromelain

This natural product is a collection of enzymes extracted from the juice and stems of pineapple. Based on research demonstrating its effectiveness in reducing swelling of the sinuses caused by injury, it is often recommended for sinusitis. Studies from the 1960s evaluated bromelain's use in the treatment of sinusitis and found favorable results.[7-9] Unfortunately, no recent studies have been published.

Once bromelain is absorbed into the bloodstream, it causes the release of kinin, a substance that has anti-inflammatory properties. The typical dose of bromelain is 80 to 320 milligrams taken two to three times per day. However, dosage will vary with the form used, so follow the manufacturer's directions.

Bromelain may cause diarrhea in some individuals and an allergic reaction in those people allergic to pineapple and wheat. Bromelain may increase your risk of bleeding if you take blood-thinning medications and herbs such as aspirin, warfarin (Coumadin®), heparin, garlic, ginger, ginkgo biloba, horse chestnut and red clover; consult your doctor before using bromelain. Taking zinc supplements concurrently with bromelain can inhibit the enzyme's action.

Nutrition Strategy Checklist for Sinusitis

- ☐ Avoid alcohol
- ☐ Fluids
- ☐ Probiotics
- ☐ Antioxidants
- ☐ Zinc
- ☐ Echinacea
- ☐ Garlic OR Ginseng
- ☐ Bromelain

Recommended Resources

www.aaaai.org
American Academy of Allergy, Asthma and Immunology
611 E Wells Street
Milwaukee, WI, USA 53202
Tel: 1-800-822-2762

www.aafa.org
Asthma and Allergy Foundation of America
1233 20th Street NW, Suite 402
Washington, DC, USA 20036
Tel: 1-800-727-8462
Fax: 202-466-8940

www.niaid.nih.gov
National Institute of Allergy and Infectious Diseases
Office of Communications, NIH, HHS
31 Center Drive, MSC 2520 Building 31, Room 7A-50
Bethesda, MD, USA 20892-2520
Tel: 301-496-5717
Fax: 301-402-0120

Stress

Contrary to popular belief, stress can be an essential and positive force in our lives. Stress generates the challenges that keep us stimulated, motivated and productive—life without some stress would be monotonous and uneventful, even boring. Many people deliver their best mental and physical performances in response to stressful situations. Stress is the energy associated with change, and it is the way we respond to change that determines whether stress will have a positive or negative influence on our lives.

While a reasonable level of stress can be beneficial, too much stress can be counterproductive. The impact of chronic, continuous stress in our lives can produce negative emotional and physical responses. Chronic stress is thought to play a role in a number of illnesses, including high blood pressure, heart attack and digestive disorders, and it has long been considered a factor in certain types of cancer. Stress weakens the immune system, making you more vulnerable to colds, flu and other infections.

Because of the strong interaction between mind and body, stress has often been known to produce physical symptoms, even though no physical disease is evident. Many times, doctors find that the causes of back pain, muscle tension and headaches can be traced directly to situations that are emotionally distressing. The psychological effect of prolonged stress can lead to feelings of anxiety, depression, loss of self-esteem, sleep disorders, eating disorders and substance abuse.

The Stress Response

Years of evolution have prepared the body to react to stressful or dangerous situations with a very specific fight-or-flight response. A stress overload triggers a series of involuntary impulses that are initiated in the brain and rapidly involve almost every body system. The adrenal glands pump adrenaline and other stress hormones into the bloodstream. The heart beats faster to send more oxygen to vital organs—blood pressure rises and muscles tense. Muscle and fat tissues release amino acids and fatty acids into the blood for fuel. The liver converts stored starch to sugars for extra energy and digestion slows down. The kidneys retain water to preserve body fluids. All these responses are designed to prepare your body to defend itself, making it swifter, stronger and poised for immediate action.

During an acute bout of stress, these reactions are normal. Once stress is removed, the body enters the adaptation/resistance stage in which energy reserves are adjusted and rebuilt. How well your body adapts to stress will depend on the extent of its nutrient stores and your personal coping ability. If stress is ongoing and

severe, your body can reach the exhaustion stage, in which its internal resources finally dwindle. At this point, stress can result in many health problems.

It is increasingly difficult to avoid situations that create prolonged stress. Our high-speed lifestyle bombards us with a steady regimen of change. Technological innovations force us to adapt instantly to new developments. Managing the ever-increasing responsibilities of work, home and play often puts excessive demands on our time and energy. When the demands of our daily environment exceed our ability to cope successfully, stress becomes a problem that can have far-reaching consequences.

Although much is known about the physical pathways of stress in our bodies, studies have indicated that it is actually the *perception* of stress that triggers our emotional and psychological response. Everyone reacts differently to stress. Why do some people cope well with major stressors, such as the death of a loved one or the loss of a job, while others fall apart when they get stuck in a traffic jam or make a simple mistake at work? Whether stress has a negative or positive impact is influenced by an individual's attitude. Those who interpret a stressful situation as an opportunity for personal growth fare much better than those who view the circumstances as daunting or fraught with tension and concern. The amount of stress that each person can handle is influenced by a number of factors, including

- *Genetic makeup* A predisposition to depression, alcoholism or heart problems in the family may make you more vulnerable to stress.

- *Learned behaviors* Learning problem-solving skills at a young age and cultivating good self-esteem may improve coping abilities.

- *Social support* Sharing problems with close relatives, friends and colleagues alleviates the pressure of daily stress.

- *A sense of belonging* Association with a religious, national or ethnic group provides ongoing support and helps with stress management.

The workplace is probably the most common source of chronic stress. Job overload, shift work, lack of promotion, role conflicts and thwarted career plans leave most people feeling exhausted, frustrated and even physically ill at the end of a day. And it's not only high-level executives who succumb to the pressures of stress. Often it is the front-line workers, the secretaries, assistants and middle management employees who have the highest level of stress, mainly because they have so little control over the daily operation of their work environment.

In addition to work problems, there are a number of life events that have been identified and ranked on a stress-rating scale. The highest stress scores were given to major events, such as the death of a spouse, divorce, personal injury or illness, unemployment and marriage. More minor stress factors included Christmas holidays, vacations, traffic tickets and a change in working or social conditions. While the circumstances that trigger stress may vary from person to person, we all feel the pressures of our demanding lives and must work to develop sensible coping strategies in order to maintain a long and healthy life.

Symptoms of Chronic Stress

There are many warning signs of chronic stress, including

- feeling tired all the time
- difficulty sleeping
- upset stomach, indigestion, gas pain
- loss of appetite
- muscle tension
- back pain
- headaches

- pounding heart
- anxiety, nervousness
- forgetfulness, difficulty concentrating
- irritability, moodiness
- reduced efficiency, difficulty making decisions
- increased susceptibility to colds and infections
- use of drugs or alcohol to cope

Who's at Risk?

Everyone is at risk for stress, it seems. Approximately 3.5 million Canadians are estimated to suffer from severe stress, and 43 percent of all adults suffer adverse health effects due to stress.[1] In fact, 75 to 90 percent of all visits to family doctors are for stress-related complaints.

Conventional Treatment

A number of simple lifestyle changes will go a long way in helping you cope with stress:

- Learn to recognize stressful situations and avoid situations you know will generate stress or try to alter the circumstances in some way to create a more positive result.

- Reduce commitments and give up responsibilities that are not rewarding or positive.

- Simplify your life: delegate tasks; learn to say no.

- Take a break: go for a walk, have a bath, go to a movie, take a weekend off work.

- Include regular, moderate exercise in your daily routine.

- Use relaxation techniques such as deep breathing or meditation to help cope with stressful situations.

- Set priorities: do only those things that you feel are truly important.

- Share problems with friends, colleagues or close relatives.

- Eat a healthy, balanced diet to maintain a high energy level.

- Get a good night's sleep (see page 391, Insomnia, for tips on how to relax before bedtime).

- Take up a hobby or develop new interests— do something you enjoy.

- Consider getting professional help with your efforts to reduce stress.

Managing Stress

The importance of good nutrition during periods of stress cannot be overemphasized. A healthy diet, together with certain nutritional supplements, provides your body with energy, vitamins and minerals for dealing with stress and can offset the negative effects of stress on the body's immune system.

Dietary Strategies

Carbohydrates

Stress affects the concentration of a brain chemical called serotonin, a compound well known for its ability to induce a calming, relaxing effect. Over the years, researchers have learned that high-carbohydrate diets result in a greater amount of serotonin being released in the brain. High-carbohydrate diets that supply little protein provide the brain with tryptophan, an amino acid that is used as a building block to synthesize serotonin.

When stress-prone individuals are placed on either a high-carbohydrate or a high-protein diet and subjected to stress, those on the high-carbohydrate diet fare better. Studies have found that, among stress-prone individuals, high-carbohydrate, low-protein diets result in increased levels of tryptophan and serotonin, reduced stress hormone levels, improved mental performance and a decreased stress-induced depression.[2-4]

To help your body respond more positively to stress, include carbohydrate-rich meals and snacks in your daily diet. Pasta, whole-grain breads and cereals, rice, legumes, fruits and vegetables should be the focus of your meals rather than meat, poultry, fish or eggs.

Caffeine

Many studies have found that the combination of caffeine and stress has detrimental effects on blood pressure, especially in those who are at high risk for hypertension.[5-9] It appears the effects of caffeine and stress are additive and lead to larger increases in stress hormones and blood pressure than if measured separately. Regular consumption of caffeine does not build up a tolerance for its effects. Both habitual and light caffeine consumers experience negative effects on the body's stress response. Research among healthy individuals has shown that avoidance of coffee does decrease heart rate in response to stress.

Individuals who have high blood pressure or are at risk for the condition should avoid caffeine, especially when work demands or other stressors are high. See page 82, Chapter 5, to learn the caffeine content of various beverages and foods.

Alcohol

During periods of prolonged stress, you would be wise to avoid alcoholic beverages. Although many people drink to relieve stress, alcohol actually induces the body's stress response by stimulating the release of various stress hormones.[10-12] Alcohol has a dehydrating effect and also interferes with sleep, two factors that can cause fatigue and suboptimal physical and mental performance. If you must drink during stressful periods, limit yourself to no more than one drink per day.

Vitamins and Minerals
Multivitamin and Mineral Supplements
The body responds to stress by mobilizing its stored energy and converting it into blood glucose for immediate fuel. This requires the help of many different nutrients, most notably the B vitamins. Vitamin B6 is also needed by the brain to synthesize serotonin, a chemical that can help avert psychological stress. Trace minerals such as zinc are needed for the production of many stress hormones.

Studies show that chronically stressed individuals have depressed levels of nutrients in their body and that the extent of these deficiencies is related to the severity and duration of stress.[13,14] Researchers have found that a multivitamin and mineral supplement can correct nutrient imbalances and result in an improved ability to tolerate stress.[15] In one study, a multivitamin in combination with calcium, magnesium and zinc resulted in reduced anxiety and perceived stress among healthy men.[16]

To increase your intake of B vitamins during periods of stress, take a high-potency multivitamin and mineral pill once daily. Such a product will supply a greater amount of B vitamins than standard formulas. Alternatively, you could use a B complex supplement in addition to a standard multivitamin and mineral. In Chapter 4, I outline food sources for each B vitamin.

Vitamin C
The body's adrenal glands concentrate vitamin C, where it is used to make two hormones involved in the stress response, noradrenaline and thyroxin. These hormones regulate the body's metabolic rate and energy metabolism, which speed up under stress. Animal studies have found that blood vitamin C levels are decreased during stress.[17,18]

Try to eat plenty of vitamin-C-rich foods each day: citrus fruit, strawberries, kiwi, cantaloupe, broccoli, bell peppers, Brussels sprouts, cabbage, tomatoes and potatoes are all good sources. Your multivitamin will supply additional vitamin C. If you use a B complex supplement, buy one with vitamin C added. If your diet lacks fruits and vegetables, consider taking a separate vitamin C supplement: 500 milligrams of Ester C once or twice daily or 1000 milligrams of time-released C once daily.

Calcium and Magnesium
The body's response to stress includes a decrease in blood levels of calcium and magnesium.[19,20] These two minerals work together to conduct nerve impulses and contract muscles. Magnesium is essential for the production of energy, and your body's needs for this mineral may be increased during prolonged stress. One study in children exposed to a stressful television program found that supplementation with calcium prevented the decline in blood calcium.[21]

During times of stress, ensure you are meeting your daily requirements for calcium and magnesium (see Chapter 4 for RDAs and food sources). If you need to supplement your diet, use a calcium citrate supplement with added magnesium (and vitamin D for bone health). If you do not take calcium supplements, take 250 to 350 milligrams of magnesium citrate daily.

Herbal Remedies
Panax Ginseng
Also known as Asian ginseng, this herb is well known for its role as an adaptogen. As such, it is believed to help the body adapt to stress via its effect on the adrenal glands. Studies in animals under stress have shown that ginseng increases endurance and causes chemical changes that may help the body adapt to stress.[22-25] In humans, ginseng has been found to improve mental performance and enhance the immune system, both of which are adversely affected by chronic stress.[26,27]

To supplement, choose a product with a statement of standardization or "G115" printed on the label, such as Ginsana® (Pharmaton® Natural Health Products). The typical dosage of a standardized extract is 100 or 200 milligrams once daily. Take ginseng for three weeks to three months, followed with a one- to two-week rest period before you resume taking the herb. In some people, ginseng may cause mild stomach upset, irritability and insomnia. To avoid overstimulation, start with 100 milligrams a day and avoid taking the herb with caffeine. Ginseng should not be used during pregnancy or breast-feeding or in individuals with poorly controlled high blood pressure.

Siberian Ginseng
(*Eleutherococcus senticosus*)

Unlike Panax ginseng, this herb has a much milder effect and fewer reported side effects. Pregnant and nursing women can safely take Siberian ginseng, and it is much less likely to cause overstimulation in sensitive individuals. To ensure quality, choose a product standardized for eleutherosides B and E. The usual dosage is 300 to 400 milligrams once daily for six to eight weeks, followed by a one- to two-week break.

Nutrition Strategy Checklist for Stress

- ☐ High-carbohydrate diet
- ☐ Avoid caffeine
- ☐ Avoid alcohol
- ☐ Multivitamin/mineral supplement OR B complex
- ☐ Vitamin C
- ☐ Calcium
- ☐ Magnesium
- ☐ Panax OR Siberian ginseng

Recommended Resources

www.stress.org
The American Institute of Stress
124 Park Avenue
Yonkers, NY, USA 10703

Tel: 914-963-1200
Fax: 914-965-6267
E-mail: stress124@earthlink.net

www.stresscanada.org
Canadian Institute of Stress
Medcan Clinic Office
150 York Street, Suite 1500
Toronto, ON, Canada M5H 3S5
Tel: 416-236-4218

www.mayoclinic.com
Mayo Foundation for Medical Education and Research

Ulcers (Peptic Ulcers)

Once thought to be the inevitable result of a highly spiced diet and a stressful lifestyle, we now know that 80 percent of all stomach ulcers and more than 90 percent of all duodenal ulcers are actually caused by a bacteria called *Helicobacter pylori* (*H. pylori*).[1] This major scientific advance has completely changed the way ulcers are treated and has allowed many people to enjoy a complete recovery.

What Causes Ulcers?

A peptic ulcer is a sore or crater that develops when the lining of the stomach or the small intestine has been eaten away by stomach acid and digestive juices. The name *peptic* comes from pepsin, an enzyme that helps to break down food for digestion. Normally, the stomach defends itself from acid erosion by secreting mucus that acts as a protective barrier and chemicals that neutralize acids. Blood circulating through the stomach lining acts to promote new cell growth and repair. Although these defense mechanisms are usually effective, sometimes a particular combination of stomach acids and digestive enzymes can burn right into the delicate tissue of the stomach.

Ulcers are often no bigger than a pencil eraser, but the pain that they cause can be unbearable. There are several different types of peptic ulcers:

- *Duodenal ulcers* are the most common type; they develop in the upper small intestine.

- *Gastric ulcers* occur along the upper curve of the stomach.

- *Esophageal ulcers* occur when stomach acid repeatedly flows back up into the esophagus.

- *Marginal ulcers* develop after surgery to remove part of the stomach; they usually appear where the stomach has been reattached to the intestine.

One in every ten people will develop an ulcer.[2] Most people with ulcers are infected with the H. pylori bacteria. But not everyone infected with H. pylori will develop ulcers. This seems to suggest that H. pylori infection, by itself, is not enough to cause a problem. Scientists suspect that the bacteria must work in combination with other factors, such as a genetic predisposition to ulcers, to create the right environment for an ulcer to develop.

Researchers think that H. pylori may be transmitted through food or water or by kissing someone who is infected. The bacteria operates by secreting an enzyme that neutralizes stomach acid. It then migrates to the stomach lining, where it burrows into the mucous lining. This weakens the protective coating, allowing acid to irritate the sensitive stomach tissue.

Another major cause of ulcers is the use of nonsteroidal anti-inflammatory drugs (NSAIDs), such as ibuprofen and aspirin. Regular use of these drugs irritates the stomach and interferes with the defensive mechanisms that protect the stomach lining. Once the drugs are stopped, the ulcer usually heals and doesn't recur unless the drugs are taken again.

Ulcers can sometimes cause serious complications that may require surgery:

- *Penetration* The ulcer can pass right through the wall of the stomach or duodenum and into a nearby organ, such as the liver.

- *Perforation* Ulcers on the duodenum and sometimes those on the stomach can burn right through the abdominal wall, creating an opening into the abdomen. The abdomen becomes very tender and intense pain spreads rapidly.

- *Bleeding* Vomiting blood or passing black or bloody stools usually indicates a bleeding ulcer, which may lead to anemia.

- *Obstruction* Swollen tissue or scarring around the ulcer may narrow the duodenum or the passageway from the stomach. Repeated vomiting, bloating and loss of appetite are symptoms of a blockage.

Symptoms

- gnawing, burning pain felt anywhere between the breastbone and the navel

- pain that tends to occur when the stomach is empty, often developing two to three hours after a meal

- moderate or mild pain that may last from a few minutes to many hours

- pain relief from drinking milk, eating or taking antacids, but the pain returns within a few hours

- worsened pain at night

- pain while eating; bloating, nausea or vomiting after eating (gastric ulcer)

- pain while swallowing or lying down (esophageal ulcer)

- poor appetite, weight loss

Who's at Risk?

Duodenal ulcers often occur between the ages of 30 and 50, whereas gastric ulcers are more common after age 60. Duodenal ulcers are twice as common in men, and gastric ulcers are more common in women. Common risk factors for developing an ulcer include

- daily use of NSAIDs

- exposure to *H. pylori* bacteria

- a family history of peptic ulcer

- cigarette smoking, which doubles the risk of ulcers, increases severity, slows healing and increases risk of recurrence

- drinking caffeinated beverages

- drinking alcohol

- race: blacks and Hispanics are at higher risk

Conventional Treatment

Usually a combination of antibiotics and acid-blocking medications is used to treat ulcers caused by H. pylori infections. Histamine H2 receptor antagonist drugs, such as Zantac® (ranitidine), Pepcid® (famotidine) and Tagamet® (cimetidine), decrease the production of stomach acid. Proton pump inhibitor drugs, such as Losec® (omeprazole), Pantoloc® (pantoprazole) and Prevacid® (lansoprazole), are used to stop the pumping of acid into the stomach.

To help an ulcer heal, stop taking NSAIDs such as ibuprofen. Use alternative medications to reduce side effects. Antacids may help relieve symptoms by temporarily neutralizing stomach acids.

Surgery may be necessary if the ulcer fails to heal, keeps recurring or leads to complications. Caffeine, smoking and alcohol should be avoided since they are all known to irritate an ulcer.

Managing Ulcers

Dietary Strategies

The traditional bland diet is no longer recommended for people with peptic ulcers as there is no evidence that it speeds the rate of healing. In view of this, only slight dietary changes are required, many of them based on an individual's tolerance to certain foods. The goal of the peptic ulcer diet is to avoid extreme elevations in stomach acid secretion and irritation of the mucosal lining. To help heal an ulcer, implement the following dietary strategies:

- Avoid caffeinated and decaffeinated beverages and alcohol; all stimulate acid secretion.

- Avoid eating frequent meals and bedtime snacks to prevent increased acid secretion.

- Avoid eating large quantities of food at one sitting.

- Avoid spices that may trigger acid secretion and cause indigestion: black pepper, red chili peppers, cloves, garlic, chili powder. You may find that other spices bother you—these should be avoided during the healing process. (While chili peppers can irritate an active ulcer, they may actually prevent an ulcer from developing in the first place.)

- Citric acid juices, such as apple juice, may cause heartburn and discomfort in some people.

Fermented Milk Products

There is some evidence that lactic acid bacteria present in yogurt, kefir and sweet acidophilus milk may prevent ulcers from occurring.[3] Such foods are referred to as probiotics, which means "to promote life." Once consumed, these lactic acid bacteria adhere to the lining of the gastrointestinal tract, where they protect the body from disease-causing microbes. In this way, they may reduce the risk of H. pylori infections. Include one serving of a fermented milk product in your daily diet. Probiotic supplements are also available (see below).

Polyunsaturated Fat

Laboratory studies suggest that polyunsaturated fats found in fish, vegetable oils, nuts and seeds may prevent a peptic ulcer by inhibiting the growth of H. pylori.[4] The body also uses polyunsaturated fats to manufacture prostaglandins, immune compounds that may affect gastric blood flow and acid secretion. Researchers have learned that people with peptic ulcer disease have lower levels of polyunsaturated fats and prostaglandins in their bloodstream.[5-7]

Include 1 to 2 tablespoons (15 to 30 ml) of flaxseed, canola or walnut oil in your daily diet. Borage oil and black currant oil, available in health food stores, are also excellent sources of health-enhancing polyunsaturated fats. Eat oily fish three times per week.

Vitamins and Minerals

Antioxidants

Free radical molecules are believed to play an important role in peptic ulcers. Vitamins C and E, beta-carotene and selenium protect the lining of the gastrointestinal tract by mopping up free radicals before they can harm cells. One study found that people with stomach ulcers had markedly lower levels of all antioxidant nutrients compared with healthy people.[8] The degree of antioxidant depletion was similar whether the ulcer was caused by H. pylori or NSAID drug use. Use the following as a guide to increase your antioxidant intake:

- *Vitamin C* The recommended dietary allowance (RDA) is 75 and 90 milligrams for women and men respectively (smokers need an additional 35 milligrams). Best food sources include citrus fruit, citrus juices, cantaloupe, kiwi, mango, strawberries, broccoli, Brussels sprouts, cauliflower, red pepper and tomato juice. To supplement, take 500 milligrams of Ester C once or twice daily. The daily upper limit is 2000 milligrams.

- *Vitamin E* The RDA is 22 international units (IU). Best food sources include wheat germ, nuts, seeds, vegetable oils, whole grains and kale. To supplement, take 200 to 800 IU of natural source vitamin E. Buy a "mixed" vitamin E supplement if possible. The daily upper limit is 1500 IU.

- *Selenium* The RDA is 55 micrograms. Best food sources are seafood, chicken, organ meats, whole grains, nuts, onions, garlic and mushrooms. To supplement, take 200 micrograms of selenium-rich yeast per day. The daily upper limit is 400 micrograms.

- *Beta-Carotene* No RDA has been established. Best food sources are orange and dark green produce, including carrots, sweet potato, winter squash, broccoli, collard greens, kale, spinach, apricots, cantaloupe, peaches, nectarines, mango and papaya. Avoid taking beta-carotene supplements if you smoke. If you are a nonsmoker, choose a multivitamin and mineral with beta-carotene added.

Vitamin B12

If you take acid-blocking medication, such as cimetidine, you need to increase your intake of vitamin B12. For vitamin B12 to be absorbed into the bloodstream, it first must be cleaved from its food sources. Stomach acid performs this task, providing the body with an absorbable form of the vitamin. Acid-blocking drugs have the potential to cause a B12 deficiency, especially in people who don't get enough of the nutrient from their diet.[9]

Vitamin B12 is found exclusively in animal foods: meat, poultry, fish, eggs and dairy products. Fortified soy and rice beverages also supply vitamin B12. If you are a strict vegetarian who eats no animal products and you don't drink fortified soy or rice beverages, take a B12 supplement. Take a high-potency multivitamin and mineral supplement or a B complex supplement that contains the whole family of B vitamins. If you take a single B12 supplement, take 500 to 1000 micrograms once daily. If you are taking a high-dose B12 supplement to correct a deficiency, don't take it with a vitamin C pill. Large amounts of vitamin C can destroy B12. Take your vitamin C supplement one hour after you take your B12.

Herbal Remedies

Garlic (*Allium sativum*)

Historically, garlic has been used around the world to treat bacterial infections. Garlic has been shown to exhibit a broad-spectrum antibiotic effect, killing many different types of bacteria. Scientists have now demonstrated that garlic kills H. pylori—even strains resistant to antibiotic therapy.[10-13] It should be noted that small studies using garlic cloves, garlic powder or garlic oil have not found an effect in people infected with H. pylori. However, the testing methods used in these studies have been criticized.

Adding garlic to your daily diet may prevent an ulcer from occurring. Use one-half to one clove of fresh garlic in cooking each day (do not use garlic when your ulcer is active). To supplement, buy a product made with aged garlic extract. Take two to six capsules a day in divided doses. Aged garlic extract (Kyolic®)is odorless and less irritating to the gastrointestinal tract than other forms of garlic supplements (garlic oil capsules, garlic powder tablets). You might also consider using Kwai® brand garlic powder tablets; take 300 milligrams three times daily.

Licorice (*Glycyrrhiza glabra*)

A special form of this herb, called deglycrrhizinated licorice (DGL), may be an effective treatment for healing ulcers. To make DGL, the por-tion of the herb that causes fluid retention, high blood pressure and potassium loss, is removed. Two studies have shown that DGL taken in combination with antacids can heal ulcers as effectively as acid-blocking drugs.[14,15] The herb does not kill H. pylori, so it should be taken on a regular basis to prevent an ulcer from recurring.

To treat an ulcer, chew two to four 380 milligram DGL tablets before each meal. The only side effect noted is its unpleasant taste. Licorice as a whole herb (not DGL) may have hormonal activity in the body and should not be used by women with breast cancer or men with low testosterone levels. It is less likely that these effects occur with DGL, but it's better to be safe and avoid the product if you fall into one of these categories.

Other Natural Health Products

Probiotic Supplements

If you don't eat yogurt or other fermented milk products on a regular basis, consider taking probiotic supplements. To supplement, buy a product that offers 1 to 10 billion live cells per dose (capsule). Take one capsule three times daily with food. Choose a product that is stable at room temperature and does not require refrigeration. This allows you to continue taking your supplement while traveling. Refer to page 137, Chapter 8, for further information on probiotics.

Nutrition Strategy Checklist for Ulcers

☐ Avoid caffeine

☐ Avoid eating often

☐ Avoid spices

☐ Fermented milk products

☐ Polyunsaturated fat

☐ Antioxidants

☐ Vitamin B12

☐ Garlic

☐ Deglycrrhizinated licorice (DGL)

☐ Probiotic supplements

Recommended Resources

www.acg.gi.org
American College of Gastroenterology
4900-B S 31st Street
Arlington, VA, USA 22206
Tel: 703-820-7400
Fax: 703-931-4520

www.mayoclinic.com
Mayo Foundation for Medical Education and Research

www.niddk.nih.gov
National Digestive Diseases Information Clearinghouse
2 Information Way
Bethesda, MD, USA 20892-3570
Tel: 301-654-3810

Urinary Tract Infections (UTIs)

Women experience the symptoms of a urinary tract infection (UTI), such as pain or a burning sensation during urination, far more often than men. In fact, Canadian women make about 500,000 visits to doctors each year because of UTIs.[1] While UTIs are distressing and uncomfortable, they are easily cured and rarely have lasting complications if treated promptly. However, if left untreated, UTIs can lead to potentially life-threatening problems. Early detection and treatment are essential to prevent a serious health risk.

What Causes Urinary Tract Infections?

The role of the urinary system is to help the body eliminate waste products in the form of urine. Your urinary tract comprises the kidneys, ureters, bladder and urethra, which work in harmony to produce, store and eliminate urine. The urinary process begins with the kidneys, which filter and remove waste products from the bloodstream. These waste products become urine, which flows from the kidneys through small tubes called the ureters into the bladder. The bladder serves as a storage tank, collecting the urine until it can be eliminated. During urination, muscles in the bladder push urine out through the urethra, which has an opening on the outside of your body to discharge this fluid waste.

Normally, the urine that flows through the urinary tract system is sterile, which means that it does not contain bacteria. UTIs usually begin when bacteria enter the urethra and travel upward through the urinary tract, producing inflammation and irritation. Most UTIs are caused by Escherichia coli (E. coli) bacteria, which migrate into the urinary tract from the rectum or the vagina. On rare occasions, bacteria may enter the urinary tract through the bloodstream.

Subtle differences in the anatomy of the male and female urinary tract make women more prone than men to develop UTIs. In women, the opening of the urethra is very close to the opening of the rectum, or anus. Because of the close proximity of these two openings, bacteria can be easily transferred from the rectum into the urinary tract, causing infection. The female urethra is also considerably shorter than it is in men, and this allows the bacteria to reach the bladder much more easily. The final difference lies in the fact that the female urethra is purely a urinary duct, whereas the male urethra also carries semen. It's thought that the male prostate gland secretes a bacteria-killing fluid into the urethra to protect the semen as it travels through this multifunctional passageway. This fluid may help prevent men from contracting UTIs.

The most common type of UTI is cystitis, which is an infection of the bladder. Cystitis may be accompanied by an inflammation of the urethra, a condition known as urethritis. Sexually transmitted diseases, such as herpes, chlamydia and gonorrhea, often cause urethritis in both men and women. If the infection is left untreated, bacteria will travel farther into the urinary tract. In some cases, the infection may even attack the kidneys, a condition that can cause permanent kidney damage if not treated promptly.

Symptoms

One of the most recognizable symptoms of a UTI is a burning sensation at the beginning or during urination. As the infection progresses, the urge to urinate may become stronger and more frequent. The urine may also appear cloudy, dark and have a strange odor.

A UTI may produce fever, chills and vomiting or may cause pain in the back or lower abdominal area. Do not ignore these symptoms because they may indicate the beginning of a kidney infection, a serious complication of a UTI.

Who's at Risk?

Sexually active girls and women are most often at risk for developing a UTI. During intercourse, friction can push bacteria from the anus into the urethra, initiating the cycle of infection.

Pregnant women are also at a higher risk for developing UTIs. Pregnancy produces hormonal changes that affect the urinary system, increasing the likelihood of infection. The urinary tract is often dislodged from its normal position by pressure from the growing fetus, which further increases susceptibility.

Urinary tract infections are also a common concern for elderly women. As women approach menopause, estrogen levels begin to fall, leaving them prone to infections and irritations of the vagina and urinary tract. In rare cases, UTIs may be the result of anatomical problems, causing obstructions within the urinary tract.

Conventional Treatment

In some cases, UTIs will clear up spontaneously, without any treatment. However, most are treated with antibiotics. The drugs may be given in a single, large dose or may be spread over a course of three to seven days. A repeat infection is treated with a second course of antibiotics. Treatment is normally continued until symptoms disappear and a urine test shows no bacteria.

As many as 80 percent of women who have a UTI will get another in 18 months.[2] Low daily doses of antibiotics for a six-month period or a single dose of antibiotic after sexual activity may prevent long-term problems. Postmenopausal women with recurrent UTIs may find some relief through estrogen replacement therapy, particularly estrogen creams that are applied to the vagina.

Preventing and Managing Urinary Tract Infections

Personal Hygiene

One of the most important methods of preventing a UTI is to practice good personal hygiene. To avoid spreading bacteria from the rectum into the urethra, wipe gently from front to back whenever you urinate or have a bowel movement. When you feel the urge to urinate, try not to resist. A regular release of fresh, sterile urine will often wash harmful bacteria out of the urethra before it has a chance to travel into the urinary tract.

It is also a wise idea to clean your genital area before having intercourse, as this will remove harmful bacteria that may be accidentally transferred into the urethra. Urinating before and after intercourse will help wash out any bacteria that has migrated into the urinary tract.

Bacteria grow best in a warm, moist environment. Wear cotton underwear or pantyhose with cotton liners for good ventilation. Avoid tight-fitting pants or other types of clothing that may trap heat, irritate tissues and promote bacterial growth. Washing your undergarments in strong soaps or bleach may cause irritations that could lead to a UTI. Avoid chemical irritants such as bubble bath, perfumed soaps, douches, feminine hygiene deodorants and deodorant tampons and pads.

Dietary Strategies

Aggravating Foods

During your recovery period, avoid coffee, alcohol and spicy foods, which may aggravate the urinary tract. You may find that other foods can also exacerbate discomfort. Refer to page 397, Interstitial Cystitis, for a list of condiments and spices that can irritate the bladder. Some of these foods and spices may also aggravate UTIs.

Cranberry Juice

Natural chemicals in cranberries, called proanthocyanins, treat UTIs by preventing E. coli bacteria from adhering to the wall of the urinary tract. As a result, bacteria are flushed out in the urine.

Studies show that a daily glass of cranberry juice may not only prevent a UTI but also may be effective at treating one.[3,4] Finnish researchers found that a 1/4 cup (60 ml) of cranberry-lignonberry juice consumed daily prevented a repeat UTI significantly better than the placebo treatments. An American study found similar results. Researchers followed 153 women who were given either 300 milliliters (10 fluid ounces) of cranberry juice or a placebo drink once daily. At the end of six months, women drinking the cranberry juice were only about one-quarter as likely as those in the placebo group to continue to have UTIs.

If you are susceptible to UTIs, drink at least 300 milliliters of cranberry juice each day. In the American study, participants drank a cranberry cocktail that was 27 percent juice. When buying cranberry juice, be sure to check the labels—most cranberry cocktails contain 10 to 33 percent cranberry juice.

Drinking large quantities (1 liter or more) of cranberry juice may aggravate kidney stones in some people. Stones made from oxalate and uric acid are more likely to form in acidic urine. Women with irritable bowel syndrome may experience diarrhea if they drink too much cranberry juice—500 milliliters or more, although this will vary from person to person.

Blueberries

Proanthocyanins, the same compounds found in cranberries that prevent E. coli bacteria from adhering to the wall of the urinary tract, are also present in blueberries. Reports from Rutgers University in New Jersey suggest that blueberries also promote urinary tract health. If you don't like cranberry juice, or you want to add variety, add 1/2 to 1 cup (125 to 250 ml) of fresh, frozen or dried blueberries to your daily diet.

Water

Drink at least 8 to 12 cups (2 to 3 liters) of water each day to help flush bacteria out of your system. Women who engage in vigorous exercise should drink 12 to 16 cups (3 to 4 liters) per day. Drink 1 to 2 cups (250 to 500 milliliters) with each meal and snack. Carry a water bottle with you when you travel.

Herbal Remedies

Cranberry Extract

If you do not want to consume the sugar and calories found in cranberry juice, you might consider taking capsules of dried cranberry. Capsules contain anywhere from 300 to 800 milligrams of dried cranberry powder and are available in health food stores and pharmacies. Take two 500 milligram capsules per day—the equivalent of 300 milliliters of cranberry juice.

Garlic (*Allium sativum*)

A daily intake of garlic can help the body fight bacterial infection. Studies have shown that garlic, in particular the allyl sulfur compounds in aged garlic extract, stimulate the body's immune system by increasing the activity of white blood cells that fight infection.[5-7]

Most scientists agree that one-half to one clove of fresh garlic consumed each day will offer health benefits. And most people can take one or two cloves a day without any problems. Add fresh garlic to salad dressings, pasta sauces and stir-fries.

The oil-soluble compounds in fresh garlic account for its odor and its potential to cause stomach upset. If you decide to supplement instead of eating fresh garlic, buy an aged garlic extract. This form of garlic has the highest concentration of the sulfur compounds that boost the immune system. Aged garlic extract is also odorless and gentler on the stomach. Take two to six capsules per day in divided doses. Since both fresh garlic and garlic supplements can thin the blood, consult your physician if you are taking blood-thinning medication such as warfarin (Coumadin®).

Uva Ursi

Studies suggest that, when taken on a short-term basis, this herb may be effective for acute, uncomplicated UTIs.[8-10] The leaf of the plant contains arbutin, tannins and hydroquinone, ingredients that have antiseptic and astringent effects in the urinary tract. Uva ursi may also reduce inflammation. Although this theory is not proven, some experts believe that foods that increase the acidity of the urine (like cranberry juice) diminish the antibacterial properties of uva ursi.

Buy a product standardized to contain 20 percent arbutin. The recommended dosage is 400 to 800 milligrams of arbutin daily, and this amount should not be exceeded. To use a tea, steep 3 grams of the dried leaf in 150 milliliters of cold water for 12 to 24 hours and then strain. Take 1 cup of tea four times a day. Prepare the tea with cold water to minimize its tannin content as tannins can cause stomach upset. Uva ursi leaves are available from a certified herbalist.

There are safety concerns associated with using uva ursi. *Do not use the herb longer than one week without medical supervision.* Tannins can irritate the stomach and limit the herb's duration of use. Hydroquinone can have toxic effects if taken in larger amounts for an extended period. Your doctor should evaluate any urinary tract symptoms that persist for longer than 48 hours after taking the herb. *Limit your use of uva ursi to five times a year.*

Do not take uva ursi if you are pregnant or breastfeeding. The herb can increase the speed of labor in pregnant women, and there is very little information available about its use during lactation. Do not use uva ursi if you have a kidney disorder.

Other Natural Health Products

Probiotic Supplements

Once consumed, friendly bacteria such as Lactobacillus acidophilus and bifidobacteria produce lactic acid and hydrogen peroxide, compounds that suppress the growth of E. coli in the intestinal tract. Research has demonstrated that these bacteria prevent E. coli from attaching to the lining of the intestine and the vagina.[11-13] One study even found that lactobacillus treatment reduced the recurrence of UTIs in women.[14] Probiotics may also enhance the body's immune system.

If you are taking an antibiotic for your UTI, consider adding a probiotic supplement to your treatment regime. Antibiotics kill all bacteria —friendly and disease-causing. Taking a probiotic supplement while on antibiotic therapy may lessen the chances of a repeat infection and decrease gastrointestinal upset caused by the drug.

The strength of a probiotic supplement is expressed in the number of live bacteria cells per capsule. To treat a UTI, take 1 to 10 billion live cells in three divided doses daily. Take your supplement with a meal.

Add probiotic foods such as yogurt, kefir and sweet acidophilus milk to your daily diet.

Nutrition Strategy Checklist for UTIs

- ☐ Avoid aggravating foods
- ☐ Cranberry juice OR Cranberry supplements
- ☐ Blueberries
- ☐ Water
- ☐ Garlic
- ☐ Uva ursi
- ☐ Probiotic supplements

Recommended Resources

www.kidney.ca
The Kidney Foundation of Canada
300-5165 Sherbrooke Street W
Montreal, PQ, Canada H4A 1T6
Tel: 514-369-4806 or 1-800-361-7494
Fax: 514-369-2472

www.mayoclinic.com
Mayo Foundation for Medical Education and Research

www.niddk.nih.gov
National Kidney and Urologic Diseases Information Clearinghouse
The National Institute of Diabetes and Digestive and Kidney Diseases
Office of Communications and Public Liaison
NIDDK, NIH, 31 Center Drive, MSC 2560
Bethesda, MD, USA 20892-2560
Tel: 1-800-622-9010

Varicose Veins

Varicose veins are quite common and affect women far more often than men. Unfortunately, varicose veins cannot be cured, but they can be managed successfully with simple preventative measures and progressive medical treatments.

Varicose veins occur most often in the legs, on the inside of the leg, at the back of the calf or around the ankles. They can also develop in the vagina during pregnancy, around the anus as hemorrhoids, and, occasionally, they may appear in other parts of the body.

What Causes Varicose Veins?

To understand how varicose veins develop, it's important to first learn how the body's circulatory system works. Within your circulatory system, your heart acts like a pump, sending nutrients and oxygen-rich blood to all your cells. This blood is pumped to your cells through a network of arteries. It then flows back to the heart along an extensive system of veins. As the blood returns from the lower parts of your body, it must fight against the natural pull of gravity, which constantly draws it backward, away from the heart. To help keep the blood moving upward toward your heart, veins are equipped with a series of tiny, one-way valves. The forward flow of the blood pushes the valves open in the direction of the heart. As gravity exerts its normal pull, the backpressure of the blood causes the valves to close, preventing any blood from flowing backward into the veins.

Varicose veins develop when these important valves become damaged, allowing blood to pool in the veins. This increased blood flow eventually stretches and weakens the veins, causing them to bulge and swell painfully. Over time, these veins lose their elasticity and stretch to become wider and longer. To fit into the same space, the veins begin to twist and bend under the skin, assuming the characteristic snake-like appearance of varicose veins. As the veins become wider, the valves inside them can no longer close tightly. Blood leaks backward into the veins and causes even more stretching and widening. This vicious cycle continues, creating a worsening condition that usually results in large, bulging blue veins that knot the surface of the skin.

Symptoms

Some people with varicose veins have no symptoms at all, but most complain of swollen feet and ankles, a dull pressure or aching heaviness in their legs, muscle cramps or itchy skin near the affected veins. The discomfort of varicose veins tends to become worse at the end of the day or after prolonged sitting or standing. Women often suffer more during the days immediately before menstruation.

If varicose veins become worse, you may experience some skin changes caused by a slowing of the blood flow through your veins. These changes include dryness, rashes, brown discolorations or ulcers (open sores). The slower blood flow may also cause a painful inflammation known as phlebitis (see page 472). It can also make you more susceptible to dangerous blood clots inside the damaged vein.

Who's at Risk?

Varicose veins usually begin to appear between the ages of 30 and 60. Several factors increase the odds of getting varicose veins, including obesity, prolonged standing and a family history of varicose veins. Women are more susceptible to varicose veins than men because pressure put on the pelvis during pregnancy and hormonal changes associated with menstruation can both interfere with vein function.

Conventional Treatment

Unfortunately, varicose veins don't get better on their own. Treatment may be undertaken for medical or cosmetic reasons and usually works to relieve symptoms, improve appearance and prevent complications.

Elastic stockings (compression or support hose) are often used to slow the progression of varicose veins. These special stockings help keep your veins from stretching and hurting by massaging the legs and stimulating blood flow. They are to be worn daily, from the moment you get out of bed until you retire in the evening.

Elevating your legs by lying down or using a footstool when sitting will also promote blood drainage and help relieve symptoms. Other ways to relieve the symptoms of varicose veins include

- Regular exercise—activities such as walking encourage blood circulation in your legs.

- Maintain a healthy weight—shedding excess weight will take unnecessary pressure off your veins.

- Avoid standing or sitting for long periods.

- Don't wear tight clothing or undergarments that restrict your waist, groin or legs.

- When traveling by air or during long car trips, get up from your seat or stop the car once every 45 minutes so that you can stretch and move around.

If a self-care approach does not relieve symptoms, your doctor may recommend one of the following medical treatments:

- *Sclerotherapy* A saline solution is injected into small or medium-sized veins, causing them to collapse and seal shut. Blood flow is diverted to stronger, healthier veins, and the body gradually reabsorbs the closed veins. The procedure is very effective, relatively painless and can be done in your doctor's office. It may take several injections before each vein is eliminated, and the injections can only be given at four- to six-week intervals.

- *Ambulatory phlebectomy* A series of small incisions are made in the skin in order to grab the vein with a tiny hook and pull it out. This is performed in the doctor's office using local or regional anesthetic.

- *Laser light therapy* A laser is targeted on the blue color of the oxygen-deprived blood in the damaged vein. It heats the blood, scalding and sealing the vein, while leaving the surrounding tissue intact. This technique is useful only on veins close to the skin surface.

- *Stripping/Ligation* This surgery is done in an operating room under general anesthetic. An incision is made at the groin and another one at your ankle in order to open that vein at each end. A fine wire is threaded through the vein and then pulled out again, removing the vein with it. Alternatively, the vein may be tied off and left in place to be absorbed by your body. The stripping/ligation procedure is lengthy and will leave visible scars.

Preventing and Managing Varicose Veins

Dietary Strategies

Dietary Fiber

Eat high-fiber foods such as whole grains, bran cereal and fresh fruit and vegetables to promote regular bowel function. Research suggests that constipation can contribute to varicose veins.[1] Straining to evacuate small, firm stools puts pressure on the abdominal muscles, which can be transmitted to the veins in the leg. To avoid constipation, consume 25 to 35 grams of fiber per day.

Foods contain varying amounts of insoluble fibers and soluble fibers. Foods that have a greater proportion of insoluble fibers, such as wheat bran, whole grains, nuts, seeds and certain fruits and vegetables, are used to treat and prevent constipation. Once consumed, insoluble fibers make their way to the intestinal tract, where they absorb water, help form larger, softer stools and speed evacuation. Psyllium, a type of soluble fiber, also adds bulk to stools and can be used to treat constipation. Refer to page 243, Constipation, for more on psyllium.

Fiber needs plenty of fluid so that it can swell and promote the passage of large, soft stools through the bowel. Drink at least 8 cups (2 liters) of fluid each day. If you exercise regularly, drink an additional 4 cups (1 liter).

Sodium

Reduce your salt intake to prevent swelling that may damage veins. Consume no more than 2400 milligrams of sodium per day (about 1 teaspoon worth of salt). Avoid the saltshaker at the table, minimize the use of salt when you cook and buy commercial food products that are low in added salt. Instead of salt, season your foods with herbs, spices, flavored vinegars and fruit juices. Most of the salt we consume every day comes from processed and prepared foods. You'll find the sodium content of selected foods on page 80, Chapter 5.

Herbal Remedies

Bilberry (*Vaccinium myrtillus*)

This herb contains anthocyanins, a compound that belongs to the flavonoids family. Anthocyanins help form strong connective tissue and blood capillaries. Most research on bilberry has been in eye health, but one controlled study found it to be effective at relieving leg pain and swelling in people with varicose veins.[2] Buy a product standardized to 25 to 36 percent anthocyanins. Take 120 to 240 milligrams twice daily. No adverse effects have been reported with bilberry use.

Gotu Kola (*Centella asiatica*)

This herb has long been used in India and Indonesia to promote wound healing and treat skin diseases. Since the 1970s it has been used in Europe to treat venous insufficiency disorders. Studies have shown that taking the herb for four weeks can reduce leg heaviness, discomfort, foot and ankle swelling, and fluid leakage in the veins.[3-7] Gotu kola seems to promote the formation of healthy connective tissue.

Buy a product standardized to 40 percent asiaticoside, 30 percent Asiatic acid, 30 percent madecassic acid and 1 to 2 percent madecassoside. Take 20 to 40 milligrams three times daily. The herb is not associated with any side effects other than the occasional skin rash. Safety in pregnant and breastfeeding women and young children has not been established.

Horse Chestnut (*Aesculus hippocastanum*)

Evidence supports the use of horse chestnut in the treatment of varicose veins. While it does not reduce the visible appearance of varicose veins, studies have demonstrated its ability to reduce leg swelling, leg pain and heaviness.[8-10] One study even found that horse chestnut was equally effective as compression stockings, although the herb took longer to have an effect.[11]

An active compound, called aesin, in the horse chestnut seeds enhances circulation through the veins. The herb appears to constrict and promote normal tone in the veins so that blood returns to the heart. The compound also has anti-inflammatory properties and may reduce swelling in the legs.

Buy a product standardized to 16 to 21 percent aescin. Take 300 milligrams, three times daily. Once leg symptoms have improved, reduce the dose to 150 milligrams per day. The extract used in the clinical studies is sold as Venastat® (Pharmaton® Natural Health Products) in Canada and the United States. The safety of horse chestnut during pregnancy and breastfeeding has not been established; avoid using the herb at these times. Do not take horse chestnut if you have liver or kidney disease.

Other Natural Health Products

Grapeseed Extract

Like bilberry, this supplement is rich in anthocyanins, natural compounds that help keep blood vessels healthy. Grapeseed extract is thought to work by inhibiting the action of enzymes that break down connective tissue. Three studies have evaluated its use in varicose veins and found that it significantly improved symptoms compared with the placebo treatment.[12-14] Anthocyanins may also help reduce blood clots.

The recommended dose is 150 to 300 milligrams per day. Some experts recommend taking 150 to 300 milligrams for three weeks, followed by a maintenance dose of 40 to 80 milligrams daily. Grapeseed extract is considered extremely safe, although it may have blood-thinning properties when taken in high doses. Consult your doctor if you are taking an anticoagulant medication.

Nutrition Strategy Checklist for Varicose Veins

☐ Dietary fiber
☐ Fluids
☐ Low sodium
☐ Horse chestnut* OR Bilberry OR Gotu kola
☐ Grapeseed extract

*Strongest evidence—start here.

Recommended Resources

www.crha-health.ab.ca
Calgary Regional Health Authority
Communications
1035-7th Avenue SW
Calgary, AB, Canada T2P 3E9
Tel: 403-265-INFO (403-265-4636) or 1-800-
860-2742 (Alberta only)
E-mail: publicweb@crha-health.ab.ca

www.mayoclinic.com
Mayo Foundation for Medical Education and
Research

www.medicinenet.com
An online medical information site for consumers.

Endnotes

Introduction

1. IPSOS-Reid Canadian Nutritional Supplement Review, 2000.
2. The National Institute of Nutrition, *Tracking Nutrition Trends 1989–1994–1997. An Update on Canadians' Attitudes, Knowledge and Reported Actions* (Ottawa, November 1997).

Part 1: Nutrition and Diet

Chapter 5

1. Jacobs, D.R., Jr. et al. "Whole-grain intake may reduce the risk of ischemic heart disease death in postmenopausal women: The Iowa Women's Health Study," *Am J Clin Nutr* 1998; 68(2):248–257.
2. Liu, S. et al. "Whole-grain consumption and risk of coronary heart disease: results from the Nurses' Health Study," *Am J Clin Nutr* 1999; 70(3):412–419.
3. Liu, S. et al. "A prospective study of whole-grain intake and risk of type 2 diabetes mellitus in US women," *Am J Public Health* 2000; 90(9):1409–1415.
4. Thompson, L.U. et al. "Flaxseed and its lignan and oil components reduce mammary tumor growth at a late stage of carcinogenesis," *Carcinogenesis* 1996; 17(6):1373–1376.
5. Thompson, L.U. et al. "Antitumorigenic effect of a mammalian lignan precurser from flaxseed," *Nutr Cancer* 1996; 26(2):159–165.
6. Thompson, L.U. et al. "Biological effects of dietary flaxseed in patients with breast cancer," *Breast Cancer Research and Treatment* 64(1):50.
7. Somekawa, Y. et al. "Soy intake related to menopausal symptoms, serum lipids, and bone mineral density in postmenopausal Japanese women," *Obstet Gynecol* 2001; 97(1):109–115.
8. Horiuchi, T. et al. "Effect of soy protein on bone metabolism in postmenopausal Japanese women," *Osteoporos Int* 2000; 11(8):721–724.
9. Alekel, D.L. et al. "Isoflavone-rich soy protein isolate attenuates bone loss in the lumbar spine of peri-menopausal women." Third International Symposium on the Role of Soy in Preventing and Treating Chronic Disease. Washington, DC: October 1999. [Abstract]
10. Jacobsen, B.K. et al. "Does high soy milk intake reduce prostate cancer incidence? The Adventist Health Study (United States)," *Cancer Causes and Control* 1998; 9(6)553–557.
11. Hu, F.B. et al. "Frequent nut consumption and risk of coronary heart disease in women: prospective cohort study," *Br Med J* 1998; 317(7169):1341–1345.
12. Sesso, H.D. et al. "Coffee and tea intake and the risk of myocardial infarction," *Am J Epidemiol* 1999; 149(2):162–167.
13. Hunter, D.J. et al. "A prospective study of caffeine, coffee, tea and breast cancer," *Am J Epidemiol* 1992; 136:1000–1001. [Abstract]

Part 2: Herbs and Natural Health Products

Chapter 6

1. IPSOS-Reid Canadian Nutritional Supplement Review, 2000.
2. CTV/Angus Reid Group Poll, September 1997.

Chapter 7

General

Boon, H. and M. Smith. *The Botanical Pharmacy: The Pharmacology of 47 Common Herbs* (Kingston: Quarry Press, 1999).

Chandler, F., ed. *Herbs: Everyday Reference for Health Professionals* (Ottawa: Canadian Pharmacists Association and Canadian Medical Association, 2000).

Schultz. V., R. Hansel and V.E. Tyler. *Rational Phytotherapy: A Physician's Guide to Herbal Medicine*, 3rd ed. (Berlin: Springer-Verlag, 1998).

Bilberry

1. Repossi, P. et al. "The role of anthocyanosides on vascular permeability in diabetic retinopathy," *Ann Ottamol Clin Ocul* 1987; 113(4):357–361. [Italian]

2. Perossini, M. et al. "Diabetic and hypertensive retinopathy with Vaccinium myrtillus," *Ann Ottamol Clin Ocul* 1987; 113(12):1173–1190. [Italian]

3. Colombo, D. and R. Vescovini. "Controlled clinical trial on the use of Vaccinium myrtillus in primary dysmenorrhea," *G Ital Ostet Ginecol* 1985; 7(12):1033–1038. [Italian]

Black Cohosh

1. Düker, E.M. et al. "Effects of extracts from *Cimicifuga racemosa* on gonadotropin release in menopausal women and ovariectomized rats," *Planta Medica* 1991; 57:420–424.

2. Wuttke, W. "*Cimicifuga racemosa*: pharmacological and clinical profile of BNO 1055," First International Symposium on Health Phytotherapies, Rio de Janerio, April 6, 2001. [Abstract]

3. Foster, S. "Black cohosh: a literature review," *Herbalgram* 1999; 45:35–49.

Chasteberry

1. Loch, E.G. et al. "Treatment of premenstrual syndrome with a phytopharmaceutical formulation containing Vitex angus castus," *J Women's Health Gend Based Med* 2000; 9(3):315–320.

Dong Quai

1. Chang, H.M. and P.P.H. But. *Pharmacology and application of Chinese material medica* (Singapore: World Scientific Press, 1987).

2. He, Z.P. et al. "Treating amenorrhea in vital energy-deficient patients with Angelica sinensis–Astragalus membranaceus menstruation-regulating decoction," *J Tradit Chin Med* 1986; 6(3):187–190.

3. Hudson, T.S. et al. "Clinical and endocrinological effects of a menopausal botanical formula," *J Naturopath Med* 1997; 7(1):73–77.

4. Hirata, J.D. et al. "Does dong quai have estrogenic effects in postmenopausal women? A double-blind, placebo-controlled trial," *Fertil Steril* 1997; 68(6):981–986.

Echinacea

1. Steinmuller, C. et al. "Polysaccharides isolated from plant cell cultures of Echinacea pupurea enhance the resistance of immunosuppressed mice against systemic infections with Candida albicans and Listeria monocytogenes," *Int J Immunopharmacol* 1993; 15(5):605–614.

2. Grimm, M. et al. "A randomized controlled trial of the effect of fluid extract of Echinacea purpurea on the incidence and severity of colds and respiratory tract infections," *Am J Med* 1999; 106:138–143.

3. Mechart, D. et al. "Echinacea root extracts for the prevention of upper respiratory tract infections," *Arch Fam Med* 1998; 7:541–545.

4. Dorn, M. et al. "Placebo-controlled, double-blind study of Echinacea pallidae radix in upper respiratory tract infections," *Complement Ther Med* 1997; 5:40–42.

5. Melchart, D. et al. "Results of five randomized studies on the immunomodulatory activity of preparations of Echinacea," *J Alt Complement Med* 1995; 1:145–160.

6. Melchart, D. et al. "Echinacea for preventing and treating the common cold," *Cochrane Database Syst Rev* 2000; 44(2):CD000530.

Evening Primrose

1. Gateley, C.A. et al. "Drug treatments for mastalgia: 17 years experience in the Cardiff Mastalgia Clinic," *J R Soc Med* 1992; 85(1):12–15.

2. Morse, P.F. et al. "Meta analysis of placebo controlled studies of the efficacy of Epogram in treatment of atopic eczema: relationship between plasma essential fatty acid changes and response," *Br J Dermatol* 1989; 121:75–90.

3. Belch, J.J. and A. Hill. "Evening primrose oil in rheumatologic conditions," *Am J Clin Nutr* 2000; 71(1):352S–356S.

4. Meehan, E. et al. "Influence of an n-polyunsaturated fatty acid-enriched diet on the development of tolerance during chronic ethanol administration in rats," *Alcohol Clin Exp Res* 1995; 19(6):1141–1146.

5. Corbett, R. et al. "The effects of chronic administration of ethanol on synpatosomal fatty acid composition: modulation by oil enriched with gamma-linolenic acid," *Alcohol Alcohol* 1992; 27(1):11–14.

6. Vaddadi, K.S. and C.J. Gilleard. "Essential fatty acids, tardive dyskinesia and schizophrenia," in *Omega-6 essential fatty acids: pathophysiology and roles in clinical medicine*, ed. Horrobin D.F. (New York: Wiley-Liss, 1990).

Feverfew

1. Murphy, J.J. et al. "Randomised double-blind placebo-controlled trial of feverfew in migraine prevention," *Lancet* 1988; 2(8604):189–192.

Garlic

1. Steiner, M. et al. "A double-blind crossover study in moderately hypercholesterolemic men that compared the effect of aged garlic extract and placebo administration on blood lipids," *Am J Clin Nutr* 1996; 64(6):866–870.
2. Hozgartner, H. et al. "Comparison of the efficacy and tolerance of a garlic preparation vs. bezafibrate," *Arzneimittelforschung* 1992; 42(12):1473–1477.
3. Bordia, A. "Effects of garlic on blood lipids in patients with coronary heart disease," *Am J Clin Nutr* 1981; 34(10):2100–2103.
4. Bordia, A. et al. "Effect of garlic (Allium sativum) on blood lipids, blood sugar, fibrinogen and fibrinolytic activity in patients with coronary artery disease," *Prostaglandins Leukot Essent Fatty Acids* 1998; 58(4):257–263.
5. Ibid.
6. Ide, N. and B.H. Lau. "Aged garlic extract attenuates intracellular oxidative stress," *Phytomedicine* 1999; 6(2):125–131.
7. Ide, N. and B.H. Lau. "Garlic compounds protect vascular endothelial cells from oxidized low-density lipoprotein-induced injury," *Journal of Pharmacy and Pharmacology* 1997; 49(9):908–911.
8. Steiner, M. et al. "A double-blind crossover study in moderately hypercholesterolemic men that compared the effect of aged garlic extract and placebo administration on blood lipids," *Am J Clin Nutr* 1996; 64(6):866–870.
9. Steinmetz, K.A. et al. "Vegetables, fruit, and colon cancer in the Iowa Women's Health Study," *Am J Epidemiol* 1994; 139(1):1–15.
10. Levi, F. et al. "Food groups and colorectal cancer risk," *Br J Cancer* 1999; 79(7–8):1283–1287.
11. Key, T.J. et al. "A case-control study of diet and prostate cancer," *Br J Cancer* 1997; 76(5):678–687.
12. Sivam, G.P. "Protection against Helicobacter pylori and other bacterial infections by garlic," *J Nutr* 2001; 131(Suppl 3):S1106–S1108.
13. Cellini. L. et al. "Inhibition of Helicobacter pylori by garlic extract (Allium sativum)," *FEMS Immunol Med Microbiol* 1996; 13(4):273–277.
14. Song, K. and J. Milner. "The influence of heating on the anticancer properties of garlic," *J Nutr* 2001; 131:1054S–1057S.

Ginger

1. Grontved, A. et al. "Ginger root against seasickness. A controlled trial on the open sea," *Acta Otolaryngol* 1988; 105:45–49.
2. Schmid, R. et al. "Comparison of seven commonly used agents for prophylaxis of seasickness," *J Travel Med* 1994; 1:203–206.
3. Stewart, J.J. et al. "Effects of ginger on motion sickness susceptibility and gastric function," *Pharmacology* 1991; 42:111–120.
4. Manno, J.E. et al. "Comparison of efficacy of ginger with various antimotion sickness drugs," *Clin Res Pract Drug Reg Aff* 1988; 6:129–136.
5. Vutyavanich, T., T. Kraisarin and R. Ruangsri. "Ginger for nausea and vomiting in pregnancy: Randomized, double-masked, placebo-controlled trial," *Obstet Gynecol* 2001; 97(4):577–582.
6. Fischer-Rasmussen, W. et al. "Ginger treatment of hyperemesis gravidarum," *Eur J Obstet Gynecol Reprod Biol* 1991; 38:19–24.
7. Ernst, E. and M.H. Pittler. "Efficacy of ginger for nausea and vomiting: a systematic review of randomized clinical trials," *Br J Anaesth* 2000; 84(3):367–371.

Ginkgo

1. Le Bars, P.L. et al. "A placebo-controlled, double-blind, randomized trial of an extract of Ginkgo biloba for dementia," North American EGb Study Group, *JAMA* 1997; 278(16):1327–1332.
2. Bauer, U. "Six month double-blind randomised clinical trial of Ginkgo biloba extract versus placebo in two parallel groups in patients suffering from peripheral artery insufficiency," *Arzneimittelforschung* 1984; 34:716–720.
3. Mouren, X. et al. "Study of the antiischemic action of Egb 761 in the treatment of peripheral arterial occlusive disease by TcPO2 determination," *Angiology* 1994; 45:413–417.
4. Balon, R. "Ginkgo biloba for antidepressant-induced sexual dysfunction?" *J Sex Marital Ther* 1999; 25(1):1–2.

Ginseng

1. Scaglione, F. et al. "Efficacy and safety of the standardized ginseng extract G 115 for potentiating vaccination against influenza syndrome and protec-

tion against the common cold," *Drugs Exp Clin Res* 1996; 22(2):65–72.

2. Vuksan, V. et al. "American ginseng (Panax *quinquefolius* L) reduces postprandial glycemia in nondiabetic subjects and subjects with type 2 diabetes mellitus," *Arch Intern Med* 2000; 160(7):1009–1113.

Horse Chestnut

1. Guillaume, M. and F. Padioleau. "Veinotonic effect, vascular protection, antiinflammatory and free radical scavenging properties of horse chestnut extract," *Arzneimittelforschung* 1994; 44(1):25–35.

2. Diehm, C. et al. "Medical edema protection—clinical benefit in patients with chronic deep vein incompetence. A placebo controlled double-blind study," *Vasa* 1992; 21(2):188–192.

3. Pittler, M.H. and E. Ernst. "Horse-chestnut seed extract for chronic venous insufficiency. A criteria-based systematic review," *Arch Dermatol* 1998; 134(11):1356–1360.

4. Rehn, D. et al. "Comparative clinical efficacy and tolerability of oxerutins and horse chestnut extract in patients with chronic venous insufficiency," *Arzneimittelforschung* 1996; 46(5):483–487.

5. Diehm, C. et al. "Comparison of leg compression stocking and oral horse-chestnut seed extract therapy in patients with chronic venous insufficiency," *Lancet* 1996; 347(8997):292–294.

Kava Kava

1. Pittler, M.H. and E. Ernst. "Efficacy of kava extract for treating anxiety: systematic review and meta-analysis," *J Clin Psychopharmacol* 2000; 20(1):84–89.

2. Volz, H.P. and M. Kieser. "Kava-kava extract WS 1490 versus placebo in anxiety disorders—a randomized placebo-controlled 25-week outpatient trial," *Pharmacopsychiatry* 1997; 30(1):1–5.

3. Lehmann, E., E. Kinzler and J. Friedemann. "Efficacy of a special Kava extract (Piper methysticum) in patients with states of anxiety, tension and excitedness of non-mental origin—a double-blind placebo-controlled study of four weeks treatment," *Phytomedicine* 1996; 3(2):113–119.

4. Woelk, H. et al. "Comparison of Kava Special Extract WS 1490 and Benzodiazepines in Patients with Anxiety," *Z Allg Med* 1993; 69:271–277.

5. Warnecke, G. "Psychosomatic dysfunctions in the female climacteric. Clinical effectiveness and toler-

ance of Kava Extract WS 1490," *Fortschr Med* 1991; 109(4):119–122. [German]

Milk Thistle

1. Schulz, V., R. Hansel and V.E. Tyler. *Rational Phytotherapy: A Physician's Guide to Herbal Medicine*, 3rd ed. (Berlin: Springer-Verlag, 1998):216.

2. Hikino, H. and Y. Kiso. "Natural products for liver disease," *Econ Med Plant Res* 1988; 2:39–72.

3. Muzes, G. et al. "Effects of silymarin (Legalon) therapy on the antioxidant defense mechanism and lipid peroxidation in alcoholic liver disease," *Orv Hetil* 1990; 131:863–866. [Hungarian]

4. Berenguer, J. and D. Carrasco. "Double-blind trial of silymarin vs. placebo in the treatment of chronic hepatitis," *Munch Med Wochenschr* 1977; 119:240–260.

5. Buzzelli, G. et al. "A pilot study on the liver protective effect of silybin-phosphatidylcholine complex (IdB 1016) in chronic active hepatitis," *Int J Clin Pharmacol Ther Toxicol* 1993; 31:456–460.

6. Lirussi, F. and L. Okolicsanyi. "Cytoprotection in the nineties: Experience with ursodeoxycholic acid and silymarin in chronic liver disease," *Acta Physiol Hung* 1992; 80:363–367.

7. Salmi, H.A. and S. Sarna. "Effect of silymarin on chemical, functional and morphological alterations of the liver. A double-blind controlled study," *Scand J Gastroenterol* 1982; 17:517–521.

8. Feher, J. et al. "Liver protective action of silymarin therapy in chronic alcoholic liver diseases," *Orv Hetil* 1989; 130:2723–2727. [Hungarian]

9. Fintelmann, V. and A. Albert. "Proof of the therapeutic efficacy of Legalon® for toxic liver illnesses in a double-blind trial," *Therapiewoche* 1980; 30:5589–5594. [Translated from German]

10. Ferenci, P. et al. "Randomized controlled trial of silymarin treatment in patients with cirrhosis of the liver," *J Hepatol* 1989; 9:105–113.

11. Benda, L. et al. "The influence of therapy with silymarin on the survival rate of patients with liver cirrhosis," *Wein Klin Wochenschr* 1980; 92:678–683.

12. Brinker, F. *Herb Contraindications and Drug Interactions: With Appendices Addressing Specific Conditions and Medicines*, 2nd ed. (Sandy, OR: Eclectic Medical Publications; 1998):103.

St. John's Wort

1. Laakmann, G. et al. "St. John's Wort in mild to moderate depression: the relevance of hyperforin for the clinical efficacy," *Pharmacopsychiatry* 1998; 31(Suppl):S54–S59.
2. Schellenberg, R. et al. "Pharmacodynamic effects of two different hypericum extracts in healthy volunteers measured by quantitative EEG," *Pharmacopsychiatry* 1998; 31(Suppl):S44–S53.
3. Linde, K. et al. "St. John's Wort for depression—an overview and meta-analysis of randomized clinical trials," *Br Med J* 1996; 313:253–258.

Saw Palmetto

1. Wilt, T.J. et al. "Saw palmetto extracts for treatment of benign prostatic hyperplasia: a systematic review," *JAMA* 1998; 280(18):1604–1609.

Valerian

1. Lindahl, O. et al. "Double blind study of a valerian preparation," *Pharmacology Biochemistry and Behaviour* 1989; 32:1065–1066.
2. Leathwood, P.D. et al. "Aqueous extract of valerian root improves sleep quality in man," *Pharmacology Biochemistry and Behaviour* 1982; 17:65–71.
3. Leathwood, P.D. et al. "Aqueous extract of valerian root reduces latency to fall asleep in man," *Planta Medica* 1985; 51:144–148.

Chapter 8

Alpha-Lipoic Acid

1. Ziegler, D. et al. "The ALADIN III Study Group. Treatment of symptomatic diabetic polyneuropathy with the antioxidant alpha-lipoic acid: a 7-month multicenter randomized controlled trial (ALADIN III Study)," *Diabetes Care* 1999; 22:1296–1301.
2. Ziegler, D. et al. "Treatment of symptomatic diabetic peripheral neuropathy with the anti-oxidant alpha-lipoic acid. A 3-week multicentre randomized controlled trial (ALADIN Study)," *Diabetologia* 1995; 38:1425–1433.
3. Ziegler, D. and F.A. Gries. "Alpha-lipoic acid in the treatment of diabetic peripheral and cardiac autonomic neuropathy," *Diabetes* 1997; 46(Suppl 2):S62–S66.
4. Hounsom, L. et al. "A lipoic acid–gamma linolenic acid conjugate is effective against multiple indices of experimental diabetic neuropathy," *Diabetologia* 1998; 41:839–843.

5. Cameron, N.E. et al. "Effects of alpha-lipoic acid on neurovascular function in diabetic rats: Interaction with essential fatty acids," *Diabetologia* 1998; 41:390–399.
6. Jacob, S. et al. "Enhancement of glucose disposal in patients with type 2 diabetes by alpha–lipoic acid," *Arzneimittelforschung* 1995; 45:872–874.

Chondroitin Sulfate

1. McAlindon, T.E. et al. "Glucosamine and Chondroitin for Treatment of Osteoarthritis: A Systematic Quality Assessment and Meta-analysis," *JAMA* 2000; 283:1469–1475.
2. Morreale, P. et al. "Comparison of the anti-inflammatory efficacy of chondroitin sulfate and diclofenac sodium in patients with knee osteoarthritis," *J Rheumatol* 1996; 23(8):1385–1391.
3. Conrozier, T. "Anti-arthrosis treatments: efficacy and tolerance of chondroitin sulfates," *Presse Med* 1998; 27(36):1862–1865. [French]
4. Mazieres, B. et al. "Chondroitin sulfate in the treatment of gonarthrosis and coxarthrosis. 5-months result of a multicenter double-blind controlled prospective study using placebo," *Rev Rhum Mal Osteoartic* 1992; 59(7–8):466–472. [French]
5. Bucsi, L. and G. Poor. "Efficacy and tolerability of oral chondroitin sulfate as a symptomatic slow-acting drug for osteoarthritis (SYSADOA) in the treatment of knee osteoarthritis," *Osteoarthritis Cartilage* May 1998; Suppl 6.
6. Leeb, B.F. et al. "A meta-analysis of chondroitin sulfate in the treatment of osteoarthritis," *J Rheumatol* 2000; 27(1):205–211.

Coenzyme Q10

1. Khatta, M. et al. "The effect of coenzyme Q10 in patients with congestive heart failure," *Ann Intern Med* 2000; 132(8):636–640.
2. Morisco, C., B. Trimarco and M. Condorelli. "Effect of coenzyme Q10 therapy in patients with congestive heart failure: A long-term multicenter randomized study," *Clin Investig* 1993; 71(Suppl 8):S134–S136.
3. Hofman-Bang, C. et al. "Coenzyme Q10 as an adjunctive treatment of congestive heart failure," *J Card Fail* 1995; 1:101–107.
4. Baggio, E. et al. "Italian multicenter study on the safety and efficacy of coenzyme Q10 as adjunctive therapy in heart failure. CoQ10 Drug Surveillance

Investigators," *Mol Aspects Med* 1994; (Suppl 15):S287–S294.

5. Hanaki, Y. et al. "Coenzyme Q10 and coronary artery disease," *Clin Investig* 1993; 71(8 Suppl):S97–S102.

6. Greenberg, S. and W.H. Fishman. "Coenzyme Q10: A New Drug for Cardiovascular Disease," *J Clin Pharmacol* 1990; 30:596–608.

7. Folkers, K. et al. "Lovastatin decreases coenzyme Q levels in humans," *Proc Natl Acad Sci USA* 1990; 87(22):8931.

8. Mortensen, S.A. et al. "Dose-related decrease of serum coenzyme Q10 during treatment with HMG-CoA reductase inhibitors," *Mol Aspects Med* 1997; 18(Suppl):S137–S144.

9. Ghirlanda, G. et al. "Evidence of plasma CoQ10-lowering effect by HMG-CoA reductase inhibitors: A double blind, placebo-controlled study," *J Clin Pharmacol* 1993; 33(3):226–229.

10. Weis, M. et al. "Bioavailability of four oral coenzyme Q10 formulations in healthy volunteers," *Mol Aspects Med* 1994; 15:S273–S280.

11. Henriksen, J.E. et al. "Impact of ubiquinone (coenzyme Q10) treatment on glycaemic control, insulin requirement and well-being in patients with Type 1 diabetes mellitus," *Diabet Med* 1999; 16:312–318.

12. Eriksson, J.G. et al. "The effect of coenzyme Q10 administration on metabolic control in patients with type 2 diabetes mellitus," *Biofactors* 1999; 9:315–318.

13. Andersen, C.B. et al. "The effect of coenzyme Q10 on blood glucose and insulin requirement in patients with insulin dependent diabetes mellitus," *Mol Aspects Med* 1997; 18(Suppl):S307–S309.

14. Heck, A.M., B.A. DeWitt and A.L. Lukes. "Potential interactions between alternative therapies and warfarin," *Am J Health Syst Pharm* 2000; 57:1221–1227.

15. Spigset, O. "Reduced effect of warfarin caused by ubidecarenone," *Lancet* 1994; 334:1372–1373.

Conjugated Linoleic Acid (CLA)

1. Hubbard, N.E. et al. "Reduction of murine mammary tumor metastasis by conjugated linoleic acid," *Cancer Letter* 2000; 150(1):93–100.

2. Ip, C. et al. "Induction of apoptosis by conjugated linoleic acid in cultured mammary tumor cells and premalignant lesions of the rat mammary gland," *Cancer Epidemiol Biomarkers Prev* 2000; 9(7):689–696.

3. O'Shea, M. et al. "Milk fat conjugated linoleic acid (CLA) inhibits growth of human mammary MCF-7 cancer cells," *Anticancer Res* 2000; 20(5B):3591–3601.

4. Ip, C. "Review of the effects of trans fatty acids, oleic acid, n-3 polyunsaturated fatty acids, and conjugated linoleic acid on mammary carcinogenesis in animals," *Am J Clin Nutr* 1997; 66(Suppl 6):S1523–S1529.

5. Pariza, M., Y. Park and M.E. Cook. "Conjugated linoleic acid and the control of cancer and obesity," *Toxicological Sciences* 1999; 52(Suppl):S107–S110.

6. West, D.B. et al. "Effects of conjugated linoleic acid on body fat and energy metabolism in the mouse," *Am J Physiol* (Regulatory Integrative Comp Physiol) 1998; 275:R667–672.

7. DeLany, J.P. et al. "Conjugated linoleic acid rapidly reduced body fat content in mice without affecting energy intake," *Am J Physiol* (Regulatory Integrative Comp Physiol) 1999; 276:45:R1172–1179.

8. Sebedio, J.L., S. Gnaedig and J.M. Chardigny. "Recent advances in conjugated linoleic acid research," *Curr Opin Clin Nutr Metab Care* 1999; 2(6):499–506.

9. Blankson, H. et al. "Effects of conjugated linoleic acid (CLA) on body fat mass in overweight or obese human volunteers: a double-blind randomized placebo controlled study," American Chemical Society 220th National Meeting. Washington, DC; August 20–24, 2000. [Abstract 23]

10. Unknown. Linoleic Acid Supplements May Help Dieting Adults Keep Weight Off, Reuters Health, August 22, 2000. URL: **www.medscape.com/reuters/ prof/2000/08/08.22/20000822drgd003.html.**

DHEA

1. Reiter, W.J. "Serum dehydroepiandrosterone sulfate concentrations in men with erectile dysfunction," *Urology* 2000; 55:755–758.

2. Reiter, W.J. et al. "Dehydroepiandosterone in the treatment of erectile dysfunction: A prospective, double-blind, randomized, placebo-controlled study," *Urology* 1999; 53(3):590–595.

3. Arlt, W. et al. "Dehydroepiandrosterone replacement in women with adrenal insufficiency," *N Engl J Med* 1999; 341:1013–1020.

4. Oelkers, W. "Dehydroepiandosterone for adrenal insufficiency," [editorial] *N Engl J Med* 1999; 341:1073–1074.

5. Mease, P.J. et al. "GL701 (prasterone, dehydro-epiandrosterone) improves systemic lupus erythematosus," 2000 American College of Rheumatology Meeting. Philadelphia; 29 October–2 November:1230. [Abstract]

6. van Vollenhoven, R.F. "Dehydroepiandrosterone in systemic lupus erythematosus," *Rheum Dis Clin North Am* 2000; 26(2):349–362.

7. van Vollenhoven, R.F. et al. "A double-blind, placebo-controlled, clinical trial of dehydro-epiandrosterone in severe lupus erythematosus," *Lupus* 1999; 8:181–7.

8. van Vollenhoven, R.F. et al. "Treatment of Systemic Lupus Erythematosus with Dehydro-epiandrosterone: 50 Patients Treated up to 12 Months," *J Rheumatol* 1998; 25:285–289.

9. Barry, N.N., J.L. McGuire and R.F. van Vollenhoven. "Dehydroepiandrosterone in systemic lupus erythematosus: relationship between dosage, serum levels, and clinical response," *J Rheumatol* 1998; 25:2352–2356.

10. van Vollenhoven, R.F., E.G. Engleman and J.L. McGurie. "Dehydroepiandrosterone in Systemic Lupus Erythematosus," *Arth Rheum* 1995; 38(12):1826–1831.

11. van Vollenhoven, R.F., E.G. Engleman and J.L. McGuire. "Dehydroepiandrosterone in Systemic Lupus Erythematosus," *Arth Rheum* 1994; 37(9):1305–1310.

12. Bates, G.W. et al. "Dehydroepiandrosterone attenuates study-induced declines in insulin sensitivity in postmenopausal women," *Ann N Y Acad Sci* 1995; 774:291–293.

Fish Oils

1. Stark, K.D. et al. "Effect of a fish-oil concentrate on serum lipids in postmenopausal women receiving and not receiving hormone replacement therapy in a placebo-controlled, double-blind trial," *Am J Clin Nutr* 2000; 72(2):389–394.

2. Roche, H.M. and M.J. Gibney. "Effect of long-chain n-3 polyunsaturated fatty acids on fasting and post-prandial triacylglycerol metabolism," *Am J Clin Nutr* 2000; 71(Suppl 1):S232–S237.

3. Vognild, E. et al. "Effects of dietary marine oils and olive oil on fatty acid composition, platelet membrane fluidity, platelet responses, and serum lipids in healthy humans," *Lipids* 1998; 33(4):427–436.

4. Grimsgaard, S. et al. "Highly purified eicosapen-taenoic acid and docosahexaenoic acid in humans have similar triacylglycerol-lowering effects but divergent effects on serum fatty acids," *Am J Clin Nutr* 1997; 66(3):649–659.

5. Agren, J.J. et al. "Fish diet, fish oil and docosa-hexaenoic acid rich oil lower fasting and postprandial plasma lipid levels," *Eur J Clin Nutr* 1996; 50(11):765–771.

6. Sacks, F.M. et al. "Short report: the effect of fish oil on blood pressure and high-density lipoprotein-cholesterol levels in phase I of the Trials of Hypertension Prevention," *J Hypertens* 1994; 12(2):209–213.

7. Prisco, D. et al. "Effect of medium-term supplementation with a moderate dose of n-3 polyunsaturated fatty acids on blood pressure in mild hypertensive patients," *Thromb Res* 1998; 1(3):105–112.

8. Toft, I. et al. "Effects of n-3 polyunsaturated fatty acids on glucose homeostasis and blood pressure in essential hypertension. A randomized, controlled trial," *Ann Intern Med* 1995; 123(12):911–918.

9. Vandongen, R. et al. "Effects on blood pressure of omega 3 fats in subjects at increased risk of cardio-vascular disease," *Hypertension* 1993; 22(3):371–379.

10. Su, K.P., W.W. Shen and S.Y. Huang. "Are omega3 fatty acids beneficial in depression but not mania?" *Arch Gen Psychiatry* 2000; 57(7):716–717.

11. Kinrys, G. "Hypomania associated with omega3 fatty acids," *Arch Gen Psychiatry* 2000; 57(7):715–716.

12. Stoll, A.L. et al. "Omega 3 fatty acids in bipolar disorder: A preliminary double-blind, placebo-controlled trial," *Arch Gen Psychiatry* 1999; 56:407–412.

13. Burgess, J.R. et al. "Long-chain polyunsaturated fatty acids in children with attention-deficit hyper-activity disorder," *Am J Clin Nutr* 2000; 71(Suppl 1):S327–S330.

14. Navarro, E. et al. "Abnormal fatty acid pattern in rheumatoid arthritis. A rationale for treatment with marine and botanical lipids," *J Rheumatol* 2000; 27(2):298–303.

15. Lau, C.S., K.D. Morley and J.J. Belch. "Effects of fish oil supplementation on non-steroidal anti-inflammatory drug requirement in patients with mild

rheumatoid arthritis—a double-blind placebo controlled study," *Br J Rheumatol* 1993; 32:982–989.

16. Kjeldsen-Kragh, J. et al. "Dietary omega-3 fatty acid supplementation and naproxen treatment in patients with rheumatoid arthritis," *J Rheumatol* 1992; 19(10):1531–1536.

17. Astorga, G. et al. "Active rheumatoid arthritis: effect of dietary supplementation with omega-3 oils. A controlled double-blind trial," *Rev Med Chil* 1991; 119(3):267–272.

18. van der Tempel, H. et al. "Effects of fish oil supplementation in rheumatoid arthritis," *Ann Rheum Dis* 1990; 49(2):76–80.

19. Belluzzi, A. et al. "Polyunsaturated fatty acids and inflammatory bowel disease," *Am J Clin Nutr* 2000 Jan; 71(Suppl 1):339S–342S.

20. Belluzzi, A. et al. "Effect of an enteric-coated fish-oil preparation on relapses in Crohn's disease," *N Engl J Med* 1996; 334:1557–1560.

21. Lorenz-Meyer, H. et al. "Omega-3 fatty acids and low carbohydrate diet for maintenance of remission in Crohn's disease. A randomized controlled multi-center trial. Study Group Members (German Crohn's Disease Study Group)," *Scand J Gastroenterol* 1996; 31:778–785.

22. Greenfield, S.M. et al. "A randomized controlled study of evening primrose oil and fish oil in ulcerative colitis," *Aliment Pharmacol Ther* 1993; 7(2):159–166.

23. Alsan, A. and G. Triadafilopoulos. "Fish oil fatty acid supplementation in active ulcerative colitis: a double-blind, placebo-controlled crossover study," *Am J Gastroenterol* 1992; 87:432–437.

24. Hawthorne, A.B. et al. "Treatment of ulcerative colitis with fish oil supplementation: a prospective 12 month randomised controlled trial," *Gut* 1992; 33(7):922–928.

25. Mayser, P. et al. "Omega-3 fatty acid-based lipid infusion in patients with chronic plaque psoriasis: results of a double-blind, randomized, placebo-controlled, multicenter trial," *J Am Acad Dermatol* 1998; 38(4):539–547.

26. Bittiner, S.B. et al. "A double-blind, randomised placebo-controlled trial of fish oil in psoriasis," *Lancet* 1988; 1:378–380.

Glucosamine Sulfate

1. McAlindon, T.E. et al. "Glucosamine and Chondroitin for Treatment of Osteoarthritis: A Systematic Quality Assessment and Meta-analysis," *JAMA* 2000; 283:1469–1475.

2. Drovanti, A., A.A. Bignamini and A.A. Rovati. "Therapeutic activity of oral glucosamine sulfate in osteoarthrosis: a placebo-controlled double-blind investigation," *Clin Ther* 1980; 3:260–272.

3. Lopes Vaz, A.L. "Double-blind clinical evaluation of the relative efficacy of ibuprofen and glucosamine sulphate in the management of osteoarthrosis of the knee in out-patients," *Curr Med Res Opin* 1982; 8:145–149.

4. Pujalte, J.M., E.P. Llavore and F.R. Ylescupidez. "Double-blind clinical evaluation of oral glucosamine sulphate in the basic treatment of osteoarthrosis," *Curr Med Res Opin* 1980; 7:110–114.

5. Forster, K.K. et al. "Longer-term treatment of mild-to-moderate osteoarthritis of the knee with glucosamine sulfate—a randomized, controlled, double-blind clinical study," *Euro J Clin Pharmacol* 1996; 50:542.

6. Reginster, J.Y. et al. "Long-term effects of glucosamine sulfate on osteoarthritis progression: a randomized, placebo-controlled trial," *Lancet* 2001; 357:251–256.

7. Qiu, G.X. et al. "Efficacy and safety of glucosamine sulfate versus ibuprofen in patients with knee osteoarthritis," *Arzneimittelforschung* 1998; 48:469–474.

8. Mundell, E.J. Glucosamine supplements may raise diabetes risk, Reuters Health, April 19, 2000. URL: **www.reutershealth.com**.

9. Holmang, A. et al. "Induction of insulin resistance by glucosamine reduces blood flow but not interstitial levels of either glucose or insulin," *Diabetes* 1999; 48:106–111.

10. Rossetti, L. et al. "In vivo glucosamine infusion induces insulin resistance in normoglycemic but not in hyperglycemic conscious rats," *J Clin Invest* 1995; 96(1):132–140.

Grapeseed Extract

1. Thebaut, J.F. et al. "Study of endotelon in functional manifestations of peripheral venous insufficiency. *Gazette Medicale* 1985; 92:12. [Translated from French]

2. Tixier, J.M. et al. "Evidence by in vivo and in vitro studies that binding of pycnogenols to elastin affects its rate of degradation by elastases," *Biochem Pharmacol* 1984; 33:3933–3939.

3. Kuttan, R. et al. "Collagen treated with catechin becomes resistant to the action of mammalian collagenase," *Experientia* 1981; 37:221–223.

4. Masquelier, J. et al. "Stabilization of collagen by procyanidolic oligomers," *Acta Therap* 1981; 7:101–105.

5. Arcangeli, P. "Pycnogenol® in chronic venous insufficiency," *Fitoterapia* 2000; 71(3):236–244.

6. Delacroix, P. et al. "Double-blind study of endotelon in chronic venous insufficiency," *La Revue de Medecine* 1981; 31:1793–1802.

7. Bagchi, D. et al. "Oxygen free radical scavenging abilities of vitamins C and E, and a grapeseed proanthocyanidin extract in vitro," *Res Commun Mol Pathol Pharmacol* 1997; 95(2):179–189.

8. Frankel, E.N. et al. "Inhibition of oxidation of human low-density lipoprotein by phenolic substances in red wine," *Lancet* 1993; 341:454–457.

9. Chang, W.C. et al. "Inhibition of platelet aggregation and arachidonate metabolism in platelets by procyanidins," *Prostaglandins Leukot Essent Fatty Acids* 1989; 38:181–188.

10. Pütter, M. et al. "Inhibition of smoking-induced platelet aggregation by aspirin and pycnogenol," *Thromb Res* 1999; 95:155–161.

Inositol

1. Levine, J. "Controlled trials of inositol in psychiatry," *Eur Neuropsychopharmacol* 1997; 7:147–155.

2. Levine, J. et al. "Double-blind, controlled trial of inositol treatment of depression," *Am J Psychiatry* 1995; 152(5):792–794.

3. Levine, J. et al. "Follow-up and relapse analysis of an inositol study of depression," *Isr J Psychiatry Relat Sci* 1995; 32:14–21.

4. Nestler, J.E. et al. "Ovulatory and metabolic effects of D-chiro-inositol in the polycystic ovary syndrome," *N Engl J Med* 1999; 340(17):1314–1320.

Lecithin (Phosphatidylcholine)

1. Oosthuizen, W. et al. "Lecithin has no effect on serum lipoprotein, plasma fibrinogen and macro molecular protein complex levels in hyperlipidaemic men in a double-blind controlled study," *Eur J Clin Nutr* 1998; 52:419–424.

2. Stoll, A.L. et al. "Choline in the treatment of rapid-cycling bipolar disorder: clinical and neurochemical findings in lithium-treated patients," *Biol Psychiatry* 1996; 40:382–388.

3. Cohen, B.M., J.F. Lipinski and R.I. Altesman. "Lecithin in the treatment of mania: Double-blind, placebo-controlled trials," *Am J Psychiatry* 1982; 139:1162–1164.

4. Polinsky, R.J. et al. "Cholinergic treatment in the Tourette syndrome," *N Engl J Med* 1980; 302:1310.

5. Weintraub, S. et al. "Lecithin in the treatment of Alzheimer's disease," *Arch Neurol* 1983; 40:527–528.

6. Cohen, B.M. et al. "Lecithin in mania: a preliminary report," *Am J Psychiatry* 1980; 137:242–243.

7. Cohen, B.M., J.F. Lipinski and R.I. Altesman. "Lecithin in the treatment of mania: Double-blind, placebo-controlled trials," *Am J Psychiatry* 1982; 139:1162–1164.

8. Joe, S.H. et al. "Effect of lecithin on tardive dyskinesia," *Korea Univ Med J* 1985; 22:197–206.

9. Guan, R. et al. "The effect of polyunsaturated phosphatidyl choline in the treatment of acute viral hepatitis," *Ailment Pharmacol Ther* 1995; 9:699–703.

10. Schuller-Perez, A. and F. Gonzalez San Martin. "A controlled study with polyunsaturated phosphatidylcholine compared to placebo in alcoholic steatosis of the liver," *Med Welt* 1985; 36:517–521.

11. Knuchel, F. "Double-blind study in patients with alcoholic toxic fatty liver. Effect of essential phospholipids on enzyme behavior and lipid composition of the serum," *Med Welt* 1979; 30:411–416.

12. Jenkins, P.J. et al. "Use of polyunsaturated phosphatidylcholine in HBsAg negative chronic active hepatitis: results of prospective double-blind controlled trial," *Liver* 1982; 2:77–81.

13. Niederau, C. et al. "Polyunsaturated phosphatidylcholine and interferon alpha for treatment of chronic hepatitis B and C: a multi-center, randomized, double-blind, placebo-controlled trial," *Hepatogastroenterology* 1998; 45:797–804.

Lutein

1. Landrum, J.T., R.A. Bone and M.D. Kilburn. "The macular pigment: a possible role in protection from age-related macular degeneration," *Adv Pharmacol* 1997; 38:537–556.

2. Moeller, S.M. et al. "The role of dietary xanthophylls in cataract and age-related macular degeneration," *J Am Coll Nutr* 2000; 19(Suppl 5):S522–S527.

3. Berendschott, T.T. et al. "Influence of lutein supplementation on macular pigment, assessed with two objective techniques," *Invest Opthalmol Vis Sci* 2000; 41(11):3322–3326.

4. Dagnelie, G. et al. "Lutein improves visual function in some patients with retinal degeneration: a pilot study via the Internet," *Optometry* 2000; 71(3):147–164.

5. Hammond, B.R., Jr. et al. "Dietary modification of human macular pigment density," *Invest Opthalmol Vis Sci* 1997; 38(9):1795–1801.

6. Landrum, J.T. et al. "A one year study of the macular pigment: the effect of 140 days on a lutein supplement," *Exp Eye Res* 1997; 65(1):57–62.

7. Mares-Perlman, J.A. et al. "Diet and nuclear lens opacities," *Am J Epidemiol* 1995; 141:322–334.

8. Hankinson, S.E. et al. "Nutrient intake and cataract extraction in women: a prospective study," *Br Med J* 1992; 305:335–339.

9. Brown, L. et al. "A prospective study of carotenoid intake and risk of cataract extraction in US men," *Am J Clin Nutr* 1999; 70(4):517–524.

Lycopene

1. Sies, H. and W. Stahl. "Lycopene: antioxidant and biological effects and its bioavailability in the human," *Proc Soc Exp Biol Med* 1998; 218:121–124.

2. Rao, A.V. and S. Agarwal. "Bioavailability and in vivo antioxidant properties of lycopene from tomato products and their possible role in the prevention of cancer," *Nutr Cancer* 1998; 31:199–203.

3. Giovannucci, E. et al. "Intake of carotenoids and retinol in relation to risk of prostate cancer," *JNCI* 1995; 87:1767–1776.

4. Gann, P.H. et al. "Lower prostate risk in men with elevated plasma lycopene levels: results of a prospective study," *Cancer Res* 1999; 59:1225–1230.

5. Clinton, S.K. et al. "Cis-trans lycopene isomers, carotenoids, and retinal in the human prostate," *Cancer Epidemiol Biomarkers Prev* 1996; 5(10):823–833.

6. Nomura, A.M. et al. "Serum micronutrients and prostate cancer in Japanese Americans in Hawaii," *Cancer Epidemiol Biomarkers Prev* 1997; 6:487–491.

7. Paetau, I. et al. "Chronic ingestion of lycopene-rich tomato juice or lycopene supplements significantly increases plasma concentrations of lycopene and related tomato carotenoids in humans," *Am J Clin Nutr* 1998; 68(6):1187–1195.

8. Mares-Perlman, J.A. et al. "Serum antioxidants and age-related macular degeneration in a population-based case-control study," *Arch Ophthalmol* 1995; 113:1518–1523.

9. Kantesky, P.A. et al. "Dietary intake and blood levels of lycopene: association with cervical dysplasia among non-Hispanic, black women," *Nutr Cancer* 1998; 31(1):31–40.

Lysine

1. Griffith, R.S., D.C. DeLong and J.D. Nelson. "Relation of arginine-lysine antagonism to herpes simplex growth in tissue culture," *Chemotherapy* 1981; 27(3):209–213.

2. Thein, D.J. and W.C. Hurt. "Lysine as a prophylactic agent in the treatment of recurrent herpes simplex labialis," *Oral Surg Oral Med Oral Pathol* 1984; 58(6):659–666.

3. McCune, M.A. et al. "Treatment of recurrent herpes simplex infections with L-lysine monohydrochloride," *Cutis* 1984; 34(4):366–373.

4. DiGiovanna, J.J. and H. Blank. "Failure of lysine in frequently recurrent herpes simplex infection. Treatment and prophylaxis," *Arch Dermatol* 1984; 120(1):48–51.

5. Milman, N., J. Scheibel and O. Jessen. "Lysine prophylaxis in recurrent herpes simplex labialis: a double-blind, controlled crossover study," *Acta Derm Venereol* 1980; 60(1):85–87.

6. Griffith, R.S., A. Norins and C. Kagan. "A multicentered study of lysine therapy in Herpes simplex infection," *Dermatologica* 1978; 156(5):257–267.

7. Griffith, R.S. et al. "Success of L-lysine therapy in frequently recurrent herpes simplex infection. Treatment and prophylaxis," *Dermatologica* 1987; 175(4):183–190.

8. Civitelli, R. et al. "Dietary L-lysine and calcium metabolism in humans," *Nutrition* 1992; 8(6):400–405.

Melatonin

1. Brzezinski, A. "Melatonin in humans," *N Engl J Med* 1997; 336(3):186–195.

2. Dollins, A.B. et al. "Effect of inducing nocturnal serum melatonin concentrations in daytime on sleep, mood, body temperature, and performance," *Proc Natl Acad Sci USA* 1994; 91(5):1824–1828.

3. Zhdanova, I.V. et al. "Sleep-inducing effects of low doses of melatonin ingested in the evening," *Clin Pharmacol Ther* 1995; 57(5):552–558.

4. Nave, R., R. Peled and P. Lavie. "Melatonin improves evening napping," *Eur J Pharmacol* 1995; 275(2):213–216.

5. Brusco, L.I. et al. "Effect of melatonin in selected populations of sleep-disturbed patients," *Biol Signals Recept* 1999; 8(1–2):126–131.

6. Garfinkel, D. et al. "Improvement of sleep quality in elderly people by controlled-release melatonin," *Lancet* 1995; 346(8974):541–544.

7. Haimov, I. et al. "Melatonin replacement therapy of elderly insomniacs," *Sleep* 1995; 18(7):598–603.

8. Garfinkel, D. et al. "Improvement of sleep quality in elderly people by controlled-release melatonin," *Lancet* 1995; 346(8974):541–544.

9. Attenburrow, M.E., P.J. Cowen and A.L. Sharpley. "Low dose melatonin improves sleep in healthy middle-aged subjects," *Psychopharmacology* 1996; 126(2):179–181.

10. Suhner, A. et al. "Comparative study to determine the optimal melatonin dosage form for the alleviation of jet lag," *Chronobiol Int* 1998; 15(6):655–656.

11. Petrie, K. et al. "A double-blind trial of melatonin as a treatment for jet lag in international cabin crew," *Biol Psychiatry* 1993; 33(7):526–530.

12. Claustrat, B. et al. "Melatonin and jet lag: confirmatory result using a simplified protocol," *Biol Psychiatry* 1992; 32(8):705–711.

13. Petrie, K. et al. "Effect of melatonin on jet lag after long haul flights," *Br Med J* 1989; 298(6675):705–707.

14. Sanders, D.C., A.K. Chaturvedi and J.R. Hordinsky. "Melatonin: aeromedical, toxicopharmacological, and analytical aspects," *J Anal Toxicol* 1999; 23(3):159–167.

15. Carman, J.S. et al. "Negative effects of melatonin on depression," *Am J Psychiatry* 1976; 133(10):1181–1186.

Phosphatidylserine

1. Crook, T. et al. "Effects of phosphatidylserine in Alzheimer's disease," *Psychopharmacol Bull* 1992; 28(1):61–66.

2. Cenacchi, T. et al. "Cognitive decline in the elderly: a double-blind, placebo-controlled multicenter study on efficacy of phosphatidylserine administration," *Aging* (Milano) 1993; 5(2):123–133.

3. Engel, R.R. et al. "Double-blind cross-over study of phosphatidylserine vs. placebo in patients with early dementia of the Alzheimer type," *Eur Neuropsychopharmacol* 1992; 2(2):149–155.

4. Delwaide, P.J. et al. "Double-blind randomized controlled study of phosphatidylserine in senile demented patients," *Acta Neurol Scand* 1986; 73(2):136–140.

5. Crook, T.H. et al. "Effects of phosphatidylserine in age-associated memory impairment," *Neurology* 1991; 41(5):644–649.

6. van den Besselaar, A.M. "Phosphatidylethanolamine and phosphatidylserine synergistically promote heparin's anticoagulant effect," *Blood Coagul Fibrinolysis* 1995; 6:239–244.

Probiotics

1. Colombel, J.F. et al. "Yoghurt with Bifidobacterium longum reduces erythromycin-induced gastrointestinal effects," *Lancet* 1987; 2:43.

2. Surawicz, C.M. et al. "Prevention of antibiotic-associated diarrhea by Saccharomyces boulardii: a prospective study," *Gastroenterology* 1989; 96:981–988.

3. McFarland, L.V. et al. "Prevention of Beta-lactam-associated diarrhea by Saccharomyces boulardii compared with placebo," *Am J Gastroenterol* 1995; 90:439–448.

4. Surawicz, C.M. et al. "Prevention of antibiotic-associated diarrhea by Saccharomyces boulardii: a prospective study," *Gastroenterology* 1989; 96:981–988.

5. Guandalini, S. et al. "Lactobacillus GG administered in oral rehydration solution to children with acute diarrhea: a multicenter European trial," *J Pediatr Gastroenterol Nutr* 2000; 30:54–60.

6. Shornikova, A.V. et al. "Bacteriotherapy with Lactobacillus reuteri in rotavirus gastroenteritis," *Pediatr Infect Dis J* 1997; 16:1103–1107.

7. Saavedra, J.M. et al. "Feeding of Bifidobacterium bifidum and Streptococcus thermophilus to infants in hospital for prevention of diarrhoea and shedding of rotavirus," *Lancet* 1994; 344:1046–1049.

8. Scarpignato, C. and P. Rampal. "Prevention and treatment of traveler's diarrhea: a clinical pharmacological approach," *Chemotherapy* 1995; 41(Suppl 1):S48–S81.

9. Hilton, E. et al. "Efficacy of Lactobacillus GG as a diarrheal preventive in travelers," *J Travel Med* 1997; 4:41–43.

10. Oksanen, P.J. et al. "Prevention of traveller's diarrhoea by Lactobacillus GG," *Ann Med* 1990; 22:53–56.

11. Kollaritsch, V.H. et al. "Prevention of traveler's diarrhea with Saccharomyces boulardii. Results of a

placebo-controlled double-blind study," *Fortschr Med* 1993; 111:152–156.

12. Elmer, G.W., C.M. Surawicz and L.V. McFarland. "Biotherapeutic agents: A neglected modality for the treatment and prevention of selected intestinal and vaginal infections," *JAMA* 1996; 275:870–876.

13. Hilton, E. et al. "Ingestion of yogurt containing Lactobacillus acidophilus as prophylaxis for candidal vaginitis," *Ann Intern Med* 1992; 116(5):353–357.

14. Nobaek, S. et al. "Alteration of intestinal microflora is associated with reduction in abdominal bloating and pain in patients with irritable bowel syndrome," *Am J Gastroenterol* 2000; 95:1231–1238.

15. Halpern, G.M. et al. "Treatment of irritable bowel syndrome with Lacteol Fort: a randomized, double-blind, cross-over trial," *Am J Gastroenterol* 1996; 91:1579–1585.

SAMe

1. Janicak, P.G. et al. "S-adenosylmethionine in depression. A literature review and preliminary report," *Ala J Med Sci* 1988; 25(3):306–313.

2. Bressa, G.M. "S-adenosyl-l-methionine (SAMe) as antidepressant: meta-analysis of clinical studies," *Acta Neurol Scand* 1994; 154(Suppl):S7–S14.

3. Bell, K.M. et al. "S-adenosylmethionine blood levels in major depression: changes with drug treatment," *Acta Neurol Scand* 1994; 154(Suppl):S15–S18.

4. Salmaggi, P. et al. "Double-blind, placebo-controlled study of S-adenosyl-L-methionine in depressed postmenopausal women," *Psychother Psychosom* 1993; 59(1):34–40.

5. De Vanna, M. and R. Rigamonti. "Oral S-adenosyl-L-methionine in depression," *Curr Ther Res* 1992; 52(3):478–485.

6. Kagan, B.L. et al. "Oral S-adenosylmethionine in depression: a randomized, double-blind, placebo-controlled trial," *Am J Psychiatry* 1990; 147(5):591–95.

7. Rosenbaum, J.F. et al. "The antidepressant potential of oral S-adenosyl-l-methionine," *Acta Psychiatr Scand* 1990; 81(5):432–36.

8. Bradley, J.D. et al. "A randomized, double-blind, placebo-controlled trial of intravenous loading with S-adenosylmethionine (SAM) followed by oral SAM therapy in patients with knee osteoarthritis," *J Rheumatol* 1994; 21(5):905–11.

9. Domljan, Z. et al. "A double-blind trial of ademetionine vs. naproxen in activated gonarthrosis," *Int J Clin Pharmacol Ther Toxicol* 1989; 27(7):329–33.

10. Konig, B. "A long-term (two years) clinical trial with S-adenosylmethionine for the treatment of osteoarthritis," *Am J Med* 1987; 83(5a):78–80.

11. Berger, R. and H. Nowak. "A new medical approach to the treatment of osteoarthritis. Report of an open phase IV study with ademetionine (Gumbaral)," *Am J Med* 1987; 83(5A):84–88.

12. Muller-Fassbender, H. "Double-blind clinical trial of S-adenosylmethionine versus ibuprofen in the treatment of osteoarthritis," *Am J Med* 1987; 83(5A):81–83.

13. Vetter, G. "Double-blind comparative clinical trial with S-adenosylmethionine and indomethacin in the treatment of osteoarthritis," *Am J Med* 1987; 83(5A):78–80.

14. Maccagno, A. et al. "Double-blind controlled clinical trial of oral S-adenosylmethionine versus piroxicam in knee osteoarthritis," *Am J Med* 1987; 83(5A):72–77.

15. Caruso, I. and V. Pietrogrande. "Italian double-blind multicenter study comparing S-adenosylmethionine, naproxen, and placebo in the treatment of degenerative joint disease," *Am J Med* 1987; 83(5A):66–71.

16. di Padova, C. "S-adenosylmethionine in the treatment of osteoarthritis. Review of the clinical studies," *Am J Med* 1987; 83(5A):60–65.

17. Jacobsen, S., B. Danneskiold-Samsoe and R.B. Andersen. "Oral S-adenosylmethionine in primary fibromyalgia. Double-blind clinical evaluation," *Scand J Rheumatol* 1991; 20(4):294–302.

18. Tavoni, A. et al. "Evaluation of S-adenosylmethionine in primary fibromyalgia. A double-blind crossover study," *Am J Med* 1987; 83(5A):107–110.

Part 3: The Health Conditions

Acne

1. Downing, D.T. et al. "Essential fatty acids and acne," *J Am Acad Dermatol* 1986; 14(2 Pt 1):221–225.

2. Akamatsu, H. et al. "Suppressive effects of linoleic acid on neutrophil oxygen metabolism and phagocytosis," *J Invest Dermatol* 1990; 95(3):271–274.

3. Sherertz, E.F. "Acneiform eruption due to "megadose" vitamin B6 and B12," *Cutis* 1991; 48(2):119–120.

4. McCarty, M. "High-chromium yeast for acne?" *Med Hypotheses* 1984; 14(3):307–310.

5. Bruce, A. "Swedish views on selenium," *Ann Clin Res* 1986; 18(1):8–12.

6. Michaelsson, G. and L.E. Edqvist. "Erythrocyte glutathione peroxidase activity in acne vulgaris and the effect of selenium and vitamin E treatment," *Acta Derm Venereol* 1984; 64(1):9–14.

7. Michaelsson, G. and K. Ljunghall. "Patients with herpetiformis acne, psoriasis and Darier's disease have low epidermal zinc concentrations," *Acta Derm Venereol* 1990; 70(4):304–308.

8. Dreno, B. et al. "Low dose of zinc gluconate for inflammatory acne," *Acta Derm Venereol* 1989; 69(6):541–543.

9. Verma, K.C. et al. "Oral zinc sulphate therapy in acne vulgaris: a double-blind trial," *Acta Derm Venereol* 1980; 60(4):337–340.

10. Williams, L.R. et al. "The composition and bacteriocidal activity of oil of Melaleuca alternifolia (tea tree oil)," *Int J Aromather* 1988; 1:15–17.

11. Ernst, E. and A. Huntley. "Tea tree oil: a systematic review of randomized clinical trials," *Forsch Komplemetarmed* 2000; 7(1):17–20.

Alcoholism

1. *Alcohol.* Alberta Alcohol and Drug Abuse Commission, November 2000. Available at **www.gov.ab.ca/aadac/addictions/beyond/beyond_ alcohol.html**.

2. Biery, J.R. et al. "Alcohol craving in rehabilitation: assessment of nutrition therapy," *J Am Diet Assoc* 1991; 91(4):463–466.

3. The American Dietetic Association. *Manual of Clinical Dietetics,* 6th ed. (Chicago, 2000).

4. Pita, M.L. et al. "Chronic alcoholism decreases polyunsaturated fatty acid levels in human plasma, erythrocytes and platelets—influence on chronic liver disease," *Thromb Haemost* 1997; 78(2):808–812.

5. Reitz, R.C. "Dietary fatty acids and alcohol: effects on cellular membranes," *Alcohol Alcohol* 1994; 28(1):59–71.

6. Hibbeln, J.R. and N. Salem, Jr. "Dietary polyunsaturated fatty acids and depression: when cholesterol does not satisfy," *Am J Clin Nutr* 1995; 62(1):1–9.

7. Gloria, L. et al. "Nutritional deficiencies in chronic alcoholics: relation to dietary intake and alcohol consumption," *Am J Gastroenterol* 1997; 92(3):485–489.

8. Fernando, O.V. and E.W. Grimsley. "Prevalence of folate deficiency and macrocytosis in patients with

and without alcohol-related illness," *South Med J* 1998; 91(8):721–725.

9. Carney, M.W. et al. "Red cell folate concentrations in psychiatric patients," *J Affect Disord* 1990; 19(3):207–213.

10. Fernandez-Calle, P. et al. "Alcoholic cognitive deterioration and nutritional deficiencies," *Acta Neurol Scand* 1994; 89(5):384–390.

11. Harper, C. and J. Kril. "An introduction to alcohol-induced brain damage and its causes," *Alcohol Alcohol Suppl* 1994; 2:237–243.

12. Tallaksen, C.M. et al. "Blood and serum thiamin and thiamin phosphate ester concentrations in patients with alcohol dependence syndrome before and after thiamin treatment," *Alcohol Clin Exp Res* 1992; 16(2):320–325.

13. Zubaran, C. et al. "Wernicke-Korsakoff syndrome," *Postgrad Med J* 1997; 73(855):27–31.

14. Naidoo, D.P. et al. "Wernicke's encephalopathy and alcohol-related disease," *Postgrad Med J* 1991; 67(793):978–981.

15. Van Gossum, A. et al. "Deficiency in antioxidant factors in patients with alcohol-related chronic pancreatitis," *Dig Dis Sci* 1996; 41(6):1225–1231.

16. Lecomte, E. et al. "Effect of alcohol consumption on blood antioxidant nutrients and oxidative stress indicators," *Am J Clin Nutr* 1994; 60(2):255–261.

17. Siest, G. and Y. Artur. "The relation of alcohol consumption to serum carotenoid and retinal levels. Effects of withdrawal," *Int J Vitam Nutr Res* 1994; 64(3):170–175.

18. Bjorneboe, G.A. et al. "Diminished serum concentration of vitamin E in alcoholics," *Ann Nutr Metab* 1988; 32(2):56–61.

19. Bjorneboe, G.A. et al. "Effect of heavy alcohol consumption on serum concentrations of fat-soluble vitamins and selenium," *Alcohol Alcohol* 1987; (Suppl 1):S533–S537.

20. Altura, B.M. and B.T. Altura. "Role of magnesium and calcium in alcohol-induced hypertension and strokes as probed by in vivo television microscopy, digital image microscopy, optical microscopy, 31P-NMR, spectroscopy and a unique magnesium ion-selective electrode," *Alcohol Clin Exp Res* 1994; 18(5):1057–1068.

21. Abbott, L. et al. "Magnesium deficiency in alcoholism: possible contribution to osteoporosis and cardiovascular disease in alcoholics," *Alcohol Clin Exp Res* 1994; 18(5):1076–1082.

22. Gullstad, L. et al. "Oral magnesium supplementation improves metabolic variables and muscle strength in alcoholics," *Alcohol Clin Exp Res* 1992; 16(5):986–990.

23. Menzano, E. and P.L. Carlen. "Zinc deficiency and corticosteroids in the pathogenesis of alcoholic brain dysfunction—a review," *Alcohol Clin Exp Res* 1994; 18(4):895–901.

24. Feher, J. et al. "Liver protective action of silymarin therapy in chronic alcoholic liver diseases," *Orv Hetil* 1989; 130:2723–2727. [Hungarian]

25. Muzes, G. et al. "Effects of silymarin (Legalon) therapy on the antioxidant defense mechanism and lipid peroxidation in alcoholic liver disease," *Orv Hetil* 1990; 131:863–866. [Hungarian]

26. Lieber, C.S. et al. "Attenuation of alcohol-induced hepatic fibrosis by polyunsaturated lecithin," *Hepatology* 1990; 12:1390–1398.

27. Lieber, C.S. and E. Rubin. "Alcoholic fatty liver," *N Engl J Med* 1969; 280:705–708.

28. Schuller-Perez, A. and F. Gonzalez San Martin. "A controlled study with polyunsaturated phosphatidylcholine compared to placebo in alcoholic steatosis of the liver," *Med Welt* 1985; 36:517–521.

29. Chawla, R.K. et al. "Biochemistry and pharmacology of S-adenosyl-L-methionine and rationale for its use in liver disease," *Drugs* 1990; 40(Suppl 3):S98–S110.

30. Loguercio, C. et al. "Effect of S-adenosyl-L-methionine administration on red blood cell cysteine and glutathione levels in alcoholic patients with and without liver disease. *Alcohol Alcohol* 1994; 29(5):597–604.

Alzheimer's Disease

1. *What is Alzheimer's disease?* Alzheimer Society of Canada, September 2000. Available at **www.alzheimer.caalz/content/html/disease_en/disease-whatisit-eng.html**.

2. *What is Alzheimer's disease?* Alzheimer Society of Canada, September 2000. Available at **www.alzheimer.caalz/content/html/disease_en/disease-whatisit-eng.html**.

3. Poehlman, E.T. and R.V. Dvorak. "Energy expenditure, energy intake, and weight loss in Alzheimer disease," *Am J Clin Nutr* 2000; 71(2):650S–655S.

4. Kalmijn, S. et al. "Dietary fat intake and the risk of incident dementia in the Rotterdam Study," *Ann Neurol* 1997; 42(5):775–782.

5. Yehuda, S. et al. "Essential fatty acids preparation (SR-3) improves Alzheimer's patients' quality of life," *J Dev Neurosci* 1996; 87(3–4):141–149.

6. Meins, W. et al. "Subnormal serum vitamin B12 and behavioural and psychological symptoms in Alzheimer's disease," *Int J Geriatr Psychiatry* 2000; 15(5):415–418.

7. Levitt, A.J. and H. Karlinsky. "Folate, vitamin B12 and cognitive impairment in patients with Alzheimer's disease," *Acta Psychiatr Scand* 1992; 86(4):301–305.

8. Sano, M. et al. "A controlled trial of selegiline, alpha-tocopherol, or both as treatment for Alzheimer's disease. The Alzheimer's Disease Cooperative Study," *N Engl J Med* 1997; 336(17):1216–1222.

9. Grundman, M. "Vitamin E and Alzheimer's disease: the basis for additional clinical trials," *Am J Clin Nutr* 2000; 71(2):630S–636S.

10. Vatassery, G.T. et al. "High doses of vitamin E in the treatment of disorders of the central nervous system in the aged," *Am J Clin Nutr* 1999; 70(5):201–203.

11. Sato, Y. et al. "High prevalence of vitamin D deficiency and reduced bone mass in elderly women with Alzheimer's disease," *Bone* 1998; 23(6):555–557.

12. Le Bars, P.L. et al. "A placebo-controlled, double-blind, randomized trial of an extract of Ginkgo biloba for dementia. North American EGb Study Group," *JAMA* 1997; 278(16):1327–1332.

13. Wettstein, A. "Cholinesterase inhibitors and Ginkgo extracts—are they comparable in the treatment of dementia? Comparison of published placebo-controlled efficacy studies of at least six months' duration," *Phytomedicine* 2000; 6(6):393–401.

14. Oken, B.S. et al. "The efficacy of Ginkgo biloba on cognitive function in Alzheimer disease," *Arch Neurol* 1998; 55(11):1409–1415.

15. Jaggy, H. and E. Koch. "The chemistry and biology of alkylphenols from Ginkgo biloba L," *Pharmazie* 1997; 52(10):735–738.

16. Mook-Jung, I. et al. "Protective effects of asiaticoside derivatives against beta-amyloid neurotoxicity," *J Neurosci Res* 1999; 58:417–425.

17. Brooks, J.O., 3rd et al. "Acetyl-L-carnitine slows decline in younger patients with Alzheimer's disease: a reanalysis of a double-blind, placebo-controlled study using the trilinear approach," *Int Psychogeriatr* 1998; 10(2):193–203.

18. Thal, L.J. et al. "A 1-year placebo-controlled study of acetyl-L-carnitine in patients with Alzheimer's disease," *Neurology* 1996; 47(3):705–711.

19. Pettegrew, J.W. et al. "Clinical and neurochemical effects of acetyl-L-carnitine in Alzheimer's disease," *Neurobiol Aging* 1995; 16(1):1–4.

20. Tettamanti, M. et al. "Long-term acetyl-L-carnitine treatment in Alzheimer's disease," *Neurology* 1991; 41(11):1726–1732.

21. Rai, G. et al. "Double-blind, placebo controlled study of acetyl-L-carnitine in patients with Alzheimer's dementia," *Curr Med Res Opin* 1990; 11(10):638–647.

22. Higgins, J.P. and L. Flicker. "Lecithin for dementia and cognitive impairment," *Cochrane Database Syst Rev* 2000; (2):CD001015.

23. Holford, N.H. and K. Peace. "The effect of tacrine and lecithin in Alzheimer's disease: A population pharmacodynamic analysis of five clinical trials," *Eur J Clin Pharmacol* 1994; 47(1):17–23.

24. Crook, T. et al. "Effects of phosphatidylserine in Alzheimer's disease," *Psychopharmacol Bull* 1992; 28(1):61–66.

25. Engel, R.R. et al. "Double-blind cross-over study of phosphatidylserine vs. placebo in patients with early dementia of the Alzheimer type," *Eur Neuropsychopharmacol* 1992; 2(2):149–155.

26. Delwaide, P.J. et al. "Double-blind randomized controlled study of phosphatidylserine in senile dementia patients," *Acta Neurol Scand* 1986; 73(2):136–140.

Anemia

1. Kuzminski, A.M. et al. "Effective treatment of cobalamin deficiency with oral cobalamin," *Blood* 1998; 92(4):1191–1198.

Angina

1. Rimm, E.B. et al. "Vitamin E consumption and the risk of coronary heart disease in men," *New Eng J Med* 1993; 328(20):1450–1456.

2. Stampfer, M.J. et al. "Vitamin E consumption and the risk of coronary heart disease in women," *New Eng J Med* 1993; 328(20):1444–1449.

3. Yusut, S. et al. "Vitamin E Supplementation and cardiovascular events in high-risk patients. The Heart Outcomes Prevention Evaluation Study Investigators," *New Eng J Med* 2000; 342:154–160.

4. Satake, K. et al. "Relation between severity of magnesium deficiency and frequency of anginal attacks in men with variant angina," *J Am Coll Cardiol* 1996; 28(4):897–902.

5. Teragawa, H. et al. "The preventative effect of magnesium of coronary spasm in patients with vasospastic angina," *Chest* 2000; 118(6):1690–1695.

6. Lasserre, B. et al. "Should magnesium therapy be considered for the treatment of coronary heart disease? II. Epidemiological evidence in outpatients with and without coronary heart disease," *Magnes Res* 1994; 7(2):145–153.

7. Shechter, M. et al. "Oral magnesium therapy improves endothelial function in patients with coronary artery disease," *Circulation* 2000; 102:2353–2358.

8. Upton, R., ed. *Hawthorn Leaf with Flower: quality control, analytical and therapeutic monograph* (Santa Cruz: American Herbal Pharmacopoeia, 1999):1–29.

9. Kamikawa, T. et al. "Effects of coenzyme Q10 on exercise tolerance in chronic stable angina pectoris," *Am J Cardiol* 1985; 56(4):247–251.

10. Iyer, R.N. et al. "L-carnitine moderately improves the exercise tolerance in chronic stable angina," *J Assoc Physicians India* 2000; 48(11):1050–1052.

11. Cacciatore, L. et al. "The therapeutic effect of L-carnitine in patients with exercise-induced stable angina: a controlled study," *Drugs Exp Clin Res* 1991; 17:225–235.

12. Cherchi, A. et al. "Effects of L-carnitine on exercise tolerance in chronic stable angina: a multicenter, double-blind, randomized, placebo-controlled crossover study," *Int J Clin Pharmacol Ther Toxicol* 1985; 23:569–572.

13. Bartels, G.L. et al. "Effects of L-propionylcarnitine on ischemia-induced myocardial dysfunction in men with angina pectoris," *Am J Cardiol* 1994; 74:125–130.

14. Bartels, G.L. et al. "Additional anti-ischemic effects of long-term L-propionylcarnitine in anginal patients treated with conventional antianginal therapy," *Cardiovasc Drugs Ther* 1995; 9:749–753.

15. Bartels, G.L. et al. "Anti-ischaemic efficacy of L-propionyl-carnitine—a promising novel metabolic approach to ischaemia?" *Eur Heart J* 1996; 17:414–420.

16. Lagioia, R. et al. "Propionyl-L-carnitine: a new compound in the metabolic approach to the treat-

ment of effort angina," *Int J Cardiol* 1992; 34:167–172.

Asthma

1. *Quick Facts and Statistics.* The Canadian Lung Association, 2001. Available at **www.lung.ca/ statistics.**

2. *Asthma.* The Canadian Lung Association, 2001. Available at **www.lung.ca/asthma/asthma1.html**.

3. Monteleonem, C.A. and A.R. Sherman. "Nutrition and asthma," *Arch Intern Med* 1997; 157(1):23–34.

4. La Vecchia, C. et al. "Vegetable consumption and the risk of chronic disease. *Epidemiology* 1998; 9(2):208–210.

5. Forastiere, F. et al. "Consumption of fresh fruit in vitamin C and wheezing symptoms in children," *Thorax* 2000; 55(4):283–288.

6. Lindahl, O. et al. "Vegan regimen with reduced medication in the treatment of bronchial asthma," *J Asthma* 1985; 22(1):45–55.

7. Camargo, C.A., Jr. et al. "Prospective study of body mass index, weight change, and risk of adult-onset asthma in women," *Arch Intern Med* 1999; 159(21):2582–2588.

8. Chen, Y. et al. "Increased effects of smoking and obesity on asthma among female Canadians," *Am J Epidemiol* 1999; 150(3):255–262.

9. Stenius-Aarniala, B. et al. "Immediate and long-term effects of weight reduction in obese people with asthma: randomized controlled study," *Br Med J* 2000; 320(7238):827–832.

10. Schwartz, J. "Role of polyunsaturated fatty acids in lung function," *Am J Clin Nutr* 2000; 71(Suppl 1):S393–S396.

11. Medici, T.C. et al. "Are asthmatics salt-sensitive? A preliminary controlled study," *Chest* 1993; 104(4):1138–1143.

12. Pistelli, R. et al. "Respiratory symptoms and bronchial responsiveness are related to dietary salt intake and urinary potassium excretion in male children," *Eur Respir J* 1993; 6(4):517–522.

13. Carey, O.J. et al. "Effect of alterations of dietary sodium on the severity of asthma in men," *Thorax* 1993; 48(7):714–718.

14. Collipp, P.J. et al. "Pyridoxine treatment of child-hood bronchial asthma," *Ann Allergy* 1975; 35:93–97.

15. Sur, S. et al. "Double-blind trial of pyridoxine (vita-min B6) in the treatment of steroid-dependent asthma," *Ann Allergy* 1993; 70:147–152.

16. Kelly, F.J. et al. "Altered lung antioxidant status in patients with mild asthma," *Lancet* 1999; 354(9177):482–483.

17. Bielory, L. and R. Gandhi. "Asthma and vitamin C," *Ann Allergy* 1994; 73:89–99.

18. Cohen, H.A. et al. "Blocking effect of vitamin C in exercise-induced asthma," *Arch Pediatr Adolesc Med* 1997; 151(32):103–109.

19. Caruso, C. "Bronchial reactivity and intracellular magnesium: a possible mechanism for the bron-chodilating effects of magnesium in asthma," *Clin Sci* 1998; 95(2):137–142.

20. Hashimoto, Y. et al. "Assessment of magnesium status in patients with bronchial asthma," *J Asthma* 2000; 37(6):489–496.

21. Hill, J. et al. "Investigation of the effects of short-term change in dietary magnesium intake in asthma," *Eur Respir J* 1997; 10(10):2225–2229.

22. Gupta, I. et al. "Effects of Boswellia serrata gum resin in patients with bronchial asthma: results of a double-blind, placebo-controlled, 6-week clinical study," *Eur J Med Res* 1998; 3:511–514.

23. Arm, J.P. and T.H. Lee. "The use of fish oil in bronchial asthma," *Allergy Proc* 1989; 10(3):185–187.

24. Dry, J. and D. Vincent. "Effect of fish oil diet on asthma: results of a 1-year double-blind study," *Int Arch Allergy Appl Immunol* 1991; 95(2–3):156–157.

25. Villani, F. et al. "Effect of dietary supplementation with polyunsaturated fatty acids on bronchial hyperactivity in subjects with seasonal asthma," *Respiration* 1998; 65(4):265–269.

Attention Deficit Hyperactivity Disorder (ADHD)

1. *About Attention Deficit Hyperactivity Disorder (ADHD).* The Clarke Institute of Psychiatry (Toronto, Canada). Available at **www.camh.net/ CLARKEPages/about_illnesses/about_adhd.html**.

2. *The Disability Named AD/HD. CHADD Facts. Children and Adults with Attention-Deficit/ Hyperactivity Disorder.* CHADD, 1996–2001. Available at **www.chadd.org/facts/add_facts01.htm**.

3. Bornstein, R.A. et al. "Plasma amino acids in atten-tion deficit disorder," *Psychiatry Res* 1990; 33(3):301–306.

4. Eisenberg, J. et al. "Effect of tyrosine on attention deficit disorder with hyperactivity," *J Clin Psychiatry* 1988; 49(5):193–195.

5. Reimherr, F.W. et al. "An open trial of L-tyrosine in the treatment of attention deficit disorder, residual type," *Am J Psychiatry* 1987; 144(8):1071–1073.

6. Smith, A. et al. "Effects of breakfast and caffeine on cognitive performance, mood and cardiovascular functioning," *Appetite* 1994; 22(1):39–55.

7. Burgess, J.R. et al. "Long-chain polyunsaturated fatty acids in children with attention-deficit hyperactivity disorder," *Am J Clin Nutr* 2000; 71(Suppl 1):S327–S330.

8. Stevens, L.J. et al. "Essential fatty acid metabolism in boys with attention-deficit hyperactivity disorder," *Am J Clin Nutr* 1995; 62(4):761–768.

9. Mitchell, E.A. et al. "Clinical characteristics and serum essential fatty acid levels in hyperactive children," *Clin Pediatr* 1987; 26(8):406–411.

10. Wender, D.H. "The food additive-free diet in the treatment of behaviour disorders: a review," *J Dev Behav Pediatr* 1986; 7(1):35–42.

11. Rowe, K.S. "Synthetic food colourings and 'hyperactivity': a double-blind crossover study," *Aust Paediatr J* 1988; 24(2):143–147.

12. Rippere, V. "Food additives and hyperactive children: a critique of Conners," *Br J Clin Psychol* 1983; 22(Pt 1):19–32.

13. Adams, W. "Lack of behavioural effects from Feingold diet violations," *Percept Mot Skills* 1981; 52(1):307–313.

14. Mattes, J.A. and R. Gittleman. "Effects of artificial food colourings in children with hyperactive symptoms: A critical review and results of a controlled study," *Arch Gen Psychiatry* 1981; 38(6):714–718.

15. Salamay, J. et al. "Physiological changes in hyperactive children following the ingestion of food additives," *J Neurosci* 1982; 16(3–4):241–246.

16. Kaplan, B.J. et al. "Dietary replacement in preschool-aged hyperactive boys," *Pediatrics* 1989; 83(1):7–17.

17. Egger, J. et al. "Controlled trial of oligoantigenic diet treatment in the hyperkinetic syndromes," *Lancet* 1985; 1(8428):540–545.

18. Bamforth, K.J. et al. "Common food additives are potent inhibitors of human liver 17 alpha-ethinyloestradiol and dopamine sulphotransferases," *Biochem Pharmacol* 1993; 46(10):1713–1720.

19. Weinshilboum, R.M. "Phenol sulfotransferase in humans: properties, regulation, and function," *Fed Proc* 1986; 45(8):2223–2228.

20. Harris, R.M. and R.H. Waring. "Dietary modulation of human platelet phenolsulphotransferase activity," *Xenobiotica* 1996; 26(12):1241–1247.

21. Krummel, D.A. et al. "Hyperactivity: is candy causal?" *Crit Rev Food Sci Nutr* 1996; 36(1):31–47.

22. Wolraich, M.L. et al. "The effect of sugar on behaviour or cognition in children. A meta-analysis," *JAMA* 1995; 274(20):1617–1621.

23. Kanarek, R.B. "Does sucrose or aspartame cause hyperactivity in children?" *Nutr Rev* 1994; 52(5):173–175.

24. Roshon, M.S. and R.L. Hagen. "Sugar consumption, task orientation, and learning in preschool children," *J Abnorm Child Psychol* 1989; 17(3):349–357.

25. Wender, E.H. and M.V. Solanto. "Effects of sugar on aggressive and inattentive behavior in children with attention deficit disorder with hyperactivity and normal children," *Pediatrics* 1991; 88(5):960–966.

26. Kozielec, T. and B. Starobrat-Hermelin. "Assessment of magnesium levels in children with attention deficit hyperactivity disorder (ADHD)," *Magnes Res* 1997; 10(2):143–148.

27. Starobrat-Hermelin, B. and T. Kozielec. "The effects of magnesium supplementation on hyperactivity in children with attention deficit hyperactivity disorder (ADHD). Positive response to a magnesium oral loading test," *Magnes Res* 1997; 10(2):149–156.

28. Bekaroglu, M. et al. "Relationships between serum free fatty acids and zinc, and attention deficit hyperactivity disorder: a research note," *J Child Psychol Psychiatry* 1996; 37(2):225–227.

29. Arnold, L.E. et al. "Does hair zinc predict amphetamine improvement in ADD/hyperactivity?" *Int J Neurosci* 1990; 50(1–2):103–107.

30. Arnold, L.E. et al. "Gamma-linolenic acid for attention-deficit hyperactivity disorder: placebo-controlled comparison to D-amphetamine," *Biol Psychiatry* 1989; 25(2):222–228.

31. Aman, M.G. et al. "The effects of fatty acid supplementation by Efamol in hyperactive children," *J Abnorm Child Psychol* 1987; 15(1):75–90.

32. Richardson, A.J. et al. "Reduced behavioural and learning problems in children with specific learning difficulties after supplementation with highly unsaturated fatty acids: a randomized double-blind placebo-controlled trial," presented at the 2nd Forum of European Neuroscience Societies, July 24–28, 2000, Brighton, United Kingdom.

Breast Cancer

1. Holmes, M.D. et al. "Association of dietary fat and fatty acids with risk of breast cancer," *JAMA* 1999; 281(10):914–920.

2. Boyd, N.F. et al. "Effects at two years of a low fat, high carbohydrate diet on radiologic features of the breast: results from a randomized trial. Canadian Diet and Breast Cancer Prevention Study Group," *JNCI* 1997; 89(7):488–496.

3. Boyd, N.F. et al. "Effects of a low-fat high-carbohydrate diet on plasma sex hormones in premenopausal women: results from a randomized controlled trial. Canadian Diet and Breast Cancer Prevention Study Group, *Br J Cancer* 1997; 76(1):127–135.

4. Zheng, W. et al. "Well-done meat intake and the risk of breast cancer," *JNCI* 1998; 90(22):1724–1729.

5. Rose, D.P. et al. "Effect of omega-3 fatty acids on the progression of metastases after surgical excision of human breast cancer cell solid tumors growing in nude mice," *Clinical Cancer Research* 1996; 2(10):1751–1756.

6. Thompson, L.U. et al. "Flaxseed and its lignan and oil components reduce mammary tumor growth at a late stage of carcinogenesis," *Carcinogenesis* 1996; 17(6):1373–1376.

7. Thompson, L.U. et al. "Antitumorigenic effect of a mammalian lignan precurser from flaxseed," *Nutr Cancer* 1996; 26(2):159–165.

8. Thompson, L.U. et al. "Biological effects of dietary flaxseed in patients with breast cancer," *Breast Cancer Research and Treatment* 2000; 64(1):50.

9. Hunter, D.J. et al. "A prospective study of intake of vitamin C, E and A and the risk of breast cancer," *N Engl J Med* 1993; 329:234–240.

10. Freudenheim, J.L. et al. "Premenopausal breast cancer risk and intake of vegetables, fruits and related nutrients," *JNCI* 1996; 88(6):340–348.

11. Howe, G.R. et al. "Dietary factors and risk of breast cancer: combined analysis of 12 case-control studies," *JNCI* 1990; 82:561–569.

12. Hunter, D.J. et al. "A prospective study of caffeine, coffee, tea and breast cancer," *Am J Epidemiol* 1992; 136:1000–1001. [Abstract]

13. Longnecker, M.P. et al. "Alcoholic beverage consumption in relation to risk of breast cancer: meta analysis and review," *Cancer Causes and Control* 1994; 5:73–82.

14. Hankinson, S.E. et al. "Alcohol, height, and adiposity in relation to estrogen and prolactin levels in post-menopausal women," *JNCI* 1995; 87(17):1297–1302.

15. Hirose, K. et al. "Effect of body size on breast cancer risk among Japanese women," *Int J Cancer* 1999; 80(3):349–355.

16. Huang, Z. et al. "Dual effects of weight and weight gain on breast cancer risk," *JAMA* 1997; 278(17):1407–1411.

17. La Vecchia, C. et al. "Body mass index and post-menopausal breast cancer: an age-specific analysis," *Br J Cancer* 1997; 75(3):441–444.

18. Rohan, T.E. et al. "Dietary fibre, vitamins A, C, and E and the risk of breast cancer: a cohort study," *Cancer Causes and Control* 1993; 4:29–37.

19. Zhang, S. et al. "Dietary carotenoids and vitamins A, C, and E and risk of breast cancer," *JNCI* 1999; 91(6):547–556.

20. Wu, K. et al. "A prospective study on folate, B12, and pyridoxal-5'-phosphate (B6) and breast cancer," *Cancer Epidemiol Biomarkers Prev* 1999; 8(3):209–217.

21. Zhang, S. et al. "A prospective study of folate intake and the risk of breast cancer," *JAMA* 1999; 281(17):1632–1637.

Bronchitis

1. La Vecchia, C. et al. "Vegetable consumption and risk of chronic disease," *Epidemiology* 1998; 9(2):208–210.

2. Mylek, D. "ALCAT test results in the treatment of respiratory and gastrointestinal symptoms, arthritis, skin and central nervous system," *Rocz Akad Med Bialymst* 1995; 40(3):625–629.

3. Morabia, A. et al. "Vitamin A, cigarette smoking, and airway obstruction," *Am Rev Respir Dis* 1989; 140(5):1312–1316.

4. Hemila, H. and R.M. Douglas. "Vitamin C and acute respiratory infections," *Int J Tuberc Lung Dis* 1999; 3(9):756–761.

5. Schwartz, J. and S.T. Weiss. "Dietary factors and their relation to respiratory symptoms," *Am J Epidemiol* 1990; 132(1):67–76.

6. Hunt, C. et al. "The clinical effects of vitamin C supplementation in elderly hospitalized patients with acute respiratory infections," *Int J Vitam Nutr Res* 1994; 64(3):221–219.

7. Britton, J. et al. "Dietary magnesium, lung function, wheezing, and airway hyperreactivity in a random adult population sample," *Lancet* 1994; 344(8919):357–362.

8. Schwartz, J. and S.T. Weiss. "Dietary factors and their relation to respiratory symptoms," *Am J Epidemiol* 1990; 132(1):67–76.

9. Matthys, H. et al. "Efficacy and tolerability of myrtol standardized in acute bronchitis. A multi-centre, randomised, double-blind, placebo-controlled parallel group clinical trial vs. cefuroxime and ambroxol," *Arzneimittelforschung* 2000; 50(8):700–711.

10. Meister, R. et al. "Efficacy and tolerability of myrtol standardized in long-term treatment of chronic bronchitis. A double-blind, placebo-controlled study. Study Group Investigators," *Arzneimittelforschung.* 1999; 49(4):351–358.

11. Grandjean, E.M. et al. "Efficacy of oral long-term N-acetylcysteine in chronic bronchopulmonary disease: a meta-analysis of published double-blind, placebo-controlled clinical trials," *Clin Ther* 2000; 22(2):209–221.

12. Holdiness, M.R. "Clinical pharmacokinetics of N-acetylcysteine," *Clin Pharmacokinet* 1991; 20(2):123–134.

Burns

1. Cunningham, J.J. et al. "Calorie and protein provision for recovery from severe burns in infants and young children," *Am J Clin Nutr* 1990; 51(4):553–557.

2. Wolfe, R.R. "Herman Award Lecture 1996: relation of metabolic studies to clinical nutrition—the example of burn injury," *Am J Clin Nutr* 1996; 64(5):800–808.

3. Pasulka, P.S. and T.L. Wachtel. "Nutritional considerations for the burned patient," *Surg Clin North Am* 1987; 67(1):109–131.

4. Garrel, D.R. et al. "Improved clinical status and length of care with low-fat nutrition support in burn patients," *JPEN* 1995; 19(6):482–491.

5. Alexander, J.W. and M.M. Gottschlich. "Nutritional immunomodulation in burn patients," *Crit Care Med* 1990; 18(Suppl 2):S149–S153.

6. Gerster, M. "The use of n-3 PUFAs (fish oil) in enteral nutrition," *Int J Vitam Nutr Res* 1995; 65(1):3–20.

7. Tashiro, T. et al. "N-3 versus n-6 polyunsaturated fatty acids in critical illness," *Nutrition* 1998; 14(6):551–553.

8. Tanaka, H. et al. "Reduction of resuscitation fluid volumes in severely burned patients using ascorbic acid administration: a randomized, prospective study," *Arch Surg* 2000; 135(3):326–331.

9. Zhang, M.J. et al. "Comparative observation of the changes in serum lipid peroxides influenced by the supplementation of vitamin E in burn patients and healthy controls," *Burns* 1992; 18(1):19–21.

10. Haberal, M. et al. "The stabilizing effect of vitamin E, selenium, and zinc on leucocyte membrane permeability: a study in vitro," *Burns Incl Therm Inj* 1987; 13(2):118–122.

11. Berger, M.M. et al. "Trace element supplementation modulates pulmonary infection rates after major burns: a double-blind, placebo-controlled trial," *Am J Clin Nutr* 1998; 68(2):365–371.

12. Berger, M.M. et al. "Influence of large intakes of trace elements on recovery after major burns," *Nutrition* 1994; 10(4):327–334.

13. Shukla, A. et al. "In vitro and in vivo wound healing activity of asiaticoside isolated from *Centella asiatica*," *J Ethnopharmacol* 1999; 65:1–11.

14. Schmidt, J.M. and J.S. Greenspoon. "Aloe vera dermal wound gel is associated with a delay in wound healing," *Obstet Gynecol* 1991; 78:115–117.

15. Klein, A.D. and N.S. Penneys. "Aloe vera," *J Am Acad Dermatol* 1988; 18(4 Pt 1):714–720.

16. Visuthikosol, V. et al. "Effect of aloe vera gel to healing of burn wound: a clinical and histological study," *J Med Assoc Thai* 1995; 78(8):403–409.

17. Coudray-Lucas, C. et al. "Ornithine alpha-ketoglutarate improves wound healing in severe burn patients: a prospective randomized double-blind trial versus isonitrogenous controls," *Crit Care Med* 2000; 28(6):1772–1776.

18. Donati, L. et al. "Nutritional and clinical efficacy of ornithine alpha-ketoglutarate in severe burn patients," *Clin Nutr* 1999; 18(5):307–311.

19. De Bandt, J.P. et al. "A randomized controlled trial of the influence of the mode of enteral ornithine alpha-ketoglutarate administration in burn patients," *J Nutr* 1998; 128(3):563–569.

Candidiasis

1. Pizzo, G. et al. "Effect of dietary carbohydrates on the in vitro epithelial adhesion of Candida albicans, Candida tropicalis, and Candida krusei," *New Microbiol* 2000; 23(1):63–71.
2. Samaranayake, Y.H. et al. "The in vitro proteolytic and saccharolytic activity of Candida species cultured in human saliva," *Oral Microbiol Immunol* 1994; 9(4):229–235.
3. Elmer, G.W. et al. "Biotherapeutic agents. A neglected modality for the treatment and prevention of selected intestinal and vaginal yeast infections," *JAMA* 1996; 275(11):870–876.
4. Hawes, S.E. et al. "Hydrogen peroxide-producing lactobacilli and acquisition of vaginal infections," *J Infec Dis* 1996; 174(5):1058–1063.
5. Hilton, E. et al. "Ingestion of yogurt containing Lactobacillus acidophilus as a prophylaxis for candidal vaginitis," *Ann Intern Med* 1992; 116(5):353–357.
6. Reid, G. et al. "Is there a role for Lactobacilli in prevention of urogenital and intestinal infections?" *Clin Microbiol Rev* 1990; 3:335–344.
7. Collins, E.B. and P. Hardt. "Inhibition of Candida albicans by Lactobacillus acidophilus," *J Dairy Scientific* 1980; 63:830–832.
8. Ankri, S. and D. Mirelman. "Antimicrobial properties of allicin from garlic," *Microbes Infect* 1999; 1(2):125–129.
9. Ghannoum, M.A. "Studies on the anticandidal mode of action of Allium sativum (garlic)," *J Gen Microbiol* 1988; 134 (Pt 11):2917–2924.
10. Yoshida, S. et al. "Antifungal activity of ajoene derived from garlic," *Appl Environ Microbiol* 1987; 53(3):615–617.
11. Adetumbi, M., G.T. Javor and B.H. Lau. "Allium sativum (garlic) inhibits lipid synthesis by Candida albicans," *Antimicrob Agents Chemother* 1986; 30(3):499–501.

Canker Sores

1. Nolan, A. et al. "Recurrent aphthous ulceration and food sensitivity," *J Oral Pathol Med* 1991; 20(10):473–475.
2. Raiha, I. and S. Syrjanen. "Oral mucosal changes in celiac patients on a gluten-free diet," *Eur J Oral Sci* 1998; 106(5):899–906.
3. McCartan, B.E. and D.G. Weir. "Gliadin antibodies identify gluten-sensitive oral ulceration in the absence of villous atrophy," *J Oral Pathol Med* 1991; 20(10):476–468.
4. Porter, S.R. et al. "Hematologic status in recurrent aphthous stomatitis compared with other oral disease," *Oral Surg Oral Med Oral Pathol* 1988; 66(1):41–44.
5. Weusten, B.L. and A. Weil. "Aphthous ulcers and vitamin B12 deficiency," *Neth J Med* 1998; 53(4):172–175.
6. Haisraeli-Shalish, M. et al. "Recurrent aphthous stomatitis and thiamine deficiency," *Oral Surg Oral Med Oral Pathol Oral Radiol Endod* 1996; 82(6):634–636.
7. Nolan, A. et al. "Recurrent aphthous ulceration: vitamin B1, B2 and B6 status and response to replacement therapy," *J Oral Pathol Med* 1991; 20(8):389–391.
8. Porter, S.R. et al. "Hematologic status in recurrent aphthous stomatitis compared with other oral disease," *Oral Surg Oral Med Pathol* 1988; 66(1):41–44.
9. Das, S.K. et al. "Deglycyrrhizinated licorice in aphthous ulcers," *J Assoc Physicians India* 1989; 37:647.

Cataracts

1. Hiller, R. et al. "Cigarette smoking and the risk of development of lens opacities: the Framingham studies," *Arch Ophthalmol* 1997; 115(9):1113–1118.
2. Christen, W.G. et al. "Smoking cessation and risk of age-related cataract in men," *JAMA* 2000; 284(6):713–716.
3. Glynn, R.J. et al. "Body mass index. An independent predictor of cataract," *Arch Ophthalmol* 1995; 113(9):1131–1137.
4. Schaumberg, D.A. et al. "Relations of body fat distribution and height with cataract in men," *Am J Clin Nutr* 2000; 72(6):1495–1502.
5. Hiller, R. et al. "A longitudinal study of body mass index and lens opacities: the Framingham studies," *Ophthalmol* 1998; 105(7):1244–1250.
6. Cumming, R.G. et al. "Dietary sodium intake and cataract: the Blue Mountain Eye Study," *Am J Epidemiol* 2000; 151(6):624–626.
7. Manson, J.E. et al. "A prospective study of alcohol consumption and risk of cataract," *Am J Prev Med* 1994; 10(3):156–161.
8. Klein, B.E. et al. "Incident cataract after a five-year interval and lifestyle factors: the Beaver Dam eye study," *Ophthalmic Epidemiol* 1999; 6(4):247–255.

9. Munoz, B. et al. "Alcohol use and risk of posterior subscapular opacities," *Arch Ophthalmol* 1993; 111(1):110–112.

10. Chasan-Taber, L. et al. "A prospective study of alcohol consumption and cataract extraction among U.S. women," *Ann Epidemiol* 2000; 10(6):347–353.

11. Brown, L. et al. "A prospective study of carotenoid intake and risk of cataract extraction in US men," *Am J Clin Nutr* 1999; 70(4):517–524.

12. Chasan-Taber, L. et al. "A prospective study of carotenoid and vitamin A intakes and risk of cataract extraction in US women," *Am J Clin Nutr* 1999; 70(4):509–516.

13. Mares-Perlman, J.A. et al. "Vitamin supplement use and incident cataracts in a population-based study," *Arch Ophthalmol* 2000; 118(11):1556–1563.

14. Leske, M.C. et al. "Antioxidant vitamins and nuclear opacities: the longitudinal study of cataract," *Ophthalmol* 1998; 105(5):831–836.

15. Seddon, J.M. et al. "The use of vitamin supplements and the risk of cataract among US male physicians," *Am J Public Health* 1994; 84(5):788–792.

16. Simon, J.A. and E.S. Hudes. "Serum ascorbic acid and other correlates of self-reported cataract among older Americans," *J Clin Epidemiol* 1999; 52(12):1207–1211.

17. Tessier, F. et al. "Decrease in vitamin C concentration in human lenses during cataract progression," *Int J Vitam Nutr Res* 1998; 68(5):309–315.

18. Jacques, P.F. et al. "Long-term vitamin C supplement use and prevalence of early age-related lens opacities," *Am J Clin Nutr* 1997; 66(4):911–916.

19. Rouhianinen, P. et al. "Association between low plasma vitamin E concentration and progression of early cortical lens opacities," *Am J Epidemiol* 1996; 144(5):496–500.

20. Leske, M.C. et al. "Antioxidant vitamins and nuclear opacities: the longitudinal study of cataract," *Ophthalmol* 1998; 105(5):831–836.

21. Robertson, J.M. et al. "Vitamin E intake and risk of cataracts in humans," *Ann N Y Acad Sci* 1989; 570:372–382.

22. Teikari, J.M. et al. "Long-term supplementation with alpha-tocopherol and beta-carotene and age-related cataract," *Acta Ophthalmol Scand* 1997; 75(6):634–640.

23. Repossi, P. et al. "The role of anthocyanosides on vascular permeability in diabetic retinopathy," *Ann Ottamol Clin Ocul* 1987; 113(4):357–361. [Italian]

24. Perossini, M. et al. "Diabetic and hypertensive retinopathy with Vaccinium myrtillus," *Ann Ottamol Clin Ocul* 1987; 113(12):1173–1190. [Italian]

Celiac Disease

1. Mariani, P. et al. "The gluten-free diet: a nutritional risk factor for adolescents with celiac disease?" *J Pediatr Gastroenterol Nutr* 1998; 27(5):519–523.

2. Kemppainen, T. et al. "Osteoporosis in adult patients with celiac disease," *Bone* 1999; 24(3):249–255.

3. Mora, S. et al. "Reversal of low bone density with a gluten-free diet in children and adolescents with celiac disease," *Am J Clin Nutr* 1998; 67(3):477–481.

4. Kemppainen, T. et al. "Bone recovery after a gluten-free diet: a 5-year follow-up study," *Bone* 1999; 25(3):355–360.

5. Sategna-Guidetti, C. et al. "The effects of 1-year gluten withdrawal on bone mass, bone metabolism and nutritional status in newly-diagnosed adult celiac disease patients," *Aliment Pharmacol Ther* 2000; 14(1):35–43.

6. Rude, R.K. and M. Olerich. "Magnesium deficiency: possible role in osteoporosis associated with gluten-sensitive enteropathy," *Osteoporos Int* 1996; 6(6):453–461.

Cervical Dysplasia

1. Schiffman, M.H. "New epidemiology of human papillomavirus infection and cervical neoplasia," *JNCI* 1995; 87:1345–1347.

2. Palefsky, J.M. and E.A. Holly. "Molecular virology and epidemiology of human papillomavirus and cervical cancer," *Cancer Epidemiol Biomarkers Prev* 1995; 4:415–428.

3. Nagata, C. et al. "Serum retinal level and risk of cervical cancer in cases with cervical dysplasia," *Cancer Invest* 1999; 17(4):253–258.

4. Romney, S.L. et al. "Effects of beta-carotene and other factors on outcome of cervical dysplasia and human papillomavirus infection," *Gynecol Oncol* 1997; 65(3):483–492.

5. Mackerras, D. et al. "Randomized double-blind trial of beta-carotene and vitamin C in women with minor cervical abnormalities," *Br J Cancer* 1999; 79(9–10):1448–1453.

6. Kantesky, P.A. et al. "Dietary intake and blood levels of lycopene: association with cervical dysplasia among non-Hispanic, black women," *Nutr Cancer* 1998; 31(1):31–40.

7. Basu, J. et al. "Plasma ascorbic acid and beta-carotene levels in women evaluated for HPV infection, smoking, and cervix dysplasia," *Cancer Detec Prev* 1991; 15(3):165–170.

8. Goodman, M.T. et al. "The association of plasma micronutrients with the risk of cervical dysplasia in Hawaii," *Cancer Epidemiol Biomarkers Prev* 1998; 7(6):537–544.

9. McPherson, R.S. "Nutritional factors and the risk of cervical dysplasia," proceedings and abstracts of papers presented at the 22nd annual meeting of the Society for Epidemiological Research, June 14–16, 1989; Birmingham, AL, *Am J Epidemiol* 1989; 130(4):830. [Abstract]

10. Whitehead, N. et al. "Megaloblastic changes in the cervical epithelium: association with oral contraceptive therapy," *JAMA* 1973; 226:1421–1424.

11. Butterworth, C. et al. "Improvement in cervical dysplasia associated with folic acid therapy in users of oral contraceptives," *Am J Clin Nutr* 1982; 35:73–82.

12. Childers, J.M. et al. "Chemoprevention of cervical cancer with folic acid: a phase 111 Southwest Oncology Group Intergroup Study," *Cancer Epidemiol Biomarkers Prev* 1995; 4:155–159.

Chronic Fatigue Syndrome (CFS)

1. Sibbald, B. "Chronic Fatigue Syndrome comes out of the closet," *CMAJ* 1998; 159:537–541.

2. The facts about Chronic Fatigue Syndrome. US Department of Health and Human Services, March 1995, Atlanta, GA.

3. Gray, J.B. and A.M. Martinovic. "Eicosanoids and essential fatty acid modulation in chronic disease and the chronic fatigue syndrome," *Med Hypotheses* 1994; 43(1):32–42.

4. Heap, L.C. et al. "Vitamin B status in patients with chronic fatigue syndrome," *J R Soc Med* 1999; 92(4):183–185.

5. Regland, B. et al. "Increased concentrations of homocysteine in the cerebrospinal fluid in patients with fibromyalgia and chronic fatigue syndrome," *Scand J Rheumatol* 1997; 26(4):301–307.

6. Werbach, M.R. "Nutritional strategies for treating chronic fatigue syndrome," *Altern Med Rev* 2000; 5(2):93–108.

7. Jacobson, W. et al. "Serum folate and chronic fatigue syndrome," *Neurology* 1993; 43(12):2645–2647.

8. Moorkens, G. et al. "Magnesium deficit in a sample of the Belgian population presenting with chronic fatigue syndrome," *Magnes Res* 1997; 10(4):329–337.

9. Cox, I.M. et al. "Red blood cell magnesium and chronic fatigue syndrome," *Lancet* 1991; 337(8744):757–760.

10. See D.M. et al. "In vitro effects of Echinacea and ginseng on natural killer and antibody-dependent cell cytotoxicity in healthy subjects and chronic fatigue syndrome or acquired immunodeficiency syndrome patients," *Immunopharmacology* 1997; 35(3):229–235.

11. Behan, P.O. et al. "Effects of high doses of essential fatty acids on the postviral fatigue syndrome," *Acta Neurol Scand* 1990; 82(3):209–216.

12. Warren, G. et al. "The role of essential fatty acids in chronic fatigue syndrome. A case-controlled study of red-cell membrane essential fatty acids (EFA) and a placebo-controlled treatment study with high dose of EFA," *Acta Neurol Scand* 1999; 99(2):112–116.

13. Plioplys, A.V. and S. Plioplys. "Serum levels of carnitine in chronic fatigue syndrome: clinical correlates," *Neuropsychobiology* 1995; 32(3):132–138.

14. Kuratsune, H. et al. "Acylcarnitine deficiency in chronic fatigue syndrome," *Clin Infec Dis* 1994; 18(Suppl 1):S62–S67.

15. Plioplys, A.V. and S. Plioplys. "Amantadine and L-carnitine treatment of Chronic Fatigue Syndrome," *Neuropsychobiology* 1997; 35(1):16–23.

Cirrhosis of the Liver

1. The American Dietetic Association. *Manual of Clinical Dietetics,* 6th ed. (Chicago, 2000).

2. Jensen, M.G. "Long-term oral refeeding of patients with cirrhosis of the liver," *Br J Nutr* 1995; 74(4):557–567.

3. Bianchi, G.P. et al. "Vegetable versus animal protein diet in cirrhotic patients with chronic encephalopathy," *J Intern Med* 1993; 233(5):385–392.

4. Verboeket-van de Venne, W.P. et al. "Energy expenditure and substrate metabolism in patients with cirrhosis of the liver: effects of the pattern of food intake," *Gut* 1995; 36(10):110–116.

5. Marchesini, G. et al. "Nutritional treatment with branched-chain amino acids in advanced liver cirrhosis," *J Gastroenterol* 2000; 35(Suppl):S7–S12.

6. Okita, M. et al. "Nutritional treatment of liver cirrhosis by branched chain amino acids," *J Nutr Sci Vitaminol* 1985; 31(3):291–303.

7. Maddrey, W.C. "Branched chain amino acid therapy in liver disease," *J Am Coll Nutr* 1985; 4(6):639–650.

8. Jenkins, D.J. et al. "Low glycemic index foods and reduced glucose, amino acid, and endocrine responses in cirrhosis," *Am J Gastroenterol* 1989; 84(7):732–739.

9. Runyon, B.A. "Management of adult patients with ascites caused by cirrhosis," *Hepatology* 1998; 27(1):264–272.

10. Wong, F. et al. "The effect of posture on central blood flow volume in patients with preascitic cirrhosis on a sodium-restricted diet," *Hepatology* 1996; 23(5):1141–1147.

11. Gauthier, A. et al. "Salt or no salt in the treatment of cirrhotic ascites: a randomized study," *Gut* 1986; 27(6):705–709.

12. Nalini, G. et al. "Oxidative stress in alcoholic liver disease," *Ind J Med Res* 1999; 110:200–203.

13. Britton, R.S. and B.R. Bacon. "Role of free radicals in liver diseases and hepatic fibrosis," *Hepatogastroenterology* 1994; 41(4):343–348.

14. Ward, R.J. and T.J. Peters. "The antioxidant status of patients with either alcohol-induced liver damage or myopathy," *Alcohol Alcohol* 1992; 27(4):359–365.

15. Ferro, D. et al. "Vitamin E reduces monocyte tissue factor expression in cirrhotic patients," *Blood* 1999; 93(9):2945–2950.

16. Van Gossum, A. and J. Neve. "Low selenium status in alcoholic cirrhosis is correlated with aminopyrine breath test. Preliminary effects of selenium supplementation," *Biol Trace Elem Res* 1995; 47(1–3):201–207.

17. Muzes, G. et al. "Effects of silymarin (Legalon) therapy on the antioxidant defense mechanism and lipid peroxidation in alcoholic liver disease," *Orv Hetil* 1990; 131:863–866. [Hungarian]

18. Ferenci, P. et al. "Randomized controlled trial of silymarin in patients with cirrhosis of the liver," *J Hepatol* 1989; 9(1):105–113.

19. Feher, J. et al. "Liver protective action of silymarin therapy in chronic alcoholic liver diseases," *Orv Hetil* 1989; 130:2723–2727. [Hungarian]

20. Leiber, C.S. "Prevention and treatment of liver fibrosis based on pathogenesis," *Alcohol Clin Exp Res* 1999; 23(5):944–949.

21. Schuller-Perez, A. and F. Gonzalez San Martin. "A controlled study with polyunsaturated phosphatidylcholine compared to placebo in alcoholic steatosis of the liver," *Med Welt* 1985; 36:517–521.

22. Mato, J.M. et al. "S-adenosyl-L-methionine synthetase and methionine metabolism deficiencies in cirrhosis," *Adv Exp Med Biol* 1994; 368(1):113–117.

23. Almasio, P. et al. "Role of S-adenosyl-L-methionine in the treatment of intrahepatic cholestasis," *Drugs* 1990; 40(Suppl 3):S111–S123.

24. Loguercio, C. et al. "Effect of S-adenosyl-L-methionine administration on red blood cell cysteine and glutathione levels in alcoholic patients with and without liver disease," *Alcohol Alcohol* 1994.; 29(5):597–604.

25. Kakimoto, H. et al. "Changes in lipid composition of erythrocyte membranes with administration of S-adenosyl-L-methionine in chronic liver disease," *Gastroenterol Jpn* 1992; 27(4):508–513.

26. Mato, J.M. et al. "S-adenosyl-L-methionine in alcoholic liver cirrhosis: a randomized, placebo-controlled, double-blind, multicenter clinical trial," *J Hepatol* 1999; 30:1081–1089.

Colorectal Cancer

1. *Prevention of colorectal cancer.* CancerNet, a service of the National Cancer Institute. Available at **www.cancernet.nci.nih.gov**.

2. Shike, M. "Diet and lifestyle in the prevention of colorectal cancer: an overview," *Am J Med* 1999; 106(1A):11S–15S.

3. Slattery, M.L. et al. "Lifestyle and colon cancer: an assessment of factors associated with risk," *Am J Epidemiol* 1999; 159(8):868–877.

4. Ford, E.S. "Body mass index and colon cancer in a national sample of adult US men and women," *Am J Epidemiol* 1999; 150(4):390–398.

5. Reddy, B.S. et al. "Effect of quality and quantity of dietary fat and dimethylhydrazine in colon carcinogenesis in rats," *Proc Soc Exp Biol Med* 1976; 151(2):237–239.

6. Nauss, K.M. et al. "Effect of alterations in the quality and quantity of dietary fat on 1,2-dimethylhydrazine-induced colon tumorigenesis in rats," *Cancer Res* 1983; 43(9):4083–4090.

7. Hirayama, T. et al. "A large scale cohort study on the relationship between diet and selected cancers of the digestive organs," *Banbury Report* 1981; 7:409–429.

8. Bjelke, E. "Epidemiology of colorectal cancer, with emphasis on diet," *Int Cong Series* 1980; 484:158–174.

9. Goldbohm, R.A. et al. "A prospective cohort study on the relation between meat consumption and the risk of colon cancer," *Cancer Res* 1994; 54(3):718–723.

10. Singh, P.N. and G.E. Fraser. "Dietary risk factors for colon cancer in a low-risk population," *Am J Epidemiol* 1998; 148(8):761–774.

11. World Cancer Research Fund/American Institute for Cancer Research. *Food Nutrition and the Prevention of Cancer: A Global Perspective* (Washington, DC, 1997).

12. de Deckere, E.A. "Possible beneficial effect of fish and fish n-3 polyunsaturated fatty acids in breast and colorectal cancer," *Eur J Can Prev* 1999; 8(3):213–221.

13. Bartsch, H. et al. "Dietary polyunsaturated fatty acids and cancers of the breast and colorectum: emerging evidence of their role as risk modifiers," *Carcinogenesis* 1999; 20(12):2209–2218.

14. Rose, D.P. and J.M. Connolly. "Omega-3 fatty acids as cancer chemopreventative agents," *Pharmcol Ther* 1999; 83(3):217–244.

15. Anti, M. et al. "Effects of different doses of fish oil on rectal cell proliferation in patients with sporadic colonic adenomas," *Gastroenterology* 1994; 107(6):1709–1718.

16. Purasiri, P. et al. "Modulation of cytokine production in vivo by dietary essential fatty acids in patients with colorectal cancer," *Clin Sci (Colch)* 1994; 87(6):711–717.

17. Macquart-Moulin, G. et al. "Colorectal polyps and diet: a case-control study in Marseilles," *J Cancer* 1987; 40:179–188.

18. Sandler, R.S. et al. "Diet and risk of colorectal adenomas: macronutrients, cholesterol, and fiber," *JNCI* 1993; 85:884–891.

19. McKeown-Eyssen, G.E. et al. "A randomized trial of a low fat high fibre diet in the recurrence of colorectal polyps," *J Clin Epidemiol* 1994; 47:525–536.

20. Giovanucci, E. et al. "Physical activity, obesity, and risk for colon cancer and adenoma in men," *Ann Intern Med* 1995; 122:327–334.

21. Howe, G.R. et al. "Dietary intake of fiber and decreased risk of cancers of the colon and rectum: evidence from the combined analysis of 13 case-control studies," *J Nat Canc Inst* 1992; 84(24):1187–1896.

22. Schatzkin, A. et al. "Lack of effect of a low-fat, high-fiber diet on the recurrence of colorectal adenomas. Polyp Prevention Trial Study Group," *N Engl J Med* 2000; 342(16):1149–1155.

23. Alberts, D.S. et al. "Lack of effect of a high-fiber cereal supplement on the recurrence of colorectal adenomas," *N Engl J Med* 2000; 342(16):1156–1162.

24. Fuchs, C.S. et al. "Dietary fiber and the risk of colorectal cancer and adenoma in women," *N Engl J Med* 1999; 340(3):169–176.

25. Thun, M.J. et al. "Risk factors for fatal colon cancer in a large prospective study," *JNCI* 1992; 84:1491–1500.

26. Slattery, M.L. et al. "Carotenoids and colon cancer," *Am J Clin Nutr* 2000; 71(2):575–582.

27. August, D.A. et al. "Ingestion of green tea rapidly decreases prostaglandin E2 levels in rectal mucosa in humans," *Cancer Epidemiol Biomarkers Prev* 1999; 8(8):709–713.

28. Ji, B.T. et al. "Green tea consumption and the risk of pancreatic and colorectal cancers," *Int J Cancer* 1997; 70(3):255–258.

29. Longnecker, M.P. et al. "A meta-analysis of alcoholic beverage consumption in relation to risk of colorectal cancer," *Cancer Causes and Control* 1990:1(1):59–68.

30. Kune, G.A. et al. "Alcohol consumption and the etiology of colorectal cancer: a review of the scientific evidence from 1957 to 1991," *Nutr Cancer* 1992; 18(2):97–111.

31. Boutron, M.C. et al. "Diet and the adenoma-cancer sequence," *Eur J Can Prev* 1993:2(Suppl 2):S95–S98.

32. Bostick, R.M. et al. "Reduced risk of colon cancer with high intake of vitamin E: the Iowa Women's Health Study," *Cancer Res* 1993; 53(18):4230–4237.

33. Albanes, D. et al. "Effects of supplemental alpha-tocopherol and beta-carotene on colorectal cancer: results from a controlled trial (Finland)," *Cancer Causes and Control* 2000; 11(3):197–205.

34. Pappalardo, G. et al. "Antioxidant and colorectal carcinogenesis: role of beta-carotene, vitamin E and vitamin C," *Tumori* 1996; 82(1):6–11.

35. Giovannucci, E. et al. "Multivitamin use, folate, and colon cancer in women in the Nurses' Health Study," *Ann Intern Med* 1998; 129(7):517–524.

36. Kampman, E. et al. "Calcium, vitamin D, sunshine exposure, dairy products and colon cancer risk (United States)," *Cancer Causes and Control* 2000; 11(5):459–466.

37. Holt, P.R. "Dairy foods and prevention of colon cancer: human studies," *J Am Coll Nutr* 1999; 18(Suppl 5):S379–S391.

38. Whelan, R.L. et al. "Vitamin and calcium supplement use is associated with decreased adenoma recurrence in patients with a previous history of neoplasia," *Dis Colon Rectum* 1999; 42(2):212–217.

39. La Vecchia, C. et al. "Intake of selected nutrients and risk of colorectal cancer," *Int J Cancer* 1999; 73(4):525–530.

40. Welberg, J.W. et al. "Effects of oral calcium supplementation on intestinal bile acids and cytolytic activity of fecal water in patients with adenomatous polyps of the colon," *Eur Clin Invest* 1993; 23(1):63–68.

41. Scieszka, M. et al. "Plasma selenium concentration in patients with stomach and colon cancer," *Neoplasma* 1997; 44(6):395–397.

42. Russo, M.W. et al. "Plasma selenium levels and the risk of colorectal adenomas," *Nutr Cancer* 1997; 28(2):125–129.

43. Psathakis, D. et al. "Blood selenium and glutathione peroxidase status in patients with colorectal cancer," *Dis Colon Rectum* 1998; 41(3):328–335.

44. Combs, G.F., L.C. Clark and B.W. Turnbull. "Reduction of cancer risk with an oral selenium supplement," *Biomed Environ Sci* 1997; 19(2–3):227–234.

45. Fleischauer, A.T., C. Poole and L. Arab. "Garlic consumption and cancer prevention: meta-analyses of colorectal and stomach cancers," *Am J Clin Nutr* 2000; 72(4):1047–1052.

46. Steinmetz, K.A. et al. "Vegetables, fruit, and colon cancer in the Iowa Women's Health Study," *Am J Epidemiol* 1994; 139(1):1–15.

Common Cold

1. Saketkhoo, K., A. Januszkiewicz and M.A. Sackner. "Effects of drinking hot water, cold water, and chicken soup on nasal mucus velocity and nasal airflow resistance," *Chest* 1978; 74(4):408–410.

2. Kopp-Hoolihan, L. "Prophylactic and therapeutic uses of probiotics: a review," *J Am Diet Assoc* 2001; 101(2):229–238.

3. Isolauri, E. et al. "Probiotics: effects on immunity," *Am J Clin Nutr* 2001; 73(Suppl 2):S444–S450.

4. Lykova, E.A. et al. "Disruption of microbiocenosis of the large intestine and the immune and interferon status in children with bacterial complications of acute viral infections of the respiratory tract and their correction by high doses of bifidumbacterin forte," *Antibiot Khimioter* 2000; 45(10):22–27. [Russian]

5. Douglas, R.M., E.B. Chalker and B. Tracey. "Vitamin C for preventing and treating the common cold," *Cochrane Database Syst Rev* 2000; 34(2):CD000980.

6. Hemila, H. "Vitamin C supplementation and common cold symptoms: factors affecting the magnitude of benefit," *Med Hypotheses* 1999; 52(2):171–178.

7. Hemila, H. and R.M. Douglas. "Vitamin C and acute respiratory infections," *Int J Tuberc Lung Dis* 1999; 3(9):756–761.

8. Meydani, S.N. et al. "Vitamin E supplementation enhances cell-mediated immunity in healthy elderly subjects," *Am J Clin Nutr* 1990; 52(3):557–563.

9. Ravaglia, G. et al. "Effect of micronutrient status in natural killer cell immune function in healthy free living subjects aged >/=90 y," *Am J Clin Nutr* 2000; 71(2):590–598.

10. Prasad, A.S. et al. "Duration of symptoms and plasma cytokine levels in patients with the common cold treated with zinc actetate. A randomized, double-blind, placebo-controlled trial," *Ann Intern Med* 2000; 133(4):245–252.

11. Petrus, E.J. et al. "Randomized, double-masked, placebo-controlled clinical study of the effectiveness of zinc acetate lozenges on common cold symptoms in allergy tested subjects," *Curr Ther Res* 1998; 59:595–607.

12. Mossad, S.B. et al. "Zinc gluconate lozenges for treating the common cold. A randomized, double-blind, placebo-controlled study," *Ann Intern Med* 1996 15; 125(2):81–88.

13. Jackson, J.L. et al. "Zinc and the common cold: a meta-analysis revisited," *J Nutr* 2000; 139(Suppl 5):S1512–S1515.

14. Eby, G.A. "Zinc ion availability—the determinant of efficacy in zinc lozenge treatment of common colds," *J Antimicrob Chemother* 1997; 40(4):483–493.

15. Melchart, D. et al. "Echinacea for preventing and treating the common cold," *Cochrane Database Syst Rev* 2000; 44(2):CD000530.

16. Kyo, E. et al. "Immunomodulatory effects of aged garlic extract," *J Nutr* 2001; 131(Suppl 3):S1075–S1079.

17. Amagase, H. et al. "Intake of garlic and its bioactive components," *J Nutr* 2001; 131(Suppl 3):S955–S962.

18. Salman, H. et al. "Effect of a garlic derivative (alliin) on peripheral blood cell immune responses," *Int J Immunopharmacol* 1999; 21(9):589–597.

19. Scaglione, F. et al. "Efficacy and safety of the standardized ginseng extract G115 for potentiating vaccination against the influenza syndrome and protection against the common cold," *Drugs Exp Clin Res* 1996; 22:65–72.

Congestive Heart Failure

1. Hambrecht, R. et al. "Effects of exercise training on left ventricular function and peripheral resistance in patients with chronic heart failure: A randomized trial," *JAMA* 2000; 283(23):3095–3101.

2. Oka, R.K. et al. "Impact of a home-based walking program and resistance training program on quality of life in patients with heart failure," *Am J Cardiol* 2000; 85(3):365–369.

3. Kiilavuori, K. et al. "The effect of physical training on skeletal muscle in patients with chronic heart failure," *Eur J Heart Fail* 2000; 2(1):53–63.

4. Kostis, J.B. et al. "Nonpharmacologic therapy improves functional and emotional status in congestive heart failure," *Chest* 1994; 106(4):996–1001.

5. Waldenstrom, A. "Alcohol and congestive heart failure," *Alcohol Clin Exp Res* 1998; 22(Suppl 7):S315–S317.

6. Singal, P.K. et al. "Oxidative stress in congestive heart failure," *Curr Cardiol Rep* 2000; 2(3):206–211.

7. Hoeschen, R.J. "Oxidative stress and cardiovascular disease," *Can J Cardiol* 1997; 13(11):1021–1025.

8. Ball, A.M. and M.J. Sole. "Oxidative stress and the pathogenesis of heart failure," *Cardiol Clin* 1998; 16(4):665–675.

9. Watanabe, H. et al. "Randomized, double-blind, placebo-controlled study of ascorbate on the preventative effect of nitrate intolerance in patients with congestive heart failure," *Circulation* 1998; 97(9):886–891.

10. Chandra, M. "Oxy free radical system in heart failure and therapeutic role of oral vitamin E," *J Cardiol* 1996; 57(2):119–127.

11. Brady, J.A. et al. "Thiamin status, diuretic medications, and the management of congestive heart failure," *J Am Diet Assoc* 1995; 95(5):541–545.

12. Suter, P.M. et al. "Diuretic use: a risk for subclinical thiamine deficiency in elderly patients," *J Nutr Health Aging* 2000; 4(2):69–71.

13. Seligmann, H. et al. "Thiamine deficiency in patients with congestive heart failure receiving long-term furosemide therapy: a pilot study," *Am J Med* 1991; 91(2):151–155.

14. Motro, M. et al. "Improved left ventricular function after thiamine supplementation in patients with congestive heart failure receiving long-term furosemide therapy," *Am J Med* 1995; 98(5):485–490.

15. Crippa, G. et al. "Magnesium and cardiovascular drugs: interactions and therapeutic role," *Ann Ital Med Int* 1999; 14(1):40–45.

16. Douban, S. et al. "Significance of magnesium in congestive heart failure," *Am Heart J* 1996; 132(3):664–671.

17. Hix, C.D. "Magnesium in congestive heart failure, acute myocardial infarction and dysrhythmias," *J Cardiovasc Nurs* 1993; 8(1):19–31.

18. Ceremuzynski, L. et al. "Hypomagnesemia in heart failure with ventricular arrhythmias. Beneficial effects of magnesium supplementation," *J Intern Med* 2000; 247(1):78–86.

19. Sueta, C.A. et al. "Antiarrhythmic action of pharmacological administration of magnesium in heart failure: a critical review of new data," *Magnes Res* 1995; 8(4):389–401.

20. Dorup, I. et al. "Oral magnesium supplementation restores the concentrations of magnesium, potassium and sodium-potassium pumps in skeletal muscle of patients receiving diuretic treatment," *J Intern Med* 1993; 233(2):117–123.

21. Upton, R., ed. *Hawthorn Leaf with Flower: quality control, analytical and therapeutic monograph* (Santa Cruz: American Herbal Pharmacopoeia; 1999):1–29.

22. Schwinger, R.H. et al. "Crataegus special extract WS 1442 increases force of contraction in human myocardium camp-independently," *J Cardiovasc Pharmacol* 2000; 35(5):700–707.

23. Miller, A.L. "Botanical influences on cardiovascular diseases," *Altern Med Rev* 1998; 3(6):422–431.

24. Khatta, M. Alexander B.S. et al. "The effect of coenzyme Q10 in patients with congestive heart failure," *Ann Intern Med* 2000; 132(8):636–640.

25. Soja, A.M. and S.A. Mortensen. "Treatment of congestive heart failure with coenzyme Q10 illuminated by meta-analysis of clinical trials," *Mol Aspects Med* 1997; 18(Suppl 1):S159–S168.

26. Morisco, C., B. Trimarco and M. Condorelli. "Effect of coenzyme Q10 therapy in patients with congestive heart failure: A long-term multicenter randomized study," *Clin Investig* 1993; 71(Suppl 8): S134–S136.

27. Hofman-Bang, C. et al. "Coenzyme Q10 as an adjunctive treatment of congestive heart failure," *J Card Fail* 1995; 1:101–107.

28. Baggio, E. et al. "Italian multicenter study on the safety and efficacy of coenzyme Q10 as adjunctive therapy in heart failure. CoQ10 Drug Surveillance Investigators," *Mol Aspects Med* 1994; (Suppl 15):S287–S294.

29. Arsenian, M.A. "Carnitine and its derivatives in cardiovascular disease," *Prog Cardiovasc Dis* 1997; 40(3):265–286.

30. Anand, I. et al. "Acute and chronic effects of propionyl-L-carnitine on the hemodynamics, exercise capacity, and hormones in patients with congestive heart failure," *Cardiovasc Drugs Ther* 1998; 12(3):291–299.

31. Ferrari, R. and F. De Giuli. "The propionyl-L-carnitine hypothesis: an alternative approach to treating heart failure," *J Card Fail* 1997; 3(3):217–224.

32. Mancini, M. et al. "Controlled study on the therapeutic efficacy of propionyl-L-carnitine in patients with congestive heart failure," *Arzneimittelforschung* 1992; 42(9):1101–1104.

33. Kobayashi, A. et al. "L-carnitine treatment of congestive heart failure—experimental and clinical study," *Jpn Circ J* 1992; 56(10):86–94.

34. Azuma, J. et al. "Double-blind randomized crossover trial of taurine in congestive heart failure," *Curr Ther Res* 1983; 34:543–557.

35. Azuma, J. et al. "Double-blind randomized crossover trial of taurine in congestive heart failure," *Clin Cardiol* 1985; 8:276–282.

Constipation

1. Voderholzer, W.A. et al. "Clinical response to dietary fiber in the treatment of chronic constipation," *Am J Gastroenterol* 1997; 92(1):95–98.

2. Tramonte, S.M. et al. "The treatment of chronic constipation in adults. A systematic review," *J Gen Intern Med* 1997; 12(1):15–24.

3. Hillemeier, C. "An overview of the effects of dietary fiber on gastrointestinal transit," *Pediatrics* 1995; 96(5 Pt 2):997–999.

4. Jenkins, D.J. et al. "Fiber and starchy foods; gut function and implications in disease," *Am J Gastroenterol* 1986; 81(10):920–930.

5. Muller-Lissne, S.A. "Effect of wheat bran on weight of stool and gastrointestinal transit time: a meta analysis," *Br J Med* 1988; 296(6622):615–617.

6. Slavin, J.L. "Implementation of dietary modifications," *Am J Med* 1999; 106(1A):46S–49S.

7. Marlett, J.A. et al. "Comparative laxation of psyllium with and without senna in an ambulatory constipated population," *Am J Gastroenterol* 1987; 82(4):333–337.

8. Ashraf, W. et al. "Effects of psyllium therapy on stool characteristics, colon transit and anorectal function in chronic idiopathic constipation," *Aliment Pharmacol Ther* 1995; 9(6):639–647.

9. McRorie, J.W. et al. "Psyllium is superior to docusate sodium for treatment of chronic constipation," *Aliment Pharmacol Ther* 1998; 12(5):491–497.

10. Hull, C. et al. "Alleviation of constipation in the elderly by dietary fiber supplementation," *J Am Geriatr Soc* 1980; 28(9):410–414.

11. Roberfroid, M.B. "Prebiotics and probiotics: are they functional foods?" *Am J Clin Nutr* 2000; 71(Suppl 6):S1682–S1687.

12. Salminen, S. and E. Salminen. "Lactulose, lactic acid bacteria, intestinal microecology and mucosal protection," *Scand J Gastroenterol Suppl* 1997; 222(2):45–48.

Cystic Fibrosis

1. Roulet, M. et al. "Essential fatty acid deficiency in well nourished young cystic fibrosis patients," *Eur J Pediatr* 1997; 156(12):952–956.

2. Strandvik, B. et al. "Effect on renal function of essential fatty acid supplementation in cystic fibrosis," *J Pediatr* 1989; 115(2):242–250.

3. Strandvik, B. and R. Hultcrantz. "Liver function and morphology during long-term fatty acid supplementation in cystic fibrosis," *Liver* 1994; 14(1):32–36.

4. Christophe, A. et al. "Effect of administration of gamma-linolenic acid on the fatty acid composition of serum phospholipids and cholesteryl esters in patients with cystic fibrosis," *Ann Nutr Metab* 1994; 38(1):40–47.

5. Lucarelli, S. et al. "Food allergy in cystic fibrosis," *Minerva Pediatr* 1994; 46(12):543–548.

6. Hill, S.M. et al. "Cow's milk sensitive enteropathy in cystic fibrosis," *Arch Dis Child* 1989; 64(9):1251–1255.

7. Ansari, E.A. et al. "Ocular signs and symptoms and vitamin A status in patients with cystic fibrosis treated with daily vitamin A supplements," *Br J Ophthalmol* 1999; 83(6):688–691.

8. Huet, F. et al. "Vitamin A deficiency and nocturnal vision in teenagers with cystic fibrosis," *Eur J Pediatr* 1997; 156(12):949–951.

9. Rayner, R.J. et al. "Night blindness and conjunctional xerosis caused by vitamin A deficiency in patients with cystic fibrosis," *Arch Dis Child* 1989; 64(8):1151–1156.

10. Duggan, C. et al. "Vitamin A status in acute exacerbations of cystic fibrosis," *Am J Clin Nutr* 1996; 64(4):635–639.

11. Conway, S.P. et al. "Osteoporosis and osteopenia in adults and adolescents with cystic fibrosis: prevalence and associated factors," *Thorax* 2000; 55(9):798–804.

12. Donovan, D.S. et al. "Bone mass and vitamin D deficiency in adults with advanced cystic fibrosis lung disease," *Am J Respir Crit Care Med* 1998; 157(6 Pt 1):1892–1899.

13. Haworth, C.S. et al. "Low bone mineral density in adults with cystic fibrosis. *Thorax* 1999; 54(11):961–967.

14. Hendersen, R.C. and G. Lester. "Vitamin D levels in children with cystic fibrosis," *South Med J* 1997; 90(4):378–383.

15. Grey, V. et al. "Monitoring of 25-OH vitamin D levels in children with cystic fibrosis," *J Pediatr Gastroenterol Nutr* 2000; 30(3):314–319.

16. Dominguez, C. et al. "Enhanced oxidative damage in cystic fibrosis patients," *Biofactors* 1998; 8(1–2):149–153.

17. Brown, R.K. et al. "Pulmonary dysfunction in cystic fibrosis is associated with oxidative stress," *Eur Respir J* 1996; 9(2):334–339.

18. Portal, B.C. et al. "Altered antioxidant status and increased lipid peroxidation in children with cystic fibrosis," *Am J Clin Nutr* 1995; 61(4):843–847.

19. Sitrin, M.D. et al. "Vitamin E deficiency and neurologic disease in adults with cystic fibrosis," *Ann Intern Med* 1987; 107(1):51–54.

20. Kelleher, J. et al. "The clinical effect of correction of vitamin E depletion in cystic fibrosis," *Int J Vitam Nutr Res* 1987; 57(3):253–259.

21. Winklhofer-Roob, B.M. et al. "Impaired resistance to oxidation of low density lipoprotein in cystic fibrosis: improvement during vitamin E supplementation," *Free Radic Biol Med* 1995; 19(6):725–733.

22. Peters, S.A. and F.J. Kelly. "Vitamin E supplementation in cystic fibrosis," *J Pediatr Gastroenterol Nutr* 1996; 22(4):341–345.

23. Cornelissen, E.A. et al. "Vitamin K status in cystic fibrosis. *Acta Pediatr* 1992; 81(9):658–661.

24. Beker, L.T. et al. "Effect of vitamin K1 supplementation on vitamin K status in cystic fibrosis patients," *J Pediatr Gastroenterol Nutr* 1997; 24(5):512–517.

25. Rust, P. et al. "Effects of long-term oral beta-carotene supplementation on lipid peroxidation in patients with cystic fibrosis," *Int J Vit Nutr Res* 1998; 68(2):83–87.

26. Lepage, G. et al. "Supplementation with carotenoids corrects increased lipid peroxidation in children with cystic fibrosis," *Am J Clin Nutr* 1997; 64(1):87–93.

27. Winklhofer-Roob, B.M. et al. "Response to oral beta-carotene supplementation in patients with cystic fibrosis: a 16-month follow-up study," *Acta Pediatr* 1995; 84(10):1132–1136.

28. Winklhofer-Roob, B.M. et al. "Plasma vitamin C concentrations in patients with cystic fibrosis: evidence of associations with lung inflammation," *Am J Clin Nutr* 1997; 65(6):1858–1866.

29. Lambert, J.P. "Osteoporosis: a new challenge in cystic fibrosis," *Pharmacotherapy* 2000; 20(1):34–51.

30. Hendersen, R.C. and C.D. Madsen. "Bone mineral content and body composition in children and young adults with cystic fibrosis," *Pedatri Pulmonol* 1999; 27(2):80–84.

31. Mocchegiani, E. et al. "Role of low zinc bio-availability on cellular immune effectiveness in cystic fibrosis," *Clin Immunol Immunopathol* 1995; 75(3):214–224.

32. Easley, D. et al. "Effect of pancreatic enzymes on zinc absorption in cystic fibrosis," *J Pediatr Gastroenterol Nutr* 1998; 26(2):136–139.

33. Safai-Kutti, S. et al. "Zinc therapy in children with cystic fibrosis," *Beitr Infusionther* 1991; 27:104–114.

34. Percival, S.S. et al. "Altered copper status in adult men with cystic fibrosis," *J Am Coll Nutr* 1999; 18(6):614–619.

35. Percival, S.S. et al. "Reduced copper enzyme activities in blood cells of children with cystic fibrosis," *Am J Clin Nutr* 1995; 62(3):633–638.

Depression

1. *Health Facts: What is Depression?* Ontario Ministry of Health and Long-Term Care, March 2000. Available at **www.gov.on.ca:80/MOH/english/pub/mental/depression.html**.
2. Blum, I. et al. "The influence of meal composition on plasma serotonin and norepinephrine concentrations," *Metabolism* 1992; 41(2):137–140.
3. Sayegh, R. et al. "The effect of a carbohydrate-rich beverage on mood, appetite, and cognitive function in women with premenstrual syndrome," *Obstet Gynecol* 1995; 86(4 Pt 1):520–528.
4. Su, K.P., W.W. Shen and S.Y. Huang. "Are omega3 fatty acids beneficial in depression but not mania?" *Arch Gen Psychiatry* 2000; 57(7):716–717.
5. Kinrys, G. "Hypomania associated with omega3 fatty acids," *Arch Gen Psychiatry* 2000; 57(7):715–716.
6. Stoll, A.L. et al. "Omega 3 fatty acids in bipolar disorder: A preliminary double-blind, placebo-controlled trial," *Arch Gen Psychiatry* 1999; 56:407–412.
7. Wyatt, K.M. et al. "Efficacy of vitamin B6 in the treatment of premenstrual syndrome: systematic review," *Br J Med* 1999; 318(7195):1375–1381.
8. Pennix, B.W. et al. "Vitamin B(12) deficiency and depression in physically disabled older women: epidemiologic evidence from the Women's Health and Aging Study," *Am J Psychiatry* 2000; 157(5):715–721.
9. Ebly, E.M. et al. "Folate status, vascular disease and cognition in elderly Canadians," *Age Ageing* 1998; 27(4):485–491.
10. Fava, M. et al. "Folate, vitamin B12, and homocysteine in major depressive disorder," *Am J Psychiatry* 1997; 154(3):426–428.
11. Bell, I.R. et al. "B complex vitamin patterns in geriatric and young adult inpatients with major depression," *J Am Geriatr Soc* 1991; 39(3):252–257.
12. Bell, I.R. et al. "Vitamin B12 and folate status in acute geropsychiatric inpatients: affective and cognitive characteristics of a vitamin nondeficient population," *Biol Psychiatry* 1990; 27(2):125–137.
13. Linde, K. et al. "St. John's Wort for depression—an overview and meta-analysis of randomized clinical trials," *Br Med J* 1996; 313:253–258.
14. Eckmann, F. "Cerebral insufficiency treatment with *Ginkgo biloba* extract: time of onset of effect in a double-blind study with 60 inpatients," *Fortschr Med* 1990; 108:557–560.
15. Schubert, H. et al. "Depressive episode primarily unresponsive to therapy in elderly patients: efficacy of *Ginkgo biloba* (EGb 761) in combination with antidepressants," *Geriatr Forsch* 1993; 3:45–53.
16. Huguet, F. et al. "Decreases cerebral 5-HT receptors during aging: reversal by *Ginkgo biloba* extract (EGb 761)," *J Pharm Pharmacol* 1994; 46:316–318.
17. Balon, R. "*Ginkgo biloba* for antidepressant-induced sexual dysfunction?" *J Sex Marital Ther* 1999; 25(1):1–2.
18. Levine, J. et al. "Follow-up and relapse analysis of an inositol study of depression," *Isr J Psychiatry Relat Sci* 1995; 32:14–21.
19. Levine, J. "Controlled trials of inositol in psychiatry," *Eur Psychopharmacol* 1997; 7:147–155.
20. Benjamin, J. et al. "Inositol treatment in psychiatry," *Psychopharmacol Bull* 1995; 31:167–175.
21. Bressa, G.M. "S-adenosyl-l-methionine (SAMe) as antidepressant: meta-analysis of clinical studies," *Acta Neurol Scand Suppl* 1994; 154:7–14.
22. Bell, K.M. et al. "S-adenosylmethionine blood levels in major depression: changes with drug treatment," *Acta Neurol Scand Suppl* 1994; 154:15–18.
23. Salmaggi, P. et al. "Double-blind, placebo-controlled study of S-adenosyl-L-methionine in depressed postmenopausal women," *Psychother Psychosom* 1993; 59(1):34–40.
24. De Vanna, M. and R. Rigamonti. "Oral S-adenosyl-L-methionine in depression," *Curr Ther Res* 1992; 52(3):478–485.
25. Kagan, B.L. et al. "Oral S-adenosylmethionine in depression: a randomized, double-blind, placebo-controlled trial," *Am J Psychiatry* 1990; 147(5):591–595.
26. Rosenbaum, J.F. et al. "The antidepressant potential of oral S-adenosyl-l-methionine," *Acta Psychiatr Scand* 1990; 81(5):432–436.

Dermatitis and Eczema

1. *Atopic Dermatitis.* National Institutes of Health. Available at **www.nih.gov.niams/healthinfo/dermatitis/atophandout_breakks.html**.
2. *15 Million American Kids and Adults Are Itchy...* American Academy of Dermatology. Available at **www.aad.org.**

3. Sampson, H.A. "Food hypersensitivity and dietary management in atopic dermatitis," *Pediatr Dermatol* 1992; 9(4):376–369.

4. Lever, R. et al. "Randomized controlled trial of advice on egg exclusion diet in young children with atopic eczema and sensitivity to eggs," *Pediatr Allergy Immunol* 1998; 9(1):13–19.

5. Majamaa, H. et al. "Wheat allergy: diagnostic accuracy of skin prick and patch tests and specific IgE," *Allergy* 1999; 54(8):851–856.

6. Niggemann, B. et al. "Outcome of double-blind, placebo-controlled food challenge tests on 107 children with atopic dermatitis," *Clin Exp Allergy* 1999; 29(1):91–96.

7. Horrobin, D.F. "Essential fatty acid metabolism and its modification in atopic eczema," *Am J Clin Nutr* 2000; 71(Suppl 1):S367–S372.

8. Horrobin, D.F. "Fatty acid metabolism in health and disease: the role of delta-6-desaturase," *Am J Clin Nutr* 1993; 57(Suppl 5):S732–S736.

9. Wright, S. and T.A. Sanders. "Adipose tissue essential fatty acid composition in patients with atopic eczema," *Eur J Clin Nutr* 1991; 45(10):501–505.

10. Saarinen, U.M. and M. Kajosaari. "Breastfeeding as prophylaxis against atopic disease: prospective follow-up study until 17 years old," *Lancet* 1995; 346(8982):1065–1069.

11. Sandstead, H.H. "Zinc deficiency. A public health problem?" *Am J Dis Child* 1991; 145(8):853–859.

12. Prasad, A.S. "Zinc in growth and development and spectrum of human zinc deficiency," *J Am Coll Nutr* 1988; 7(5):377–384.

13. Di Toro R. et al. "Zinc and copper status of allergic children," *Acta Pediatr Scand* 1987; 76(4):612–617.

14. Fiocchi, A. et al. "The efficacy and safety of gamma-linolenic acid in the treatment of infantile dermatitis," *J Int Med Res* 1994; 22(1):24–32.

15. Hederos, C.A. and A. Berg. "Epogam evening primrose oil treatment in atopic dermatitis and asthma," *Arch Dis Child* 1996; 75(6):494–497.

16. Biagi, P.L. et al. "A long-term study on the use of evening primrose oil (Efamol) in atopic children," *Drugs Exp Clin Res* 1988; 14(4):285–290.

17. Schalin-Karrila, M. et al. "Evening primrose oil in the treatment of atopic eczema: effect on clinical status, plasma phospholipid fatty acids and circulating blood prostaglandins," *Br J Dermatol* 1987; 117(1):11–19.

18. Aertgeerts, P. et al. "Comparison of Kamillosan® cream (2 g ethanolic extract from chamomile flowers in 100g cream) versus steroid (0.25% hydrocortisone, 0.75% flucortin butyl ester) and non-steroid (5% bufexamec) external agents in the maintenance therapy of eczema," *Z Hautkr* 1985; 60:270–277. [German]

19. Patzelt-Wenczler, R. and E. Ponce-Poschl. "Proof of efficacy of Kamillosan® cream in atopic eczema," *Eur J Med Res* 2000; 5(4):171–175.

20. Isolauri, E. et al. "Probiotics in the management of atopic eczema," *Clin Exp Allergy* 2000; 30(11):1604–1610.

21. Majamaa, H. and E. Isolauri. "Probiotics: a novel approach in the management of food allergy," *J Allergy Clin Immunol* 1997; 99(2):179–185.

Diabetes Mellitus

1. *Diabetes.* Available at **www.altmed.com/conditions/conditions.cfm?ID=13**.

2. The DCCT Research Group. "The effect of intensive insulin treatment of diabetes on the development and progression of long-term complications in insulin-dependent diabetes," *N Eng J Med* 1993; 329:977–986.

3. UK Prospective Diabetes Study Group. "Intensive blood-glucose control with sulphonylureas or insulin compared with conventional treatment and risk of complications in patients with type 2 diabetes (UKPDS 33)," *Lancet* 1998; 352(9131):837–853.

4. The American Dietetic Association. *Manual of Clinical Dietetics*, 6th ed. (Chicago, 2000).

5. Wolever, T. et al. *Guidelines for the Nutritional Management of Diabetes Mellitus in the New Millennium. A Position Statement by the Canadian Diabetes Association*, National Nutrition Committee, Canadian Diabetes Association. Available at **www.diabetes.ca**.

6. Franz, M.J. et al. "Effectiveness of medical nutrition therapy provided by dietitians in the management of non-insulin-dependent diabetes mellitus: a randomized, controlled clinical trial," *J Am Diet Assoc* 1995; 95(9):1009–1117.

7. Jenkins, D.J., T.M. Wolever and A.L. Jenkins. "Starchy foods and the glycemic index," *Diabetes Care* 1988; 11(2):149–159.

8. Jenkins, D.J. et al. "Low-glycemic-index starchy foods in the diabetic diet," *Am J Clin Nutr* 1988; 48(2):248–254.

9. Tsihlias, E.B. et al. "Comparison of high- and low-glycemic-index breakfast cereals with monounsaturated fat in the long-term dietary management of type 2 diabetes," *Am J Clin Nutr* 2000; 72(2):439–449.

10. Emanuele, M.A. et al. "A crossover trial of high and low sucrose-carbohydrate diets in type II diabetics with hypertriglyceridemia," *J Am Coll Nutr* 1986; 5(5):429–437.

11. Braaten, J.T. et al. "High beta-glucan oat bran and oat gum reduce postprandial blood glucose and insulin in subjects with and without type 2 diabetes," *Diabet Med* 1994; 11(3):312–318.

12. Del Toma, E. et al. "Soluble and insoluble dietary fibre in diabetic diets," *Eur J Clin Nutr* 1988; 42(4):313–319.

13. Jenkins, D.J.A. et al. "Effect on serum lipids of very high fiber intakes in diets low in saturated fat and cholesterol," *N Eng J Med* 1993; 329:21–26.

14. Lichtenstein, A.H. and U.S. Schwab. "Relationship of fat to glucose metabolism," *Atherosclerosis* 2000; 150(2):227–243.

15. Thomsen, C. et al. "Comparison of the effects on the diurnal blood pressure, glucose and lipid levels of a diet rich in monounsaturated fatty acids with a diet rich in polyunsaturated fatty acids in type 2 diabetic subjects," *Diabet Med* 1995; 12(7):600–606.

16. Sharma, A. et al. "Evaluation of oxidative stress before and after control of glycemia and after vitamin E supplementation in diabetic patients," *Metabolism* 2000; 49(2):160–162.

17. Abahusain, M.A. et al. "Retinol, alpha-tocopherol and carotenoids in diabetes," *Eur J Clin Nutr* 1999; 53(8):630–635.

18. Davi, G. et al. "In vivo formation of 8-iso-prostaglandin falpha and platelet activation in diabetes mellitus: effects of improved metabolic control and vitamin E supplementation," *Circulation* 1999; 99(2):224–229.

19. Tutuncu, N.B. et al. "Reversal of defective nerve conduction with vitamin E supplementation in type 2 diabetes: a preliminary study," *Diabetes Care* 1998; 21(11):1915–1918.

20. Paolisso, G. et al. "Plasma vitamin C affects glucose homeostasis in healthy subjects and in non-insulin-dependent diabetics," *Am J Physiol* 1994; 266(2 Pt 1):E261–E268.

21. Cunningham, J.J. "The glucose/insulin system and vitamin C: implications in insulin-dependent diabetes mellitus," *J Am Coll Nutr* 1998; 17(2):105–108.

22. Paolisso, G. et al. "Changes in glucose turnover parameters and improvement of glucose oxidation after 4-week magnesium administration in elderly noninsulin-dependent (type II) diabetic patients," *J Clin Endocrinol Metab* 1994; 78(6):1510–1514.

23. Saggese, G. et al. "Hypomagnesemia and the parathyroid hormone-vitamin D endocrine system in children with insulin-dependent diabetes mellitus: effects of magnesium administration," *J Pediatr* 1991; 118(2):220–225.

24. Mertz, W. "Chromium in human nutrition: a review," *J Nutr* 1993; 123(4):626–633.

25. Ding, W. et al. "Serum and urine chromium concentration in elderly diabetics," *Biol Trace Elem Res* 1998; 63(3):231–237.

26. Morris, B.W. et al. "Chromium homeostasis in patients with type II (NIDDM) diabetes," *I Trace Elem Med Biol* 1999; 13(1–2):57–61.

27. Anderson, R.A. "Nutritional factors influencing the glucose/insulin system: chromium," *J Am Coll Nutr* 1997; 16(5):404–410.

28. Vuskan, V. et al. "Similar postprandial glycemic reductions with escalation of dose and administration time of American ginseng in type 2 diabetes," *Diabetes Care* 2000; 23(9):1221–1226.

29. Vuksan, V. et al. "American ginseng (Panax quinquefolius L) reduced postprandial glycemia in nondiabetic subjects and subjects with type 2 diabetes mellitus," *Arch Intern Med* 2000; 160(7):1009–1113.

30. Androne L. et al. "In vivo effect of lipoic acid on lipid peroxidation in patients with diabetic neuropathy," *In Vivo* 2000; 14(2):327–330.

31. Jain, S.K. and G. Lim. "Lipoic acid decreases lipid peroxidation and protein glycosylation and increases $(Na(+) + K(+))$- and $Ca (++)$-ATPase activities in high glucose-treated human erythrocytes," *Free Radic Biol Med* 2000; 29(11):1122–1128.

32. Ziegler, D. et al. "Treatment of symptomatic diabetic polyneuropathy with the antioxidant alpha-lipoic acid: a 7-month multicenter randomized controlled trial (ALADIN III Study). ALADIN III Study Group. Alpha-Lipoic Acid in Diabetic Neuropathy," *Diabetes Care* 1999; 22(8):1296–1301.

33. Jacob, S. et al. "Enhancement of glucose disposal in patients with type 2 diabetes by alpha-lipoic acid," *Arzneimittelforschung* 1995; 45(8):872–874.

34. Jacob, S. et al. "Oral administration of RAC-alpha-lipoic acid modulates insulin sensitivity in patients with type 2 diabetes: a placebo-controlled trial," *Free Radic Biol Med* 1999; 27(3–4):309–314.

Diarrhea

1. *Diarrhea.* The National Digestive Diseases Information Clearinghouse. Available at **www.niddk.nih.gov/health/digest/pubs/diarrhea/diarrhea.html**.

2. Dennison, B.A. "Fruit juice consumption by infants and children: a review," *J Am Coll Nutr* 1996; 15(Suppl 5):S4–S11.

3. Hoekstra, J.H. et al. "Apple juice malabsorption: fructose or sorbitol?" *J Pediatr Gastroenterol Nutr* 1993; 16(1):39–42.

4. Hoekstra, J.H. et al. "Fluid intake and industrial processing in apple juice induced chronic and non-specific diarrhoea," *Arch Dis Child* 1995; 73(2):126–130.

5. Smith, M.M. and F. Lifshitz. "Excess fruit juice consumption as a contributing factor in nonorganic failure to thrive," *Pediatrics* 1994; 93(3):438–443.

6. Rolfe, R.D. "The role of probiotic cultures in the control of gastrointestinal health," *J Nutr* 2000; 130(Suppl 2):S396–S402.

7. Vanderhoof, J.A. et al. "Lactobacillus GG in the prevention of antibiotic-associated diarrhea in children," *J Pediatr* 1999; 135(5):564–568.

8. Phuapradit, P. et al. "Reduction of rotavirus infection in children receiving bifidobacteria-supplemented formula," *J Med Assoc Thai* 1999; 82(4)(Suppl 1):S43–S48.

9. Guarino, A. et al. "Oral bacteria therapy reduces the duration of symptoms and of viral excretion in children with mild diarrhea," *J Pediatr Gastroenterol Nutr* 1997; 25(5):516–517.

10. Vanderhoof, J.A. "Food hypersensitivity in children," *Curr Opin Clin Nutr Metab Care* 1998; 1(5):419–422.

11. Ahmed, T. et al. "Humoral immune and clinical responses to food antigens following acute diarrhoea in children," *J Paediatr Child Health* 1998; 34(3):229–232.

12. Snyder, J.D. "Dietary protein sensitivity: is it an important risk factor for persistent diarrhea?" *Acta Paediatr Suppl* 381(3):78–81.

13. Wapnir, R.A. "Zinc deficiency, malnutrition and the gastrointestinal tract," *J Nutr* 2000; 130(Suppl 5):S1388–S1392.

14. Faker, P.J. et al. "The dynamic link between the integrity of the immune system and zinc status," *J Nutr* 2000; 130(Suppl 5):S1399–S1406.

15. Roy, S.K. et al. "Impact of zinc supplementation on subsequent growth and morbidity in Bangladeshi children with acute diarrhoea," *Eur J Clin Nutr* 1999; 53(7):529–534.

16. Sazawal, S. et al. "Efficacy of zinc supplementation in reducing the incidence and prevalence of acute diarrhea—a community-based, double-blind, controlled trial," *Am J Clin Nutr* 1997; 66(2):413–418.

17. Unknown. "Berebine," *Altern Med Rev* 2000; 5(2):175–177.

18. Akhter, M.H. et al. "Possible mechanism of antidiarrheal effect of berebine," *Ind J Med Res* 1979; 70:233–241.

19. Desai, A.B. et al. "Berebine in the treatment of diarrhea," *Ind Pediatr* 1971; 8:462–465.

20. Khin-Maung, U. et al. "Clinical trial of berebine in acute watery diarrhea," *Br Med J* 1985; 291:1601–1605.

21. Gupte, S. "Use of berebine in treatment of giardiasis," *Am J Dis Child* 1975; 129:866.

22. Rabbani, G.H. et al. "Randomized controlled trial of berebine sulfate therapy for diarrhea due to enterotoxigenic *Escherichia coli* and *Vibrio cholerae*," *J Inf Dis* 1987; 155:979–984.

Diverticulosis and Diverticulitis

1. *Diverticulosis and Diverticulitis.* National Digestive Diseases Information Clearinghouse, November 1998. Available at **www.niddk.nih.gov/health/digest/pubs/divert/divert.htm**.

2. O'Keefe, S.J. "A.R.P. Lecture: Food and the gut," *S Afr Med J* 1995; 85(4):261–268.

3. Cheskin, L.J. and R.D. Lamport. "Diverticular disease. Epidemiology and pharmacological treatment," *Drugs Aging* 1995; 6(1):55–63.

4. Kay, R.M. "Dietary fibre," *J Lipid Res* 1982; 23(2):221–242.

5. Walker, A.R. "Diet and bowel diseases—past history and future prospects," *S Afr Med J* 1985; 68(3):148–152.

6. Leahy, A.L. et al. "High fibre diet in symptomatic diverticular disease of the colon," *Ann R Coll Surg Eng* 1985; 67(3):173–174.

7. Aldoori, W.H. et al. "A prospective study of diet and risk of symptomatic diverticular disease in men," *Am J Clin Nutr* 1994; 60(5):757–764.

Ear Infections (Otitis Media)

1. *What is an Ear Infection?* Mayo Foundation for Medical Education and Research, April 2001. Available at **www.mayoclinic.com/home?id=DS00303**.

2. Ibid.

3. Damoiseaux, R.A. et al. "Primary care based randomized, double blind trial of amoxicillin versus placebo for acute otitis media in children aged under 2 years," *Br Med J* 2000; 320:350–354.

4. Del Mar, C. et al. "Are antibiotics indicated as initial treatment for children with acute otitis media? A meta analysis," *Br Med J* 1997; 314:1526–1529.

5. Nsouli, T.M. et al. "Role of food allergy in serious otitis media," *Ann Allergy* 1994; 73(3):215–219.

6. Juntii, H. et al. "Cow's milk allergy is associated with recurrent otitis media during childhood," *Acta Otolaryngol* 1999; 119(8):867–873.

7. Hurst, D.S. "Allergy management of refractory serious otitis media," *Otolaryngol Head Neck Surg* 1990; 102(6):664–669.

8. Bernstein, J.M. "Role of allergy in eustachian tube blockage and otitis media with effusion: a review," *Otolaryngol Head Neck Surg* 1996; 114(4):562–568.

9. Host, A. "Mechanisms of adverse reactions to food. The ear," *Allergy* 1995; 50(Suppl 20):S64–S67.

10. Lykova, E.A. et al. "Disruption of microbiocenosis of the large intestine and the immune and interferon status in children with bacterial complications of acute viral infections of the respiratory tract and their correction by high doses of bifidumbacterin forte," *Antibiot Khimioter* 2000; 45(10):22–27. [Russian]

11. Roos, K., E.G. Hakansson and S. Holm. "Effect of recolonisation with 'interfering' alpha streptococci on recurrences of acute and secretory otitis media in children: randomized placebo controlled trial," *Br Med J* 2001; 322(7280):210–222.

12. Karabaev, K.E., V.F. Antoniv and R.U. Bekmuradov. "Pathogenetic validation of optimal antioxidant therapy in suppurative inflammatory otic diseases in children," *Vestn Otorinolaringol* 1997; (1):5–7. [Russian]

13. Coulehan, J.L. et al. "Vitamin C and acute illness in Navajo school children," *N Engl J Med* 1976; 295(18):973–977.

14. Khakimov, A.M., S.S. Arifov and F.N. Faizulaeva. "Efficacy of antioxidant therapy in patients with acute and chronic purulent otitis media," *Vestn Otorinolaringol* 1997; (5):16–19. [Russian]

15. Bondestam, M., T. Foucard and M. Gebre-Medhin. "Subclinical trace element deficiency in children with undue susceptibility to infections," *Acta Paediatr Scand* 1985; 74(4):515–520.

16. Mark, J.D. K.L. Grant and L.L. Barton. "The use of dietary supplements in pediatrics: a study of echinacea," *Clin Pediatr (Phila)* 2001; 40(5):265–269.

17. Klein, J.O. "Management of acute otitis media in an era of increasing antibiotic resistance," *Int J Pediatr Otorhinolaryngol* 1999; 49(Suppl 1):S15–S27.

18. Uhari, M. et al. "A novel use of xylitol sugar in preventing otitis media," *Pediatrics* 1998; 102(4 Pt 1):879–884.

19. Uhari, M. et al. "Xylitol chewing gum in prevention of acute otitis media: double blind randomized trial," *Br Med J* 1996; 313(7066):1180–1184.

Endometriosis

1. *What is Endometriosis?* Endometriosis Association ENDOnline. Available at **www.endometriosisassn.org/endo.html**.

2. "Endometriosis," *The Merck Manual Home Edition, 1995–2000,* Merck and Co. Ltd. Available at **www.merck.com/pubs/mmanual_home/sec22/237.htm**.

3. Wu, M.Y. et al. "Increase in the production of interleukin-6, interleukin-10, and interleukin-12 by lipoploysaccharide-stimulated peritoneal macrophages from women with endometriosis," *Am J Reprod Immunol* 1999; 41(1):106–111.

4. Karck, U. et al. "PGE2 and PGF2 alpha release by human peritoneal macrophages in endometriosis," *Prostaglandins* 1996; 51(1):49–60.

5. Nabekura, H. et al. "Fallopian tube prostaglandin production with and without endometriosis," *Int J Fertil Menopausal Stud* 1994; 39(1):57–63.

6. Koike, H. et al. "Eicosanoids production in endometriosis," *Prostaglandins Leukot Essent Fatty Acids* 1992; 45(4):331–317.

7. Koike, H. et al. "Correlation between dysmenorrheic severity and prostaglandin production in women with endometriosis," *Prostaglandins Leukot Essent Fatty Acids* 1992; 46(2):133–137.

8. Benedetto, C. "Eicosanoids in primary dysmenorrhea, endometriosis and menstrual migraine," *Gynecol Endocrinol* 1989; 3(1):71–94.

9. Mathias, J.R. et al. "Relation of endometriosis and neuromuscular disease of the gastrointestinal tract: new insights," *Fertil Steril* 1998; 70(1):81–88.

10. Grodstein, F. et al. "Relation of female infertility to consumption of caffeinated beverages," *Am J Epidemiol* 1993; 137(12):1353–1360.

11. Grodstein, F. et al. "Infertility in women and moderate alcohol use," *Am J Public Health* 1994; 84(9):1429–1432.

12. Murphy, A.A. et al. "Endometriosis: a disease of oxidative stress?" *Semin Reprod Endocrinol* 1998; 16(4):263–273.

13. Dawood, M.Y. "Hormonal therapies for endometriosis: implications for bone metabolism," *Acta Obstet Gynecol Scand Suppl* 1994; 159:22–34.

Fibrocystic Breast Conditions

1. Boyd, N.F. et al. "Clinical trial of a low-fat, high-carbohydrate diet in subjects with mammographic breast dysplasia: report of early outcomes," *JNCI* 1988; 80(15):1244–1248.

2. Rose, D.P. "Effect of a low-fat diet on hormone levels in women with cystic breast disease. I. Serum steroids and gonodotropins," *JNCI* 1987; 78(4):623–626.

3. Rose, D.P. et al. "Effect of a low fat diet on hormone levels in women with cystic breast disease. II. Serum radioimmunoassayable prolactin and growth hormone and bioactive lactogenic hormones," *JNCI* 1987; 78(4):627–631.

4. Rose, D.P. et al. "Effects of diet supplementation with wheat bran on serum estrogen levels in the follicular and luteal phases of the menstrual cycle," *Nutrition* 1997; 13:535–539.

5. Rose, D.P. et al. "High-fiber diet reduces serum estrogen concentrations in premenopausal women," *Am J Clin Nutr* 1991; 24:520–524.

6. Xu, X. et al. "Effects of soy isoflavones on estrogen and phytoestrogens metabolism in premenopausal women," *Cancer Epidemiol Biomarkers Prev* 1998; 7:1101–1108.

7. Nagata, C. et al. "Decreased serum estradiol concentration associated with high dietary intake of soy products in premenopausal Japanese women," *Nutr Cancer* 1997; 29:228–233.

8. Cassidy, A. et al. "Biological effects of a diet of soy protein rich isoflavones on the menstrual cycle of premenopausal women," *Am J Clin Nutr* 1994; 60:333–340.

9. Petrakis, N.L. et al. "Stimulatory influence of soy protein isolate on breast secretion in pre and post menopausal women," *Cancer Epidemiol Biomarkers Prev* 1996; 5:785–794.

10. Russell, L.C. "Caffeine restriction as initial treatment of breast pain," *Nurse Pract* 1989; 14(2):36–37.

11. Meyer, E.C. et al. "Vitamin E and benign breast disease," *Surgery* 1990; 107(5):549–551.

12. Ernster, V.L. et al. "Vitamin E and benign breast "disease": a double-blind, randomized clinical trial," *Surgery* 1985; 97(4):490–494.

13. Pye, J.K. et al. "Clinical experience of drug treatments for mastalgia," *Lancet* 1985; 2(8451):373–377.

14. Tamborini, A. and R. Taurelle. "Value of standardized Ginkgo biloba extract (EGb 761) in the management of congestive symptoms of premenstrual syndrome," *Rev Fr Gynecol Obstet* 1993; 88(7–9):447–457. [French]

Fibromyalgia

1. *Fibromyalgia.* The Arthritis Society, January 2001. Available at **www.arthritis.ca/types/%20of%20arthritis/fibro myalgia/default.asp?s=1.**

2. Dykman, K.D. et al. "The effects of nutritional supplements on the symptoms of fibromyalgia and chronic fatigue syndrome," *Integr Physiol Behav Sci* 1998; 33(1):61–71.

3. Swezey, R.L. and J. Adams. "Fibromyalgia: a risk factor for osteoporosis," *J Rheumatol* 1999; 26(12):2642–2644.

4. Eisinger, J. et al. "Selenium and magnesium status in fibromyalgia," *Magnes Res* 1994; 7(3–4):285–288.

5. Ng, S.Y. "Hair calcium and magnesium levels in patients with fibromyalgia: a case center study," *J Manipulative Physiol Ther* 1999; 22(9):586–593.

6. Russell, I.J. et al. "Treatment of fibromyalgia syndrome with Super Malic: a randomized, double

blind, placebo controlled, crossover pilot study," *J Rheumatol* 1995; 22(5):953–958.

7. McCarty, D.J. et al. "Treatment of pain due to fibromyalgia with topical capsaicin: A pilot study," *Semin Arth Rheum* 1994; 23(Suppl 3):S41–S47.

8. Caruso, I. et al. "Double-blind study of 5-hydroxy-tryptophan versus placebo in the treatment of primary fibromyalgia syndrome," *J Int Med Res* 1990; 18:201–210.

9. Abraham, G.E. and J.D. Flechas. "Management of fibromyalgia: rationale for the use of magnesium and malic acid," *J Nutr Med* 1992; 3:49–59.

10. Jacobsen, S. et al. "Oral S-adenosylmethionine in primary fibromyalgia. Double-blind clinical evaluation," *Scand J Rheumatol* 1991; 20:294–302.

Food Allergies

1. *Food Allergy and Intolerances.* National Institute of Allergy and Infectious Disease, June 2001. Available at **www.niaid.nih.gov/factsheets/food.htm**.

2. Wetzig, H. et al. "Associations between duration of breast-feeding, sensitization to hens' egg and eczema infantum in one and two year old children at high risk of atopy," *Int J Hyg Environ Health* 2000; 203(1):17–21.

3. Chandra, R.K. "Five-year follow-up of high-risk infants with family history of allergy who were exclusively breast-fed or fed partial whey hydrolysate, soy and conventional cow's milk formulas," *J Pediatr Gastroenterol Nutr* 1997; 24(4):380–388.

4. Saarinen, U.M. and M. Kajosaari. "Breastfeeding as prophylaxis against atopic disease: prospective follow-up study until 17 years old," *Lancet* 1995; 346(8982):1065–1069.

5. Casas, R. et al. "Detection of IgA antibodies to cat, beta-lactoglobulin, and ovalbumin allergens in human milk," *J Allergy Clin Immunol* 2000; 105(6 Pt 1):1236–1240.

6. *Food Allergies.* Mayo Foundation for Medical Education and Research, July 2000. Available at **www.mayoclinic.com/home?id=DS00082**.

Gallstones

1. *Gallstones.* Mayo Foundation for Medical Education and Research, November 2000. Available at **www.mayoclinic.com/home?id=DS00165**.

2. Ibid.

3. Ibid.

4. Kern, F., Jr. "Effects of dietary cholesterol on cholesterol and bile acid homeostasis in patients with cholesterol gallstones," *J Clin Invest* 1994; 93(3):1186–1194.

5. Narain, P.K. et al. "Cholesterol enhances membrane-damaging properties of model bile by increasing the intervesicular-intermixed micellar concentration of hydrophobic bile salts," *J Surg Res* 1999; 84(1):112–119.

6. Caroli-Bosc, F.X. et al. "Cholelithiasis and dietary risk factors: an epidemiologic investigation in Vidaubanm Southeast France. General Practitioner's Group of Vidauban," *Dig Dis Sci* 1998; 43(9):2131–2137.

7. Festi, D. et al. "Gallbladder motility and gallstone formation in obese patients following very low calorie diets. Use it (fat) or lose it (well)," *Int J Obes Relat Metab Disord* 1998; 22(6):592–600.

8. Gebhard, R.L. et al. "The role of gallbladder emptying in gallstone formation during diet-induced rapid weight loss," *Hepatology* 1996; 24(3):544–548.

9. Vezina, W.C. et al. "Similarity in gallstone formation from 900 kcal/day diets containing 16 g vs 30 g of daily fat: evidence that fat restriction is not the main culprit of cholelithiasis during rapid weight reduction," *Dig Dis Sci* 1998; 43(3):554–561.

10. Heshka, S. et al. "Obesity and risk of gallstone development on a 1200 kcal/d (5025 Kj/d) regular food diet," *Int J Obes Relat Metab Disord* 1996; 20(5):450–454.

11. Syngal, S. et al. "Long-term weight patterns and risk for cholecystectomy in women," *Ann Intern Med* 1999; 130(6):471–477.

12. Leitzmann, M.F. et al. "The relation of physical activity to risk for symptomatic gallstone disease in men," *Ann Intern Med* 1998; 128(6):417–425.

13. Nair, P. and J.F. Mayberry. "Vegetarianism, dietary fibre and gastro-intestinal disease," *Dig Dis Sci* 1994; 12(3):177–185.

14. Ortega, R.M. et al. "Differences in diet and food habits between patients with gallstones and controls," *J Am Coll Nutr* 1997; 16(1):88–95.

15. Sichieri, R. et al. "A prospective study of hospitalization and gallstone disease among women: role of dietary factors, fasting period, and dieting," *Am J Public Health* 1991; 81(7):880–884.

16. Leitzmann, M.F. et al. "A prospective study of coffee consumption and the risk of symptomatic gallstone disease in men," *JAMA* 1999; 281(22):2106–2112.

17. Simon, J.A. "Ascorbic acid and cholesterol gallstones," *Med Hypotheses* 1993; 40(2):81–84.

18. Simon, J.A. and E.S. Hudes. "Serum ascorbic acid and other correlates of gallbladder disease among US adults," *Am J Public Health* 1998; 88(8):1208–1212.

19. Gustafsson, U. et al. "The effect of vitamin C in high doses on plasma and biliary lipid composition in patients with cholesterol gallstones: prolongation of nucleation time," *Eur J Clin Invest* 1997; 27(5):387–391.

20. Moerman, C.J. et al. "Dietary risk factors for clinically diagnosed gallstones in middle-aged men. A 25-year follow-up study (the Zutphen Study)," *Ann Epidemiol* 1994; 4(3):248–254.

21. Nassuato, G. et al. "Effect of silibinin on biliary lipid composition: experimental and clinical study," *J Hepatol* 1991; 12:290–295.

Glaucoma

1. Zang, E.A. and E.L. Wynder. "The association between body mass index and the relative frequencies of disease in a sample of hospitalized patients," *Nutr Cancer* 1994; 21(3):247–261.

2. Cellini, M. et al. "Fatty acid use in glaucomatous optic nerve neuropathy treatment," *Acta Ophthalmol Scand Suppl* 1998; 14(227):41–42.

3. Ritch, R. "Neuroprotection: is it really applicable to glaucoma therapy?" *Curr Opin Ophthalmol* 2000; 11(2):78–84.

4. Jampel, H.D. "Ascorbic acid is cytotoxic to dividing human Tenon's capsule fibroblasts. A possible but contributing factor in glaucoma filtration surgery success," *Arch Ophthalmol* 1990; 108(9):1323–1325.

5. Wendt, M.D. et al. "Ascorbate stimulates type I and type II collagen in human Tenon's fibroblasts," *J Glaucoma* 1997; 6(6):402–407.

6. Haas, A.L. et al. "Vitamin E inhibits proliferation of human Tenon's capsule fibroblasts in vitro," *Ophthalmic Res* 1996; 28(3):171–175.

7. Gaspar, A.Z. et al. "The influence of magnesium in visual field and peripheral vasospasm in glaucoma," *Ophthalmologica* 1995; 209(1):11–13.

8. Repossi, P. et al. "The role of anthocyanosides on vascular permeability in diabetic retinopathy," *Ann Ottamol Clin Ocul* 1987; 113(4):357–361. [Italian]

9. Perossini, M. et al. "Diabetic and hypertensive retinopathy with Vaccinium myrtillus," *Ann Ottamol Clin Ocul* 1987; 113(12):1173–1190. [Italian]

10. Ritch, R. "Potential role for Ginkgo biloba extract in the treatment of glaucoma," *Med Hypotheses* 2000; 54(2):221–235.

11. Chung, H.S. et al. "Ginkgo biloba extract increases ocular blood flow velocity," *J Ocul Pharmacol Ther* 1999; 15(3):233–240.

Gout

1. *Gout.* The Arthritis Society, April 2001. Available at **www.arthritis.ca/types%20of%20arthritis/gout/default.asp?mode=static**.

2. Dessein, P.H. et al. "Beneficial effects of weight loss associated with moderate calorie/carbohydrate restriction, and increased proportional intake of protein and unsaturated fat on serum urate and lipoprotein levels in gout: a pilot study," *Ann Rheum Dis* 2000; 59(7):539–543.

3. Loenen, H.M. et al. "Serum uric acid correlates in elderly men and women with special reference to body composition and dietary intake (Dutch Nutrition Surveillance System)," *J Clin Epidemiol* 1990; 43(12):1297–1303.

4. Heyden, S. "The workingman's diet. II. Effect of weight reduction in obese patients with hypertension, diabetes, hyperuricemia and hyperlipidemia," *Nutr Metab* 1978; 22(3):141–159.

5. Scott, J.T. and R.A. Sturge. "The effect of weight loss on plasma and urinary uric acid and lipid levels," *Adv Exp Med Biol* 1977; 76B(1):274–277.

6. The American Dietetic Association. *Manual of Clinical Dietetics*, 6th ed. (Chicago, 2000).

7. Eastmond, C.J. et al. "The effects of alcoholic beverages on urate metabolism in gout sufferers," *Br J Rheumatol* 1995; 34(8):756–769.

8. Gibson, T. et al. "Beer drinking and its effect on uric acid," *Br J Rheumatol* 1984; 23(3):203–209.

9. Sharpe, C.R. "A case-control study of alcohol consumption and drinking behaviour in patients with gout," *Can Med Assoc J* 1984; 131(6):563–567.

10. Gibson, T. et al. "A controlled study of diet in patients with gout," *Ann Rheum Dis* 1983; 42(2):123–127.

11. Tofler, O.B. and T.L. Woodings. "A 13-year follow-up of social drinkers," *Med J Aust* 1981; 2(9):479–481.

12. Ford-Hutchinson, A.W. "Leukotrienes: their formation and role as inflammatory mediators," *Fed Proc* 1985; 44(1 Pt 1):25–29.

13. Goetzl, E.J. et al. "Immunpathogenic roles of leukotrienes in human diseases," *J Clin Immunol* 1984; 4(2):79–84.

14. European Scientific Cooperative on Phytotherapy. "Harpagophyti radix (devil's claw)," Exeter, UK: ESCOP; 1996–1997. Monographs on the Medicinal Uses of Plant Drugs. Fascicule 2.

Gum Disease

1. Engle, June, ed. "Eye, Ear and Tooth Care," in *The Complete Canadian Health Guide* (Toronto: Key Porter Books, 1993):165.

2. *Brushing up on Gum Disease.* US Food and Drug Administration, May 1990. Available at **www.fdc.gov/bbs/topics/CONSUMER/CON0006S.html**.

3. Requirand, P. et al. "Serum fatty acid imbalance in bone loss: example with periodontal disease," *Clin Nutr* 2000; 19(4):271–276.

4. Campan, P. et al. "Pilot study on n-3 polyunsaturated fatty acids in the treatment of human experimental gingivitis," *J Clin Periodontol* 1997; 24(12):907–913.

5. Nishida, M. et al. "Dietary vitamin C and the risk for periodontal disease," *J Periodontol* 2000; 71(8):1215–1223.

6. Rubinoff, A.B. et al. "Vitamin C and oral health," *J Can Dent Assoc* 1989; 55(9):705–707.

7. Leggott, P.J. et al. "Effects of ascorbic acid depletion and supplementation on periodontal health and subgingival microflora in humans," *J Dent Res* 1991; 70(12):1531–1536.

8. Kumpusalo, E.A. "Periodontal health related to plasma ascorbic acid," *Proc Finn Dent Soc* 1993; 89(1–2):51–59.

9. Holmes, L.G. "Effects of smoking and/or vitamin C on crevicular fluid flow in clinically healthy gingival," *Quintessence Int* 1990; 21(3):191–195.

10. Zachariasen, R. "Oral manifestations of metabolic bone disease: vitamin D and osteoporosis," *Compendium* 1990; 11(10):612, 614–618.

11. Nishida, M. et al. "Calcium and risk for periodontal disease," *J Periodontol* 2000; 71(7):1057–1066.

12. Hanioka, T. et al. "Effect of topical application of coenzyme Q10 on adult periodontitis," *Mol Aspects Med* 1994; 15(Suppl):S241–S248.

Heart Disease and High Blood Cholesterol

1. Willett, W.C. et al. "Intake of trans fatty acids and risk of coronary heart disease among women," *Lancet* 1993; 341(8845):581–585.

2. Hu, F.B. et al. "A prospective study of egg consumption and risk of cardiovascular disease in men and women," *JAMA* 1999; 281(15):1387–1394.

3. Anderson, J.W. et al. "Meta-analysis of the effects of soy protein intake on serum lipids," *New Engl J Med* 1995; 333(5):276–282.

4. MacKay, S. and M.J. Ball. "Do beans and oat bran add to the effectiveness of a low fat diet?" *European Journal of Clinical Nutrition* 1992; 46(9):641–648.

5. Olson, B.H. et al. "Psyllium-enriched cereals lower blood total cholesterol and LDL cholesterol, but not HDL cholesterol, in hypercholesterolemic adults: results of a meta-analysis," *J Nutr* 1997; 127(10):1973–1980.

6. Liu, S. et al. "Whole-grain consumption and risk of coronary heart disease: results from the Nurses' Health Study," *Am J Clin Nutr* 1999; 70(3):412–419.

7. Jacobs, D.R., Jr. et al. "Whole-grain intake may reduce the risk of ischemic heart disease death in postmenopausal women: the Iowa Women's Health Study," *Am J Clin Nutr* 1998; 68(2):248–257.

8. Hu, F.B. et al. "Frequent nut consumption and risk of coronary heart disease in women: prospective cohort study," *Br Med J* 1998; 14; 317(7169):1341–1345.

9. Sesso, H.D. et al. "Coffee and tea intake and the risk of myocardial infarction," *Am J Epidemiol* 1999; 149(2):162–167.

10. Hankinson, S.E. et al. "Alcohol consumption and mortality among women," *N Eng J Med* 1995; 332(19):1245–1250.

11. Rimm, E.B. et al. "Folate and vitamin B6 from diet and supplements in relation to risk of coronary heart disease among women," *JAMA* 1998; 279(5):359–364.

12. Simon, J.A. et al. "Serum ascorbic acid and cardiovascular disease prevalence," *Epidemiology* 1998; 9(3):316–321.

13. Lopes, C. et al. "Diet and risk of myocardial infarction. A case-control community-based study," *Acta Med Port* 11(4):311–317.

14. Stampfer, M.J. et al. "Vitamin E consumption and the risk of coronary heart disease in women," *N Eng J Med* 1993; 328(20):1444–1449.

15. Rimm, E.B. et al. "Vitamin E consumption and the risk of coronary heart disease in men," *N Engl J Med* 1993; 328(20):1450–1456.

16. Agawal, S. and A.V. Rao. "Tomato lycopene and low density lipoprotein oxidation: a human dietary intervention study," *Lipids* 1998; 33(10):981–984.

17. Steiner, M. et al. "A double-blind crossover study in moderately hypercholesterolemic men that compared the effect of aged garlic extract and placebo administration on blood lipids," *Am J Clin Nutr* 1996; 64(6):866–870.

Hemorrhoids

1. Perez-Miranda, M. et al. "Effect of fiber supplements on internal bleeding hemorrhoids," *Hepatogastroenterology* 1996; 43(12):1504–1507.

2. Andersson, H. et al. "Colonic transit after fibre supplementation in patients with haemorrhoids," *Hum Nutr Appl Nutr* 1985; 39(2):101–107.

3. Misra, M.C. and R. Parshad. "Randomized clinical trial of micronized flavonoids in the early control of bleeding from acute internal hemorrhoids," *Br J Surg* 2000; 87(7):868–872.

4. Ho, Y.H. et al. "Micronized purified flavonidic fraction compared favorably with rubber band ligation and fibre alone in the management of bleeding hemorrhoids," *Dis Colon Rectum* 2000; 43(1):66–69.

5. Ho, Y.H. et al. "Prospective randomized controlled trial of a micronized flavonidic fraction in reduced bleeding after haemorrhoidectomy," *Br J Surg* 1995; 82(8):1034–1035.

6. Godeberge, P. "Daflon 500 mg in the treatment of hemorrhoidal disease: a demonstrated efficacy in comparison with placebo," *Angiology* 1994; 45(6 Pt 2):574–578.

7. Cospite, M. "Double-blind, placebo-controlled evaluation of clinical activity and safety of Daflon 500 mg in the treatment of acute hemorrhoids," *Angiology* 1994; 45(6 Pt 2):566–573.

8. Thanapongsathorn, W. and T. Vajrabukka. "Clinical trial of oral diosmin (Daflon) in the treatment of hemorrhoids," *Dis Colon Rectum* 1992; 35(11):1085–1088.

9. Wijayanegara, H. et al. "A clinical trial of hydroxyethylrutosides in the treatment of haemorrhoids of pregnancy," *J Int Med Res* 1992; 20(1):54–60.

10. Tixier, J.M. et al. "Evidence by in vivo and in vitro studies that binding of pycnogenols to elastin affects its rate of degradation by elastases," *Biochem Pharmacol* 1984; 33:3933–3939.

11. Kuttan, R. et al. "Collagen treated with catechin becomes resistant to the action of mammalian collagenase," *Experientia* 1981; 37:221–223.

12. Masquelier, J. et al. "Stabilization of collagen by procyanidolic oligomers," *Acta Therap* 1981; 7:101–105.

13. Arcangeli, P. Pycnogenol® in chronic venous insufficiency," *Fitoterapia* 2000; 71(3):236–244.

14. Delacroix, P. et al. "Double-blind study of endotelon in chronic venous insufficiency," *La Revue de Medecine* 1981; 31:1793–1802.

Hepatitis

1. *Hepatitis B.* Canadian Liver Foundation. Available at **www.liver.ca/english/liverdisease/ hepatitis_b.html**.

2. Ibid.

3. *Chronic Hepatitis C: Current Disease Management.* National Digestive Disorders Information Clearinghouse, November 2000. Available at **www.niddk.nih.gov/health/digest/pubs/chrnhepc/ chrnhedc/htm**.

4. Imai, K. and K. Nakachi. "Cross sectional study of effects of drinking green tea on cardiovascular and liver disease," *Br Med J* 1995; 310(6981):693–696.

5. Wada, S. et al. "Suppression of D-galactosamine-induced rat liver injury by glycosidic flavonoids-rich fraction from green tea," *Biosc Biotechnol Biochem* 1999; 63(3):570–572.

6. Beck, M.A. and O.A. Levander. "Dietary oxidative stress and the potentiation of viral infection," *Annu Rev Nutr* 1998; 18(8):93–116.

7. Yamamoto, Y. et al. "Oxidative stress in patients with hepatitis, cirrhosis, and hepoma evaluated by plasma antioxidants," *Biochem Biophys Res Commun* 1998; 247(1):116–170.

8. Yu, S.Y. et al. "Protective role of selenium against hepatitis B virus and primary liver cancer," *Biol Trace Elem Res* 1997; 56(1):117–124.

9. Look, M.P. et al. "Interferon/antioxidant combination therapy from chronic hepatitis C—a controlled pilot trial," *Antiviral Res* 1999; 43(2):113–122.

10. Berkson, B.M. "A conservative triple antioxidant approach to the treatment of hepatitis C. Combination of alpha lipoic acid (thioctic acid), silymarin, and selenium: three case histories," *Med Klin* 1999; 94(22)(Suppl 3):S84–S89.

11. Buzzelli, G. et al. "A pilot study on the liver protective effect of silybin-phosphatidylcholine complex (IdB1016) in chronic active hepatitis," *Int J Clin Pharmacol Ther Toxicol* 1993; 31(9):456–460.

12. Barbieri, B. et al. "Coenzyme Q10 administration increases antibody titer in hepatitis B vaccinated volunteers—a single blind placebo-controlled and randomized clinical study," *Biofactors* 1999; 9(2–4):351–357.

13. Yamamoto, Y. et al. "Plasma ratio ubiquinol and ubiquinone as a marker of oxidative stress," *Mol Aspects Med* 1997; 18(6)(Suppl):S79–S84.

14. Bonkovsky, H.L. "Therapy for hepatitis C: other options," *Hepatology* 1997; 26(3)(Suppl 1): S143–S151.

15. Niederau, C. et al. "Polyunsaturated phosphatidyl-choline and interferon alpha for treatment of chronic hepatitis B and C: a multi-center, randomized, double-blind, placebo-controlled trial," *Hepatogastroenterology* 1998; 45(21):797–804.

Herpes (Cold Sores and Genital Herpes)

1. Mostad, S.B. et al. "Cervical shedding of herpes simplex virus in human immunodeficiency virus-infected women: effects of hormonal contraception, pregnancy, and vitamin A deficiency," *J Infect Dis* 2000; 181(1):58–63.

2. Terezhalmy, G.T. et al. "The use of water-soluble bioflavonoid-ascorbic acid complex in the treatment of recurrent herpes labialis," *Oral Surg Oral Med Oral Pathol* 1978; 45:56–62.

3. Syed, T.A. et al. "Management of genital herpes in men with 0.5% Aloe vera extract in a hydrophilic cream: a placebo-controlled, double-blind study," *J Dermatol Treat* 1997; 8:99–102.

4. Koytchev, R. et al. "Balm mint extract (Lo-701) for topical treatment of recurring herpes labialis," *Phytomedicine* 1999; 6(4):225–230.

5. Wobling, R. and L. Leonhardt. "Local therapy of herpes simplex virus with dried extract from *Melissa officinalis*," *Phytomedicine* 1994; 1(1):25–31.

6. Dimitrova, Z. et al. "Antiherpes effect of *Melissa officinalis* L. extracts," *Acta Microbiol Bulg* 1993; 29:65–72.

7. Williams, M. "Immuno-protection against herpes simplex type II infection by eleutherococcus root extract," *Int J Alt Complement Med* 1995; 13:9–12.

8. McCune, M.A. et al. "Treatment of recurrent herpes simplex infections with L-lysine monohydrochloride," *Cutis* 1984; 34(4):366–373.

9. Griffith, R.S. et al. "Success of L-lysine therapy in frequently recurrent simplex infection. Treatment and prophylaxis," *Dermatologica* 1987; 175(4):183–190.

10. Walsh, D.E. et al. "Subjective response to lysine in therapy of herpes simplex," *J Antimicrob Chemother* 1983; 12(5):489–496.

Hiatal Hernia (Gastroesophageal Reflux Disease)

1. Engle, June, ed. "Some Specific Diseases and Disorders" in *The Complete Canadian Health Guide* (Toronto: Key Porter Books, 1993):476.

2. Wilson, L.J. et al. "Association of obesity with hiatal hernia and esophagitis," *Am J Gastroenterol* 1999; 94(10):2840–2844.

3. Ruhl, C.E. and J.E. Everhart. "Overweight, but not high dietary fat intake, increases risk of gastroesophageal reflux disease hospitalization: the NHANES I Epidemiologic Followup Study. First National Health and Nutrition Examination Survey," *Ann Epidemiol* 1999; 9(7):424–435.

4. Stene-Larsen, G. et al. "Relationship of overweight to hiatus hernia and reflux oesophagitis," *Scand J Gastroenterol* 1988; 23(4):427–432.

5. Ruhl, C.E. and J.E. Everhart. "Relationship of iron-deficiency anemia with esophagitis and hiatal hernia: hospital findings from a prospective, population-based study," *Am J Gastroenerol* 2001; 96(2):322–326.

6. Moskovitz, M. et al. "Large hiatal hernias, anemias, and linear gastric erosion: studies of etiology and medical therapy," *Am J Gastroenterol* 1992; 87(5):622–626.

High Blood Pressure (Hypertension)

1. *Facts about Heart Disease and Women: Preventing and Controlling High Blood Pressure.* The National Heart, Lung, and Blood Institute (NHLBI), August 1996. Available at **www.nhlbi.nih.gov/health/public/heart/hbp/hdwmnhbp.htm**.

2. *What is High Blood Pressure?* Mayo Foundation for Medical Education and Research, September 2000. Available at **www.mayoclinic.com/home?id=DS00100**.

3. Mertens, I.L. and L.F. Van Gaal. "Overweight, obesity and blood pressure: the effects of modest weight reduction," *Obes Res* 2000; 8(3):270–278.

4. Ascherio, A. et al. "Prospective study of nutritional factors, blood pressure and hypertension among US women," *Hypertension* 1996; 27(5):1065–1072.

5. Yamori, Y. et al. "Nutritional factors for stroke and major cardiovascular diseases: international epidemiological comparison on dietary prevention," *Health Rep* 1004; 6(1):22–27.

6. Mulrow, C.D. et al. "Dieting to reduce body weight for controlling hypertension in adults," *Cochrane Database Syst Rev* 2000; 23(2):CD000484.

7. Little, P. et al. "A controlled trial of a low sodium, low fat, high fibre diet in treated hypertensive patients: effect of antihypertensive drug requirement in clinical practice," *J Hum Hypertens* 1991; 5(3):175–181.

8. Appel, L.J. et al. "A clinical trial of the effects of dietary patterns on blood pressure," *N Engl J Med* 1997; 65(Suppl):S643–S651.

9. Conlin, P.R. et al. "The effect of dietary patterns on blood pressure control in hypertensive patients: results from the Dietary Approaches to Stop Hypertension (DASH) trial," *Am J Hypertens* 2000; 13(9):949–955.

10. Resnick, L.M. et al. "Factors affecting blood pressure responses to diet: the Vanguard study," *Am J Hypertens* 2000; 13(9):956–965.

11. Mori, T.A. et al. "Dietary fish as a major component of a weight-loss diet: effect on serum lipids, glucose, and insulin metabolism in overweight hypertensive subjects," *Am J Clin Nutr* 1999; 70(5):817–825.

12. Bao, D.Q. et al. "Effects of dietary fish and weight reduction on ambulatory blood pressure in overweight hypertensives," *Hypertension* 1998; 32(4):710–717.

13. Pauletto, P. et al. "Blood pressure and atherogenic lipoprotein profiles of fish-diet and vegetarian villagers in Tanzania: the Lugalawa study," *Lancet* 1996; 348(9030):784–788.

14. Nakanishi, N. et al. "Association of alcohol consumption with increase in aortic stiffness: a 9-year longitudinal study in middle-aged Japanese men," *Ind Health* 2001; 39(1):24-28.

15. Nanchahal, K. et al. "Alcohol consumption, metabolic cardiovascular risk factors and hypertension in women," *Int J Epidemiol* 2000; 29(1):57–64.

16. Tsuruta, M. et al. "Association between alcohol intake and development of hypertension in Japanese normotensive men: 12-year follow-up study," *Am J Hypertens* 2000; 13(5 Pt 1):482–487.

17. Sung, B.H. et al. "Caffeine elevates blood pressure response to exercise in mild hypertensive men," *Am J Hypertens* 1995; 8(12 Pt 1):1184–1188.

18. Lovallo, W.R. et al. "Caffeine and behavioural stress effects on blood pressure in borderline hypertensive Caucasian men," *Health Psychol* 1996; 15(1):11–17.

19. Rakic, V. et al. "Effects of coffee on ambulatory blood pressure in older men and women: A randomized controlled trial," *Hypertension* 1999; 33(3):869–873.

20. Rachima-Maoz, C. et al. "The effect of caffeine on ambulatory blood pressure in hypertensive patients," *Am J Hypertens* 1998; 11(12):1426–1432.

21. Carr, A. and B. Frei. "The role of natural antioxidants in preserving the biological activity of endothelium-derived nitric oxide," *Free Radic Biol Med* 2000; 28(12):1806–1814.

22. Frei, B. "On the role of vitamin C and other antioxidants in atherogenesis and vascular dysfunction," *Proc Soc Exp Biol Med* 1999; 222(3):196–204.

23. Galley, H.F. et al. "Combination oral antioxidant supplementation reduces blood pressure," *Clin Sci (Colch)* 1997; 92(4):361–365.

24. Jeserich, M. et al. "Vitamin C improves endothelial function or epicardial coronary arteries in patients with hypercholesterolemia or essential hypertension—assessed by cold pressor testing," *Eur Heart J* 1999; 20(22):1676–1680.

25. Duffy, S.J. et al. "Treatment of hypertension with ascorbic acid," *Lancet* 1999; 354(9195):2048–2049.

26. Bates, C.J. et al. "Does vitamin C lower blood pressure? Results of a large study of people aged 65 or older," *J Hypertens* 1998; 16(7):925–932.

27. Allender, P.S. et al. "Dietary calcium and blood pressure: A meta-analysis of randomized clinical trials," *Ann Intern Med* 1996; 124:825–831.

28. Bucher, H.C. et al. "Effects of dietary calcium supplementation on blood pressure: A meta-analysis of randomized controlled trials," *J Am Med Assoc* 1996; 275:1016–1022.

29. Burgess, E. et al. "Lifestyle modifications to prevent and control hypertension. 6. Recommendations on potassium, magnesium and calcium. Canadian Hypertension Society, Canadian Coalition for High Blood Pressure Prevention and Control, Laboratory

Centre for Disease Control at Health Canada, Heart and Stroke Foundation of Canada," *CMAJ* 1999; 160(Suppl 9):S35–S45.

30. Ma, J. et al. "Associations of serum and dietary magnesium with cardiovascular disease, hypertension, diabetes, insulin, and carotoid arterial wall thickness: the AIRC study," *J Clin Epidemiol* 1995; 48(7):927–940.

31. Laurant P. and R.M. Touyz. "Physiological and pathophysiological role of magnesium in the cardiovascular system: implications in hypertension," *J Hypertens* 2000; 18(9):1177–1191.

32. Sacks, F.M. et al. "Combinations of potassium, calcium and magnesium supplements in hypertension," *Hypertension* 1995; 26(6 Pt 1):950–956.

33. Krishna, G.G. "Role of potassium in the pathogenesis of hypertension," *Am J Med Sci* 1994; 307(2)(Suppl 1):S21–S25.

34. Whelton, P.K. et al. "Effects of oral potassium on blood pressure. Meta-analysis of randomized controlled clinical trials," *JAMA* 1997; 277(20):1624–1632.

35. Barri, Y. and C.S. Wingo. "The effects of potassium depletion and supplementation on blood pressure: a review," *Am J Med Sci* 1997; 314(1):37–40.

36. Preuss, H.G. "Diet, genetics and hypertension," *J Am Coll Nutr* 1997; 16(4):296–305.

37. Sacks, F.M. et al. "Effects on blood pressure of reduced dietary sodium and the Dietary Approaches to Stop Hypertension (DASH) diet. DASH-Sodium Collaborative Group," *N Eng J Med* 2001; 344(1):3–10.

38. Silagy, C.A. and H.A. Neil. "A meta-analysis of the effect of garlic on high blood pressure," *J Hypertens* 1994; 12(4):463–468.

39. McMahon, F.G. and R. Vargas. "Can garlic lower blood pressure? A pilot study," *Pharmacotherapy* 1993; 13(4):406–407.

40. Steiner, M. et al. "A double-blind crossover study in moderately hypercholesterolemic men that compared the effect of aged garlic extract and placebo administration on blood lipids," *Am J Clin Nutr* 1996; 64(6):866–870.

41. McCarty, M.F. "Coenzyme Q versus hypertension: does CoQ decrease endothelial superoxide generation?" *Med Hypotheses* 1999; 53(4):300–304.

42. Digiesi, M. et al. "Coenzyme Q10 in essential hypertension," *Mol Aspects Med* 1994; 15(Suppl): S257–S263.

43. Toft, I. et al. "Effects of n-3 polyunsaturated fatty acids on glucose homeostasis and blood pressure in essential hypertension. A randomized, controlled trial," *Ann Intern Med* 1995; 123(12):911–918.

44. Prisco, D. et al. "Effect of medium-term supplementation with a moderate dose on n-3 polyunsaturated fatty acids on blood pressure in milk hypertensive patients," *Thromb Res* 1998; 91(3):105–112.

45. Yosevy, C. et al. "Repeated fasting and refeeding with 20:5, n-3 eicosapentanoic acid (EPA): a novel approach for rapid fatty acid exchange and its effect on blood pressure," *J Hum Hypertens* 1996; 10(2)(Suppl 3):S135–S139.

46. Salvig, J.D. et al. "Effects of fish oil supplementation in late pregnancy on blood pressure: a randomized controlled trial," *Br J Obstet Gynaecol* 1996; 103(6):529–533.

47. Onwude, J.L. et al. "A randomised double blind placebo controlled trial of fish oil in high risk pregnancy," *Br J Obstet Gynaecol* 1995; 102(2):95–100.

Hyperthyroidism (Graves' Disease)

1. *A Major Women's Health Issue.* American Autoimmune Related Diseases Association, Inc. 2001. Available at **www.aarda.org/women_health_art.html**.

2. *What is Hyperthyroidism?* The Thyroid Society, 1996. Available at **www.the-thyroid-society.org/faq**.

3. *Graves' Hyperthyroidism.* The Thyroid Foundation of Canada, 2000. Available at **www.thyroid.ca/Guides/HG06.html**.

4. Yoshiuchi, K. et al. "Stressful life events and smoking were associated with Graves' disease in women, but not in men," *Psychosom Med* 1998; 60(2):182–185.

5. Jansson, S. et al. "Overweight—a common problem among women treated for hyperthyroidism," *Postgrad Med* 1993; 69(808):107–111.

6. Abid, M. et al. "Thyroid function and energy intake during weight gain following treatment of hyperthyroidism," *J Am Coll Nutr* 1999; 18(2):189–193.

7. Bianchi, G. et al. "Oxidative stress and anti-oxidant metabolites in patients with hyperthyroidism: effect of treatment," *Horm Metab Res* 1999; 31(11):620–624.

8. Costantini, F. et al. "Effect of thyroid function on LDL oxidation," *Arterioscler Thromb Vasc Biol* 1998; 18(5):732–737.

9. Goswami, U.C. and S. Choudhury. "The status of retinoids in women suffering from hyper- and hypothyroidism: interrelationship between vitamin A, beta-carotene and thyroid hormones," *Int J Vitam Nutr Res* 1999; 69(2):132–135.

10. Mano, T. et al. "Vitamin E and coenzyme Q10 concentrations in the thyroid of patients with various thyroid disorders," *Am J Med Sci* 1998; 315(4):230–232.

11. Seven, A. et al. "Biochemical evaluation of oxidative stress in propylthiouricil treated hyperthyroid patients. Effect of vitamin C supplementation," *Clin Chem Lab Met* 1998; 36(10):767–770.

12. Uzzan, B. et al. "Effects on bone mass of long term treatment with thyroid hormones: a meta-analysis," *J Clin Endocrinol Metab* 1996; 81(12):4278–4289.

13. Yamashita, H. et al. "Seasonal changes in calcium homeostasis affect the incidence of postoperative tetany in patients with Graves' disease," *Surgery* 2000; 127(4):377–382.

14. Solomon, B.L. et al. "Remission rates with antithyroid drug therapy: continuing influence of iodine intake?" *Ann Intern Med* 1987; 107(4):510–512.

Hypoglycemia

1. *Hypoglycemia.* Discovery Health, April 2001. Available at **www.health.discovery.com/ diseasesandcond/encyclopedia1568.html**.

2. Kerr, D. et al. "Effect of caffeine on the recognition of and response to hypoglycemia in humans," *Ann Intern Med* 1993; 119(8):799–804.

3. Anderson, R.A. et al. "Effects of supplemental chromium on patients with symptoms of reactive hypoglycemia," *Metabolism* 1987; 36(4):351–355.

4. Clausen, J. "Chromium induced clinical improvement in symptomatic hypoglycemia," *Biol Trace Elem Res* 1988; 17:229–236.

Hypothyroidism

1. *Hypothyroidism.* The Thyroid Foundation of Canada, 2000. Available at **www.thyroid.ca/Guides/HG03.html**.

2. Faughnan, M. et al. "Screening for thyroid disease at the menopausal clinic," *Clin Invest Med* 1995; 18(1):11–18.

3. Pucci, E. et al. "Thyroid and lipid metabolism," *Int J Obes Relat Metab Disord* 2000; (Suppl2):S109–S112.

4. Vierhapper, H. et al. "Low-density lipoprotein cholesterol in subclinical hypothyroidism," *Thyroid* 2000; 10(11):981–984.

5. Hak, A.E. et al. "Subclinical hypothyroidism is an independent risk factor for atherosclerosis and myocardial infarction in elderly women: the Rotterdam Study," *Ann Intern Med* 2000; 132(4):270–278.

6. Bindels, A.J. et al. "The prevalence of subclinical hypothyroidism at different total plasma cholesterol levels in middle aged men and women: a need for case-finding?" *Clin Endocrinol* 1999; 50(2):217–220.

7. Becerra, A. et al. "Lipoprotein(a) and other lipoproteins in hypothyroid patients before and after thyroid replacement therapy," *Clin Nutr* 1999; 18(5):319–322.

8. Diekman, T. et al. "Increased oxidizability of low-density lipoproteins in hypothyroidism," *J Clin Endocrinol Metab* 1998; 83(5):1752–1755.

9. Costantini, F. et al. "The effect of thyroid function on LDL oxidation," *Arteriosclero Thromb Vasc Biol* 1998; 18(5):732–737.

10. Nedrebo, B.G. et al. "Plasma total homocysteine levels in hyperthyroid and hypothyroid patients," *Metabolism* 1998; 47(1):89–93.

11. Tajiri, J. et al. "Studies of hypothyroidism in patients with high iodine intake," *J Clin Endocrinol Metab* 1986; 63(2):412–417.

12. Olivieri, O. et al. "Low selenium status in the elderly influences thyroid hormones," *Clin Sci (Colch)* 1995; 89(6):637–642.

13. Shakir, K.M. et al. "Ferrous sulfate-induced increase in requirement for thyroxine in a patient with primary hypothyroidism," *South Med J* 1997; 90(6):637–639.

14. Campbell, N.R. et al. "Ferrous sulfate reduces thyroxine efficacy in patients with hypothyroidism," *Ann Intern Med* 1992; 117(12):1010–1013.

Impotence (Erectile Dysfunction)

1. *Impotence.* National Kidney and Urologic Diseases Information Clearinghouse, September 1995. Available at **www.health/urology/pubs/impotence/ impotence.htm**.

2. *Erectile Dysfunction.* Mayo Foundation for Medical Education and Research, October 16, 2000. Available at **www.mayoclinic.com/home?id= DS00162**.

3. Sexual Function Health Council of the American Foundation for Urologic Disease Inc. Available at **www.impotence.org/confront/index.asp**.

4. *What should I know about impotence?* Canadian Health Network, May 1999. Available at **www.canadian-health-network.ca/faq-faq/men-hommes/9e.html**.

5. *Impotence.* National Kidney and Urologic Diseases Information Clearinghouse, September 1995. Available at **www.health/urology/pubs/impotence/impotence.htm**.

6. Feldman, H.A. et al. "Erectile dysfunction and coronary risk factors: prospective results from the Massachusetts Male Aging Study," *Prev Med* 2000;30(4):328–338.

7. Derby, C.A. et al. "Modifiable risk factors and erectile dysfunction: can lifestyle changes modify risk?" *Urology* 2000; 56(2):302–306.

8. Feldman, H.A. et al. "Erectile dysfunction and coronary risk factors: prospective results from the Massachusetts Male Aging Study," *Prev Med* 2000:30(4):328–338.

9. Khedun, S.M. et al. "Zinc, hydrochlorothiazide and sexual dysfunction," *Cent Afr J Med* 1995; 41(10):312–315.

10. Sikora, R. et al. "Ginkgo biloba extract in the therapy of erectile dysfunction," *J Urol* 1989; 142:188A.

11. Cohen, A.J. and B. Bartlik. "Ginkgo biloba for antidepressant-induced sexual dysfunction," *J Sex Marital Ther* 1998; 24(2):139–143.

12. Choi, H.K, D.H. Seong and K.H. Rha. "Clinical efficacy of Korean red ginseng for erectile dysfunction," *Int J Impot Res* 1995; 7(3):181–186.

13. Personal communication with Dr. David Saul, April 2001.

14. Reiter, W.J. et al. "Serum dehydroepiandrosterone sulfate concentrations in men with erectile dysfunction," *Urology* 2000; 55(5):755–758.

15. Reiter, W.J. et al. "Dehydroepiandrosterone in the treatment of erectile dysfunction: a prospective, double blind, randomized, placebo-controlled study," *Urology* 1999; 53:590–595.

16. Chen, J. et al. "Effect of oral administration of high-dose nitric oxide donor L-arginine in men with organic erectile dysfunction: results of a double blind, randomized placebo-controlled study," *BJU Int* 1999; 83:269–273.

Infertility

1. Stoppard, Miriam, M.D., and Catherine Younger-Lewis M.D., eds. " Infertility" in *Woman's Body* (Westmount, PQ: The Reader's Digest Association (Canada) Ltd., 1995):162.

2. Gulden, K.D. "Pernicious anemia, vitiligo and infertility," *J Am Board Fam Pract* 1990; 3(3):217–220.

3. Sanfilippo, J.S. and Y.K. Liu. "Vitamin B12 deficiency and infertility: a case report," *Int J Fertil* 1991; 36(1):36–38.

4. Gerhard, I. et al. "Mastodynon® bei weiblicher Sterilitat," *Forsch Komplemetarmed* 1998; 5:272–278. [German; English Abstract]

5. Geva, E. at al. "The effect of antioxidant treatment on human spermatozoa and fertilization rate in an in vitro fertilization program," *Fertil Steril* 1996; 66(3):430–434.

6. Suleiman, S.A. et al. "Lipid peroxidation and human sperm motility: protective role of vitamin E," *J Androl* 1996; 17(5):530–537.

7. Hansen, J.C. and Y. Deguchi. "Selenium and fertility in animals and man—a review," *Acta Vet Scand* 1996; 37(1):19–30.

8. Scott, R. et al. "The effect of oral selenium supplementation on human sperm motility," *Br J Urol* 1998; 82(1):76–80.

9. Kumamoto, Y. et al. "Clinical efficacy of mecobalamin in treatment of oligozoospermia: results of a double-blind comparative clinical study," *Acta Urol Jpn* 1998; 34:1109–1132.

10. Netter, A. et al. "Effect of zinc administration on plasma testosterone, dihydrotestosterone, and sperm count," *Arch Androl* 1981; 7:69–73.

11. Matalliotakis, I. et al. "L-carnitine levels in the seminal fluid of fertile and infertile men: correlation with sperm quality," *Int J Fertil Womens Med* 2000; 45(3):236–240.

12. Vitali, G. et al. "Carnitine supplementation in human idiopathic asthenospermia: clinical results," *Drugs Exp Clin Res* 1995; 21(4):157–159.

Inflammatory Bowel Disease: Ulcerative Colitis and Crohn's Disease

1. *Ulcerative colitis.* Altmed.com, 2000. Available at **www.altmed.com/conditions/conditions.cfm?ID=624**.

2. Mishkin, B. et al. "Increased prevalence of lactose malabsorption in Crohn's disease patients at low risk for lactose malabsorption based on ethnic origin," *Am J Gastroenterol* 1997; 92(7):1148–1153.

3. Mishkin, S. "Dairy sensitivity, lactose malabsorption, and elimination diets in inflammatory bowel disease," *Am J Clin Nutr* 1997; 65(2):564–567.

4. Bernstein, C.N. et al. "Milk intolerance in adults with ulcerative colitis," *Am J Gastroenterol* 1994; 89(6):872–877.

5. Joachim, G. "The relationship between habits of food consumption and reported reactions to food in people with inflammatory bowel disease—testing the limits," *Nutr Health* 1999; 13(2):69–83.

6. Ejderhamn, J. et al. "Long-term double-blind study on the influence of dietary fibres on faecal bile acid excretion in juvenile ulcerative colitis," *Scand J Clin Lab Invest* 1992; 52(7):697–706.

7. Pearson, M. et al. "Food intolerance and Crohn's disease," *Gut* 1993; 34(6):783–787.

8. Miura, S. et al. "Modulation of intestinal immune system by dietary fat intake: relevance to Crohn's disease," *J Gastroenterol Hepatol* 1998; 13(12):1183–1190.

9. Buffinton, G.D. and W.F. Doe. "Depleted mucosal antioxidant defences in inflammatory bowel disease," *Free Radical Biol Med* 1995; 19(6):911–918.

10. Lih-Brody, L. et al. "Increased oxidative stress and decreased antioxidant defenses in mucosa of inflammatory bowel disease," *Dig Dis Sci* 1996; 41(10):2078–2086.

11. Reimund, J.M. et al. "Antioxidant and immune status in active Crohn's disease. A possible relationship," *Clin Nutr* 2000; 19(1):43–48.

12. Hoffenberg, E.J. et al. "Circulating antioxidant concentrations in children with inflammatory bowel disease," *Am J Clin Nutr* 1997; 65(5):1482–1488.

13. Rumi, G. et al. "Decrease of serum carotenoids in Crohn's disease," *J Physiol Paris* 2000; 94(2):159–161.

14. Sturniolo, G.C. et al. "Altered plasma and mucosal concentrations of trace elements and antioxidants in active ulcerative colitis," *Scand J Gastroenterol* 1998; 33(6):644–649.

15. Rannem, T. et al. "Selenium status in patients with Crohn's disease," *Am J Clin Nutr* 1992; 56(5):933–937.

16. Cravo, M.L. et al. "Microsatellite instability in non-neoplastic mucosa of patients with ulcerative colitis," *Am J Gastroenterol* 1998; 93(11):2060–2064.

17. *Ulcerative Colitis.* National Disease Information Clearinghouse, April 2000. Available at **www.niddk.nih.gov/health/digest/pubs/colitis/colitis.htm**.

18. Lashner, B.A. et al. "The effect of folic acid supplementation on the risk for cancer or dysplasia in ulcerative colitis," *Gastroenterology* 1997; 112(1):29–32.

19. Lashner, B.A. "Red blood cell folate is associated with the development of dysplasia and cancer in ulcerative colitis," *J Cancer Res Clin Oncol* 1993; 119(9):549–554.

20. Behrend, C. et al. "Vitamin B12 absorption after ileorectal anastomosis for Crohn's disease: effect of ileal resection and time span after surgery," *Eur J Gastroenterol Hepatol* 1995; 7(5):397–400.

21. Delpre, G. et al. "Sublingual therapy for cobalamin deficiency as an alternative to oral and parenteral cobalamin supplementation," *Lancet* 1999; 354(9180):740–741.

22. Buchman, A.L. "Bones and Crohn's: problems and solutions," *Inflamm Bowel Dis* 1999; 5(3):212–227.

23. Silvennoinen, J. et al. "Dietary calcium intake and its relation to bone mineral density in patients with inflammatory bowel disease," *J Intern Med* 1996; 240(5):285–292.

24. Pigot, F. et al. "Low bone mineral density in patients with inflammatory bowel disease," *Dig Dis Sci* 1992; 37(9):1396–1403.

25. Bernstein, C.N. et al. "A randomized, placebo-controlled trial of calcium supplementation for decreased bone density in corticosteroid-using patients with inflammatory bowel disease: a pilot study," *Ailment Pharmacol Ther* 1996; 10(5):777–786.

26. Greenfield, S.M. et al. "A randomized controlled study of evening primrose oil and fish oil in ulcerative colitis," *Ailment Pharmacol Ther* 1993; 7(2):159–166.

27. Kim, Y.I. "Can fish oil maintain Crohn's disease in remission?" *Nutr Rev* 1996; 54(8):248–252.

28. Loeschke, K. et al. "n-3 fatty acids only delay early relapse of ulcerative colitis in remission," *Dig Dis Sci* 1996; 41(10):1087–1094.

29. Hawthorne, A.B. et al. "Treatment of ulcerative colitis with fish oil supplementation: a prospective 12

month randomized controlled trial," *Gut* 1992; 33(7):922–928.

30. Schultz, M. and R.B. Sartor. "Probiotics and inflammatory bowel disease," *Am J Gastroenterol* 2000; 95(Suppl 1):S19–S21.

31. Shanahan, F. "Probiotics and inflammatory bowel disease: is there a scientific rationale?" *Inflamm Bowel Dis* 2000; 6(2):107–115.

32. Rembacken, B.J. et al. "Non-pathogenic Esherichia coli versus mesalazine for the treatment of ulcerative colitis: a randomized trial," *Lancet* 1999; 354(9179):635–639.

33. Venturi, A. et al. "Impact on the composition of the faecal flora by a new probiotic preparation: preliminary data on the maintenance treatment of patients with ulcerative colitis," *Ailment Pharmacol Ther* 1999; 13(8):1103–1108.

34. Gionchetti, P. et al. "Oral bacteriotherapy as maintenance treatment in patients with chronic pouchitis: A double-blind, placebo-controlled trial," *Gastroenterology* 2000; 119:305–309.

Insomnia

1. "Sleep Disorders," *The Merck Manual of Geriatrics, 1995–2000*, Merck and Co. Ltd. Available at **www.merck.com/pubs/mm_geriatrics/sec6/ch47.htm**.

2. *Insomnia*. The College of Physicians and Surgeons of Ontario. Available at **www.cpso.on.ca/sleepmed/sleepmed_whois.htm#Insomnia**.

3. Curless, R. et al. "Is caffeine a factor in subjective insomnia of elderly people?" *Age Ageing* 1993; 22(10):41–45.

4. Bliwise, N.G. "Factors related to sleep quality in healthy elderly women," *Psychol Aging* 1992; 7(1):83–88.

5. Shirlow, M.J. and C.D. Mathers. "A study of caffeine consumption and symptoms: indigestion, palpitations, tremor, headache and insomnia," *Int J Epidemiol* 1985; 14(2):239–248.

6. Landolt, H.P. et al. "Caffeine intake (200 mg) in the morning affects human sleep and EEG power spectra at night," *Brain Research* 1995; 675(1–2):67–74.

7. Landolt, H.P. et al. "Caffeine reduces low-frequency delta activity in the human sleep EEG," *Neuropsychopharmacology* 1995; 12(3):229–238.

8. Dufour, M.C. et al. "Alcohol and the elderly," *Clin Geriatr Med* 1992; 8(1):127–141.

9. Okawa, M. et al. "Vitamin B12 treatment for sleep-wake rhythm disorders," *Sleep* 1990; 13(1):15–23.

10. Mayer, G. et al. "Effects of vitamin B12 on performance and circadian rhythm in normal subjects," *Neuropsychopharmacology* 1996; 15(5):456–464.

11. Lindahl, O. et al. "Double blind study of a valerian preparation," *Pharmacology Biochemistry and Behaviour* 1989; 32:1065–1066.

12. Leathwood, P.D. et al. "Aqueous extract of valerian root improves sleep quality in man," *Pharmacology Biochemistry and Behaviour* 1982; 17:65–71.

13. Leathwood, P.D. et al. "Aqueous extract of valerian root reduces latency to fall asleep in man," *Planta Medica* 1985; 51:144–148.

Interstitial Cystitis

1. Pelikan, Z. et al. "The role of allergy in interstitial cystitis," *Ned Tijdschr Geneeskd* 1999; 143(25):1289–1292. [Dutch]

2. Whitmore, K. et al. "Survey of the effect of Prelief® on food-related exacerbation of interstitial cystitis symptoms," Philadelphia, 1998–1999, unpublished. Available at **www.akpharma.com/Icrews/food_survey.htm**.

3. Whitmore, K. et al. "The Therapeutic Effects of Prelief® in Interstitial Cystitis," Philadelphia, January 2000, unpublished. Available at **www.akpharma.com/Icrews/food_survey.htm**.

4. Blumenthal, M. et al., eds. *The Complete German Commission E Monographs: Therapeutic Guide to Herbal Medicines*, Trans. by S. Klein (Boston: American Botanical Council, 1998).

5. Smith, S.D. et al. "Urinary nitric oxide synthase activity and cyclic GMP levels are decreased with interstitial cystitis and increased with urinary tract infections," *J Urol* 1996; 155(4):1432–1435.

6. Cartledge, J.J. et al. "A randomized double-blind placebo-controlled crossover trial of the efficacy of L-arginine in the treatment of interstitial cystitis," *BJU Int* 2000; 85(4):421–426.

7. Smith, S.D. et al. "Improvement in interstitial cystitis symptom scores during treatment with oral L-arginine," *J Urol* 1997; 158(3 Pt 1):703–708.

8. Korting, G.E. et al. "A randomized double-blind trial of oral L-arginine for treatment of interstitial cystitis," *J Urol* 1999; 161(2):558–565.

9. Wheeler, M.A. et al. "Effect of long term oral L-arginine on the nitric oxide synthase pathway in the

urine from patients with interstitial cystitis," *J Urol* 1997; 158(6):2045–2050.

Irritable Bowel Syndrome (IBS)

1. "Bowel Movement Disorders," *The Merck Manual Home Edition, 1995–2001.* Merck and Co. Ltd. Available at **www.merck.com/pubs/mmanual_home/sec9/107.htm**.

2. *Irritable Bowel Syndrome.* The American College of Gastroenterology. Available at **www.acg.gi.org/acg-dev/patientinfo/frame_giproblems.html**.

3. Niec, A.M. et al. "Are adverse food reactions linked to irritable bowel syndrome?" *Am J Gastroenterol* 1998; 93(11):2184–2190.

4. Stefanini, G.F. et al. "Oral cromolyn solution in comparison with elimination diet in the irritable bowel syndrome, diarrheic type. Multicenter study of 428 patients," *Scand J Gastroenterol* 1995; 30(6):535–541.

5. Bischoff, S.C. et al. "Prevalence of adverse reactions to food in patients with gastrointestinal disease," *Allergy* 1996; 51(11):811–818.

6. Lessof, M.H. "Food intolerance," *Scand J Gastroenterol Suppl* 1985; 109:117–121.

7. Freidman, G. "Diet and the irritable bowel syndrome," *Gastroenterol Clin North Am* 1991; 20(2):313–324.

8. Gremse, D.A. et al. "Irritable bowel syndrome and lactose maldigestion in recurrent abdominal pain in childhood," *South Med J* 1999; 92(8):778–781.

9. Bohmer, C.J. and H.A. Tuynman. "The clinical relevance of lactose malabsorption in irritable bowel syndrome," *Eur J Gastroenterol* 1996; 8(10):1013–1016.

10. Vernia, P. et al. "Lactose malabsorption and irritable bowel syndrome. Effect of a long-term lactose-free diet," *Ital J Gastroenterol* 1995; 27(3):117–121.

11. Halpern, G.M. et al. "Treatment of irritable bowel syndrome with Lacteol-Fort: a randomized double-blind, cross-over trial," *Am J Gastroenterol* 1996; 91(8):1579–1585.

12. Goldstein, R. et al. "Carbohydrate malabsorption and the effect of dietary restriction on symptoms of irritable bowel syndrome and functional bowel complaints," *Isr Med Assoc J* 2000; 2(8):583–587.

13. Evans, P.R. et al. "Fructose-sorbitol malabsorption and symptom provocation in irritable bowel syndrome," *Scand J Gastroenterol* 1998; 33(11):1158–1163.

14. Symons, P. et al. "Symptom provocation in irritable bowel syndrome: Effects of differing doses of fructose-sorbitol," *Scand J Gastroenterol* 1992; 27(11):940–944.

15. Fernandez-Banares, F. et al. "Sugar malabsorption in functional bowel disease: clinical implications," *Am J Gastroenterol* 1993; 88(12):2044–2050.

16. Symons, P. et al. "Symptom provocation in irritable bowel syndrome. Effects of differing doses of fructose-sorbitol," *Scand J Gastroenterol* 1992; 27(11):940–944.

17. Nelis, G.F. et al. "Role of fructose-sorbitol malabsorption in the irritable bowel syndrome," *Gastroenterology* 1990; 99(4):1016–1020.

18. Lambert, J.P. et al. "The value of prescribed 'high fibre' diets for the treatment of irritable bowel syndrome," *Eur J Clin Nutr* 1991; 45(12):601–609.

19. Kruis, W. et al. "Comparisons of the therapeutic effect of wheat bran, mebervine and placebo in patients with the irritable bowel syndrome," *Digestion* 1986; 34(3):196–201.

20. Arffmann, S. et al. "The effect of wheat bran in the irritable bowel syndrome. A double-blind crossover study," *Scand J Gastroenterol* 1985; 20(3):295–298.

21. Francis, C.Y. and P.J. Whorwell. "Bran and irritable bowel syndrome: time for reappraisal," *Lancet* 1994; 344(8914):39–40.

22. Pittler, M.H. and E. Ernst. "Peppermint oil for irritable bowel syndrome: a critical review and metaanalysis," *Am J Gastroenterol* 1998; 93(7):1131–1135.

23. Lui, J.H. et al. "Enteric-coated peppermint-oil capsules in the treatment of irritable bowel syndrome: a prospective, randomized trial," *J Gastroenterol* 1997; 32(6):765–768.

24. Tarpila, S. et al. "Ground flaxseed is an effective hypolipodemic bulk laxative," *Gastroenterology* 1997; 112:A836. [Abstract]

25. Nobaek, S. et al. "Alternation of intestinal microflora is associated with reduction in abdominal bloating and pain in patients with irritable bowel syndrome," *Am J Gastroenterol* 2000; 95(5):1231–1238.

Kidney Stones

1. *Kidney Stones.* The Kidney Foundation of Canada. Available at **www.kidney.ca/stone-e.htm**.

2. *Kidney Stones.* Digital Urology Journal. Available at **www.duj.com/kidneystones.html**.

3. *Kidney Stones*. The Kidney Foundation of Canada. Available at **www.kidney.ca/stone-e.htm**.

4. Bellizi, V. et al. "Effects of water hardness on urinary risk factors for kidney stones in patients with idiopathic nephrolithiasis," *Nephron* 1999; 81(Suppl 1):S66–S70.

5. Caudarella, R. et al. "Comparative study of the influence of 3 types of mineral water in patients with idiopathic calcium lithiasis," *J Urol* 1998; 159(3):658–663.

6. Curhan, G.C. et al. "Beverage use and risk for kidney stones in women," *Ann Intern Med* 1998; 128(7):534–540.

7. Hirvonen, T. et al. "Nutrient intake and use of beverages and the risk of kidney stones among male smokers," *Am J Epidemiol* 1999; 150(2):187–194.

8. Curhan, C.G. et al. "Prospective study of beverage use and the risk of kidney stones," *Am J Epidemiol* 1996; 143(3):240–247.

9. Seltzer, M.A. et al. "Dietary manipulation with lemonade to treat hypocitraturic calcium nephrolithiasis," *J Urol* 1996; 156(3):907–909.

10. Laminski, N.A. et al. "Hyperoxaluria in patients with recurrent calcium oxalate calculi: dietary and other risk factors," *Br J Urol* 1991; 68(5):454–458.

11. Massey, L.K. et al. "Effect of dietary oxalate and calcium on urinary oxalate and the risk of formation of calcium oxalate kidney stones," *J Am Diet Assoc* 1993; 93(8):901–906.

12. The American Dietetic Association. *Manual of Clinical Dietetics*, 6th ed. (Chicago, 2000).

13. Martini, L.A. and R.J. Wood. "Should dietary calcium and protein be restricted in patients with nephrolithiasis?" *Nutr Rev* 2000; 58(4):111–117.

14. Curhan, C.G. et al. "Family history and the risk of kidney stones," *J Am Soc Nephrol* 1997; 8(10):1568–1573.

15. Hess, B. "Low calcium diet in hypercalciuric nephrolithiasis: first do no harm," *Scanning Microsc* 1996; 10(2):554–556.

16. Curhan, G.C. "Dietary calcium, dietary protein, and kidney stone formation," *Miner Electrolyte Metab* 1997; 23(3–6):261–264.

17. Curhan, G.C. et al. "Comparison of dietary calcium with supplemental calcium and other nutrients as factors affecting risk for kidney stones in women," *Ann Intern Med* 1997; 126(7):497–504.

18. Curhan, G.C. et al. "A prospective study of dietary calcium and other nutrients and the risk of symptomatic kidney stones," *N Eng J Med* 1993; 328(12):833–838.

19. Coe, F.L. et al. "Stone-forming potential of milk or calcium-fortified orange juice in idiopathic hypercalciuric adults," *Kidney Int* 1992; 41(1):139–142.

20. Messa, P. et al. "Different dietary calcium intake and relative supersaturation of calcium oxalate in the urine of patients forming renal stones," *Clin Sci (Colch)* 1997; 93(3):257–263.

21. Lemann, J., Jr. et al. "Urinary oxalate excretion increases with body size and decreases with increasing dietary calcium intake among healthy adults," *Kidney Int* 1996; 49(1):200–208.

22. Giannini, S. et al. "Acute effects of moderate dietary protein restriction in patients with idiopathic hypercalciuria and calcium nephrolithiasis," *Am J Clin Nutr* 1999; 69(2):267–271.

23. Liatsikos, E.N. and G.A. Barbalias. "The influence of a low protein diet in idiopathic hypercalciuria," *Int Urol Nephrol* 1999; 31(3):271–276.

24. Rotily, M. et al. "Effects of low animal protein or high-fiber diets on urine composition in calcium nephrolithiasis," *Kidney Int* 2000; 57(3):1115–1123.

25. Auer, B.L. et al. "Relative hyperoxaluria, crystalluria and haematuria after megadose ingestion of vitamin C," *Eur J Clin Invest* 1998; 28(9):695–700.

26. Urivetszky, M. et al. "Ascorbic acid overdosing: a risk factor for calcium oxalate nephrolithiasis," *J Urol* 1992; 147(5):1215–1218.

27. Curhan, G.C. et al. "Intake of vitamin B6 and C and the risk of kidney stones in women," *J Am Soc Nephrol* 1999; 10(4):840–845.

28. Simon, J.A. and E.S. Hudes. "Relation of serum ascorbic acid to serum vitamin B12, serum ferritin, and kidney stones in US adults," *Arch Intern Med* 1999; 159(6):619–624.

29. Curhan, G.C. et al. "Comparison of dietary calcium with supplemental calcium and other nutrients affecting the risk for kidney stones in women," *Ann Intern Med* 1997; 126(7):497–504.

30. Chansirikam, S. et al. "Risk of calcium oxalate nephrolithiasis after calcium or combined calcium and calcitrol supplementation in postmenopausal women," *Osteoporos Int* 2000; 11(6):486–492.

Lactose Intolerance

1. *What is Lactose Intolerance?* Mayo Foundation for Medical Education and Research, August 1999. Available at **www.mayoclinic.com/home?id=HQ00979**.

2. *Lactose Intolerance.* The National Digestive Diseases Information Clearinghouse (NDDIC), November 1998. Available at **www.niddk.nih.gov/health/digest/pubs/lactose/lactose.htm**.

3. Hertzler, S.R. et al. "Colonic adaptation to the daily lactose feeding in lactose maldigesters reduces lactose intolerance," *Am J Clin Nutr* 1996; 64:1232–1236.

4. Vesa, T.H. et al. "Tolerance to small amounts of lactose in lactose maldigesters," *Am J Clin Nutr* 1996; 64:197–201.

5. Martini, M.C. et al. "Reduced intolerance to symptoms from lactose consumed during a meal," *Am J Clin Nutr* 1988; 47:57–60.

6. Hertzler, S.R. et al. "How much lactose is low lactose?" *J Am Diet Assoc* 1996; 96:243–246.

Lung Cancer

1. Canadian Cancer Statistics 2001. National Cancer Institute of Canada, 2001. Available at **www.cancer.ca/stats/highle.htm**.

2. Surgeon General. *Reducing the health consequences of smoking: 25 years of progress.* (Washington, DC: US Government Printing Office, 1989).

3. *Lung Cancer in Canada.* Health Canada, June 1998. Available at **www.hc-sc.gc.ca/hpb/lcdc/bc/updates/lung_e.html**.

4. Peto, R. et al. "Smoking, smoking cessation, and lung cancer in the UK since 1950: combination of national statistics with two case-control studies," *Br Med J* 2000; 321(7257):323–329.

5. Potter, J.D. et al. "Alcohol, beer and lung cancer in postmenopausal women: the Iowa Women's Health Study," *Ann Epidemiol* 1992; 2:587–595.

6. Pollack, E.S. et al. "Prospective study of alcohol consumption and cancer," *N Eng J Med* 1984; 310:617–621.

7. Kvale, G. et al. "Dietary habits and lung cancer risk," *Int J Cancer* 1983; 31:397–405.

8. Klatsky, A.I. et al. "Alcohol and mortality: a ten year Kaiser-Permanente experience," *Ann Inter Med* 1981; 95:139–145.

9. De Stefani, E. et al. "Dietary fat and lung cancer: a case-control study in Uruguay," *Cancer Causes and Control* 1997; 8(6):913–921.

10. De Stefani, E. et al. "Fatty foods and the risk of lung cancer: a case-control study from Uruguay," *Int J Cancer* 1997; 71(5):760–766.

11. Alavanja, M.C. et al. "Estimating the effect of dietary fat on the risk of lung cancer in nonsmoking women," *Lung Cancer* 1996; 14(Suppl 1): S63–S74.

12. Alavanja, M.C. et al. "Saturated fat intake and lung cancer risk among nonsmoking women in Missouri," *JNCI* 1993; 85(23):1886–1887.

13. Knept, P. et al. "Dietary cholesterol, fatty acids, and the risk of lung cancer among men," *Nutr Cancer* 1991; 16:267–275.

14. Goodman, M.T. et al. "The effect of dietary fat and cholesterol on the risk of lung cancer in Hawaii," *Am J Epidemiol* 1988; 128:1241–1255.

15. Byers, T.E. et al. "Diet and lung cancer risk: findings from the Western New York Diet Study," *Am J Epidemiol* 1987; 125:351–363.

16. Wu, Y. et al. "Dietary cholesterol, fat and lung cancer incidence among older women: the Iowa Women's Health Study," *Cancer Causes and Control* 1994; 5(5):395–400.

17. Zhang, J. et al. "Fish consumption is inversely associated with male lung cancer mortality in countries with high levels of cigarette smoking or animal fat consumption," *Int J Epidemiol* 2000; 29(4):615–621.

18. Yam, D. et al. "Suppression of tumor growth and metastasis by dietary fish oil combined with vitamins E and C and cisplatin," *Cancer Chemother Pharmacol* 2001; 47(1):34–40.

19. Kvale, G. et al. "Dietary habits and lung cancer risk," *Int J Cancer* 1983; 31:397–405.

20. Feskanich, D. et al. "Prospective study of fruit and vegetable consumption and risk of lung cancer among men and women," *JNCI* 2000; 92(22):1812–1823.

21. Brennan, P. et al. "A multicenter case-control study of diet and lung cancer among non-smokers. *Cancer Causes and Control* 2000; 11(1):49–58.

22. Nyberg, F. et al. "Dietary factors and risk of lung cancer in never-smokers," *Int J Cancer* 1998; 78(4):430–436.

23. Steinmetz, K. et al. "Vegetables, fruit, and lung cancer in the Iowa Women's Health Study," *Cancer Res* 1993; 53(3):536–543.

24. Shibata, A. et al. "Dietary [beta]-carotene, cigarette smoking, and lung cancer in men," *Cancer Causes and Control* 1992; 3:207–214.

25. Kromhout, D. et al. "Essential micronutrients in relation to carcinogenesis," *Am J Clin Nutr* 1987; 45:1361–1367.

26. Long-de, W. et al. "Lung cancer, fruit, green salad and vitamin pills," *Chin Med J* 1985; 98:206–210.

27. Speizer, F.E. et al. "Prospective study of smoking, antioxidant intake, and lung cancer in middle-aged women," *Cancer Causes and Control* 1999; 10(5):475–482.

28. Knekt, P. et al. "Dietary flavonoids and the risk of lung cancer and other malignant neoplasms," *Am J Epidemiol* 1997; 146(3):223–230.

29. Le Marchand, L. et al. "Intake of flavonoids and lung cancer," *JNCI* 2000; 92(2):154–160.

30. Yang, G.Y. et al. "Effect of black and green tea polyphenols on c-jun phosphorylation and H(2)O(2) production in transformed and non-transformed human bronchila cell lines: possible mechanisms of cell growth inhibition and apoptosis induction," *Carcinogenesis* 2000; 21(11):2035–2039.

31. Yang, C.S. et al. "Tea and tea polyphenols inhibit cell hyperproliferation, lung tumerogenesis, and tumor progression," *Exp Lung Res* 1998; 24(4):629–639.

32. Leanderson, P. et al. "Green tea polyphenols inhibit oxidant-induced DNA strand breakage in cultured cell lines," *Free Radic Biol Med* 1997; 23(2):235–242.

33. Shim, J.S. et al. "Chemopreventative effect of green tea (Camellia sinensis) among cigarette smokers," *Cancer Epidemiol Biomarkers Prev* 1995; 4(4):387–391.

34. Mukhtar, H. and N. Ahmad. "Tea polyphenols: prevention of cancer and optimizing health," *Am J Clin Nutr* 2000; 71(Suppl 6):S1698–S1702.

35. Voorrips, L.E. et al. "A prospective cohort study on antioxidant and folate intake and male lung cancer risk," *Cancer Epidemiol Biomarkers Prev* 2000; 9(4):357–365.

36. Jatoi, A. et al. "A cross-sectional study of vitamin intake in postoperative non-small cell lung cancer patients," *J Surg Oncol* 68(4):231–236.

37. Stefani, E.D. et al. "Dietary antioxidants and lung cancer risk: a case-control study in Uruguay," *Nutr Cancer* 1999; 34(1):100–110.

38. Yong, L.C. et al. "Intakes of vitamins E, C, and A and the risk of lung cancer. The NHANES I epidemiologic followup study. First National Health and Nutrition Examination Survey," *Am J Epidemiol* 1997; 146(3):231–243.

39. Woodson, K. et al. "Serum alpha-tocopherol and subsequent risk of lung cancer among male smokers," *JNCI* 1999; 91(20):1738–1743.

40. Knekt, P. et al. "Is low selenium status a risk factor for lung cancer?" *Am J Epidemiol* 1998; 148(10):975–982.

41. Comstock, G.W. et al. "The risk of developing lung cancer associated with antioxidants in the blood: ascorbic acid, carotenoids, alpha-tocopherol, selenium, and total peroxyl radical absorbing capacity," *Cancer Epidemiol Biomarkers Prev* 1997; 6(11):907–916.

42. Goodman, G.E. et al. "The association between participant characteristics and serum concentrations of beta-carotene, retinal, retinyl palmitate, and alpha-tocopherol among participants in the Carotene and Retinol Efficacy Trial (CARET) for prevention of lung cancer," *Cancer Epidemiol Biomarkers Prev* 1996; 5(10):815–821.

43. Cook, N.R. et al. "Effects of beta-carotene supplementation on cancer incidence by baseline characteristics in the Physician's Health Study (United States)," *Cancer Causes and Control* 2000; 11(7):617–626.

44. Omenn, G.S. et al. "Risk factors for lung cancer and for intervention effects in CARET, the Beta-Carotene and Retinol Efficacy Trial," *JNCI* 1996; 88(21):1550–1559.

45. Albanes, D. et al. "Effects of alpha-tocopherol and beta-carotene supplements on cancer incidence in the Alpha-Tocopherol Beta-Carotene Cancer Prevention Study," *Am J Clin Nutr* 1995; 62(Suppl 6):S1427–S1430.

Lupus

1. Morimoto, I. "A study on immunological effects of L-canavanine," *Kobe J Med Sci* 1989; 35(5–6):287–298.

2. Alcocer-Varela, J. et al. "Effects of L-canavanine on T cells may explain the induction of systemic lupus erythematosus by alfalfa," *Arth Rheum* 1985; 28(1):52–57.

3. Philbrick, D.J. and B.J. Holub. "Flaxseed: a potential treatment for lupus nephritis," *Kidney Int* 1995; 48(2):475–480.

4. Serban, M.G. et al. "Lipid peroxidase and erythro-cyte redox system in systemic vasculitides treated with corticoids. Effect of vitamin E administration," *Rom J Intern Med* 1994; 32(4):283–289.

5. Comstock, G.W. et al. "Serum concentrations of alpha tocopherol, beta carotene, and retinal preceding the diagnosis of rheumatoid arthritis and systemic lupus erythematosus," *Ann Rheum Dis* 1997; 56(5):323–325.

6. Weinmann, B.J. and D. Hermann. "Inhibition of autoimmune deterioration in MRL/lpr mice by vitamin E," *Int J Vitam Nutr Res* 1999; 69(4):255–261.

7. Tanaseanu, S. et al. "Lipid peroxidation and the activity of some antioxidant enzymes in patients with systemic vesculitides treated with corticoids," *Rom J Intern Med* 1994; 32(1):47–50.

8. Muller, K. et al. "Vitamin D3 metabolism in patients with rheumatic diseases: low serum levels of 25-hydroxyvitamin D3 in patients with systemic lupus erythematosus," *Clin Rheumatol* 1995; 14(4):397–400.

9. Barry, N.N. et al. "Dehydroepiandrosterone in systemic lupus erythematosus: relationship between dosage, serum levels, and clinical response," *J Rheumatol* 1998; 25(12):2352–2356.

10. van Vollenhoven, R.F. et al. "A double-blind, place-bo-controlled, clinical trial of dehydroepiandrosterone in severe systemic lupus erythematosus," *Lupus* 1999; 8(3):181–187.

11. van Vollenhoven, R.F. et al. "Treatment of systemic lupus erythematosus with dehydroepiandrosterone: 50 patients treated up to 12 months," *J Rheumatol* 1998; 25(2):285–289.

12. van Vollenhoven, R.F. et al. "Dehydroepiandrosterone in systemic lupus erythematosus. Results of a double-blind, placebo-controlled, randomized clinical trial," *Arth Rheum* 1995; 38(12):1826–1831.

13. van Vollenhoven, R.F. et al. "An open trial of dehydroepiandrosterone in systemic lupus erythematosus," *Arth Rheum* 1994; 37(9):1305–1310.

14. Howite, N.T. et al. "Effects of dietary modification and fish oil supplementation on dyslipoproteinemia in pediatric systemic lupus erythematosus," *J Rheumatol* 1995; 22(7):1347–1351.

15. Das, U.N. "Beneficial effect of eicosapentanoic and docosahexaenoic acids in the management of systemic lupus erythematosus and its relationship to the cytokine network," *Prostaglandins Leukot Essent Fatty Acids* 1994; 51(3):207–213.

16. Clark, W.F. and A. Parbtani. "Omega-3 fatty acid supplementation in clinical and experimental lupus nephritis," *Am J Kidney Dis* 1994; 23(5):644–647.

17. Clark, W.F. et al. "Fish oil in lupus nephritis: clinical findings and methodological implications," *Kidney Int* 1993; 44(1):75–86.

18. Walton, A.J. et al. "Dietary fish oil and the severity of symptoms in patients with systemic lupus erythematosus," *Ann Rheum Dis* 1991; 50(7):463–466.

19. Mohan I.K. and U.N. Das. Oxidant stress, anti-oxidants and essential fatty acids in systemic lupus erythematosus," *Prostaglandins Leukot Essent Fatty Acids* 1997; 56(3):193–198.

Macular Degeneration

1. *Macular Degeneration.* The Canadian National Institute for the Blind, 1997. Available at **www.cnib.ca/pamphlets_publications/bviic/cospubs/mclrdegn.htm**.

2. *Don't Lose Sight of Age-Related Macular Degeneration.* The National Eye Institute, National Institutes of Health, April 2000. Available at **www.nei.nih.gov/publications/armd.htm**.

3. Ibid.

4. Mares-Perlman, J.A. et al. "Dietary fat and age-related maculopathy," *Arch Ophthalmol* 1996; 114(2):235–236.

5. Smith, W. et al. "Dietary fat and fish intake and age-related maculopathy," *Arch Ophthalmol* 2000; 118(3):401–404.

6. Ibid

7. Seddon, J.M. et al. "Dietary carotenoids, vitamins A, C and E, and advanced age-related macular degeneration," *JAMA* 1994; 272(18):1413–1420.

8. Bone, R.A. et al. "Lutein and zeaxanthin in the eyes, serum and diet of human subjects," *Exp Eye Res* 2000; 71(3):239–245.

9. Berendschott, T.T. et al. "Influence of lutein supplementation on macular pigment, assessed with two objective techniques," *Invest Ophthalmol Vis Sci* 2000; 41(11):3322–3326.

10. Hammond, B.R., Jr. et al. "Dietary modification of human macular pigment density," *Invest Ophthalmol Vis Sci* 1997; 38(9):1795–1801.

11. Landrum, J.T. et al. "A one year study of the macular pigment: the effect of 140 days of a lutein supplement," *Exp Eye Res* 1997; 65(1):57–62.

12. Richer, S. "ARMD—pilot (case series) environmental intervention data," *J Am Optom Assoc* 1999; 70(1):24–36.

13. Reed Mangels, A. et al. "Carotenoid content of fruits and vegetables: An evaluation of analytic data," *J Am Diet Assoc* 1993; 93(3):284–296.

14. Moss, S.E. et al. "Alcohol consumption and the 5-year incidence of age-related maculopathy: the Beaver Dam Eye study," *Ophthalmology* 1998; 105(5):789–794.

15. Ritter, L.L. et al. "Alcohol use and age-related maculopathy in the Beaver Dam Eye Study," *Am J Ophthalmol* 1995; 120(2):190–196.

16. Cho, E. et al. "Prospective study of alcohol consumption and the risk of age-related macular degeneration," *Arch Ophthalmol* 2000; 118(5):681–688.

17. Delcourt, C. et al. "Age-related macular degeneration and antioxidant status in the POLA study," *Arch Ophthalmol* 1999; 117(10):1384–1390.

18. Belda, J.I. et al. "Serum vitamin E levels negatively correlate with severity of age-related macular degeneration," *Mech Ageing Dev* 1999; 107(2):159–164.

19. VandenLangenberg, G.M. et al. "Associations between antioxidant and zinc intake and the 5-year incidence of early age-related maculopathy in the Beaver Dam Eye Study," *Am J Epidemiol* 1998; 148(2):204–214.

20. Mayer, M.J. et al. "Whole blood selenium and exudative age-related maculopathy," *Acta Ophthalmol Scand* 1998; 76(1):62–67.

21. Mares-Perlman, J.A. et al. "Serum antioxidants and age-related macular degeneration in a population-based case-control study," *Arch Ophthalmol* 1995; 113(12):1518–1523.

22. Eye Disease Case-Control Study Group. "Antioxidant status and neovascular age-related macular degeneration, Eye Disease Case-Control Study Group," *Arch Ophthalmol* 1993; 111(1):104–109.

23. Christen, W.G. et al. "Prospective cohort study of antioxidant vitamin supplement use and the risk of age-related maculopathy," *Am J Epidemiol* 1999; 149(5):476–484.

24. Richer, S. "Multicenter ophthalmic and nutritional age-related macular degeneration study—part 2: antioxidant intervention and conclusions," *J Am Optom Assoc* 1996; 67(1):30–49.

25. Mares-Perlman, J.A. "Association of zinc and antioxidant nutrients with age-related maculopathy," *Arch Ophthalmol* 1996; 114(8):991–997.

26. Stur, M. et al. "Oral zinc and the second eye in age-related macular degeneration," *Invest Ophthalmol Vis Sci* 1996; 37(7):1225–1235.

27. Newsome, D.A. et al. "Oral zinc in macular degeneration," *Arch Ophthalmol* 1988; 106:192–198.

28. Scharrer, A. and M. Ober. "Anthocyanosides in the treatment of retinopathies," *Klin Monatsbl Augenheilkd* 1981; 178:386–389. [German]

29. Caselli, L. "Clinical and electroretinographic study on activity of anthocyanosides," *Arch Med Intern* 1985; 37:29–35.

30. Evans, J.R. "Ginkgo biloba extract for age-related macular degeneration," *Cochrane Database Syst Rev* 2000; 125(2):CD001775.

31. Diamond, B.J. et al. "Ginkgo biloba extract: mechanisms and clinical indications," *Arch Phys Med Rehabil* 2000; 81(5):668–678.

32. Lebuisson, D.A. et al. "Treatment of senile macular degeneration with Ginkgo biloba extract. A preliminary double-blind, drug versus placebo study," *Presse Med* 1986; 15:1556–1558. [French]

Migraine Headaches

1. The Migraine Society of Canada, 2001. Available at **www.migraine.ca**.

2. William, E.M. et al. "Guidelines for the diagnosis and management of migraine in clinical practice," *CMAJ* 1997; 156:1273–1287.

3. "Migraine," *The Merck Manual, 1995–2000,* Merck and Co. Ltd. Available at **www.merck.com/pubs/ mmanual/section14/chapter168/168b.htm**.

4. Littlewood, J.T. et al. "Red wine as a cause of migraine," *Lancet* 1988; 1(8585):558–559.

5. Monro, J. et al. "Food allergy in migraine. Study of dietary exclusion and RAST," *Lancet* 1980; 2(8184):1–4.

6. Grant, E.C. "Food allergies and migraine," *Lancet* 1979; 1(8123):966–969.

7. Mansfield, L.E. et al. "Food allergy and adult migraine: double-blind and mediator confirmation of an allergic etiology," *Ann Allergy* 1985; 55(2):126–129.

8. Schoenen, J. et al. "Effectiveness of high-dose riboflavin in migraine prophylaxis. A randomized controlled trial," *Neurology* 1998; 50(2):466–470.

9. Mauskop, A. and B.M. Altura. "Role of magnesium in the pathogenesis and treatment of migraines," *Clin Neurosci* 1998; 5(1):24–27.

10. Lodi, R. et al. "Deficit of brain and skeletal muscle bioenergetics and low brain magnesium in juvenile migraine: an in vivo 31P magnetic resonance spectroscopy," *Pediatr Res* 1997; 42(6):866–871.

11. Aloisi, P. et al. "Visual evoked potentials and serum magnesium levels in juvenile migraine patients," *Headache* 1997; 37(6):383–385.

12. Peikert, A. et al. "Prophylaxis of migraine with oral magnesium: results from a prospective, multi-center, placebo-controlled and double-blind randomized study," *Cephalalgia* 1996; 16(4):257–263.

13. Murphy, J.J. et al. "Randomised double-blind placebo-controlled trial of feverfew in migraine prevention," *Lancet* 1988; 2(8604):189–192.

Motion Sickness and Vertigo

1. *Motion Sickness in Children.* Medscape.com, 2001. Available at **www.medscape.com/adis/DTP/2001/v17.n01/dtp1701.02/dtp1701.02-01.html**.

2. Gordon, C.R. and A. Shupak. "Prevention and treatment of motion sickness in children," *CNS Drugs* 1999; 12(5):369–381.

3. Proctor, C.A. "Abnormal insulin levels and vertigo," *Laryngoscope* 1981; 91(10):1657–1662.

4. Lindseth, G. and P.D. Lindseth. "The relationship of diet to airsickness," *Aviat Space Environ Med* 1995; 66(6):537–541.

5. Mowrey, D.B. et al. "Motion sickness, ginger, and psychophysics," *Lancet* 1982; 1:655–657.

6. Grontved, A. et al. "Ginger root against seasickness. A controlled trial on the open sea," *Acta Otolaryngol* 1988; 105(1–2):45–49.

7. Grontved, A. and E. Hentzer. "Vertigo-reducing effect of ginger root. A controlled clinical study," *ORL J Otorhinolaryngol Relat Spec* 1986; 48(5):282–286.

8. Holtman, S. et al. "The anti-motion sickness mechanism of ginger. A comparative study with placebo and dimenhydrinate," *Acta Otolaryngol* 1989; 108(3–4):168–174.

9. Haguenauer, J.P. et al. "Treatment of balance disorders using Ginkgo biloba extract. A multicentre, double-blind, drug versus placebo study," *Presse Med* 1986; 15:1569–1572. [French]

10. Cesarani, A. et al. "Ginkgo biloba (EGb 761) in the treatment of equilibrium disorders," *Adv Ther* 1998; 15(5):291–304.

Multiple Sclerosis (MS)

1. *MS Information.* Multiple Sclerosis Society of Canada, 2001. Available at **www.mssociety.ca/en/information/faq.htm**.

2. *Multiple Sclerosis.* Mayo Foundation for Medical Education and Research, 2001. Available at **www.mayoclinic.com/home?id=DS00188**.

3. *Your Health: Multiple Sclerosis.* Calgary Regional Health Authority, August 2000. Available at **www.crha-health.ab.ca/hlthconn/items/ms.htm**.

4. Ghadirian, P. et al. "Nutritional factors in the aetiology of multiple sclerosis: a case-control study in Montreal, Canada," *Int J Epidemiol* 1998; 27(5):845–852.

5. Esparza, M.L. et al. "Nutrition, latitude, and multiple sclerosis mortality: an ecologic study," *Am J Epidemiol* 1995; 142(7):733–737.

6. Tola, M.R. et al. "Dietary habits and multiple sclerosis. A retrospective study in Ferra, Italy," *Acta Neurol (Napoli)* 1994; 16(4):189–197.

7. Sepcic, J. et al. "Nutritional factors and multiple sclerosis in Gorski Kotar, Croatia," *Neuroepidemiology* 1993; 12(4):234–240.

8. Swank, R.L. and B.B. Dugan. "Effects of low saturated fat diet in early and late cases of multiple sclerosis," *Lancet* 1990; 336(8706):37–39.

9. Bates, D. et al. "Polyunsaturated fatty acids in the treatment of acute remitting multiple sclerosis," *Br Med J* 1978; 2:1390–1391.

10. Millar, J.H.D. et al. "Double-blind trial of linoleate supplementation of the diet in multiple sclerosis," *Br Med J* 1973; 1:765–768.

11. Syburra, C. and S. Passi. "Oxidative stress in patients with multiple sclerosis," *WMJ* 1999; 71(3):112–115.

12. Glabinski, A. et al. "Increased generation of super-oxide radicals in the blood of MS patients," *Acta Neurol Scand* 1993; 88(3):174–177.

13. Langemann, H. et al. "Measurement of low-molecular-weight antioxidants, uric acid, tyrosine and tryptophan in plaques and white matter from patients with multiple sclerosis," *Eur Neurol* 1992; 32(5):248–252.

14. Sandyk, R. and G.I. Awerbuch. "Vitamin B12 and its relationship to age of onset of multiple sclerosis," *Int J Neurosci* 1993; 71(1–4):93–99.

15. Reynolds, E.H. et al. "Vitamin B12 metabolism in multiple sclerosis," *Arch Neurol* 1992; 39(6):649–652.

16. Reynolds, E.H. et al. "Multiple sclerosis associated with vitamin B12 deficiency," *Arch Neurol* 1991; 48(8):808–811.

17. Kira, J. et al. "Vitamin B12 metabolism and mas-sive-dose methyl vitamin B12 therapy in Japanese patients with multiple sclerosis. *Intern Med* 1994; 33(2):82–86.

18. Cantorna, M.T. et al. "1,25-Dihydroxyvitamin D3 reversibly blocks the progression of relapsing encephalomyelitis, a model of multiple sclerosis," *Proc Natl Acad Sci USA* 1996; 93(15):7861–7864.

19. Pennsylvania State University. "Study Points to Positive Results from Vitamin D Supplements for MS Sufferers," April 3, 2001. Available at **www.psu.edu/ur/2001/msandvitamind.html**. [Press release]

20. Cosman, F. et al. "Fracture history and bone loss in patients with MS," *Neurology* 1998; 51(4):1161–1165.

21. Nieves, J. et al. "High prevalence of vitamin D defi-ciency and reduced bone mass in multiple sclero-sis," *Neurology* 1994; 44(9):1687–1692.

22. Nightingale, S. et al. "Red blood cell and adipose tissue fatty acids in mild active multiple sclerosis. *Acta Neurol Scand* 1990; 82:43–50.

23. Cunnane, S.C. et al. "Essential fatty acid and lipid profiles in plasma and erythrocytes in patients with multiple sclerosis," *Am J Clin Nutr* 1989; 50:801–806.

24. Nordvik, I. et al. "Effects of dietary advice and n-3 supplementation in newly diagnosed MS patients," *Acta Neurol Scand* 2000; 102(3):143–149.

25. Lee, A. and V. Patterson. "A double-blind study of L-threonine in patients with spinal spasticity," *Acta Neurol Scand* 1993; 88(5):334–338.

26. Hauser, S.L. et al. "An antispasticity effect of threo-nine in multiple sclerosis," *Acta Neurol* 1992; 49(9):923–926.

Obesity and Weight Loss

1. *National Population Health Survey, 1994–1995.* Ottawa: Statistics Canada, 1995. Catalogue no. 82-F0001XCB. [CD-ROM version]

2. Tremblay, M.S. and J.D. Willms. "Secular trends in the body mass index of Canadian children," *CMAJ* 2000; 163(11):1429–1433.

3. Kaats, G.R. et al. "A randomized, double-masked, placebo-controlled study of the effects of chromi-um picolinate supplementation on body composi-tion: a replication and extension of a previous study," *Curr Ther Res* 1998; 59:379–388.

4. Grant, K.E. et al. "Chromium and exercise training: effect on obese women," *Med Sci Sports Exerc* 1997; 29(8):992–998.

5. Colker, C.M. et al. "Effects of *Citrus aurantium* extract, caffeine, and St. John's Wort on body fat loss, lipid levels, and mood states in overweight healthy adults," *Current Ther Res* 1999; 60(3):145–153.

6. Mattes, R.D. and L. Bormann. "Effect of (-)-hydrox-ycitric acid on appetite variables," *Physiol Behav* 2000; 71(1–2):87–94.

7. Kriketos, A.D. et al. "(-)-hydroxycitric acid does not affect energy expenditure and substrate oxidation in adult males in post absorptive state," *Int J Obes Relat Metab Disord* 1999; 23(8):867–873.

8. Heymsfield, S.B. et al. "*Garcinia cambogia* (hydrox-ycitric acid) as a potential antiobesity agent: a ran-domized controlled trial," *JAMA* 1998; 280(18):1596–1600.

9. Blankson, H. et al. "Effects of conjugated linoleic acid (CLA) on body fat mass in overweight or obese human volunteers: a double-blind random-ized placebo controlled study," Abstract 23, American Chemical Society 220th National Meeting, August 20–24, 2000, Washington, DC.

10. Anon. "Linoleic Acid Supplements May Help Dieting Adults Keep Weight Off," Reuters Health. URL: **www.medscape.com/reuters/prof/2000/08/08.22/20000822drgd003.html** (August 22, 2000).

11. Cangiano, C. et al. "Eating behaviour and adherence to dietary prescriptions in obese adult subjects treated with 5-hydroxytryptophan," *Am J Clin Nutr* 1992; 56(5):863–867.

12. Ceci, F. et al. "The effects of oral 5-hydroxytryptophan administration on feeding behaviour on obese adult female subjects," *J Neural Transm* 1989; 76(2):109–117.

Osteoarthritis

1. *Osteoarthritis*. The Arthritis Society of Canada, March 2001. Available at **www.arthritis.ca/ types%20of%20arthritis/osteoarthritis/default. asp?mode=static**.

2. White-O'Connor, B. and J. Sobal. "Nutrient intake and obesity in a multidisciplinary assessment of osteoarthritis," *Clin Ther* 1986; 9(Suppl B):S30–S42.

3. Toda, Y. et al. "Change in body fat, but not body weight or metabolic correlates of obesity, is related to symptomatic relief of obese patients with knee osteoarthritis after a weight control program," *J Rheumatol* 1998; 25(11):2181–2186.

4. McAlindon, T.E. et al. "Do antioxidant micronutrients protect against the development and progression of knee osteoarthritis?" *Arth Rheum* 1996; 39(4):648–656.

5. McAlindon, T.E. et al. "Relation of dietary intake and serum levels of vitamin D to progression of osteoporosis of the knee among participants in the Framingham Study," *Ann Intern Med* 1996; 125(5):353–359.

6. Lane, N.E. et al. "Serum vitamin D levels and incident changes of radiographic hip osteoarthritis: a longitudinal study. Study of Osteoporotic Fractures Research Group," *Arth Rheum* 1999; 42(5):854–860.

7. McCleane, G. "The analgesic efficacy of topical capsaicin is enhanced by glyceryl trinitrate in painful osteoarthritis: a randomized, double blind placebo controlled study," *Eur J Pain* 2000; 4(4):355–360.

8. Zhang, W.Y. and A. Li Wan Po. "The effectiveness of topically applied capsaicin cream. A meta-analysis," *Eur J Clin Pharmacol* 1994; 46(6):517–522.

9. Mazieres, B. et al. "Chondroitin sulfate in osteoarthritis of the knee: a prospective, double blind, placebo controlled multicenter clinical study," *J Rheumatol* 2001; 28(1):173–181.

10. Leeb, B.F. et al. "A meta-analysis of chondroitin sulfate in the treatment of osteoarthritis," *J Rheumatol* 2000; 27(1):205–211.

11. Bucsi, L. and G. Poor. "Efficacy and tolerability of oral chondroitin sulfate as a symptomatic slow-acting drug for osteoarthritis (SYSADOA) in the treatment of knee osteoarthritis," *Osteoarthritis Cartilage* 1998; 6(Suppl A):S31–S36.

12. Uebelhart, D. et al. "Effects of oral chondroitin sulfate on the progression of knee osteoarthritis: a pilot study," *Osteoarthritis Cartilage* 1998; 6(Suppl A):S39–S46.

13. Conrozier, T. "Anti-arthrosis treatments: efficacy and tolerance of chondroitin sulfates," *Presse Med* 1998; 27(36):1862–1865. [French]

14. Morreale, P. et al. "Comparison of the anti-inflammatory efficacy of chondroitin sulfate and diclofenac sodium in patients with knee osteoarthritis," *J Rheumatol* 1996; 23(8):1385–1391.

15. Verbruggen, G. et al. "Chondroitin sulfate: S/DMOAD (structure/disease modifying anti-osteoarthritis drug) in the treatment of finger joint OA," *Osteoarthritis Cartilage* 1998; 6(Suppl A):S37–S38.

16. Mazieres, B. et al. "Chondroitin sulfate in osteoarthritis of the knee: a prospective, double blind, placebo controlled multicenter clinical study," *J Rheumatol* 2001; 28(1):173–181.

17. Bourgeois, P. et al. "Efficacy and tolerability of chondroitin sulfate 1200 mg/day vs chondroitin sulfate 3 x 400 mg/day vs placebo," *Osteoarthritis Cartilage* 1998; 6(Suppl A):S25–S30.

18. McAlindon, T.E. et al. "Glucosamine and chondroitin for treatment of osteoarthritis: a systematic quality assessment and meta-analysis," *JAMA* 2000; 283(11):1469–1475.

19. Qiu, G.X. et al. "Efficacy and safety of glucosamine sulfate versus ibuprofen in patients with knee osteoarthritis," *Arzneimittelforschung* 1998; 48:469–474.

20. Forster, K.K. et al. "Longer-term treatment of mild-to-moderate osteoarthritis of the knee with glucosamine sulfate—a randomized, controlled, double-blind clinical study," *Euro J Clin Pharmacol* 1996; 50:542.

21. Lopes Vaz, A.L. "Double-blind clinical evaluation of the relative efficacy of ibuprofen and glucosamine sulphate in the management of osteoarthritis of the knee in out-patients," *Curr Med Res Opin* 1982; 8:145–149.

22. Drovanti, A., A.A. Bignamini and A.A. Rovati. "Therapeutic activity of oral glucosamine sulfate in

osteoarthritis: a placebo-controlled double-blind investigation," *Clin Ther* 1980; 3:260–272.

23. Pujalte, J.M. E.P. Llavore and F.R. Ylescupidez. "Double-blind clinical evaluation of oral glucosamine sulphate in the basic treatment of osteoarthritis," *Curr Med Res Opin* 1980; 7:110–114.

24. Reginster, J.Y. et al. "Long-term effects of glucosamine sulfate on osteoarthritis progression: a randomized, placebo-controlled trial," *Lancet* 2001; 357:251–256.

25. Konig, B. "A long-term (two years) clinical trial with S-adenosylmethionine for the treatment of osteoarthritis," *Am J Med* 1987; 83(5A):78–80.

26. Berger, R. and H. Nowak. "A new medical approach to the treatment of osteoarthritis. Report of an open phase IV study with ademetionine (Gumbaral)," *Am J Med* 1987; 83(5A):84–88.

27. Muller-Fassbender, H. "Double-blind clinical trial of S-adenosylmethionine versus ibuprofen in the treatment of osteoarthritis," *Am J Med* 1987; 83(5A):81–83.

28. Vetter, G. "Double-blind comparative clinical trial with S-adenosylmethionine and indomethacin in the treatment of osteoarthritis," *Am J Med* 1987; 83(5A):78–80.

29. Maccagno, A. et al. "Double-blind controlled clinical trial of oral S-adenosylmethionine versus piroxicam in knee osteoarthritis," *Am J Med* 1987; 83(5A):72–77.

30. Caruso, I. and V. Pietrogrande. "Italian double-blind multicenter study comparing S-adenosylmethionine, naproxen, and placebo in the treatment of degenerative joint disease," *Am J Med* 1987; 83(5A):66–71.

31. di Padova, C. "S-adenosylmethionine in the treatment of osteoarthritis. Review of the clinical studies," *Am J Med* 1987; 83(5A):60–65.

32. Glorioso, S. et al. "Double-blind multicentre study of the activity of S-adenosylmethionine in hip and knee osteoarthritis," *Int J Clin Pharmacol Res* 1985; 5(1):39–49.

Osteoporosis

1. *What is Osteoporosis?* Osteoporosis Society of Canada, 2001. Available at **www.osteoporosis.ca/OSTEO/D01-01.html**.

2. Cauley, J.A. et al. "The effect of HRT on Fracture Risk: Results of a 4-Year Randomized Trial of 2,763 Postmenopausal Women," *American Society for Bone and Mineral Research* June 1998. [Abstract T394]

3. Alekel, D.L. et al. "Isoflavone-rich soy protein isolate exerts significant bone sparing effect in the lumbar spine of perimenopausal women," Third International Symposium on the Role of Soy in Preventing and Treating Chronic Disease, October 1999. [Abstract]

4. Schieber, M.D. et al. "Dietary soy isoflavones favorably influence lipids and bone turnover in healthy postmenopausal women," Third International Symposium on the Role of Soy in Preventing and Treating Chronic Disease, October 1999. [Abstract]

5. Munger, R.G. et al. "Prospective study of dietary protein intake and risk of hip fracture in postmenopausal women," *Am J Clin Nutr* 1999; 69(1):147–152.

6. Schurch, M.A. et al. "Protein supplements increase serum insulin-like growth factor-I levels and attenuate proximal femur bone loss in patients with recent hip fracture. A randomized, double-blind, placebo-controlled trial," *Ann Intern Med* 1998; 128(10):801–809.

7. Lloyd, T. et al. "Dietary caffeine intake and bone status of postmenopausal women," *Am J Clin Nutr* 1997; 65(6):1826–1830.

8. Harris, S.S. and B. Dawson-Hughes. "Caffeine and bone loss in healthy menopausal women," *Am J Clin Nutr* 1994; 60(4):573–578.

9. Devine, A. et al. "A longitudinal study of the effect of sodium and calcium intakes on regional bone density in postmenopausal women," *Am J Clin Nutr* 1995; 62(4):740–745.

10. Sakhaee, K. et al. "The effect of calcium citrate on bone density in the early and mid-postmenopausal period: a randomized, placebo-controlled study," The Second Joint Meeting of the American Society for Bone and Mineral Research and the International Bone and Mineral Society, 1998. Mission Pharmacal Company. [Abstract]

11. Baran, D.T. et al. "A placebo-controlled study of pre-menopausal women: calcium supplementation and bone density," Annual Meeting of the American Society for Bone and Mineral Research, 1999. [Abstract]

12. Harris, S.S. and B. Dawson-Hughes. "Seasonal changes in plasma 25-hydroxyvitamin D concentra-

tions of young American black and white women," *Am J Clin Nutr* 1998; 67(6):1232–1236.

13. Leveille, S.G. et al. "Dietary vitamin C and bone mineral density: results from the PEPI study," *Calcif Tissue Int* 1998; (63)3:183–189.

14. Feskanich, D. et al. "Vitamin K intake and hip fractures in women: a prospective study," *Am J Clin Nutr* 1999; 69(1):74–79.

15. Strause, L. et al. "Spinal bone loss in postmenopausal women supplemented with calcium and trace minerals," *J Nutr* 1994; 124(7):1060–1064.

16. Ohta, H. et al. "Effects of 1-year ipriflavone treatment on lumbar bone mineral density and bone metabolic markers in postmenopausal women with low bone mass," *Horm Res* 1999; 51(4):178–183.

17. Adami, S. et al. "Ipriflavone prevents radial bone loss in postmenopausal women with low bone mass over 2 years," *Osteoporos Int* 1997; 7(2):119–125.

18. Gennari, C. et al. "Effect of ipriflavone—a synthetic derivative of natural isoflavones—on bone mass loss in the early years after menopause," *Menopause* 1998; 5(1):9–15.

19. Gennari, C. et al. "Effects of chronic treatment with ipriflavone in postmenopausal women with low bone mass," *Calcif Tissue Int* 1997; 61(Suppl 1):S19–S22.

20. Gambacciani, M. et al. "Effects of combined low dose of the isoflavone derivative ipriflavone and estrogen replacement on bone mineral density and metabolism in postmenopausal women," *Maturitas* 1997; 28(1):75–81.

21. Norkus, K. et al. "Bioavailability of two different formulations that [sic] ipriflavone," Biomedical Research Analytical Group, January 24, 2000, Bronx, NY.

22. Alexandersen, P. et al. "Ipriflavone in the treatment of postmenopausal osteoporosis. A randomized controlled trial," *JAMA* 2001; 285(11):1482–1488.

23. Dalsky, G.P. et al. "Weight-bearing exercise training and lumbar bone mineral content in postmenopausal women," *Ann Intern Med* 1988 Jun; 108(6):824–828.

Parkinson's Disease

1. Kontakos, N. and J. Stokes. "Monograph Series on Aging-related Diseases: XII," *Parkinson's Disease— Recent Developments and New Directions* 1999; 20(2). Available at **www.hc-sc.gc.ca/hpb/lcdc/ pulicat/cdic/cdic202/cd202b_3.html**.

2. *Parkinson's Disease*. Mayo Foundation for Medical Education and Research, 2001. Available at **www.mayoclinic.com/home?id=DS00295**.

3. Ibid.

4. Johnson, C.C. et al. "Adult nutrient intake as a risk factor for Parkinson's disease," *Int J Epidemiol* 1999; 28(6):1102–1109.

5. Anderson, C. et al. "Dietary factors in Parkinson's disease: the role of food groups and specific foods," *Mov Disord* 1999; 14(1):21–27.

6. Logroscino, G. et al. "Dietary iron, animal fats, and risk of Parkinson's disease," *Mov Disord* 1998; 13(Suppl 1):S13–S16.

7. Logroscino, G. et al. "Dietary lipids and antioxidants in Parkinson's disease: a population-based, case-control study," *Ann Neurol* 1996; 39(1):89–94.

8. Karstaedt, P.J. and J.H. Pincus. "Protein redistribution diet remains effective in patients with fluctuating parkinsonism," *Arch Neurol* 1992; 49(2):149–151.

9. Pare, S. et al. "Effect of daytime protein restriction on nutrient intakes of free-living Parkinson's disease patients," *Am J Clin Nutr* 1992; 55(3):701–707.

10. Bracco, F. et al. "Protein redistribution diet and antiparkinsonian response to levadopa," *Eur Neurol* 1991; 31(2):68–71.

11. Astarloa, R. et al. "Clinical and pharmacokinetic effects of a diet rich in insoluble fibre on Parkinson's disease," *Clin Neuropharmacol* 1992; 15(5):375–380.

12. Benedetti, M.D. et al. "Smoking, alcohol, and coffee consumption preceding Parkinson's disease: a case-control study," *Neurology* 2000; 55(9):1350–1358.

13. Ross, G.W. et al. "Association of coffee and caffeine intake with the risk of Parkinson disease," *JAMA* 2000; 283(20):2674–2679.

14. Jenner, P. et al. "Oxidative stress as a cause of nigral cell death in Parkinson's disease and incidental Lewy body disease. The Royal Kings and Queens Parkinson's Disease Research Group," *Ann Neurol* 1992; 32(Suppl 2):S82–S87.

15. de Rijk, M.C. et al. "Dietary antioxidants and Parkinson disease. The Rotterdam Study," *Arch Neurol* 1997; 54(6):762–765.

16. Abbott, R.A. et al. "Diet, body size, and micronutrient status in Parkinson's disease," *Eur J Clin Nutr* 1992; 46(12):879–884.

17. Shoulson, I. "DATATOP: a decade of neuroprotective inquiry. Parkinson Study Group. Deprenyl and

Tocopherol Antioxidative Therapy of Parkinsonism," *Ann Neurol* 1998; 44(3) (Suppl 1):S160–S166.

18. Puca, F.M. "Clinical pharmacodynamics of acetyl-L-carnitine in patients with Parkinson's disease," *Int J Clin Pharmacol Res* 1990; 19(1–2):139–143.

Perimenopause

1. McKinlay, S.M. et al. "The menopausal syndrome," *Br J Prev Soc Med* 1974; 28:108–115.

2. Thompsom, B. et al. "Menopausal age and symptomatology in a general practice," *J Biosoc Sci* 1973; 5:71–82.

3. Tang, G.W.K. "The climacteric of Chinese factory workers," *Maturitas* 1994; 19:177–182.

4. Murkies, A.L. et al. "Dietary flour supplementation decreases postmenopausal hot flushes: effect of soy and wheat," *Maturitas* 1995; 21:189–195.

5. Brzezinski, A. et al. "Short-term effects of phyto-estrogens-rich diet on postmenopausal women," *Menopause* 1997; 4:89–94.

6. Albertazzi, P. et al. "The effect of dietary soy supplementation on hot flushes," *Obstet Gynecol* 1998; 91(1):6–11.

7. Greenwood, S. et al. "The role of isoflavones in menopausal health: consensus opinion of The North American Menopause Society," *Menopause* 2000; 7(2):215–229.

8. Nicklas, T.A. et al. "Breakfast consumption with and without vitamin-mineral supplement use favorably impacts daily nutrient intake of ninth-grade students," *J Adolesc Health* 2000; 27(5):314–321.

9. Smith, A.P. et al. "Breakfast cereal and caffeinated coffee: effects on working memory, attention, mood, and cardiovascular function," *Physiol Behav* 1999; 67(1):9–17.

10. Benton, D. and P.Y. Parker. "Breakfast, blood glucose, and cognition," *Am J Clin Nutr* 1998; 67(4):772S–778S.

11. Akata, T. et al. "Successful combined treatment with vitamin B12 and bright artificial light of one case with delayed sleep phase syndrome," *Jpn J Psychiatry Neurol* 1993; 47(2):439–440.

12. Maeda, K. et al. "A multicenter study of the effects of vitamin B12 on sleep-waking rhythm disorders: in Shizuoka Prefecture," *Jpn J Psychiatry Neurol* 1992; 46(1):229–230.

13. Ohta, T. et al. "Treatment of persistent sleep-wake schedule disorders in adolescents with methylcobalamin (vitamin B12)," *Sleep* 1991; 14(5):414–418.

14. Okawa, M. et al. "Vitamin B12 treatment for sleep-wake rhythm disorders," *Sleep* 1990; 13(1):15–23.

15. Wuttke, W. "*Cimicifuga racemosa*: pharmacological and clinical profile of BNO 1055," First International Symposium on Health Phytotherapies, Rio de Janeiro, April 6, 2001. [Abstract]

16. Freudenstein, J. et al. "Influence of an isolated aqueous extract of *Cimicifugae racemosa* rhizoma on the proliferation of MCF-7 cells," Abstracts of the 23rd International LOF-Symposium on Phyto-Estrogens 1999, University of Gent, Belgium.

17. Stoll, W. et al. "Phytopharmacon influences atrophic vaginal epithelium: double-blind study— *Cimicifuga* vs. estrogenic substances," *Therapeuticum* 1987; 1:23–31.

18. Lehmann-Willenbrock, E. and H.H. Reidel. "Clinical and endocrinological examinations concerning therapy of climacteric symptoms following hysterectomy with remaining ovaries," *Zentrallblatt für Gynäkologie* 1988; 110(10):611–618.

19. Düker, E.M. et al. "Effects of extracts from *Cimicifuga racemosa* on gonadotropin release in menopausal women and ovariectomized rats," *Planta Medica* 1991; 57:420–424.

20. Foster, S. "Black cohosh: a literature review," *Herbalgram* 1999; 45:35–49.

21. Wuttke, W. "*Cimicifuga racemosa*: pharmacological and clinical profile of BNO 1055," First International Symposium on Health Phytotherapies, Rio de Janeiro, April 6, 2001. [Abstract]

22. Einer-Jensen, J. et al. "*Cimicifuga* and Melbrosia lack estrogenic effects in mice and rats," *Maturitis* 1996; 25:149–153.

23. Lindahl, O. et al. "Double blind study of a valerian preparation," *Pharmacology Biochemistry and Behaviour* 1989; 32:1065–1066.

24. Leathwood, P.D. et al. "Aqueous extract of valerian root improves sleep quality in man," *Pharmacology Biochemistry and Behaviour* 1982; 17:65–71.

25. Leathwood, P.D. et al. "Aqueous extract of valerian root reduces latency to fall asleep in man," *Planta Medica* 1985; 51:144–148.

26. Warnecke, G. "Psychosomatic dysfunctions in the female climacteric. Clinical effectiveness and tolerance of Kava Extract WS 1490," *Fortschr Med* 1991; 109(4):119–122. [German]

Phlebitis

1. Schulman, S. et al. "Influence of changes in lifestyle on fibrinolytic parameters and recurrence rate in patients with venous thromboembolism," *Blood Coagul Fibrinolysis* 1995; 6(4):311–316.

2. Eklof, B. et al. "Venous thromboembolism in association with prolonged air travel," *Dermatol Surg* 1996; 22(7):637–641.

3. Kozarevic, D. et al. "Drinking habits and other characteristics: the Yugoslavia Cardiovascular Disease Study," *Am J Epidemiol* 1982; 116(2):287–301.

4. Burkitt, D.P. "Varicose veins: facts and fantasy," *Arch Surg* 1976; 111(12):1327–1332.

5. Taussig, S.J. et al. "Bromelain: a proteolytic enzyme and its clinical application: A review," *Hiroshima J Med Sci* 1975; 24(2–3):185–193.

6. Seligman, B. "Oral bromelains as adjuncts in the treatment of acute thrombophlebitis," *Angiology* 1960; 20(1):22–26.

7. Scondotto, G. et al. "Use of mesoglycan in venous pathology," *Minerva Cardioangiol* 1997; 88(12):537–541. [Italian]

8. Agrati, A.M. et al. "Heparin sulfate: efficacy and safety in patients with chronic venous insufficiency," *Minerva Cardioangiol* 1991; 39(10):395–400. [Italian]

9. Scondotto, G. et al. "Use of minor fibrinolytic drug (mesoglycan) in phlebitis," *Minerva Med* 1984; 75(28–29):1733–1738.

10. Petruzzellism, V. and A. Velon. "Therapeutic action of oral mesoglycan in the pharmacologic treatment of the varicose syndrome and its complications," *Minerva Med* 1985; 76(12):543–548.

11. Prandoni, P. et al. "Long-term sequelae of deep venous thrombosis of the legs. Experience with mesoglycan," *Ann Ital Med Int* 1989; 4(4):378–385.

Polycystic Ovary Syndrome (PCOS)

1. *Polycystic Ovary Syndrome.* Vanderbilt Medical Center, 1998. Available at **www.mc.vanderbilt.edy/ peds/pidl/adolesc/polycysov.htm**.

2. Legro, R.S. "Polycystic ovary syndrome: current and future treatment paradigms," *Am J Obstet Gynecol* 1998; 179(6 Pt 2):S101–S108.

3. Taylor, A.E. "Systemic adversities of ovarian failure," *J Soc Gynecol Investig* 2001; (1 Suppl Proceedings):S7–S9.

4. Wahrenberg, H. et al. "Divergent effects of weight reduction and oral anticonception treatment on adrenergic lipolysis in obese women with the polycystic ovary syndrome," *J Clin Endocrinol Metab* 1999; 84(6):2182–2187.

5. Jakubowicz, D.J. and J.E. Nestler. "17 alpha-Hydroxyprogesterone response to leuprolide and serum androgens in obese women with and without polycystic ovary syndrome after dietary weight loss," *J Clin Endocrinol Metab* 1997; 82(2):556–560.

6. Andersen, P. et al. "Increased insulin sensitivity and fibrinolytic capacity after dietary intervention in obese women with polycystic ovary syndrome," *Metabolism* 1995; 44(5):611–616.

7. Franks, S. et al. "The role of nutrition and insulin in the regulation of sex hormone binding globulin," *J Steroid Biochem Mol Biol* 1991; 39(5B):835–838.

8. Franks, S. et al. "Obesity and polycystic ovary syndrome," *Ann NY Acad Sci* 1991; 626:201–206.

9. Kiddy, D.S. et al. "Improvement in endocrine and ovarian function during dietary treatment of obese women with polycystic ovary syndrome," *Clin Endocrinol* (Oxf) 1992; 36(10):105–111.

10. Moghetti, P. et al. "Spironolactone, but not flutamide, administration prevents bone loss in hyperandrogenic women treated with gonadotropin-releasing hormone agonist," *J Clin Endocrinol Metab* 1999; 84(4):1250–1254.

11. Mertz, W. "Chromium in human nutrition: a review," *J Nutr* 1993; 123(4):626–633.

12. Gambacciani, M. et al. "Ipriflavone prevents the loss of bone mass in pharmacological menopause induced by GnRH-agonists," *Calcif Tissue Int* 1997; 61(Suppl 1):S15–S18.

13. Norkus, K. et al. "Bioavailability of two different formulations that [sic] ipriflavone," Biomedical Research Analytical Group, January 24, 2000, Bronx, NY.

14. Nestler, J.E. et al. "Ovulatory and metabolic effects of D-chiro-inositol in the polycystic ovary syndrome," *N Engl J Med* 1999; 340(17):1314–1320.

Premenstrual Syndrome (PMS)

1. *Premenstrual Syndrome (PMS).* Discovery Health, January 2000. Available at **www.health.discovery.com/diseasesand cond/encyclopedia/2088.html**.

2. *Premenstrual Syndrome.* Mayo Foundation for Medical Education and Research, August 2000.

Available at **www.mayohealth.org/home?id= 5.1.1.16.11**.

3. Deuster, P.A. et al. "Biological, social, and behav- ioural factors associated with premenstrual syn- drome," *Arch Fam Med* 1999; 8:122–128.

4. Blum, I. et al. "The influence of meal composition on plasma serotonin and norepinephrine concen- trations," *Metabolism* 1992; 41(2):137–140.

5. Sayegh, R. et al. "The effect of a carbohydrate-rich beverage on mood, appetite, and cognitive function in women with premenstrual syndrome," *Obstet Gynecol* 1995; 86(4 Pt 1):520–528.

6. Jones, D.Y. "Influence of dietary fat on self-reported menstrual symptoms," *Physiol Behav* 1987; 40(4):483–487.

7. Boyd, N.F. et al. "Effect of a low-fat high-carbohy- drate diet on symptoms of cyclical mastopathy," *Lancet* 1988; 2(8603):128–132.

8. Barnard, N.D. et al. "Diet and sex-hormone globu- lin, dysmenorrhea, and premenstrual symptoms," *Obstet Gynecol* 2000; 95(2):245–250.

9. Wyatt, K.M. et al. "Efficacy of vitamin B6 in the treatment of premenstrual syndrome: systematic review," *Br J of Med* 1999; 318(7195):1375–1381.

10. De Souza, M.C. et al. "A synergistic effect of a daily supplement for 1 month of 200 mg magnesium plus 50 mg vitamin B6 for the relief of anxiety- related premenstrual symptoms: a randomized, double-blind, crossover study," *J Women's Health Gend Based Med* 2000; 9(2):131–139.

11. London, R.S. et al. "Efficacy of alpha-tocopherol on premenstrual symptomology: A double-blind study. II Endocrine correlates," *J Am Coll Nutr* 1984; 3:351–356.

12. London, R.S. et al. "Efficacy of alpha-tocopherol on premenstrual symptomology: A double-blind study," *J Reprod Med* 1987; 32(6):400–404.

13. London, R.S. et al. "Efficacy of alpha-tocopherol on premenstrual symptomology: A double-blind study," *J Am Coll Nutr* 1983; 2:115–122.

14. Thys-Jacobs, S. et al. "Calcium carbonate and the premenstrual syndrome: effects on premenstrual and menstrual symptoms. Premenstrual Syndrome Study Group," *Am J Obstet Gynecol* 1998; 179(2):444–452.

15. Walker, A.F. et al. "Magnesium supplementation alleviates premenstrual symptoms of fluid reten- tion," *J Women's Health* 1998; 7(9):1157–1165.

16. Facchinetti, F. et al. "Oral magnesium successfully relieves premenstrual mood changes," *Obstet Gynecol* 1991; 78(2):177–181.

17. Posaci, C. et al. "Plasma copper, zinc and magne- sium levels in patients with premenstrual tension syndrome," *Acta Obstet Gynecol Scand* 1994; 73(6):452–455.

18. Rosenstein, D.L. et al. "Magnesium measures across the menstrual cycle in premenstrual syndrome," *Biol Psychiatry* 1994; 35(8):557–561.

19. Loch, E.G. et al. "Treatment of premenstrual syn- drome with a phytopharmaceutical formulation containing Vitex angus castus," *J Women's Health Gend Based Med* 2000; 9(3):315–320.

20. Gateley, C.A. et al. "Drug treatments for mastalgia: 17 years experience in the Cardiff Mastalgia Clinic," *J R Soc Med* 1992; 85(1):12–15.

21. Tamborini, A. and R. Taurelle. "Value of standard- ized Ginkgo biloba extract (EGb 761) in the man- agement of congestive symptoms of premenstrual syndrome," *Rev Fr Gynecol Obstet* 1993; 88(7–9):447–457. [French]

22. Linde, K. et al. "St. John's Wort for depression—an overview and meta-analysis of randomized clinical trials," *Br Med J* 1996; 313:253–258.

23. Stevison, C. and E. Ernst. "A pilot study of Hypericum perforatum for the treatment of pre- menstrual syndrome," *BJOG* 2000; 107(7):870–876.

24. Pittler, M.H. and E. Ernst. "Efficacy of kava extract for treating anxiety: systematic review and meta- analysis," *J Clin Psychopharmacol* 2000; 20(1):84–89.

25. Warnecke, G. "Psychosomatic dysfunctions in the female climacteric. Clinical effectiveness and toler- ance of Kava Extract WS 1490," *Fortschr Med* 1991; 109(4):119–122. [German]

Prostate Cancer

1. *Canadian Cancer Statistics 2001*. National Cancer Institute of Canada, 2001. Available at **www.cancer.ca/stats/highle.htm**.

2. *Prostate Cancer*. Mayo Foundation for Medical Education and Research, October 2000. Available at **www.mayoclinic.com/home?id=DS00043**.

3. Ibid.

4. Ramon, J.M. et al. "Dietary fat intake and prostate cancer risk: a case-control study in Spain," *Cancer Causes and Control* 2000; 11(8):679–685.

5. Hayes, R.B. et al. "Dietary factors and risk for prostate cancer among blacks and whites in the United States," *Cancer Epidemiol Biomarkers Prev* 1999; 8(1):25–34.

6. Deneo-Pellegrini, H. et al. "Foods, nutrients and prostate cancer: a case-control study in Uruguay," *Br J Cancer* 1999; 80(3–4):591–597.

7. Bairati, I. et al. "Dietary fat and advanced prostate cancer," *I Urol* 1987; 159(4):1271–1275.

8. Barvo, M.P. et al. "Dietary factors and prostatic cancer. *Urol Int* 1991; 46(2):163–166.

9. West, W.D. et al. "Adult dietary intake and prostate cancer risk in Utah: a case-control study with special emphasis on aggressive tumors," *Cancer Causes and Control* 1991; 2(2):85–94.

10. Kolonel, L.N. et al. "Vegetables, fruits, legumes and prostate cancer: a multiethnic case-control study," *Cancer Epidemiol Biomarkers Prev* 2000; 9(8):795–804.

11. Schuurman, A.G. et al. "Vegetable and fruit consumption and prostate cancer risk: a cohort study in The Netherlands," *Cancer Epidemiol Biomarkers Prev* 1998; 7(8):673–680.

12. Norrish, A.E. et al. "Prostate cancer risk and consumption of fish oils: a dietary biomarker-based case-control study," *Br J Cancer* 1999; 81(7):1238–1242.

13. Herbert, J.R. et al. "Nutritional and socioeconomic factors in relation to prostate cancer mortality: a cross-national survey," *JNCI* 1998; 90(21):1637–1647.

14. Kolonel, L.N. et al. "Vegetables, fruits, legumes and prostate cancer: a multiethnic case-control study," *Cancer Epidemiol Biomarkers Prev* 2000; 9(8):795–804.

15. Putnam, S.D. et al. "Lifestyle and anthropometric risk factors for prostate cancer in a cohort of Iowa men," *Ann Epidemiol* 2000; 10(6):361–369.

16. Giovannucci, E. et al. "Intake of carotenoids and retinol in relation to risk of prostate cancer," *JNCI* 1995; 87(23):1767–1776.

17. Norrish, A.E. et al. "Prostate cancer and dietary carotenoids," *Am J Epidemiol* 2000; 151(2):119–123.

18. Tzonou, A. et al. "Diet and cancer of the prostate: a case-control study in Greece," *Int J Cancer* 1999; 80(5):704–708.

19. Grant, W.B. "An ecologic study of dietary links to prostate cancer," *Altern Med Rev* 1999; 4(3):162–169.

20. Lu, Q.Y. et al. "Inverse Associations between Plasma Lycopene and Other Carotenoids and Prostate Cancer," *Cancer Epidemiol Biomarkers Prev* 2001; 10(7):749–756.

21. Rao, A.V. et al. "Serum and tissue lycopene and biomarkers of oxidation in prostate cancer patients: a case-control study," *Nutr Cancer* 1999; 33(2):159–164.

22. Gann, P.H. et al. "Lower prostate cancer risk in men with elevated plasma lycopene levels: results of a prospective analysis," *Cancer Res* 1999; 59(6):1225–1230.

23. Jacobsen, B.K. et al. "Does high soymilk intake reduce prostate cancer incidence? The Adventist Health Study (United States)," *Cancer Causes and Control* 1998; 9(6):553–557.

24. Hlezlsouer, K.J. et al. "Association between alpha-tocopherol, gamma-tocopherol, selenium, and subsequent prostate cancer," *JNCI* 2000; 92(24):2018–2023.

25. Eichholzer, M. et al. "Smoking, plasma vitamins C, E, retinal, and carotene, and fatal prostate cancer: seventeen-year follow-up of the prospective Basel study," *Prostate* 1999; 38(3):189–198.

26. Heinonen, O.P. et al. "Prostate cancer and supplementation with alpha-tocopherol and beta-carotene: incidence and mortality in a controlled trial," *JNCI* 1998; 90(6):440–446.

27. Chan, J.M. et al. "Supplemental vitamin E intake and prostate cancer risk in a large cohort of men in the United States," *Cancer Epidemiol Biomarkers Prev* 1999; 8(10):893–899.

28. Hartman, T.J. et al. "Effects of long-term alpha-tocopherol supplementation on serum hormones in older men," *Prostate* 2001; 46(1):33–38.

29. Hlezlsouer, K.J. et al. "Association between alpha-tocopherol, gamma-tocopherol, selenium, and subsequent prostate cancer," *JNCI* 2000; 92(24):2018–2023.

30. Clark, L.C. et al. "Decreased risk of prostate cancer with selenium supplementation: results of a double-blind cancer prevention trial," *Br J Urol* 1998; 81(5):730–734.

31. Key, T.J. et al. "A case-control study of diet and prostate cancer," *Br J Cancer* 1997; 76(5):678–687.

32. Sigounas, G. et al. "S-allylmercaptocysteine inhibits cell proliferation and reduces the viability of erythroleukemia, breast, and prostate cancer cell lines," *Nutr Cancer* 1997; 27(2):186–191.

33. Pinto, J.T. et al. "Effects of garlic thioallyl derivatives on growth, glutathione concentration, and polyamine formation of human prostate carcinoma cells in culture," *Am J Clin Nutr* 1997; 66(2):398–405.

34. de la Taille, A. et al. "Role of herbal compounds (PC-SPES) in hormone-refractory prostate cancer: two case reports," *J Altern Complement Med* 2000; 6(5):449–451.

35. Small, E.J. et al. "Prospective trial of the herbal supplement PC-SPES in patients with progressive prostate cancer," *J Clin Oncol* 2000; 18(21):3595–3603.

36. Pfeifer, B.L. et al. "PC-SPES, a dietary supplement for the treatment of hormone-refractory prostate cancer," *BJU Int* 2000; 85(4):481–485.

37. Kubota, T. et al. "PC-SPES: a unique inhibitor of proliferation of prostate cancer cells in vitro and in vivo," *Prostate* 2000; 42(3):163–171.

38. de la Taille, A. et al. "Herbal therapy PC-SPES: in vitro effects and evaluation of its efficacy in 69 patients with prostate cancer," *J Urol* 2000; 164(4):1229–1234.

39. de la Taille, A. et al. "Effects of a phytotherapeutic agent, PC-SPES, on prostate cancer: a preliminary investigation on human cell lines and patients," *BJU Int* 1999; 84(7):845–850.

Prostate Enlargement (Benign Prostatic Hyperplasia)

1. *Prostate Enlargement: Benign Prostatic Hyperplasia.* National Kidney and Urologic Diseases Information Clearinghouse, January 2000. Available at **www.niddk.nih.gov/health/urolog/pubs/prostate/index.htm**.

2. Lagiou, P. et al. "Diet and benign prostatic hyperplasia: a study in Greece," *Urology* 1999; 54(2):284–290.

3. Gu, F. "Changes in the prevalence of benign prostatic hyperplasia in China," *Chin Med J* (Engl) 1997; 110(3):163–166.

4. Yang, Y.J. et al. "Comparison of fatty acid profiles in the serum of patients with prostate cancer and benign prostatic hyperplasia," *Clin Biochem* 1999; 32(6):405–409.

5. Wilt, T.J. et al. "Saw palmetto extracts for treatment of benign prostatic hyperplasia: a systematic review," *JAMA* 1998; 280(18):1604–1609.

6. Ishani, A. et al. "Pygeum africanum for the treatment of patients with benign prostatic hyperplasia: systematic review and quantitative analysis," *Am J Med* 2000; 109(8):654–664.

7. Hartmann, R.W. et al. "Inhibition of 5 alpha-reductatse and aromatase by PHL-00801 (Prostatonin), a combination of PY 102 (Pygeum africanum) and UR 102 (Urtica dioica) extracts," *Phytomedicine* 1996; 3:121–128.

8. Krzeski, T. et al. "Combined extracts of Urtica dioica and Pygeum africanum in the treatment of benign prostatic hyperplasia: double-blind comparison of two doses," *Clin Ther* 1993; 15(6):1011–1020.

9. Wilt, T.J. et al. "Phytotherapy for benign prostatic hyperplasia," *Public Health Nutr* 2000; 3(4A):459–472.

10. Hryb, D.J. et al. "The effect of extracts of the roots of the stinging nettle (Urtica dioica) on the interaction of SHBG with its receptor on human prostatic cell membranes," *Planta Medica* 1995; 61(1):31–21.

11. Wilt, T. et al. "Cernilton for benign prostatic hyperplasia," *Cochrane Database Syst Rev* 2000; (2):CD001042.

12. Wilt, T. et al. "Beta-sitosterols for benign prostatic hyperplasia," *Cochrane Database Syst Rev* 2000; (2):CD001043.

Psoriasis

1. *Your Health: Psoriasis.* Calgary Health Regional Education Services, March 2001. Available at **www.crha-health.ab.ca/hlthconn/items/psor.htm**.

2. *What is Psoriasis?* Mayo Foundation for Medical Education and Research, March 2000. Available at **www.mayoclinic.com/home?id=DS00193**.

3. Azzini, M. et al. "Fatty acids and antioxidant micronutrients in psoriatic arthritis," *J Rheumatol* 1995; 22(1):103–108.

4. Fahrer, H. et al. "Diet and fatty acids: can fish substitute for fish oil?" *Clin Exp Rheumatol* 1991; 9(4):403–406.

5. Collier, P.M. et al. "Effect of regular consumption of oily fish compared with white fish on chronic plaque psoriasis," *Eur J Clin Nutr* 1993; 47(4):251–254.

6. Michaelsson, G. et al. "Patients with psoriasis have elevated levels of serum eosinphil cationic protein and increased numbers of EG2 positive eosinophils

in the duodenal stroma," *Br J Dermatol* 1996;
135(3):371–378.

7. Michaelsson, G. et al. "Patients with psoriasis often
have increased serum levels of IgA antibodies to
gliadin," *Br J Dermatol* 1993; 129(6):667–673.

8. Michaelsson, G. et al. "Psoriasis patients with antibodies to gliadin can be improved by a gluten-free
diet," *Br J Dermatol* 2000; 142(1):44–51.

9. Naldi, L. et al. "Dietary factors and the risk of psoriasis. Results of an Italian case-control study," *Br J
Dermatol* 1996; 134(1):101–106.

10. Tasaki, M. et al. "Analyses of serum copper and zinc
levels and copper/zinc ratios in skin diseases,"
J Dermatol 1993; 20(1):21–24.

11. Michaelsson, G. and K. Ljunghall. "Patients with
dermatitis herpetiformis, acne, psoriasis and
Darier's disease have low epidermal zinc concentrations," *Acta Derm Venereol* 1990; 70(4):304–308.

12. Burrows, N.P. et al. "A trial of oral zinc supplementation in psoriasis," *Cutis* 1994; 54(2):117–118.

13. Leibovici, V. et al. "Effect of zinc therapy on neutrophil chemotaxis in psoriasis," *Isr J Med Sci* 1990;
26(6):306–309.

14. Syed, T.A. et al. "Management of psoriasis with Aloe
vera extract in a hydrophilic cream: a placebo-
controlled, double-blind study," *Trop Med Int
Health* 1996; 1(4):505–509.

15. Gieler, U. et al. "Mahonia aquifolium—a new type
of topical treatment for psoriasis," *J Dermatol Treat*
1995; 6:31–34.

16. Kojima, T. et al. "Long-term administration of
highly purified eicosapentaenoic acid provides
improvement for psoriasis," *Dermatologica* 1991;
182(4):225–230.

17. Lassus, A. et al. "Effects of dietary supplementation
with polyunsaturated ethyl ester lipids (Angiosan)
in patients with psoriasis and psoriatic arthritis," *J
Int Med Res* 1990; 18(1):68–73.

18. Danno, K. and N. Sugie. "Combination therapy
with low-dose etretinate and eicosapentaenoic acid
for psoriasis vulgaris," *J Dermatol* 1998;
25(11):703–705.

19. Gupta, A.K. et al. "Double-blind, placebo-controlled
study to evaluate the efficacy of fish oil and low-
dose UVB in the treatment of psoriasis," *Br J
Dermatol* 1989; 129(6):801–807.

20. Stoof, T.J. et al. "Does fish oil protect renal function
in cyclosporin-treated psoriasis patients?" *J Intern
Med* 1989; 226(6):437–441.

Rheumatoid Arthritis

1. *Rheumatoid Arthritis.* The Arthritis Society of
Canada, January 2001. Available at
**www.arthritis.ca/types%20of%20arthritis/ra/
default.asp?s=1**.

2. Kjeldsen-Kragh, J. et al. "Antibodies against dietary
antigens in rheumatoid arthritis patients treated
with fasting and a one-year vegetarian diet," *Clin
Exp Rheumatol* 1995;13(2):167–172.

3. van de Laar, M.A. et al. "Food intolerance in
rheumatoid arthritis. II. Clinical and histological
aspects," *Ann Rheum Dis* 1992; 51(3):303–306.

4. van de Laar, M.A. et al. "Food intolerance in
rheumatoid arthritis. I. A double blind, controlled
trial of the clinical effects of elimination of milk
allergens and azo dyes," *Ann Rheum Dis* 1992;
51(3):298–302.

5. Denman, A.M. et al. "Joint complaints and food
allergic disorders," *Ann Allergy.* 1983;
51(2 Pt 2):260–263.

6. Felder, M. et al. "Food allergy in patients with
rheumatoid arthritis," *Clin Rheumatol* 1987;
6(2):181–184.

7. Muller, H. et al. "Fasting followed by vegetarian diet
in patients with rheumatoid arthritis: a systematic
review," *Scand J Rheumatol* 2001; 30(1):1–10.

8. Hanninen, Kaartinen K. et al. "Antioxidants in
vegan diet and rheumatic disorders," *Toxicology*
2000; 155(1–3):45–53.

9. Kjeldsen-Kragh, J. "Rheumatoid arthritis treated
with vegetarian diets," *Am J Clin Nutr* 1999;
70(Suppl 3):594S–600S.

10. Peltonen, R. et al. "Faecal microbial flora and disease activity in rheumatoid arthritis during a vegan
diet," *Br J Rheumatol* 1997; 36(1):64–68.

11. Kjeldsen-Kragh, J. et al. "Vegetarian diet for patients
with rheumatoid arthritis—status: two years after
introduction of the diet," *Clin Rheumatol* 1994;
13(3):475–482.

12. Shapiro, J.A. et al. "Diet and rheumatoid arthritis in
women: possible protective effect of fish consumption," *Epidemiology* 1996; 7(3):256–263.

13. Comstock, G.W. et al. "Serum concentrations of
alpha tocopherol, beta carotene, and retinal preceding the diagnosis of rheumatoid arthritis and systemic lupus erythematosus," *Ann Rheum Dis* 1997;
56(5):323–325.

14. Gambhir, J.K. et al. "Correlation between blood
antioxidant levels and lipid peroxidation in

rheumatoid arthritis," *Clin Biochem* 1997; 30(4):351–355.

15. Kose, K. et al. "Plasma selenium levels in rheumatoid arthritis," *Biol Trace Elem Res* 1996; 53(1–3):51–56.

16. Azzini, M. et al. "Fatty acids and antioxidant micronutrients in psoroiatic arthritis," *J Rheumatol* 1995; 22(1):103–108.

17. Heliovaara, M. et al. "Serum antioxidants and the risk of rheumatoid arthritis," *Ann Rheum Dis* 1994; 53(1):51–53.

18. O'Dell, J.R. et al. "Serum selenium concentrations in rheumatoid arthritis," *Ann Rheum Dis* 1991; 50(6):376–378.

19. Situnayake, R.D. et al. "Chain breaking antioxidant status in rheumatoid arthritis: clinical and laboratory correlates," *Ann Rheum Dis* 1991; 50(2):81–86.

20. Tarp, U. et al. "Glutathione peroxidase activity in patients with rheumatoid arthritis and in normal subjects: effects of long-term selenium supplementation," *Arth Rheum* 1987; 30(10):1162–1166.

21. Peretz, A. et al. "Selenium status in relation to clinical variables and corticosteroids treatment in rheumatoid arthritis," *J Rheumatol* 1987; 14(6):1104–1107.

22. Lunec, J. and D.R. Blake. "The determination of dehydroascorbic acid and ascorbic acid in the serum and synovial fluid of patients with rheumatoid arthritis (RA)," *Free Rad Res Commun* 1985; 1(1):31–39.

23. Edmonds, S.E. et al. "Putative analgesic activity of prepared oral doses of vitamin E in the treatment of rheumatoid arthritis. Results of a prospective placebo controlled double blind trial," *Ann Rheum Dis* 1997; 56(11):649–655.

24. Buckley, L.M. et al. "Calcium and vitamin D3 supplementation prevents bone loss in the spine secondary to low-dose corticosteroids in patients with rheumatoid arthritis. A randomized, double-blind, placebo-controlled trial," *Ann Intern Med* 1996; 125(12):961–968.

25. Etzel, R. "Special extract of Boswellia serrata (H 15) in the treatment of rheumatoid arthritis," *Phytomedicine* 1996; 3:91–94.

26. Sander, O. et al. "Is H15 (resin extract of Boswellia serrata, "incense") a useful supplement to established drug therapy of chronic polyarthritis? Results of a double-blind pilot study," *Z Rheumatol* 1998; 57:11–16. [in German; English abstract]

27. Wegner, T. "Therapy of degenerative disease of the musculoskeletal system with South African devil's claw (Harpagophytum procumbens DC)," *Wein Med Wochenschr* 1999; 149(8–10):254–257.

28. James, M.J. and L.G. Cleland. "Dietary n-3 fatty acids and therapy for rheumatoid arthritis," *Semin Arth Rheum* 1997; 27:85–97.

29. Volker, D. et al. "Efficacy of fish oil concentrate in the treatment of rheumatoid arthritis," *J Rheumatol* 2000; 27:2343–2346.

30. Fortin, P.R. et al. "Validation of a meta-analysis: the effects of fish oil in rheumatoid arthritis," *J Clin Epidemiol* 1995; 48(11):1379–1390.

31. Geusens, P. et al. "Long-term effect of omega-3 fatty acid supplementation in active rheumatoid arthritis. A 12-month, double-blind, controlled study," *Arth Rheum* 1994; 37(6):824–829.

32. Kremer, J.M. et al. "Effects of high dose fish oil on rheumatoid arthritis after stopping nonsteroidal anti-inflammatory drugs. Clinical and immune correlates," *Arth Rheum* 1995; 38(8):1107–1114.

Shingles (Herpes Zoster)

1. *The Varicella-Zoster Virus and VZV Infections.* VZV Research Foundation, 2001. Available at **www.vzvfoundation.org/VZVInfections.html**.

2. *What is Shingles?* Mayo Foundation for Education and Research, August 2000. Available at **www.mayoclinic.com/home?id=DS00098**.

3. Meydani, S.N. et al. "Vitamin E supplementation enhances cell-mediated immunity in healthy elderly subjects," *Am J Clin Nutr* 1990; 52(3):557–563.

4. Ravaglia, G. et al. "Effect of micronutrient status in natural killer cell immune function in healthy free living subjects aged >/=90 y," *Am J Clin Nutr* 2000; 71(2):590–598.

5. Frucht-Pery, J. et al. "The use of capsaicin in herpes zoster opthalmicus neuralgia," *Acta Opthalmol Scan* 1997; 75(3):311–313.

6. Watson, C.P. et al. "A randomized vehicle-controlled trial of topical capsaicin in the treatment of postherpetic neuralgia," *Clin Ther* 1993; 15(3):510–526.

7. Peikert, A. et al. "Topical 0.025% capsaicin in chronic post-herpetic neuralgia: efficacy predictors of response and long-term course," *J Neurol* 1991; 238(8):452–426.

8. Watson, C.P. et al. "The prognosis with postherpetic neuralgia," *Pain* 1991; 46(2):195–199.

9. Kleine, M.W. et al. "The intestinal absorption of

orally administered hydrolytic enzymes and their effects in the treatment of acute herpes zoster as compared with those of oral acyclovir therapy," *Phytomedicine* 1995; 2:7–15.

10. Billigmann, P. "Enzyme therapy—an alternative in treatment for herpes zoster. A controlled study of 192 patients," *Fortschr Med* 1995; 113:43–48. [German]

Sinusitis (Sinus Infection)

1. Westerveld, G.J. et al. "Antioxidant levels in the nasal mucosa of patients with chronic sinusitis and healthy controls," *Arch Otolaryngol Head Neck Surg* 1997; 123(2):201–204.

2. Melchart, D. et al. "Echinacea for preventing and treating the common cold," *Cochrane Database Syst Rev* 2000; 44(2):CD000530.

3. Kyo, E. et al. "Immunomodulatory effects of aged garlic extract," *J Nutr* 2001; 131(Suppl 3): 1075S–1079S.

4. Amagase, H. et al. "Intake of garlic and its bioactive components," *J Nutr* 2001; 131(Suppl 3):955S–962S.

5. Salman, H. et al. "Effect of a garlic derivative (alliin) on peripheral blood cell immune responses," *Int J Immunopharmacol* 1999; 21(9):589–597.

6. Scaglione, F. et al. "Efficacy and safety of the standardized ginseng extract G115 for potentiating vaccination against the influenza syndrome and protection against the common cold," *Drugs Exp Clin Res* 1996; 22:65–72.

7. Selzer, A.P. "Adjunctive use of bromelains in sinusitis: a controlled study," *Eye Ear Nose Throat Mon* 1967; 46(10):1281–1288.

8. Ryan, R.E. "A double-blind clinical evaluation of bromelains in the treatment of acute sinusitis," *Headache* 1967; 7(1):13–17.

9. Taub, S.J. "The use of bromelains in sinusitis: a double-blind clinical evaluation," *Eye Ear Nose Throat Mon* 1967; 46(3):361–362.

Stress

1. *Your Health: Stress.* Calgary Regional Health Authority. Available from **www.crha-health.ab.ca/hlthconn/items/stress.htm**.

2. Markus, R. et al. "Effects of food on cortisol and mood in vulnerable subjects under controllable and uncontrollable stress," *Physiol Behav* 2000; 70(3–4):333–342.

3. Markus, C.R. et al. "Carbohydrate intake improves cognitive performance of stress-prone individuals under controllable and uncontrollable laboratory stress," *Br J Nutr* 1999; 82(6):457–467.

4. Markus, C.R. et al. "Does carbohydrate-rich, protein-poor food prevent a deterioration of mood and cognitive performance of stress-prone subjects when subjected to a stressful task?" *Appetite* 1998; 31(1):49–65.

5. Shepard, J.D. et al. "Additive pressor effects of caffeine and stress in male medical students at risk for hypertension," *Am J Hypertens* 2000; 13(5 Pt 1): 475–481.

6. al'Absi, M. et al. "Hypothalamic-pituitary-adrenocortical responses to psychological stress and caffeine in men at high and low risk for hypertension," *Psychosom Med* 1998; 60(4):521–527.

7. Lovallo, W.R. et al. "Hypertension risk and caffeine's effect on cardiovascular activity during mental stress in young men," *Health Psychol* 1991; 10(4):236–243.

8. Lane, J.D. et al. "Caffeine effects on cardiovascular and neuroendocrine responses to acute psychological stress and their relationship to level of habitual caffeine consumption," *Psychosom Med* 1990; 52(3):320–336.

9. van Dusseldorp, M. et al. "Effects of coffee on cardiovascular responses to stress: a 14-week controlled trial," *Psychosom Med* 1992; 54(3):344–353.

10. Eskay, R.L. et al. "The effects of alcohol on selected regulatory aspects of the stress axis," in *Alcohol and the Endocrine System*, ed. Zakhari S. National Institute of Alcohol Abuse and Alcoholism Research Monograph No. 23 (Bethesda, MD, 1993).

11. Waltman, C. et al. "The effects of mild ethanol intoxication on the hypothalamic-pituitary-adrenal axis in nonalcoholic men," *J Clin Endocrin Met* 1993; 77(2):518–522.

12. Spencer, R.L. and E.S. McEwen. "Adaptation of the hypothalamic-pituitary-adrenal axis in chronic ethanol stress," *Neuroendocrinology* 1990; 52(5):481–489.

13. Earle, R. "The Third Wave of Stress Science Controlling Future Shock Trauma in Workplace Hyperchange," The Canadian Institute of Stress. Available at **www.stresscanada.org**.

14. McCarty, M.F. "High dose pyridoxine as an 'anti-stress' strategy," *Med Hypotheses* 2000; 54(5):803–807.

15. Baldewicz, T. et al. "Plasma pyridoxine deficiency is related to increased psychological distress in recently bereaved homosexual men," *Psychosom Med* 1998; 60(3):297–308.

16. Carroll, D. et al. "The effects of an oral multivita-min combination with calcium, magnesium, and zinc on psychological well-being in healthy young male volunteers: a double-blind placebo-controlled trial," *Psychopharmacology* 2000; 150(2):220–225.

17. Desole, M.S. et al. "Analysis of immobilization stress-induced changes of ascorbic acid, noradrena-line, and dopamine metabolism in discrete brain areas of the rat," *Pharmacol Res* 1990; 22(Suppl 3): 43–44.

18. Tverdokhlip, P. et al. "Effect of emotional and pain stress on the level of antioxidant vitamins in the blood of rats," *Vopr Pitan* 1987; (6):52–54. [Russian]

19. Cernak, I. et al. "Alterations in magnesium and oxidative status during chronic emotional stress," *Magnes Res* 2000; 13(1):29–36.

20. Fujita, T. et al. "Fall of blood ionized calcium on watching a provocative TV program and its preven-tion by active absorbable algal calcium (AAA Ca)," *J Bone Miner Metab* 1990; 17(2):131–136.

21. Ibid.

22. Kim, D.H. et al. "Inhibition of stress-induced plas-ma corticosterone levels by ginsenosides in mice: involvement of nitric oxide," *Neuroreport* 1998; 9(10):2261–2264.

23. Bittles, A.H. et al. "The effect of ginseng on the lifespan and stress responses in mice," *Gerontology* 1979; 25(3):125–131.

24. Dua, P.R. et al. "Adpatogenic activity of Indian Panax pseudoginseng," *Ind J Exp Biol* 1989; 27:631–634.

25. Hiai, S. et al. "Features of ginseng saponin induced corticosterone secretion," *Endocrinol Jpn* 1979; 26:737–740.

26. Scaglione, F. et al. "Efficacy and safety of the standardized ginseng extract G115 for potentiating vaccination against the influenza syndrome and protection against the common cold," *Drugs Exp Clin Res* 1996; 22:65–72.

27. Sorenson, H. and J. Sonne. "A double-masked study of the effects of ginseng on cognitive functions," *Curr Ther Res* 1996; 57:959–968.

Ulcers (Peptic Ulcers)

1. *H. pylori and Peptic Ulcer*. National Digestive Diseases Information Clearinghouse, January 1998. Available at **www.niddk.nih.gov/health/digest/pubs/hpylori/h pylori.htm.**

2. Ibid.

3. Elmstahl, S. et al. "Fermented milk products are associated to ulcer disease. Results from a cross-sectional population study," *Eur J Clin Nutr* 1998; 52(9):668–674.

4. Thompson, L. et al. "Inhibitory effect of polyunsat-urated fatty acids on the growth of Helicobacter pylori: a possible explanation of the effect of diet on peptic ulceration," *Gut* 1994; 35(11):1157–1161.

5. Manjari, V. and U.N. Das. "Oxidant stress, anti-oxidants, nitric acid and essential fatty acids in peptic ulcer disease," *Prostaglandins Leukot Essent Fatty Acids* 1998; 59(6):401–406.

6. Hollander, D. and A. Tarnawski. "Is there a role for essential fatty acids in gastroduodenal mucosal pro-tection?" *J Clin Gastroenterol* 1991; 13(Suppl 1):S72–S74.

7. Hawley, C.J. "Prostaglandins: mucosal protection and peptic ulceration," *Methods Find Exp Clin Pharmacol* 1989; 11(Suppl 1):24–51.

8. Nair, S. et al. "Micronutrients antioxidant in gastric mucosa and serum in patients with gastritis and gastric ulcer: does Helicobacter pylori infection alter the results?" *J Clin Gastroenterol* 2000; 30(4):381–385.

9. Force, R.W. and M.C. Nahata. "Effect of histamine H2-receptor antagonists on vitamin B12 absorp-tion," *Ann Pharmacother* 1992; 26(10):1283–1286.

10. O'Gara, E.A. et al. "Activities of garlic oil, garlic powder, and their diallyl constituents against Helicobacter pylori," *Appl Environ Microbiol* 2000; 66(5):2267–2273.

11. Jonkers, D. et al. "Antibacterial effect of garlic and omeprazole on Helicobacter pylori," *Antimicrob Chemother* 1999; 43(6):837–839.

12. Sivam, G.P. et al. "Helicobacter pylori—in vitro sus-ceptibility to garlic (Allium sativum) extract," *Nutr Cancer* 1997; 27(2):118–121.

13. Cellini, L. et al. "Inhibition of Helicobacter pylori by garlic extract (Allium sativum)," *FEMS Immunol Med Microbiol* 1996; 13(4):273–277.

14. Kassir, Z.A. et al. "Endoscopic controlled trial of four drug regimens in the treatment of chronic duodenal ulceration," *Ir Med J* 1985; 78:153–156.

15. Morgan, A.G. et al. "Maintenance therapy: a two-year comparison between Caved-S and cimetidine treatment in the prevention of symptomatic gastric ulcer recurrence," *Gut* 1985; 26:599–602.

Urinary Tract Infections (UTIs)

1. *Urinary Tract Infections.* The Kidney Foundation of Canada, 2001. Available at **www.kidney.ca/publications-eng.htm**.

2. *Treatment of Urinary Tract Infection (UTI).* The National Kidney and Urologic Diseases Information Clearinghouse, January 1999. Available at **www.niddk.nih.gov/health/urolog/pubs/utiadult/utiadult.htm**.

3. Kontiokari, T. et al. "Randomised trial of cranberry-lingonberry juice and Lactobacillus GG drink for the prevention of urinary tract infections in women," *Br Med J* 2001; 322(7302):1571.

4. Avron, J. et al. "Reduction of bacteriuria and pyuria after ingestion of cranberry juice," *JAMA* 1994; 271:751–754.

5. Kyo, E. et al. "Immunomodulatory effects of aged garlic extract," *J Nutr* 2001; 131(Suppl 3): 1075S–1079S.

6. Amagase, H. et al. "Intake of garlic and its bioactive components," *J Nutr* 2001; 131(Suppl 3):955S–962S.

7. Salman, H. et al. "Effect of a garlic derivative (alliin) on peripheral blood cell immune responses," *Int J Immunopharmacol* 1999; 21(9):589–597.

8. Schulz, V., R. Hansel and V.E. Tyler. "Rational Phytotherapy: A Physician's Guide to Herbal Medicine," 3rd ed. (Berlin: Springer-Verlag; 1998):223.

9. European Scientific Cooperative on Phytotherapy. "Uvae Ursi Folium (bearberry leaf)," Exeter, UK: ESCOP, 1996–1997:2. Monographs on the Medicinal Uses of Plant Drugs, Fascicule 5.

10. Kedzia, B. et al. "Antibacterial action of urine containing arbutin metabolic products," *Med Dosw Mikrobiol* 1975; 27:305–314. [in Polish; English Abstract]

11. Reid, G. "Potential preventative strategies and therapies in urinary tract infection," *World J Urol* 1999; 17(6):359–363.

12. Velraeds, M.M. et al. "Inhibition of initial adhesion of uropathogenic Enterococcus faecalis by biosurfactants from Lactobacillus isolates," *Appl Environ Micorbiol* 1996; 62(6):1958–1963.

13. Hawthorn, L.A. and G. Reid. "Exclusion of uropathogen adhesion to polymer surfaces by Lactobacillus acidophilus," *J Biomed Mater Res* 1990; 24(1):39–46.

14. Reid, G. et al. "Is there a role for lactobacilli in prevention of urogenital and intestinal functions?" *Clin Microbiol Rev* 1990; 3(4):335–344.

Varicose Veins

1. Burkitt, D.P. "Varicose veins: facts and fantasy," *Arch Surg* 1976; 111(12):1327–1332.

2. Bone, K. *Mediherb Professional Review* 1997; 59:3.

3. Cesarone, M.R. et al. "The microcirculatory activity of *Centella asiatica* in venous insufficiency: A double-blind study," *Minerva Cardioangiol* 1994; 42:299–304.

4. Cesarone, M.R. et al. "Activity of *Centella asiatica* in venous insufficiency," *Minerva Cardioangiol* 1992; 42:137–143.

5. Belcaro, G.V. et al. "Improvement of capillary permeability in patients with venous hypertension after treatment with TTFCA," *Angiology* 1990; 41:533–540.

6. Belcaro, G.V. et al. "Capillary filtration and ankle edema in patients with venous hypertension treated with TTCFA," *Angiology* 1990; 41:12–18.

7. Pointel, J.P. et al. "Titrated extract of *Centella asiatica* (TECA) in the treatment of venous insufficiency of the lower limbs," *Angiology* 1987; 38:46–50.

8. Lohr, E. et al. "Anti-edemic therapy in chronic venous insufficiency with tendency to formation of edema," *Munch Med Wsch* 1986; 128(34):579–581. [German]

9. Rudofsky, G. et al. "Antiedematous effects and clinical effectiveness of horse chestnut seed extract in double bind studies," *Phlebologie und Proktologie* 1986; 15:47–54. [German]

10. Neiss, A. et al. "Proof of the efficacy of horse chestnut seed extract in the treatment of varicose veins," *Munch Med Wsch* 1976; 118(7):213–216. [German]

11. Diehm, C. et al. "Comparison of leg compression stocking and oral horse-chestnut seed extract therapy in patients with chronic venous insufficiency," *Lancet* 1996 Feb 3; 347(8997):292–294.

12. Tixier, J.M. et al. "Evidence by in vivo and in vitro studies that binding of pycnogenols to elastin affects its rate of degradation by elastases," *Biochem Pharmacol* 1984; 33:3933–3939.

13. Masquelier, J. et al. "Stabilization of collagen by procyanidolic oligomers," *Acta Therap* 1981; 7:101–105.

14. Schwitters, B. et al. *OPC in Practice: Bioflavonols and Their Applications* (Rome: Alfa Omega, 1993).

Index